Musculoskeletal Examination

This title is also available as an e-book.
For more details, please see
www.wiley.com/buy/9781118962763
or scan this QR code:

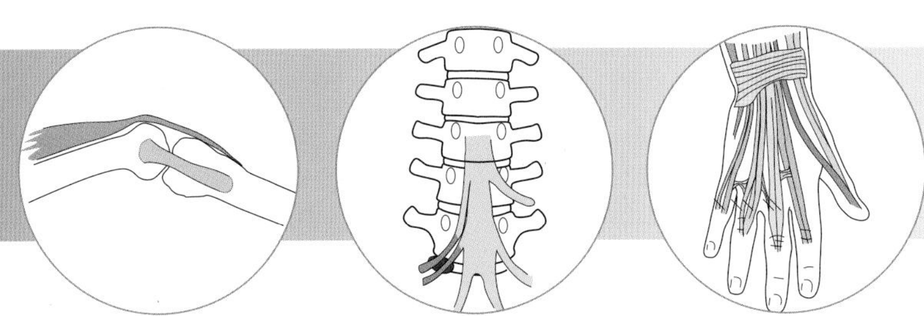

Musculoskeletal Examination

Fourth Edition

Jeffrey M. Gross, MD
Clinical Assistant Professor of Rehabilitation Medicine
Weill-Cornell Medical College
Adjunct Clinical Associate Professor of Rehabilitation Medicine
New York University School of Medicine
Medical Director
Union Square Rehabilitation and Sports Medicine
New York

Joseph Fetto, MD
Associate Professor of Orthopedic Surgery
New York University School of Medicine
Associate Professor and Consultant
Manhattan V.A. Medical Center
New York

Elaine Rosen, PT, DHSc, OCS
Associate Professor of Physical Therapy
Hunter College
City University of New York
Partner
Queens Physical Therapy Associates
Forest Hills, New York

WILEY Blackwell

This edition first published 2016 © 2016 by John Wiley & Sons, Ltd
Previous editions: 1996, 2009 by Jeffrey Gross, Joseph Fetto, Elaine Rosen

Registered office: John Wiley & Sons, Ltd, The Atrium, Southern Gate, Chichester, West Sussex, PO19 8SQ, UK

Editorial offices: 9600 Garsington Road, Oxford, OX4 2DQ, UK
The Atrium, Southern Gate, Chichester, West Sussex, PO19 8SQ, UK
111 River Street, Hoboken, NJ 07030-5774, USA

For details of our global editorial offices, for customer services and for information about how to apply for permission to reuse the copyright material in this book please see our website at www.wiley.com/wiley-blackwell

Library of Congress Cataloging-in-Publication Data

Gross, Jeffrey M., 1957–, author.
Musculoskeletal examination / Jeffrey M. Gross, Joseph Fetto, Elaine Rosen. – 4th edition.
p. ; cm.
Includes bibliographical references and index.
ISBN 978-1-118-96276-3 (pbk.)
I. Fetto, Joseph, author. II. Rosen, Elaine, author. III. Title.
[DNLM: 1. Musculoskeletal Diseases–diagnosis. 2. Musculoskeletal Physiological Phenomena. 3. Musculoskeletal System–anatomy & histology. 4. Physical Examination–methods. WE 141]
RC925.7
616.70076–dc23

2015000697

A catalogue record for this book is available from the British Library.

Wiley also publishes its books in a variety of electronic formats. Some content that appears in print may not be available in electronic books.

Cover image: istock (photo/muscles-of-the-arm-34748034) 02-09-14 (c) Eraxion

Set in 10/12pt SabonLTStd by Aptara Inc., New Delhi, India
Printed and bound in Singapore by Markono Print Media Pte Ltd

1 2016

Contents

How to Use This Book

Musculoskeletal Examination is to be used as both a teaching text and a general reference on the techniques of physical examination. This volume represents the joint authoring efforts of a physiatrist, an orthopedic surgeon, and a physical therapist and presents the information in a clear and concise format, free of any professional biases that reflect one specialty's preferences. The importance of this will be seen as we take you through each anatomical region and delineate the basic examination. Included in each chapter are the abnormalities most frequently encountered or noted while performing an examination.

The book is organized into regional anatomical sections including the spine and pelvis, the upper extremity, and the lower extremity. The book opens with two chapters that define the structures of the musculoskeletal system and discuss the basic concepts and parts of the musculoskeletal exam. A final chapter describes the examination of gait.

Each main chapter is organized in an identical manner:

- overview of the anatomical region
- observation of the patient
- subjective examination
- gentle palpation
- trigger points (where applicable)
- active movement testing
- passive movement testing
- physiological movements
- mobility testing
- resistive testing
- neurological examination
- referred pain patterns
- special tests
- radiological views

In Chapter 2, Basic concepts of the physical examination, we provide you with a framework for performing the examination, beginning with observation and ending with palpation. However, in each regional anatomy chapter, palpation follows observation and subjective examination and precedes all other sections. This is deliberate. For reasons of length, we felt it important to discuss each anatomical region and its own special anatomical structures as soon as possible in each chapter. This avoids repetition, gives you the anatomy early in each chapter, and then allows you to visualize each structure as you read the subsequent sections on testing. Hopefully, this will reinforce the anatomy and help you apply anatomy to function and function to the findings of your examination.

Each chapter includes a generous number of original line drawings, many of which are two-color. These provide clear snapshots of how to perform each examination technique. Thirty-two X-rays and MRIs have been included to help you with radiological anatomy. Paradigms and tables provide additional information that will help you understand the how and why of each examination technique.

By using *Musculoskeletal Examination* as a guide and reference, the reader will be able to perform the complete basic examination and understand common abnormalities and their pathological significance. We hope that our readers will gain an appreciation for the intimate relationship between the structure and function of the components of the musculoskeletal system. This understanding should then enable any reader to make a correct diagnosis and a successful treatment plan for each patient.

Acknowledgments

The writing of *Musculoskeletal Examination* would not have been possible without the overwhelming support and understanding of my wife, Elizabeth, and my sons, Tyler and Preston. I also want to thank my parents, Malcolm and Zelda Gross, for their guidance and efforts on my behalf.

J.G.

Thank you to my wife and family for their understanding, patience, support, and love.

J.F.

To my husband, Jed, for his unlimited patience, understanding, and encouragement.

To my business partner and friend, Sandy, for being there whenever I needed her.

To my family for their support, and to my many patients, colleagues, and friends who have helped me grow.

E.R.

About the Companion Website

Don't forget to visit the companion website for this book:

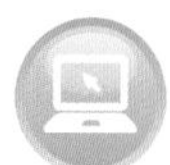

www.wiley.com/go/musculoskeletalexam

There you will find:
Hundred interactive multiple-choice questions to test your learning.
Links to the examination videos mentioned in the book.

Scan this QR code to visit the companion website

CHAPTER 1

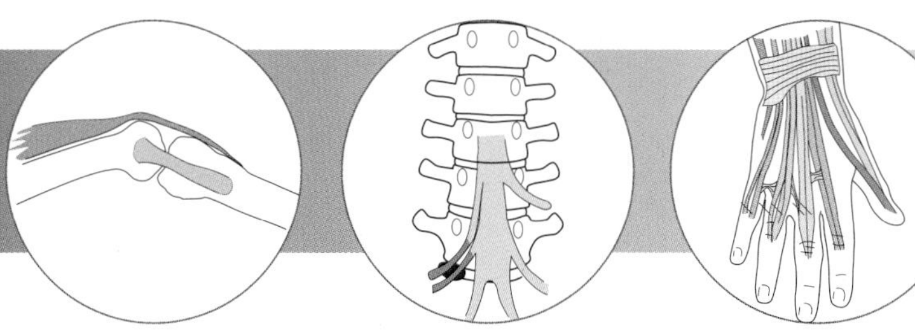

Introduction

The intention of this book is to provide the reader with a thorough knowledge of regional anatomy and the techniques of physical examination. A second and equally important intention is to describe a method for the interpretation and logical application of the knowledge obtained from a physical examination.

What Is a Physical Examination?

The physical examination is the inspection, palpation, measurement, and auscultation of the body and its parts. It is the step that follows the taking of a patient history and precedes the ordering of laboratory tests and radiological evaluation in the process of reaching a diagnosis.

What Is the Purpose of the Physical Examination?

The physical examination has two distinct purposes. The first is to localize a complaint, that is, to associate a complaint with a specific region and, if possible, a specific anatomical structure. The second purpose of a physical examination is to qualify a patient's complaints. Qualifying a complaint involves describing its character (i.e., dull, sharp, etc.), quantifying its severity (i.e., visual analog scale; grade I, II, III), and defining its relationship to movement and function.

How Is the Physical Examination Useful?

By relating a patient's complaints to an anatomical structure, the physical examination brings meaning to a patient's history and symptoms.

This, however, presupposes that the clinician possesses a thorough knowledge of anatomy. It also requires a methodology for the logical analysis and application of the information obtained from the patient's history and physical examination. This methodology is derived from a clinical philosophy based on specific concepts. These concepts are as follows:

1. If one knows the structure of a system and understands its intended function, it is possible to predict how that system is vulnerable to breakdown and failure (injury).
2. A biological system is no different from an inorganic system in that it is subject to the same laws of nature (physics, mechanics, engineering, etc.). However, the biological system, unlike the inorganic system, has the potential not only to respond but also to adapt to changes in its environment.

Such concepts lay the foundation for understanding the information obtained on physical examination. They also lead to a rationale for the treatment and rehabilitation of injuries. A correlation of this type of analysis is that it becomes possible to anticipate injuries. This in turn permits proactive planning for the prevention of injuries.

How Does the Musculoskeletal System Work?

The musculoskeletal system, like any biological system, is not static. It is in a constant state of dynamic equilibrium. This equilibrium is termed homeostasis.

As such, when subjected to an external force or stress, a biological system will respond in a very specific manner. Unlike the inorganic system (i.e., an

Musculoskeletal Examination, Fourth Edition. Jeffrey M. Gross, Joseph Fetto and Elaine Rosen.

Companion website: www.wiley.com/go/musculoskeletalexam

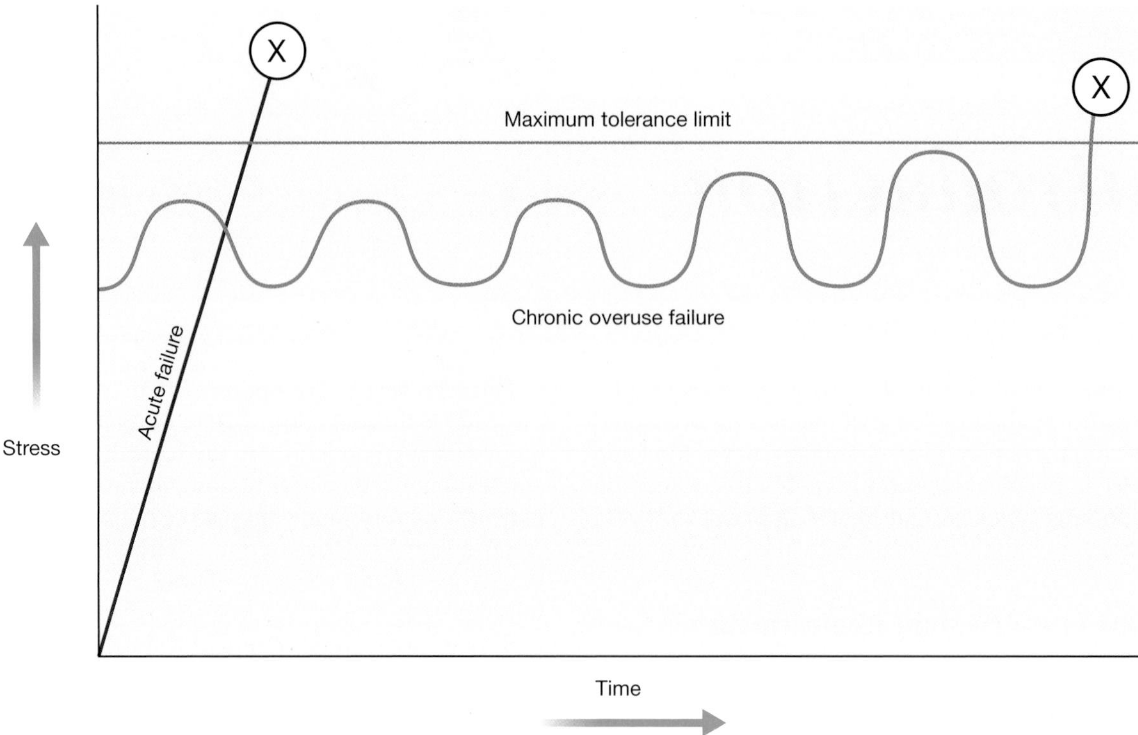

Figure 1.1 Biological systems, like inorganic systems, can fail under one of two modes: an acute single supramaximal stress or repetitive submaximal chronic loading.

airplane wing that is doomed to fail after a predictable number of cycles of load), the biological system will attempt to reestablish an equilibrium state in response to a change that has occurred in its environment. In doing so, the biological system will experience one of three possible scenarios: adaptation (successful establishment of a new equilibrium state without breakdown), temporary breakdown (injury), or ultimate breakdown (death). These scenarios can be expressed graphically. Any system can be stressed in one of the two modes: acute single supratolerance load or chronic repetitive submaximal tolerance load (Figure 1.1). In the first mode, the system that suffers acute failure is unable to resist the load applied. In the second mode, the system will function until some fatigue limit is reached, at which time failure will occur. In the biological system, either failure mode will initiate a protective-healing response, termed the inflammatory reaction. The inflammatory reaction is composed of cellular and humoral components, each of which initiates a complex series of neurological and cellular responses to the injury. An important consequence of the inflammatory reaction is the production of pain. The sole purpose of pain is to bring one's attention to the site of injury. Pain prevents further injury from occurring by causing protective guarding and limited use of the injured structure. The inflammatory response is also characterized by increased vascularity and swelling in the area of injury. These are the causes of the commonly observed physical signs (i.e., redness and warmth) associated with the site of injury.

However, the problem with pain is that although it brings protection to the area of injury (the conscious or unconscious removal of stress from the injured area), and permits healing to take place by removing dynamic stimuli from the biological system, this removal of stimuli (rest) promotes deterioration of a system's tolerance limit to a lower threshold. In this way, when the injury has resolved, the entire system, although "healed," may actually be more vulnerable to reinjury when "normal" stresses are applied to the recently repaired structures. This initiates the "vicious cycle of injury" (Figure 1.2).

Contrary to this scenario is one in which the biological system successfully adapts to its new environment before failure occurs. This situation represents conditioning of a biological system. The result is

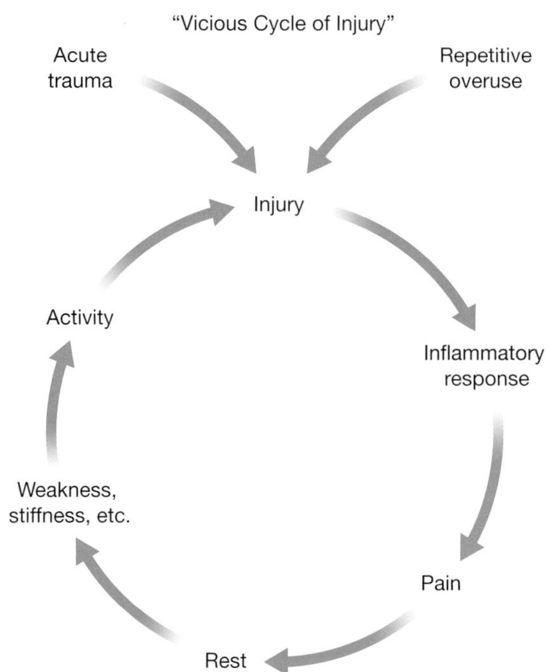

Figure 1.2 The "vicious cycle of injury" results from the reinjury of a vulnerable, recently traumatized system. This increased vulnerability occurs due to a diminishing of a system's tolerance limit as a result of adaptation to a lower level of demand during the period of rest necessitated by pain.

hypertrophy, enhanced function, and a consequent increase in the system's tolerance limit. The concept acting here is that the biological system's tolerance limit will adapt to increased demands if the demands are applied at a frequency, intensity, and duration within the system's ability to adapt (Figure 1.3).

Therefore, during the physical examination, asymmetry must be noted and analyzed as representing either adaptation or deconditioning of a given system. Any of these fundamental principles under which the musculoskeletal system functions makes it possible to organize the information obtained from a physical examination and history into general categories or pathological conditions (traumatic, inflammatory, metabolic, etc.), and the subsets of these conditions (tendinitis, ligamentous injuries, arthritis, infection, etc.). From such an approach, generalizations called paradigms can be formulated. These paradigms provide a holistic view of a patient's signs and symptoms. In this way, diagnoses are arrived at based on an analysis of the entire constellation of signs and symptoms with which a given patient presents. This method, relying on a multitude of factors and their interrelationships rather than on a single piece of information, such as the symptom of clicking or swelling, ensures a greater degree of accuracy in formulating a diagnosis.

What Are Paradigms?

Paradigms are snapshots of classic presentations of various disease categories. They are, as 19th-century clinicians would say, "augenblick," a blink-of-the-eye impression of a patient (Table 1.1). From such an impression, a comparison is made with an idealized patient, to evaluate for congruities or dissimilarities. Here is an example of a paradigm for osteoarthritis: a male patient who is a laborer, who is at least 50 years old, whose complaints are asymmetrical pain involving larger joints, and whose symptoms are in proportion to his activity. Another example might be that of rheumatoid arthritis. This paradigm would describe a female patient who is 20–40 years old, complaining of symmetrical morning stiffness involving the smaller joints of the hands, with swelling, possibly fever, and stiffness reducing with activity.

Paradigms may also be created for specific tissues (i.e., joints, tendons, muscles, etc.). The paradigm for a joint condition such as osteoarthritis would be well localized pain, swelling, stiffness on sedentary posturing, and pain increasing in proportion to use, whereas a paradigm for a mild tendon inflammation (tendinitis) may be painful stiffness after sedentary posturing that becomes alleviated with activity and gentle use. A paradigm for ligament injury would include a history of a specific traumatic event, together with the resultant loss of joint stability demonstrated on active and passive tensile loading of a joint.

The reader is encouraged to create his or her own paradigms for various conditions—paradigms that include the entire portrait of an injury or disease process with which a given patient or tissue may be compared. In this process, it will become obvious that it is not sufficient to limit one's expertise to the localization of complaints to an anatomical region. It is also necessary to be able to discriminate between the involvement of specific structures that may lie in close proximity within that region (i.e., bursae and tendons overlying a joint).

It can be concluded therefore that an accurate physical examination is as critical to the process of diagnosis as is a complete and accurate history of a patient's complaints. An accurate physical examination demands a thorough knowledge and familiarity with anatomy and function.

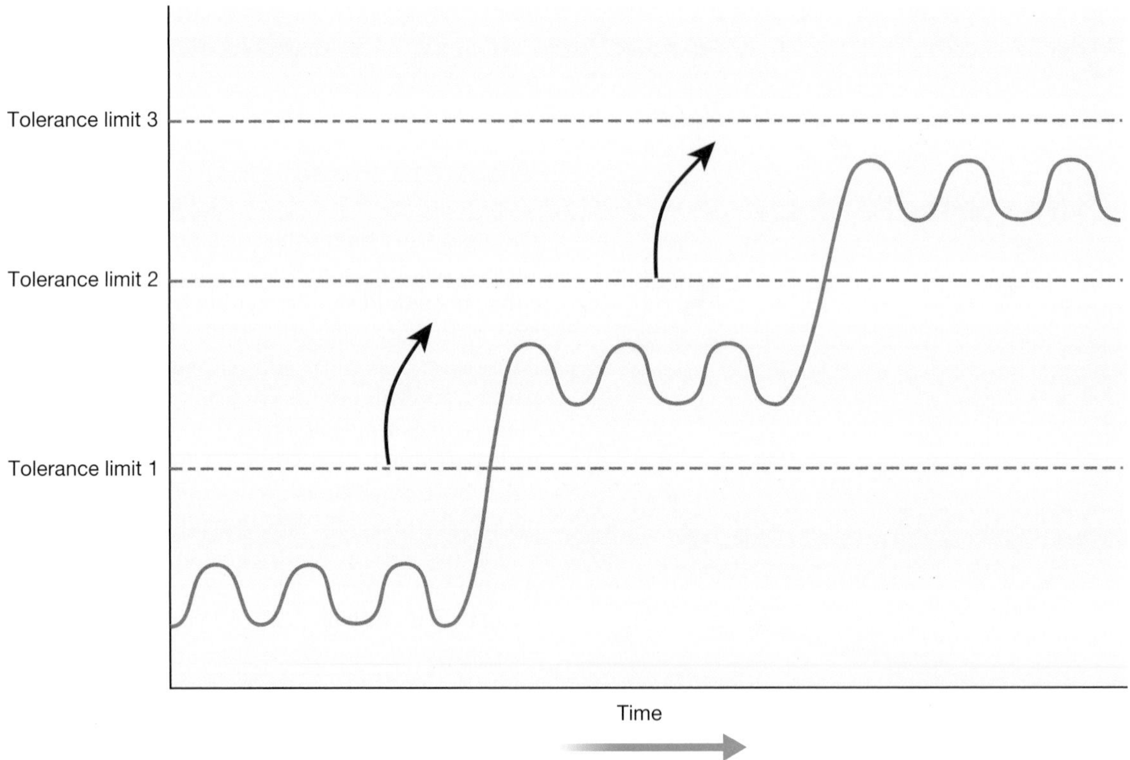

Figure 1.3 Conditioning is the adaptation of a biological system to the controlled application of increasing stress at a frequency, intensity, and duration within the system's tolerance limit, with a resultant increase in the system's tolerance limit.

What Are the Components of the Musculoskeletal System?

The musculoskeletal system is composed of bone, cartilage, ligaments, muscle, tendons, synovium, bursae, and fascia. This system is derived embryologically from the mesenchyme and is composed of soft and hard connective tissues. These tissues have evolved to serve two basic functions: structural integrity and stable mobility. The tissues are composite materials made up of cells lying within the extracellular matrix they produce.

Table 1.1 Paradigms for Osteoarthritis and Rheumatoid Arthritis

Paradigm for Osteoarthritis	Paradigm for Rheumatoid Arthritis
Male	Female
Laborer	20–40 years old
50+ years old	Symmetrical small joint involvement
Large joint involvement	Associated swelling, fever, rash, morning stiffness
Asymmetrical involvement	Abating with use
Pain in proportion to activity	

Collagen, a long linear protein (Figure 1.4a), is the most abundant of the extracellular materials found in connective tissues. The foundation of collagen is a repetitive sequence of amino acids that form polypeptide chains. Three such chains are then braided together to form a triple helical strand called tropocollagen. These strands join to make microfibrils; long linear structures specifically designed to resist tensile loading. The microfibrils are bonded together through chemical cross-linking to form collagen fibers. The degree of cross-linking determines the physical properties of a specific collagen fiber. The more cross-linking that exists, the stiffer the fiber will be. The degree of collagen cross-linking is in part genetically and in part metabolically determined. This explains why some people are much more flexible than others. Vitamin C is critical for the formation of cross-links. As such, scurvy, a clinical expression of vitamin deficiency, is characterized by "weak tissues." Hypermobility of joints (i.e., ability to extend the thumbs to the forearms, ability to hyperextend

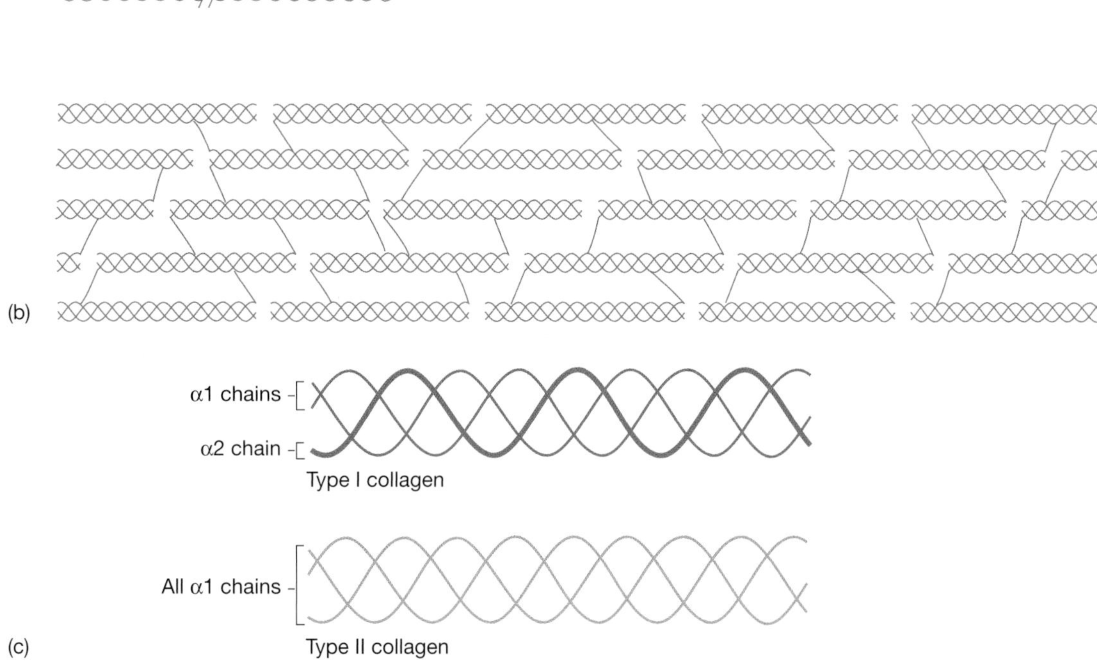

Figure 1.4 (a) Collagen is a linear protein made of α chains that wind into a triple-helix. (b) Collagen fibrils are formed by the cross-linking of collagen monomer proteins. (c) The different types of collagen are determined by the number of $\alpha 1$ and $\alpha 2$ collagen monomers that join to form a triple-helix collagen molecule. For example, two $\alpha 1$ chains and one $\alpha 2$ chain that join to form a triple-helix make type I collagen, which is found in bone, tendon, ligament, fascia, skin, arteries, and the uterus. Type II collagen, which is found in articular cartilage, contains three $\alpha 1$ chains. There are at least 12 different collagen types.

at the knees and elbows, excessive subtalar pronation with flat, splayed feet) is a clinical manifestation of genetically determined collagen cross-linking (Figure 1.4b).

Different types of collagen exist for different categories of tissues. These types are defined by the specific composition of the polypeptide chains that form the strands of the collagen molecules. Type I collagen is found in connective tissue such as bone, tendons, and ligaments. Type II is found uniquely in articular hyaline cartilage. Other collagen types exist as well (Figure 1.4c).

If collagen represents the fiber in the composite structure of connective tissue, ground substance represents the "filler" between the fibers. The main components of ground substance are aggregates of polyglycan macromolecules. An example of such a macromolecule is the proteoglycan hyaluronic acid, found in articular cartilage. Hyaluronic acid is a molecule of more than 1 million daltons. It is composed of a long central core from which are projected many protein side chains containing negatively charged sulfate radicals. It can best be visualized as a bristle brush from which many smaller bristle brushes are projected (Figure 1.5). These strongly negative sulfate radicals make the hyaluronic acid molecule highly hydrophilic (water attracting). This ability to attract and hold water allows the connective tissue ground substance to function as an excellent hydrostatic bearing surface that resists compression load.

Immobilization reduces the diffusion and migration of nutrients throughout the connective tissues. This in turn compromises cellular activity and upsets the normal homeostatic balance of collagen and ground substance turnover. The result is an atrophy of collagen fibers and a diminution of ground substance (Cantu and Grodin, 2011), with subsequent deterioration of the connective-tissue macrofunction (i.e., chondromalacia patellae).

Bone

Bone provides the structure of the body. It is the hardest of all connective tissues. One-third of bone is composed of collagen fibers and two-thirds mineral salts, primarily calcium hydroxyapatite. Bone is formed in response to stress. Although genetically

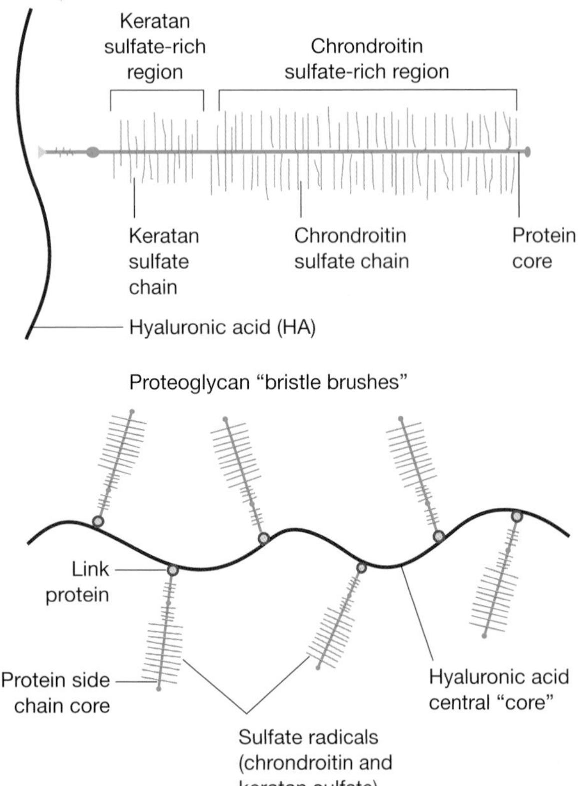

Figure 1.5 The proteoglycan aggregate is formed on a backbone of hyaluronic acid and has the appearance of a bristle brush.

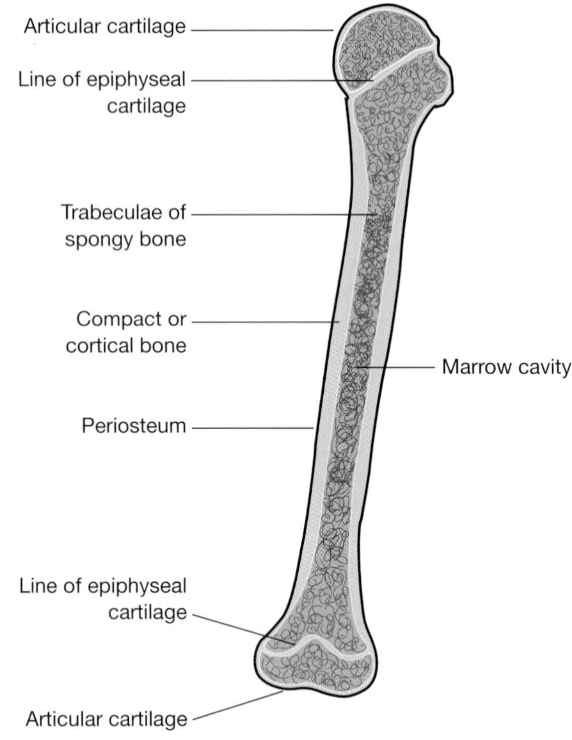

Figure 1.6 The structure of a typical long bone.

determined, the size and shape of a bone are dependent on environmental factors for its full expression. This response of bone to its loading history has been termed Wolff's law. There are two major types of bone: cortical and cancellous. All bones are covered by highly vascularized and innervated tissue called periosteum, except when they are within the synovial cavity of a joint (Figure 1.6).

Cortical bone is very dense, highly calcified, and uniquely constructed to resist compression loads. It can also resist tensile bending and torsional loads, but much more poorly. This is a direct function of cortical bone's ultrastructure, which is a composite of flexible collagen fibers and rigid mineral crystals. Cortical bone is usually found within the diaphysis of long bones. It has a hollow central cavity that is termed the medullary canal or marrow cavity.

At the end of long bones and at the sites of tendon and ligament attachments, bones tend to expand and cortical bone gives way to a more porous structure, termed cancellous or trabecular bone. The trabeculae of cancellous bones lie in the direction of transmitted loads. They act as conduits of load from the articular surface to the underlying diaphyseal cortical bone. Overload of the trabeculae will, on a microscopic scale, duplicate overload of an entire bone (i.e., fracture). This overload, because of the innervation that exists within a bone, will give rise to pain (arthritic discomfort due to mechanical overload secondary to joint deformity or erosion of articular cartilage). The resultant healing of these microfractures leads to increased calcium deposition, hence subchondral sclerosis noted around articular joints on x-ray films, and hypertrophy of stressed sites such as the midshaft of the tibia secondary to stress fractures occurring from overuse in distance running.

Cartilage

Cartilage is a connective tissue made of cells (chondroblasts and chondrocytes) that produce an extracellular matrix of proteoglycans and collagen fibers with a high water content. The tensile strength of cartilage is due to the collagen component. Its resistance to compression is due to the ability of proteoglycan to attract and hold water. Cartilage types include articular or hyaline cartilage (Figure 1.7); fibrocartilage,

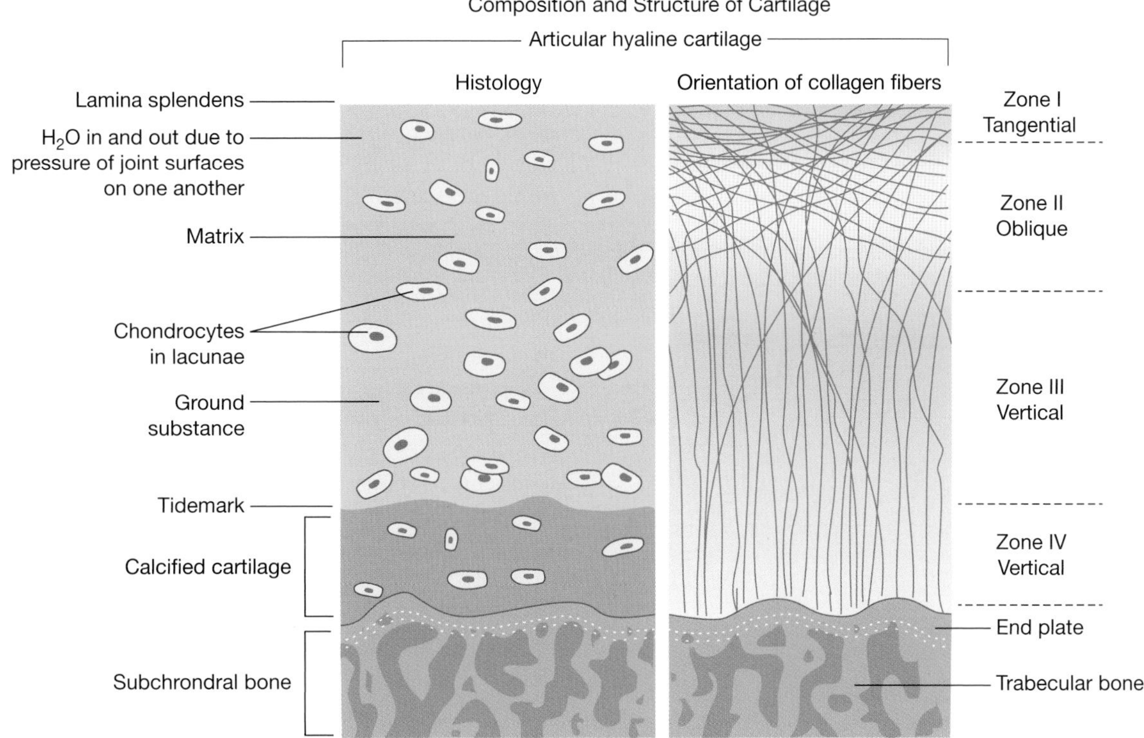

Figure 1.7 The composition and structure of articular hyaline cartilage. Water moves in and out of the cartilage due to the pressure of the joint surfaces on one another and attraction of the water by the ground substance. Note the orientation of the collagen fibers.

which exists at the attachment sites of ligaments, tendons, and bones; fibroelastic cartilage, found in menisci and intravertebral discs; and growth-plate cartilage, located in the physis of immature bones. With age, cartilage tends to decrease in water content and the number of cross-links among collagen molecules increases. The result is that cartilage tissue becomes more brittle, less supple, and less able to resist tensile, torsional, and compression loading. Hence, cartilage becomes more vulnerable to injury with age.

Articular cartilage lines the spaces in synovial joints. It is attached to the underlying bone by a complex interdigitation analogous to that of a jigsaw puzzle. Regeneration of this cartilage is slow and inconsistent in terms of restoration of articular integrity. It can be replaced by a less mechanically efficient fibrocartilage after injuries have occurred. There are no blood vessels within articular cartilage and nutrition is solely dependent on the loading and unloading of the joint, which allows water-soluble nutrients and waste products to enter and leave the cartilaginous matrix through a porous surface layer.

The fibroelastic cartilage of the intervertebral disc allows for very minimal movement between adjacent vertebrae while providing shock absorption. Because of the orientation of the fibers, they are more vulnerable to flexion and rotational forces. Fibroelastic cartilage is also present in the menisci of the knee. Here, it functions not only to absorb shock but also to increase the functional surface area of the joint, thereby providing additional stability. Because of its elastin content, fibroelastic cartilage is resilient and able to return to its prior shape following deformation.

Ligaments

Ligaments are the static stabilizers of joints. They connect bones to bones (Figure 1.8). Ligaments and other capsular structures of the joint are made of dense, organized connective tissue. Ligaments contain collagen and a variable amount of elastin. The collagen provides tensile strength to the ligaments and elastin provides suppleness. The fibers of collagen are arranged more or less parallel to the forces that the ligament is intended to resist. Most ligaments and capsular tissues enter the bone as a progression from collagen fibers to fibrocartilage to calcified cartilage

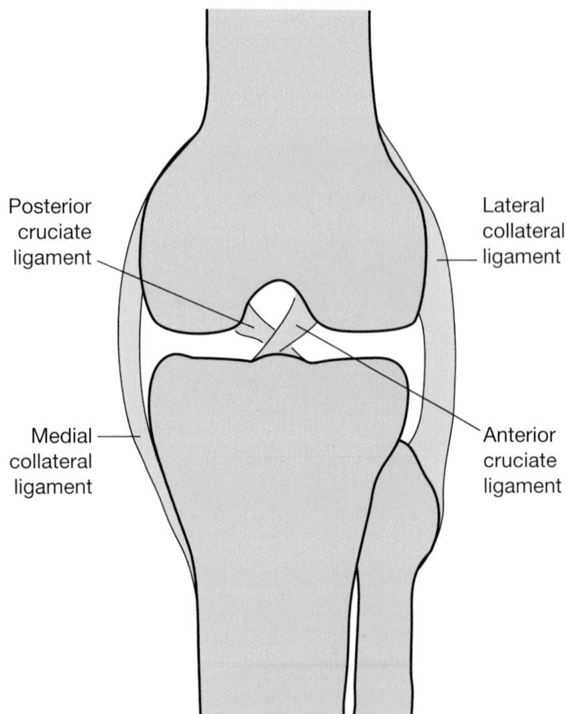

Figure 1.8 The ligaments of the knee. Because of the inherent instability of the joint, ligaments are necessary to prevent motion in all planes. They act as the primary stabilizers of the joint and are assisted by the muscles and other connective tissues.

and then finally bone. Some ligaments (and tendons) attach to the periosteum first, which then attaches to the bone. The site of ligament failure is a function of the load it experiences. Ligaments resist slow loading better than rapid loading. Therefore, rapid loading may produce an intraligamental lesion, whereas a slower pattern of loading will create injuries at or near the bone–ligament interface.

Elastin is a protein that permits elastic recoiling to occur in a tissue. Some ligaments, such as the cruciate ligament of the knee, contain almost no elastin. Other ligaments, such as the ligamentum flavum of the spine, contain large amounts of elastin. Figure 1.9 shows that because it contains more collagen than elastin, the anterior cruciate ligament can resist tensile loads with little elongation. In this way, the anterior cruciate ligament serves the knee well as a stabilizing structure. On the other hand, the ligamentum flavum of the spine, being composed mostly of elastin and little collagen, can be stretched a great deal before breaking, but can only resist very weak tensile loading.

Ligaments function to limit joint motion and to guide the bones as they move. Ligaments therefore usually have a dual internal structure, such that they may stabilize the joint at either extreme of motion.

Ligaments are most lax at midrange of joint motion. The capsule of a synovial joint is in fact a weak ligamentous structure. Disruption of a ligament can result in severe joint instability and increased frictional stresses to the articular surfaces of that joint. This will result in premature osteoarthritis. Conversely, a loss of normal capsular laxity from fibrosis following trauma will result in a severe restriction in joint motion (i.e., posttraumatic adhesive capsulitis of the shoulder).

Ligaments have very little vascularity; hence they heal poorly. However, they do have innervation, which may be useful to quantify the severity of a given ligamentous injury. When the structural integrity of a ligament has been completely compromised (grade III sprain), relatively little pain is produced on attempts to passively stretch the injured ligament. This is because no tension load can be created across a completely disrupted ligament. However, in a less severe partial tear (grade I sprain), severe and exquisite pain will be produced when tension is applied across the damaged structure. This paradoxical pain pattern (less pain equals a more severe sprain) can be a significant diagnostic clue obtained during the physical examination of a recently injured ligament. This also has dramatic import in defining a patient's prognosis and determining a treatment plan.

Muscle

Skeletal muscle is a contractile tissue made up of fibers that contain specialized proteins (Figures 1.10 and 1.11). A loose connective tissue known as endomysium fills the space between these fibers. This tissue attaches to a stronger connective tissue that surrounds the muscle vesiculae, known as perimysium. Perimysium is in turn connected to the epimysium, which encases the entire muscle. This in turn is anchored to the fascial tissues of the nearby structures. Muscles therefore are composed of two elements: contractile tissues and inert, noncontractile tissues. The forces generated by the muscles are extrinsically applied to the muscle and will affect both types of tissue.

Muscles exist in many shapes and sizes. Some of these are shown in Figure 1.12.

Muscles contain three different fiber types: I, IIa, and IIb. They are defined by the chemical machinery used to generate adenosine triphosphate (ATP). Genetic makeup, training, and neuromuscular disease

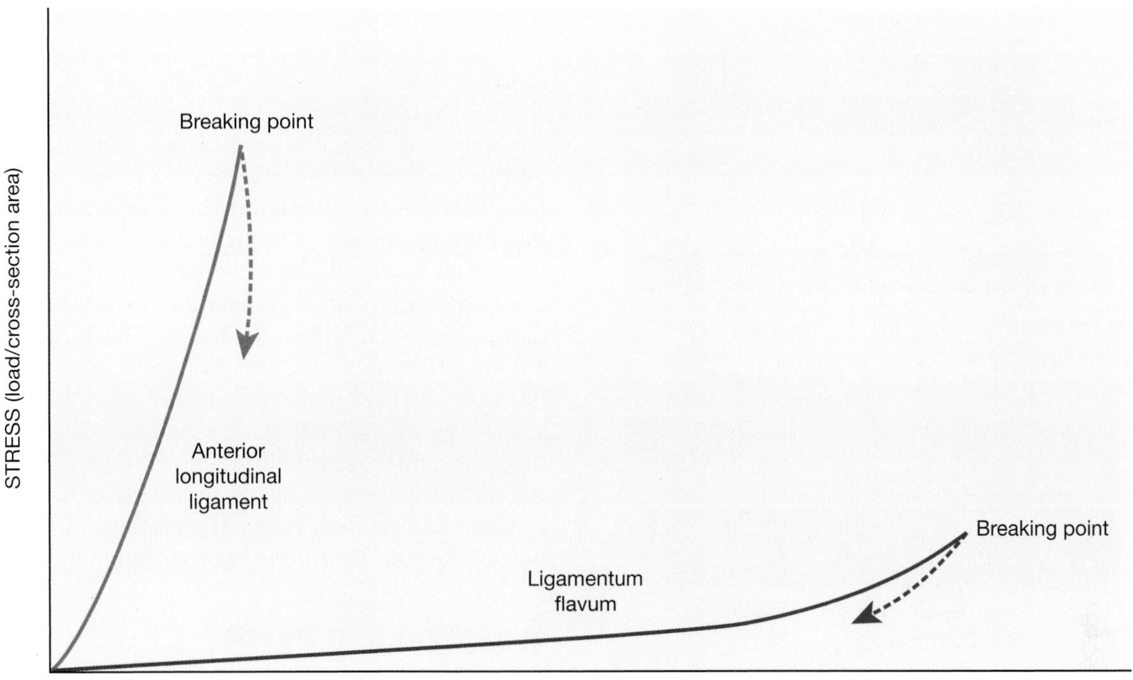

Figure 1.9 The mechanical response of stress and strain on the anterior longitudinal ligament and the ligamentum flavum. The anterior cruciate ligament, having more collagen than elastin, can handle a larger load but will only stretch a short amount before breaking. The ligamentum flava, having more elastin than collagen, cannot tolerate a very large load but can stretch a lot before breaking.

can affect the composition of a given muscle with respect to fiber type. Characteristics of these various fiber types are shown in Table 1.2.

Muscles act to move body parts or to stabilize a joint. As dynamic stabilizers of joints, muscles serve to duplicate the static stabilizing action of ligaments. Muscle fibers are capable of shortening to about 50% of their original length. The tension developed by a contracted muscle can be either active or passive. Active tension is due to the contractile components, namely, actin and myosin. Passive tension results from elastic properties of the contractile tissues within the muscle.

The strength of the muscle is proportional to its cross-sectional area and mass. The force of contraction of a muscle is related to many factors, including the length of the fibers, the velocity of contraction, and the direction in which the fiber is moving at the time of its contraction. Types of muscle contraction include concentric or shortening, eccentric or lengthening, and isometric, in which the muscle does not change length. Muscles are characterized by their function; agonists are prime movers, antagonists resist the action of prime movers, and synergists support the function of the agonists. For example, in ankle dorsiflexion, the anterior tibialis is the agonist. The extensor hallucis longus and extensor digitorum longus muscles assist the tibialis anterior muscle and therefore are synergists. The gastrocnemius and soleus and plantar flexors of the toes are antagonists of the tibialis anterior.

Muscles are described in anatomy texts as having origins and insertions. It is very important to recognize that this is an arbitrary distinction. A muscle that is referred to as a hip flexor because it brings the thigh toward the torso can function just as well to bring the torso over the thigh. In order for muscles to function normally, they must be both strong and flexible.

With respect to innervation of muscles, except for the deepest layers of the vertebral muscles, the exact innervation of the limb and trunk muscles is similar between individuals, with some variability. Tables listing segmental innervation differ from text to text.

Injuries to muscles are termed strains. Analogous to ligament injuries, they are classified by severity into three grades: grade I indicates minimal damage; grade II represents an intermediate amount of damage to the muscle structure; and grade III, complete disruption.

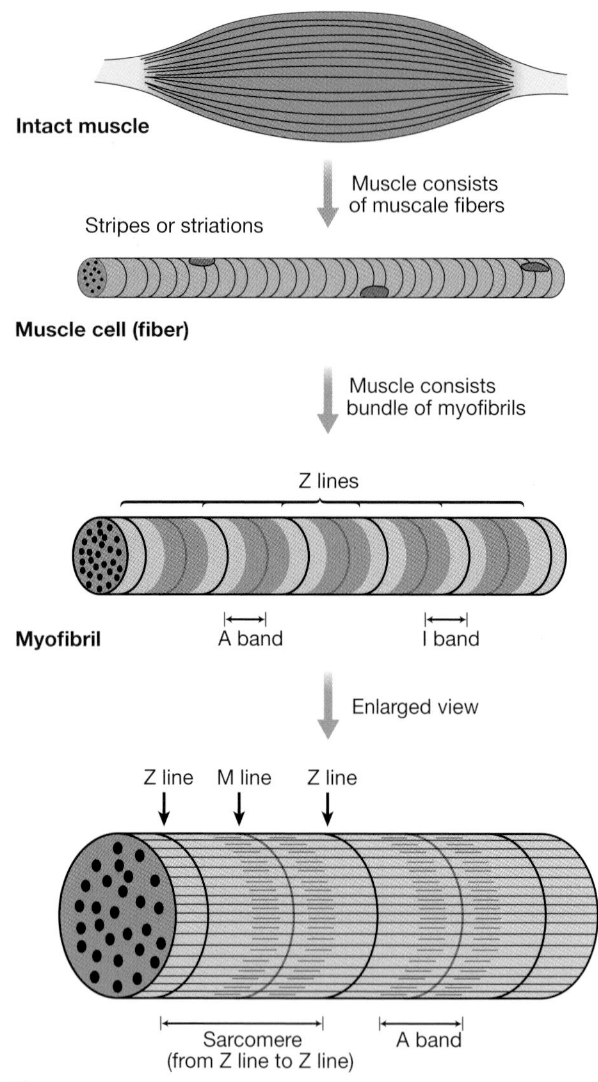

Figure 1.10 A microscopic view of muscle shows the repeated patterns of the sarcomeres and the fibrils.

Tendons

Tendons connect muscles to other structures (see Figure 1.13). Like ligaments, tendons are also composed of collagen, ground substance, and cells. The collagen of tendons is aligned in a very strict linear fashion and is always oriented in the line of the pull of the muscle. Tendons have been designed to transmit the force of the muscular contractile tissues to bone and other connective tissues, such as skin and ligaments, to which they are attached. Tendons are said to be able to withstand at least twice the maximum force that muscles can exert on them. The zone where the muscle blends into the tendinous tissues is called the musculotendinous junction. Muscle–tendon units represent tensile structures. As such, they may fail in the muscle, at the muscle–tendon junction, within the tendon, or at the tendon–bone insertion. Most commonly, however, failure occurs at the point of transition between two different materials (i.e., the musculotendinous junction). Some tendons are surrounded by a double-walled tubular covering, referred to as a tendon sheath or a peritendon (i.e., Achilles tendon or flexor tendons of the hand). This is lined with a synovial membrane. The sheath is used both to lubricate the tendon and to guide it toward the bony attachment. Tendon sheaths provide a pathway for the gliding movement of the tendon within the sheath. An inflamed tendon sheath can cause a locking or restricted movement, as in a trigger finger. Inflammation of the tendon structure is termed tendinitis.

Synovium and Bursae

Synovial tissue lies in the inner aspect of synovial joints and bursal sacs. It has two functions: to produce lubricating fluids and to phagocytize (remove) foreign debris. Synovium is highly vascularized and innervated. As such, when traumatized or inflamed, synovial tissue will rapidly enlarge and produce significant pain.

Bursal sacs serve to reduce friction. Therefore, they are located wherever there is need for movement between structures in close proximity. For example, the olecranon bursa lies between the olecranon process of the ulna and the skin overlying the posterior part of the elbow (see Figure 1.14). The subacromial bursa lies between the acromioclavicular arch above and the rotator cuff tendons below. Inflammation of synovial or bursal tissues due to trauma, inflammatory processes, or foreign materials is termed synovitis or bursitis.

Fascia

There are three kinds of fascial tissues: superficial, deep, and subserous. The fascia is composed of loose to dense connective tissue. Superficial fascia is under the skin; deep fascia is beneath the superficial and also envelops the head, trunk, and limbs. Subserous fascia surrounds organs in the thorax, abdomen, and pelvis.

Superficial fascia contains fat, blood vessels, and nerves. It is loose in consistency and very thin. It is attached to the undersurface of the skin.

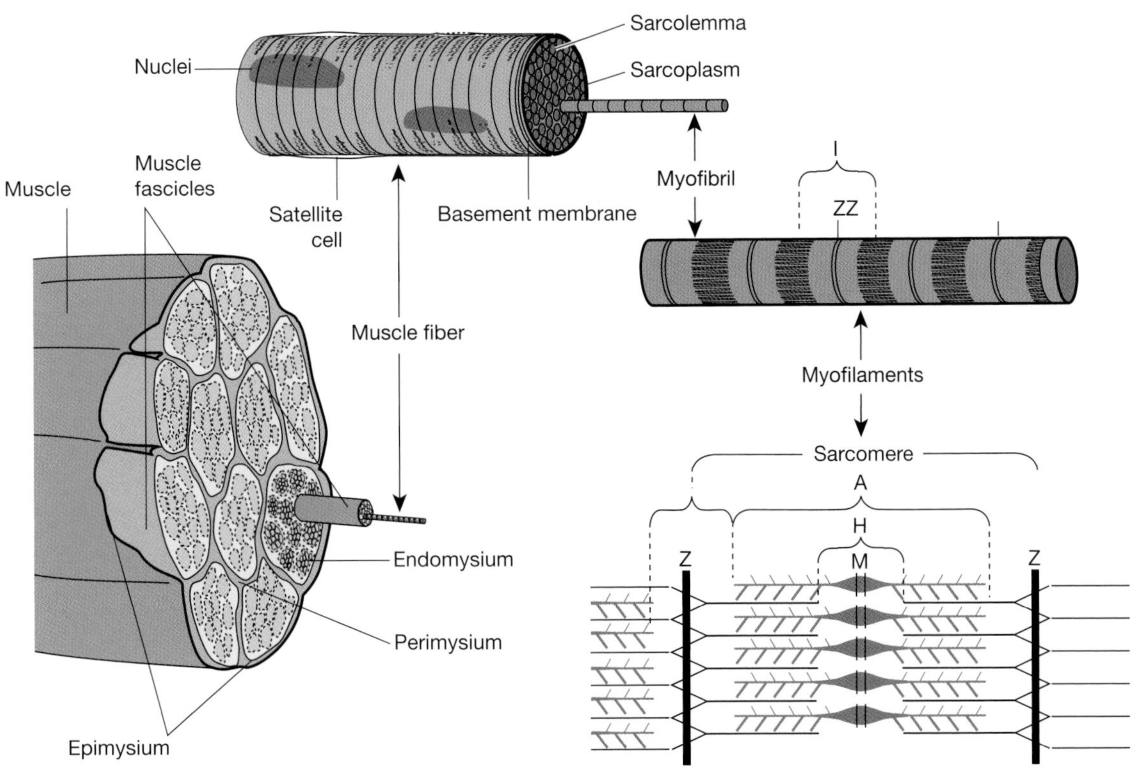

Figure 1.11 The organization of skeletal muscle tissue.

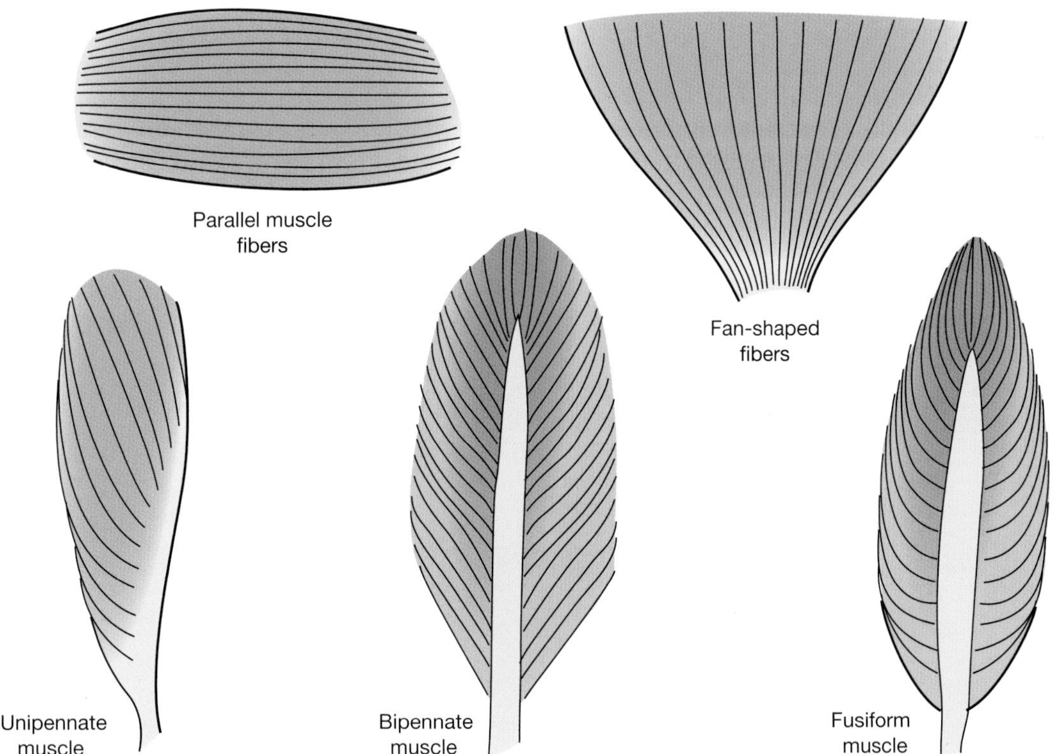

Figure 1.12 Different types of muscle–fascicle arrangements.

Table 1.2 Characteristics of Skeletal Muscle Fibers Based on Their Physical and Metabolic Properties

Property	Muscle Fiber Type Slow Twitch	Intermediate	Fast Twitch
Speed of contraction	Slow	Intermediate	Fast
Rate of fatigue	Slow	Intermediate	Fast
Other names used	Type I Slow oxidative	Type IIB Fast oxidative/glycolytic	Type IIA Fast glycolytic
Muscle fiber diameter	Small	Intermediate	Large
Color	Red	Red	White
Myoglobin content	High	High	Low
Mitochondria	Numerous	Numerous	Few
Oxidative enzymes	High	Intermediate	Low
Glycolytic enzymes	Low	Intermediate	High
Glycogen content	Low	Intermediate	High
Myosin ATPase activity	Low	High	High
Major source of ATP	Oxidative phosphorylation	Oxidative phosphorylation	Glycolysis

ATP, adenosine triphosphate.

Deep fascia is dense and tough and has two layers. It wraps around regions of the body and splits to envelop superficial muscles such as the sartorius and tensor fasciae latae. Periosteum, perimysium, and perichondrium are all elements of the deepest layer of the deep fascia. The deep fascia serves to interconnect the different muscle groups. By being continuous, it can provide tension at a distant site when pulled by a contracting muscle. Some muscles take their origin from the deep fascia. The fascia also separates groups of muscles with similar function, for example, the flexor and extensor groups of the leg. Because of the relative inelasticity of fascia, abnormally high pressure within a fascial compartment (i.e., due to injury or inflammation) can compromise the function of the nerves and blood vessels that course through that compartment. This may result in serious compromise of the tissues supplied by these nerves and vessels. Fascia may, as other tissues, experience an inflammatory reaction, fasciitis. This condition can be accompanied by moderate or even severe discomfort and scarring (fibrosis). Fibrosis can lead to stiffness and restricted movement.

The Interaction of Connective Tissues

In general, osteoarthrosis is a "wear and tear" condition. The body, although much more complex, is a machine and as such, it is subject to the same rules and laws of nature as our cars, etc. With use and in proportion to that use, it will "wear." Excluding secondary initiating causes, such as infection and inflammatory diseases, damage of an articulation (osteoarthrosis) which often becomes painful (osteoarthritis) is a manifestation of this wear and tear process. The development of osteoarthrosis should be predictable as a function of load per unit area (L/A^2) over time. However, this does not appear to be the case. For example,

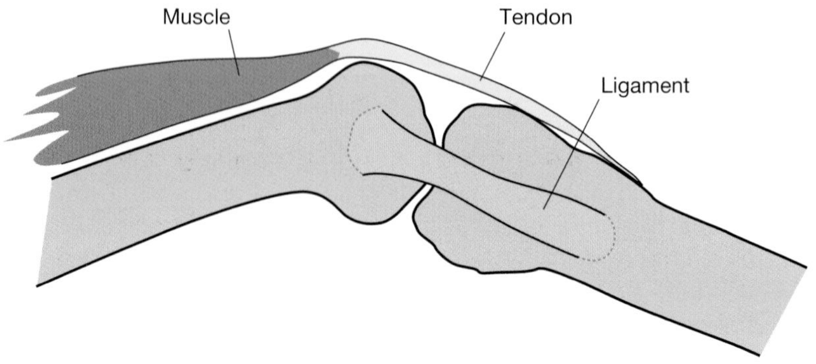

Figure 1.13 A tendon.

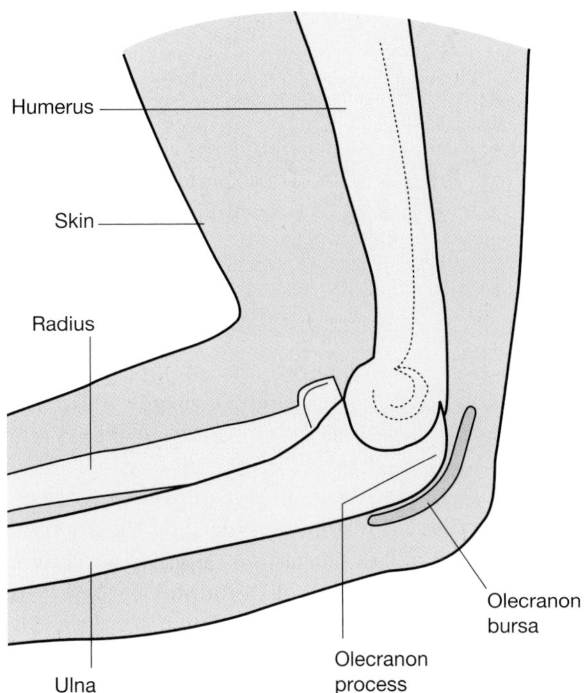

Figure 1.14 The olecranon bursa is between the skin and the olecranon process at the elbow.

consider the ankle and the knee. The talus supports the same body weight as does the tibia. The ankle experiences an equal number of loading cycles during weightbearing throughout a lifetime as does the knee. Yet the ankle is far less often afflicted with primary osteoarthrosis, than is the knee!

Since the development of osteoarthrosis is related to the degeneration and deterioration of the articular cartilage which covers the surface of a bone, it would appear that any mechanical stress which is in excess of the physiologic tolerance of the cartilage may lead to damage of that material. In general, the surface of articular cartilage is a very well-structured alignment of collagen fibers with a microporosity permitting the diffusion of nutrients and water across this barrier. Any disruption of the integrity of the surface layer will permit the large macromolecule, proteoglycan, to escape through defects in the surface layer. This would be analogous to the stuffing of a pillow escaping through a tear in the fabric on the surface of the pillow. Once the proteoglycan has escaped from the articular cartilage matrix, the ability of articular cartilage to absorb and release water as a lubricant is compromised. The loss of this self-lubricating mechanism will increase articular surface frictional wear, causing further damage and deterioration of the entire articular cartilage structure. The inevitable consequence of this process is the erosion of the articular cartilage and the eventual exposure of the underlying subchondral bone leading to the classic "bone-on-bone" seen in end-stage osteoarthrosis.

From this model, it is easy to understand that excessive frictional or shear loads on the articular cartilage surface will lead to this inevitable demise of the joint. Stability therefore plays a critical role in the maintenance and protection of articular cartilage integrity. Stability of a specific articulation is determined by a combination of factors: its geometry and the soft tissue structures crossing that joint. The geometry of an articulation determines its degrees of freedom of movement in three dimensions. The soft tissue structures provide additional joint stability and are divided into two groups. The first is comprised of static structures (ligaments), each of which has a fixed length. The second group of soft tissue stabilizers is composed of the muscle–tendon units which cross the joint. Unlike ligaments, muscle–tendons have the dynamic capability to alter their length and tension. Therefore, the development of osteoarthrosis can be predicted by an assessment of a given articulation's inherent stability provided by its architecture or geometry, and the integrity of the soft tissues crossing that articulation.

In the case of the ankle, the mortise created by the medial malleolus, tibial plafond, and lateral malleolus, into which the talus is inset, creates a very rigid structure severely restricting and limiting the degrees of freedom of talar motion. While the knee, being composed of two large condylar surfaces resting on a relatively flat tibial plateau, has no inherent geometric stability and is therefore totally dependent upon soft tissues for its stability. It is easy to understand and predict therefore that the knee being solely dependent upon soft tissues, very vulnerable to injury, would be at a significantly greater risk of developing osteoarthrosis than would the talus. This is consistent with clinical observations. The ankle appears to be relatively immune to the spontaneous development of osteoarthrosis throughout an individual's lifetime. This is true except in the case of fracture involving the articular geometry of the ankle or damage of the syndesmosis ligament connecting the tibia and fibula causing a widening of the ankle mortise. In either of those cases, an ankle will rapidly develop osteoarthrosis. In this way, connective tissues, bone, ligaments, muscles, and tendons work in synergy to not only afford proper functioning of a given articulation but also provide a primary means of protection against "wear and tear" over the course of time.

CHAPTER 2

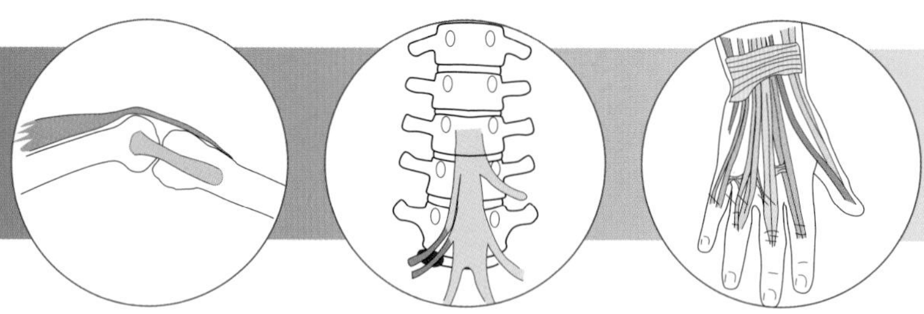

Basic Concepts of Physical Examination

Introduction

The ability to examine a joint completely and accurately is a critical part of the diagnostic process for the clinician evaluating an orthopedic problem. To accomplish this, the clinician must possess a thorough knowledge of anatomy, biomechanics, and kinesiology, as well as an understanding of the structure, purpose, and response of the various tissues. Information is obtained through observation and palpation. The clinician must be able to determine whether the patient's pathology is of musculoskeletal origin.

The examination process must be performed in a specific and logical order. This order will remain the same regardless of whether the clinician is examining the shoulder joint or the spine. It is important for the examiner to develop the habit of utilizing a set sequence in order to be as organized and efficient as possible and to avoid inadvertently omitting information.

Observation

The examination should begin in the waiting room before the patient is aware of being observed. Information regarding the degree of the patient's pain, disability, level of functioning, posture, and gait can be observed. The clinician should pay careful attention to the patient's facial expressions with regard to the degree of discomfort the patient reports that he or she is experiencing. Observing the patient sitting and coming to a standing position will provide insight into the patient's ability to tolerate flexion and to then go from flexion to extension. Observation of the patient's gait will provide information regarding the ability to bear weight, strength of push-off, balance in relationship to unilateral stance, and cadence. The information gathered in this short period could be very useful in creating a total picture of the patient's condition.

Subjective Examination (History)

The patient should be escorted to a private area to enable the clinician to begin the subjective portion of the examination. The patient will be much more comfortable and relaxed if he or she is allowed to remain dressed during this part of the examination. The clinician should pay close attention to the details of the present bout and all previous related bouts. The patient deserves and will appreciate the examiner's undivided attention, even if only for a short period. A skilled clinician must be able to listen politely while directing the interview. Concise and direct questions posed in a logical order will help to provide the appropriate information.

The clinician should begin the interview by determining the history of the present bout. Questions should include the following: When did the episode begin? What was the etiology (traumatic vs. insidious)? Are the symptoms the same or are they increasing? It is important to determine whether there were any previous episodes, and if there were, to determine when they occurred, what the etiology was, how long they lasted, and how they resolved (Box 2.1).

It is helpful to elicit whether the pain is constant or intermittent. Symptoms that are brought about by

Musculoskeletal Examination, Fourth Edition. Jeffrey M. Gross, Joseph Fetto and Elaine Rosen.

Companion website: www.wiley.com/go/musculoskeletalexam

Box 2.1 Typical Questions for the Subjective Examination

Where is the pain located?
How long have you had the pain?
How did the pain start? Was it traumatic or insidious? Is the pain constant or intermittent?
If it is intermittent, what makes it better or worse? How easy is it to bring on the complaint?
Describe the pain (nature of pain)?
What is the intensity of the pain (0–10)? Does the pain awaken you at night? What position do you sleep in?
What are your work and leisure activities? What type of mattress and pillow do you use? How many pillows do you sleep on?
Does the pain change as the day progresses?
Have you had a previous episode of this problem? If yes, how was it treated?

Past Medical History (PMH):
Thorough systems review.
Specific questions are beyond the scope of this text.

Medications:
Are you taking any medication?
For which problem (symptom) is the medication providing relief?

Special Questions:
Specific questions and concerns related to each joint are discussed in the individual chapters.

changing position may be mechanical in nature. If the symptoms remain unaltered regardless of position or activity, they may be chemical in nature, secondary to the release of noxious substances that are at a sufficient level to irritate the nerve endings. Constant pain that changes in intensity or quality is considered to be intermittent (Cyriax, 1982). It is also useful to determine what makes the symptoms better or worse and how long the symptoms remain following their onset. If a patient develops pain very quickly while performing an activity and the pain lasts a long time, the clinician would consider the patient's pain to be irritable (Maitland, 2014a,b). It would be beneficial to modify the physical portion of the examination so as not to exacerbate the symptoms. The pain can also be followed over a 24-hour period. Is the patient better or worse at times throughout the course of the day? If the patient is stiffer in the morning on arising, he or she may not be using a firm mattress, may be sleeping in an inappropriate position, or may have osteoarthritis, which presents with increased stiffness following prolonged inactivity. A pain scale (McGill Pain Scale; Melzack, 1975) may be used to gain a better understanding of the patient's perception of their pain. Easy to use visual and numerical scales exist.

To organize the information that is obtained, it is helpful to use a body chart (Figure 2.1). This chart allows information to be recorded graphically for observation and comparison. The chart also enables the recording of information concerning areas other than the one affected. If an area is examined and found to be asymptomatic (clear), a check mark can be placed over that area to indicate that it has been examined and found to be free of symptoms. For example, if the patient presents with pain in the right hip on the day of the initial examination but returns with pain in the left hip 2 weeks later, the clinician can quickly refer back to the diagram to confirm the history.

Information must be gathered regarding the primary area of the complaint and any related area(s). Areas of radiating pain, anesthesia, or paresthesia should be noted. This allows the clinician to develop a better total picture of the problem. It will also help to assess whether there is any relationship between the areas. For example, if the patient's major complaint is that of low back pain and pain in the right knee, there may or may not be a direct relationship. Perhaps the patient has radicular pain in an L3 dermatomal pattern, or perhaps that patient's injury was secondary to a fall in which the patient landed on the right knee at the same time the back was injured. The quality or description of the pain (stabbing, nagging) in the patient's own words must also be noted. If the patient complains of burning pain, the nerve root might be implicated, whereas a deep ache may be associated with muscle dysfunction.

Objective Examination

Dominant Eye

Accuracy in observation requires the use of visual discrimination. This can best be accomplished by using the dominant eye. Determination of the dominant eye is done as follows: the clinician extends both arms and uses the thumb and the index finger to make a small triangle. A distant object is then selected and aligned in the center of the triangle. The clinician then closes the left eye and checks if the object remains in the same position or if it moves. If it remains, the clinician is right-eye dominant. The procedure is repeated for the other eye. The dominant eye should be checked periodically since it may change. The dominant eye should be placed over the center of all structures as

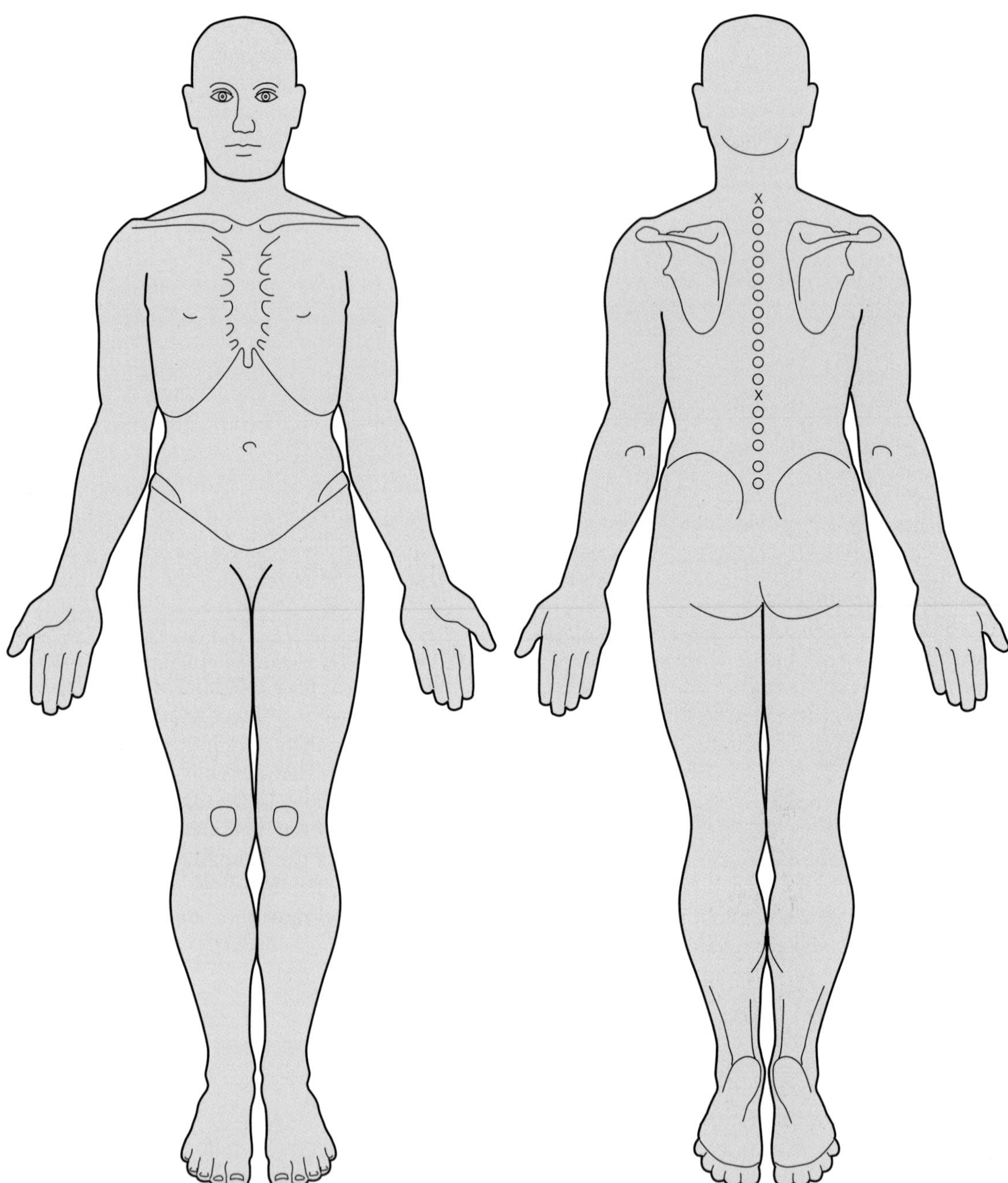

Figure 2.1 Body chart.

they are being examined to allow for more accuracy in visualization (Isaacs and Bookhout, 2002).

Structural Examination

The posture or structural examination is a static observation of the patient. This is an extremely important part of the total examination process. You can obtain a considerable amount of information regarding the patient on the basis of structure alone. Normal posture is maintained by balanced, strong, and flexible muscles, intact ligaments, freely moving fascia, healthy, properly functioning joints, a balanced line of gravity and good postural habits.

Changes in postural alignment may be secondary to structural malformation, joint degeneration, bone deterioration, joint instability, a change in the center of gravity, poor postural habits, or pain. Faulty alignment creates unnecessary stress and strain on the individual, creating either excessive elongation or adaptive shortening of muscles. Muscle elongation or shortening results in decreased efficiency while performing even the easiest of activities. The structural examination will help you gain a better understanding of the patient's predisposition to overuse or to injury.

The structural examination allows you to integrate the structure and function of all the joints. Recognize that when a person develops elongated or shortened muscles, he or she may not develop symptoms immediately. It may take many years of stress and strain for problems to reach clinical recognition.

To begin the examination, the patient is asked to disrobe and is provided with an appropriate garment, which allows you to expose the areas that are being examined. It is important that the lighting in the room is equally distributed so there are not any shadows. The patient should be instructed to stand in the middle of the examining room with their feet approximately 6 in. apart so that you can observe him or her from the anterior, posterior, and lateral views. Note whether the patient is distributing the weight equally between both feet. Most examiners prefer to have the patient remove his or her shoes to observe the feet. If, however, the patient has a known leg length discrepancy and uses a lift or wears an orthotic device, have the patient wear the shoes with the lift or orthotic device in place. Observe the patient with and without inserts or lifts. Pay particular attention to symmetry of structure including bony landmarks, muscle tone, bulk, guarding, atrophy, and alignment of the joints. The optimal, most efficient posture is symmetrical and balanced. Recognizing that no one is perfectly symmetrical, minor variations are considered to be functional. Significant differences may be secondary to anatomical malposition which is either congenital or acquired; mechanical dysfunction whether hypomobile or hypermobile; or dysfunction of the soft tissue whether hypertrophied, atrophied, taut, or slack.

The examination is approached in a logical fashion, proceeding either in a cranial or caudal direction. Here, we describe the examination from the feet first on the basis of the assumption that the weight-bearing structures will influence the structures that rest on them. It is helpful to compare any affected joints to those on the "normal" opposite side. Information from this examination can be quickly recorded on a body chart for ease of documentation and recall.

Posterior View

Normal

In a normal individual the calcaneus is in neutral alignment with the Achilles tendon vertically aligned. The feet should show 8–10 degrees of toeing out. The medial malleoli should be of equal height on both sides. The tibias should be straight without any bowing or torsion. The popliteal fossae should be of equal heights and the knee joints should show 13–18 degrees of valgus. The greater trochanters and the gluteal folds should be of equal heights. The pelvis should be the same height on both sides, with the posterior superior iliac spines level on the horizontal plane. The spine should be straight without any lateral curves. The scapulae should be equidistant from the spine and flat against the thoracic cage. The levels of the inferior angles and the spines of the scapulae should be equal in height. The shoulders should be of equal height. Patients may demonstrate a hand dominance pattern where the dominant shoulder is lower and the corresponding hip higher (Kendall *et al.*, 2005). The head and neck should be straight without any lateral tilt or rotation (Figure 2.2).

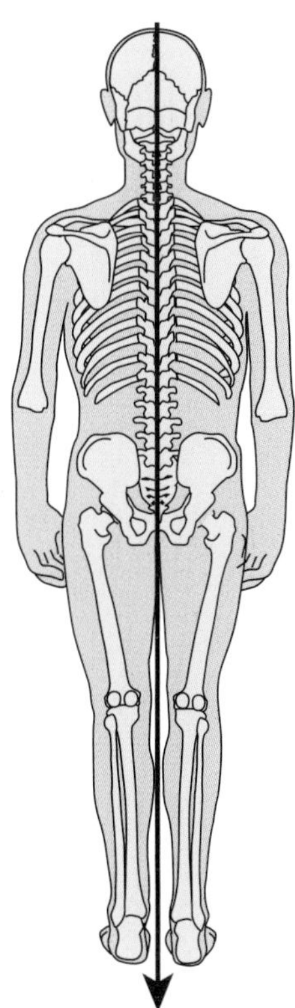

Figure 2.2 Normal posterior view.

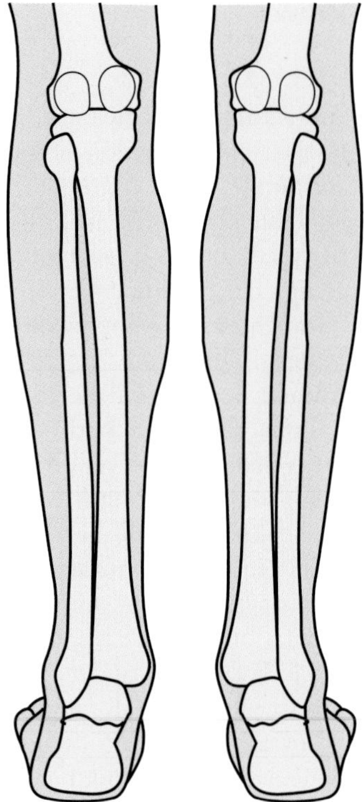

Figure 2.3 Calcaneal valgus deformity.

Possible Deviations from the Norm

Start by observing the patient's feet. Does the patient demonstrate pes planus or cavus and to what degree? Is the patient able to put the entire foot on the ground while not wearing shoes, or does he or she need a shoe with a heel because of an equinus deformity? What is the alignment of the calcaneus? Is there an excessive degree of varus or valgus (Figure 2.3)? Check the alignment of the Achilles tendon. Note the girth and symmetry of the calves. Is any atrophy or edema noted? Note the length of the leg. Does one tibia appear to be shorter than the other? Is there any bowing of the tibia or tibial torsion?

Check the alignment of the knee joints. From the posterior aspect you can observe genu recurvatum, varum, or valgum (Figure 2.4). Any of these deformities will cause a functional leg length difference unless they are symmetrical bilaterally. Note the height of the fibular heads. A difference in height may indicate an anatomical leg length difference in the tibia and fibula.

Note the alignment of the hip joint. Increased flexion may be present secondary to a hip flexion contracture (see pp. 317, 319–20, Figure 11.66). To confirm this, a Thomas test would have to be performed to test

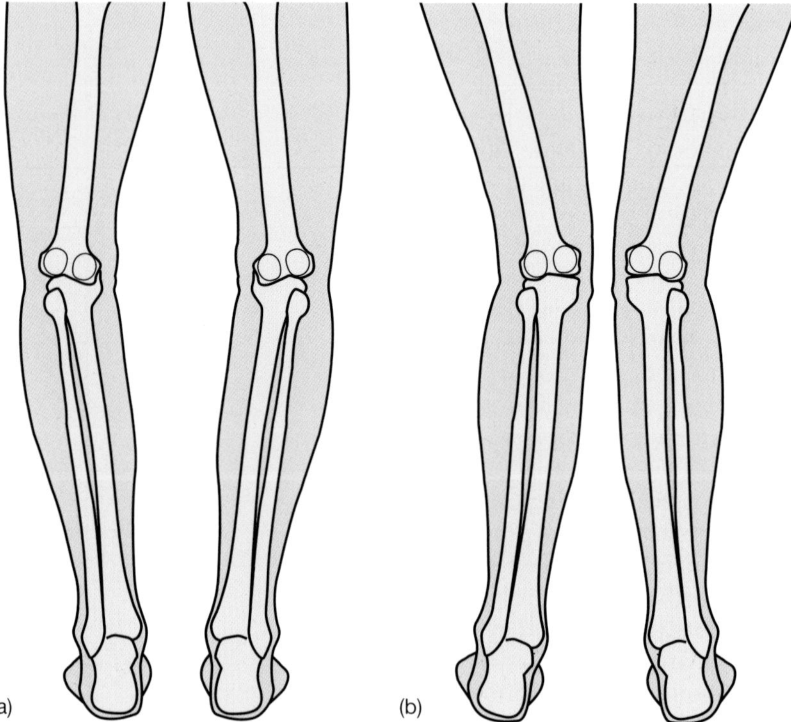

Figure 2.4 Genu varum (a) and valgum (b) deformities.

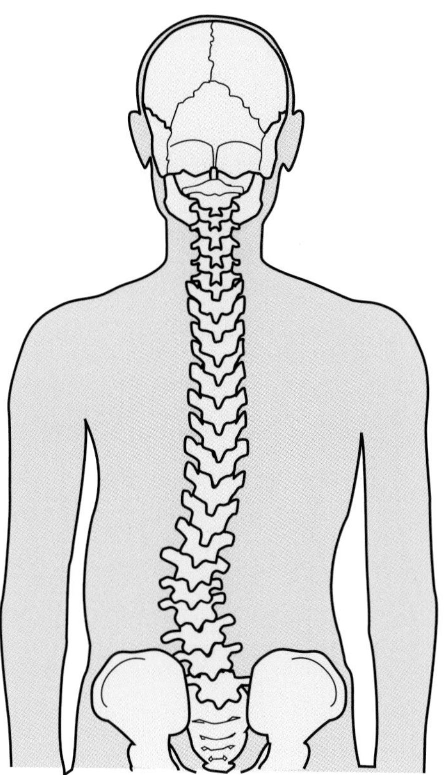
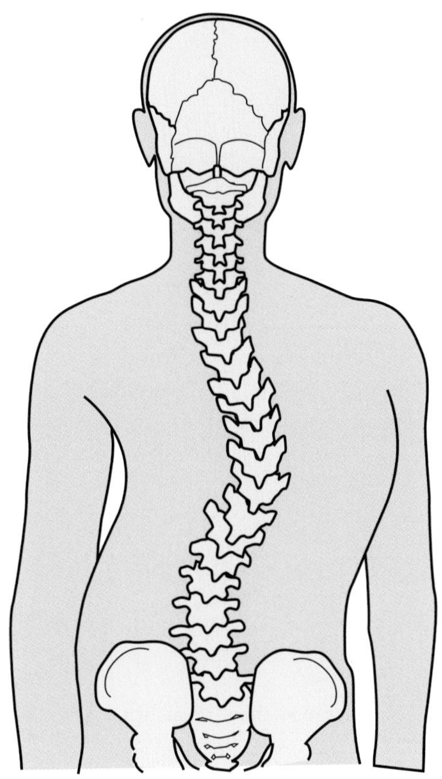

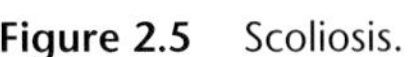
Figure 2.5 Scoliosis.

for hip flexor length. Is there excessive medial or lateral rotation? Check the relative heights of the greater trochanters. A difference in height may be secondary to a structural difference in the length of the femur.

Check the pelvis. Place your hands on the iliac crests and observe their relative heights. If one is higher than the other, it may be secondary to a pelvic torsion, a structural anomaly, or a structural or functional short leg. Place your hands on the posterior superior iliac crests and note their relative location. A change in height may be secondary to a pelvic rotation, a sacroiliac dysfunction, or a leg length discrepancy.

Observe the spine. First pay attention to the soft tissue. Are there any areas of muscle guarding or spasm? These may be secondary to a facilitated segment or surrounding an area of dysfunction. Note any differences in the skinfolds. This will allow you to better visualize lateral curves and spinal rotations. Note the alignment of the spinous processes. Is the back in straight alignment or does the patient present with a scoliosis (Figure 2.5) or kyphosis (Figure 2.6)? If scoliosis is present, note the rib cage, the degree of rotation, and the presence of any lateral humps. Is there symmetrical rib expansion both anteriorly/posteriorly and laterally? Is a lateral shift present? Is the patient

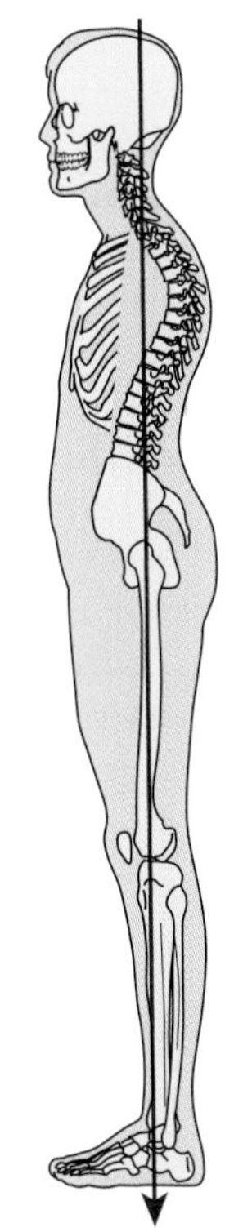
Figure 2.6 Rounded thoracic kyphosis.

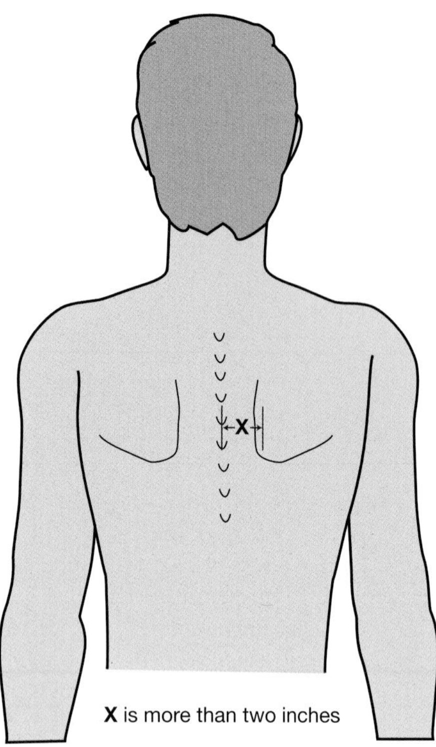

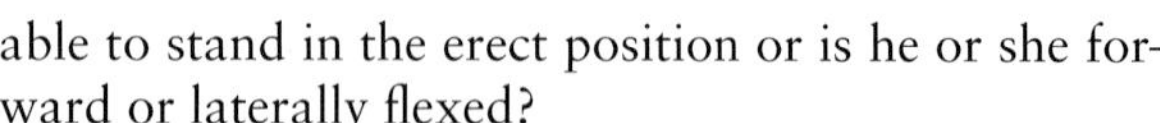

Figure 2.7 Abducted scapula.

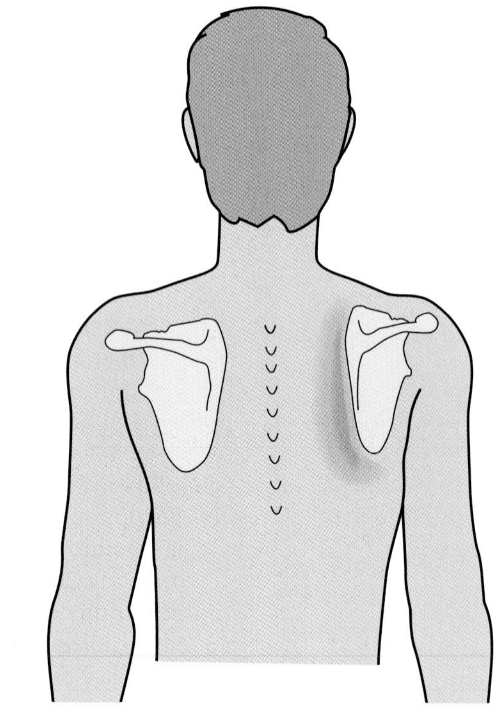

Figure 2.8 Winged scapula.

able to stand in the erect position or is he or she forward or laterally flexed?

Observe the scapulae. Are they equidistant from the spine? Are they of equal height? Are they overly abducted or adducted (Figure 2.7)? Is one side winged (Figure 2.8)? This may be secondary to weakness of the serratus anterior muscle or long thoracic nerve palsy. Is Sprengel's deformity present (Figure 2.9)? Note the muscle bellies of the infraspinatus, supraspinatus, and teres major and minor muscles over the scapula. Is there an area of atrophy? Disuse atrophy may occur in the supraspinatus or infraspinatus following a rotator cuff injury. Note the relative shoulder heights and position. Pay attention to the upper trapezius and note any hypertrophy or atrophy. Note the upper extremities. Does the patient position both arms in the same manner? Is one arm held farther away from the trunk or in either more internal or external rotation? This can be secondary to muscle shortening and imbalances or fascial restrictions.

Observe the position of the head and neck. Is the head in a forward, rotated, or laterally flexed posture? Can the patient hold the head up against gravity?

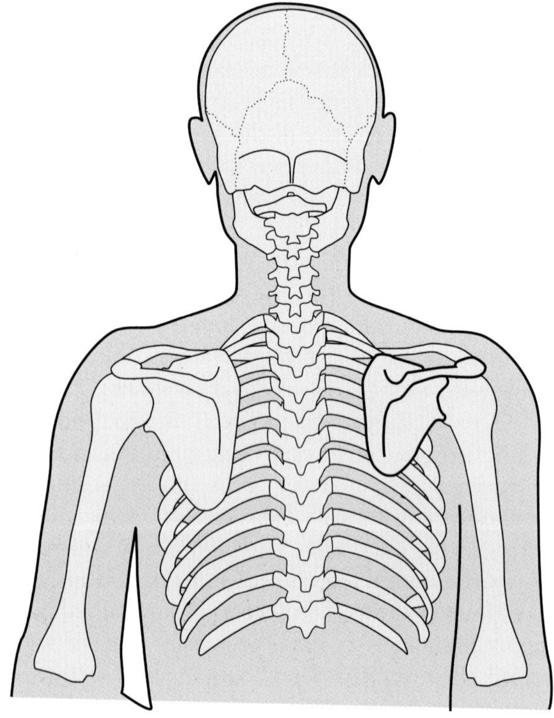

Figure 2.9 Sprengel's deformity.

Anterior View

Normal

The feet should show 8–10 degrees of toeing out. There should be a normal medial longitudinal arch that is symmetrical bilaterally. The navicular tuberosity should be located on Feiss' line (see pp. 374–5, Figures 2.19 and 13.7) (from the medial malleolus to the first metatarsophalangeal joint). The tibias should be straight without bowing or torsion. The knees should show 13–18 degrees of valgus (normal Q angle) (see Figures 12.9 and 12.12). The patellae should point straight ahead. The fibular heads should be of equal height. The pelvis should be of equal height on both sides. The anterior superior iliac spines should be level bilaterally. The spine should be straight without any lateral curves. Although the spine is not directly visible from this view, you can surmise curves by observing the anterior trunk and the pattern in which the hair grows. The rib cage should be symmetrical without any protrusion or depression of the ribs or sternum. The shoulders should be of equal height. The slope and development of the trapezii should be symmetrical. The acromioclavicular joints, the clavicles, and the sternoclavicular joints should be at equal heights and symmetrical. The arms should hang equally from the trunk with the same degree of rotation. The elbows should demonstrate equal valgus (carrying angle) (see p. 198) bilaterally. The head and neck should be straight without any rotation or lateral tilt.

The normal posture of the jaw should be where the lips are touching but relaxed and with a small space between the upper and lower teeth. The tongue should be on the hard palate behind the upper teeth (see p. 92, Figures 2.10 and 5.16).

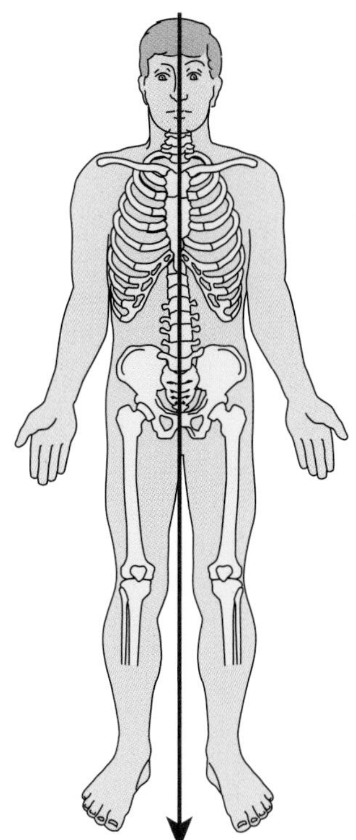

Figure 2.10 Normal anterior view.

Possible Deviations from the Norm

Starting from the feet, observe the patient's medial longitudinal arch. Does the patient have a normal arch or is a pes planus (Figure 2.11) or cavus present? Note whether the patient has hammertoes (Figure 2.12), hallux valgus (Figure 2.13), or claw toes. What is the appearance of the toenails? Are they discolored, brittle, thickened, or absent? Note the color of the patient's feet and the pattern of hair growth. This will give the information regarding the patient's peripheral vascular status by noting any deviations from normal.

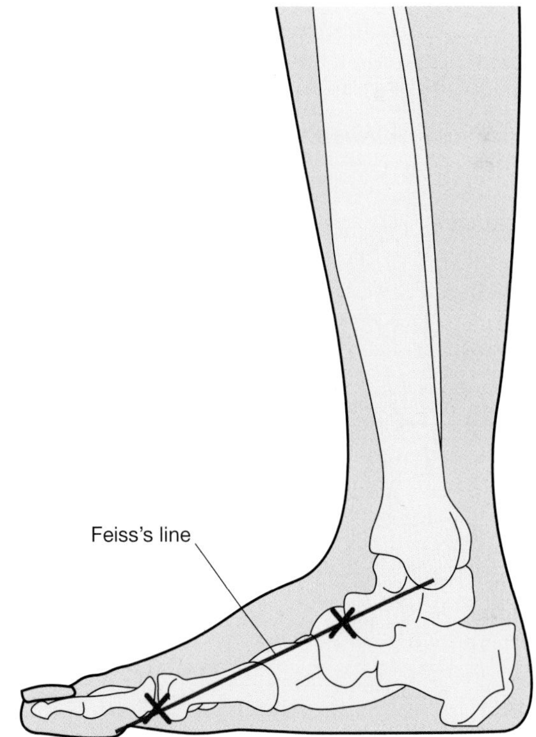

Figure 2.11 Pes planus deformity.

Observe the tibia. Note whether any bowing or tibial rotation is present. The patient may have tibial

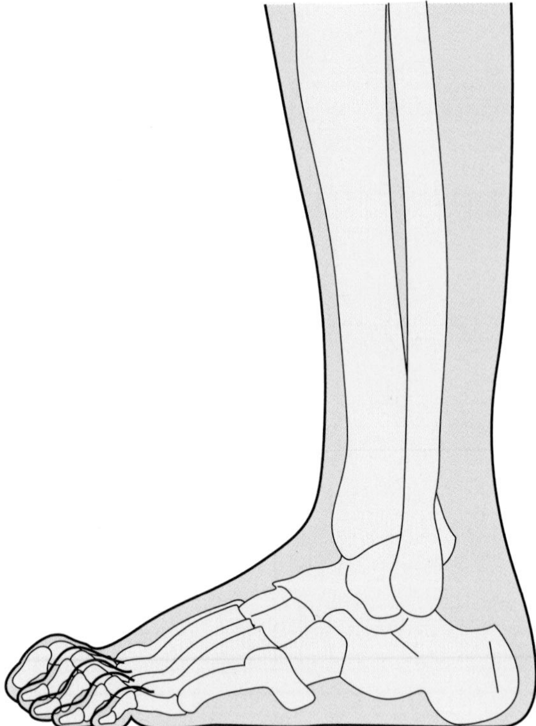

Figure 2.12 Hammertoe deformity.

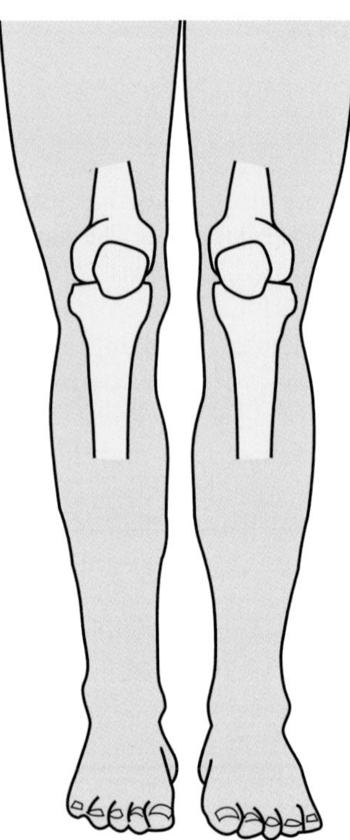

Figure 2.14 Squinting patellae. The patellae face each other.

torsion. Note the relative heights of the fibular heads. Pay attention to the patellae. Do they squint (Figure 2.14) or are they bullfrog eyes (see pp. 332–333 and Figure 12.10)? Are they of equal height? Observe the anterior aspect of the thigh and note whether

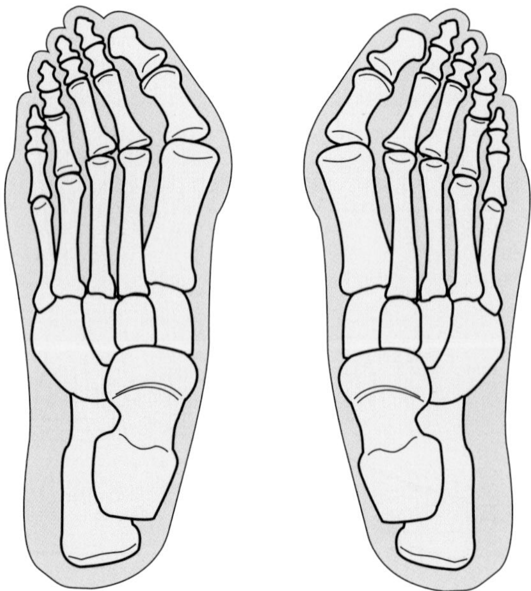

Figure 2.13 Hallux valgus deformity.

the patient presents with quadriceps atrophy. Does the patient present with genu recurvatum, valgum, or varum (Figures 2.15 and 2.20)?

Observe the hip joint. Is there excessive medial or lateral rotation? There may be an excessive amount of anteversion or retroversion present. Is a hip flexion contracture present? Is the patient's hip postured in an abnormal position? Note the heights of the greater trochanters. Place your hand over the iliac crest and check for leg length discrepancies. Place your fingers over the anterior iliac crests and note whether they are symmetrical. Changes in relative height may be secondary to pelvic rotation, sacroiliac dysfunction, or structural or functional leg length discrepancies.

Observe the patient's trunk. If the patient has chest hair, you will more easily be able to determine if a scoliosis is present by observing changes in the growth pattern. Observe the patient's chest. Note symmetry of expansion during the breathing cycle. Is there symmetrical rib expansion both anteriorly/posteriorly and laterally? If a scoliosis is present, note the rib cage, the degree of rotation, and the presence of any lateral humps. Is a lateral shift present? Is the patient able to stand in the erect position or is he or she forward or laterally flexed?

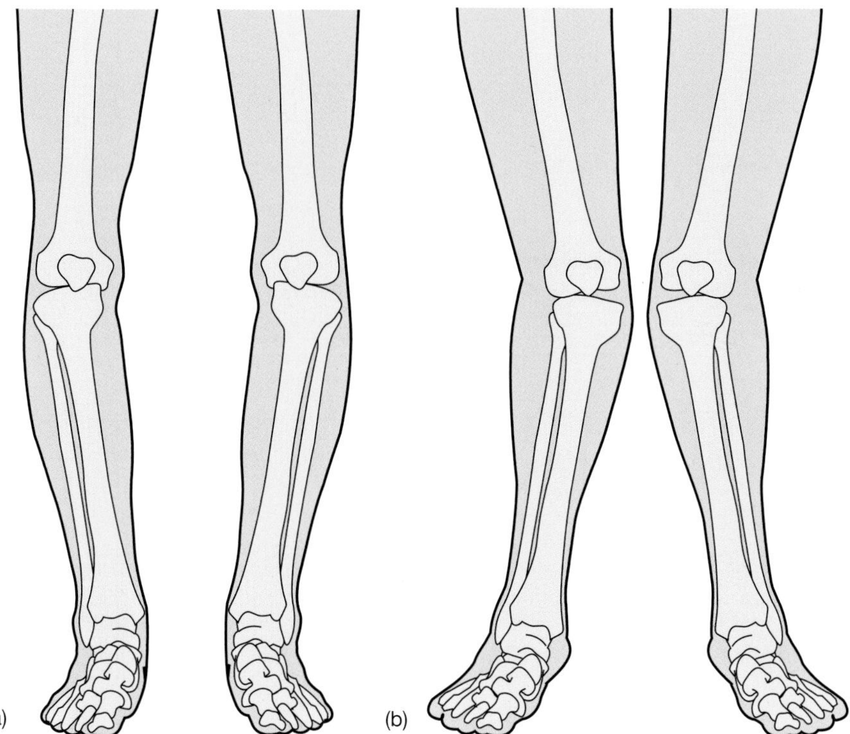

Figure 2.15 Genu varum (a) and valgum (b) deformities.

Observe the clavicles and sternum. Is one acromioclavicular or sternoclavicular joint higher than the other? Is a shoulder separation present? Does the patient demonstrate pectus excavatum, pectus carinatum, or barrel chest (Figure 2.16)? Check the sternoclavicular joints for symmetry. Note the acromioclavicular joints and observe for any separation. Note the upper extremities. Does the patient position both arms in the same manner? Is one arm held farther away from the trunk or held in more medial or lateral rotation? This can be secondary to muscle shortening and imbalances or fascial restrictions.

Does the patient present with a forward head posture? Is the head tilted to one side? Is torticollis present, with the head postured in side bending and rotation to opposite sides (Figure 2.17)?

Lateral View

Normal

It is important to observe the patient from both the right and left lateral views and compare the findings (Figure 2.18). The feet should show a normal longitudinal arch. The navicular tuberosity should be located on Feiss' line (from the medial malleolus

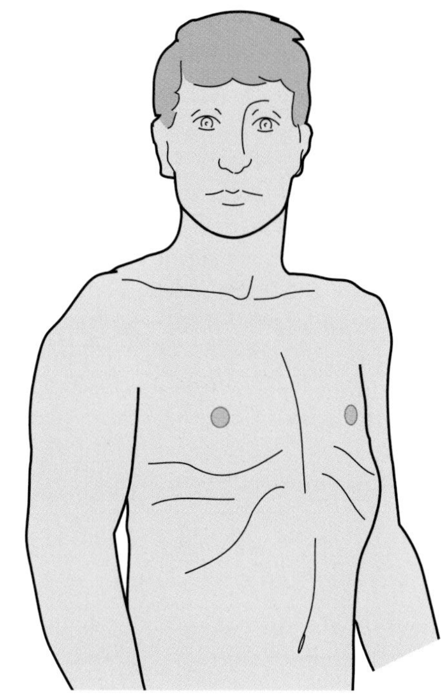

Figure 2.16 Barrel chest deformity.

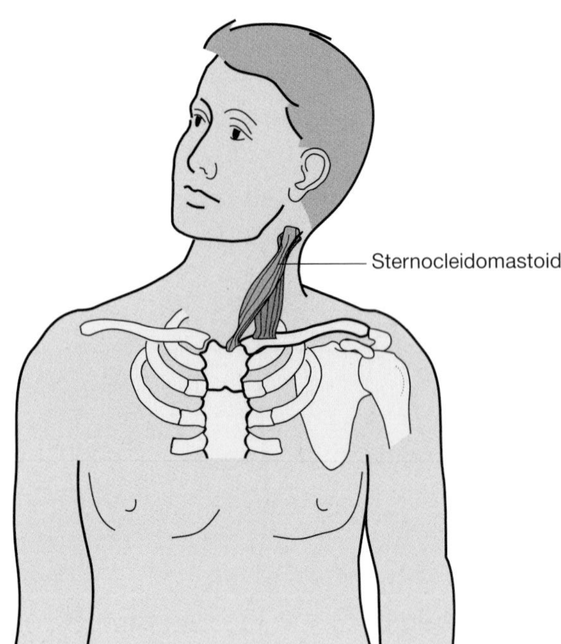

Figure 2.17 Torticollis.

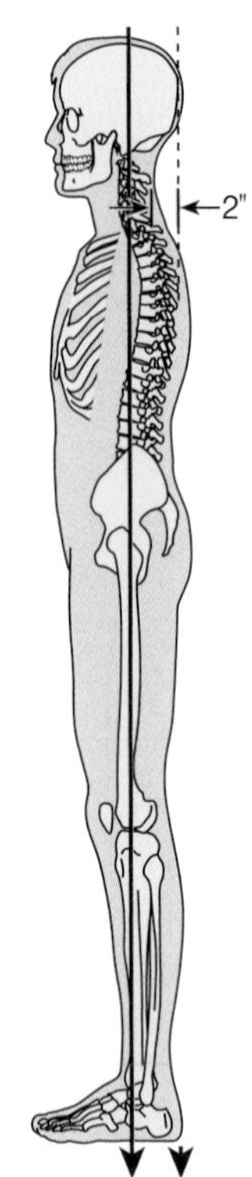

Figure 2.18 Normal lateral view.

to the first metatarsophalangeal joint). The knees should be from 0 to 5 degrees of flexion. The hips should be in 0 degrees of flexion. The pelvis should be aligned so that the anterior and posterior superior iliac spines are in the same plane horizontally, creating a normal lordosis. The pelvis should not be rotated. The anterior superior iliac spine and pubic symphysis should be in the same plane vertically. The normal posterior–anterior pelvic angle is 30 degrees from the posterior superior iliac spine to the pubic ramus. The spine should demonstrate the normal anterior–posterior curves of lumbar lordosis, thoracic kyphosis, and cervical lordosis. The chest should have a smooth contour without any areas of depression or protrusion. The shoulders should be in proper alignment without being protracted or rounded. The head should be over the shoulders with the ear lobe on a vertical line with the acromion process. Rocabado notes that the apex of the thoracic kyphosis should not be more than 2 in. posterior to the deepest point of the cervical lordosis (Figure 2.18).

Possible Deviations from the Norm

Start by observing the patient's feet. Note the medial longitudinal arch (Figure 2.19). You can observe Feiss' line and determine if a pes planus (Figure 2.11) or cavus is present. Note the alignment of the knee. The lateral view gives you the easiest way to note a knee flexion contracture or genu recurvatum (Figure 2.20).

Note the relative position of the anterior and posterior superior iliac spines. If the anterior superior iliac spine is higher, it could indicate a posterior pelvic tilt or a posterior rotation of the innominate bone. A posterior pelvic tilt will cause a decrease in the lumbar lordosis or a flat back (Figure 2.21). Is a sway back present (Figure 2.22)? If the posterior superior iliac spine is relatively higher, this could indicate an anterior pelvic tilt or an anterior rotation of the innominate bone. An anterior pelvic tilt will cause an increase in the lumbar lordosis.

Observe the trunk. The lateral view allows you to observe the anterior and posterior curves. Does the patient present with a rounded (Figure 2.6) or a flattened thoracic kyphosis? Is a Dowager's hump present (Figure 2.23)?

Note the position of the shoulders. Does the patient present with anteriorly displaced rounded shoulders (Figure 2.24)? Where are the upper extremities in relation to the trunk? Observe the head and neck. Does the patient present with a forward head posture (Figure 2.25)?

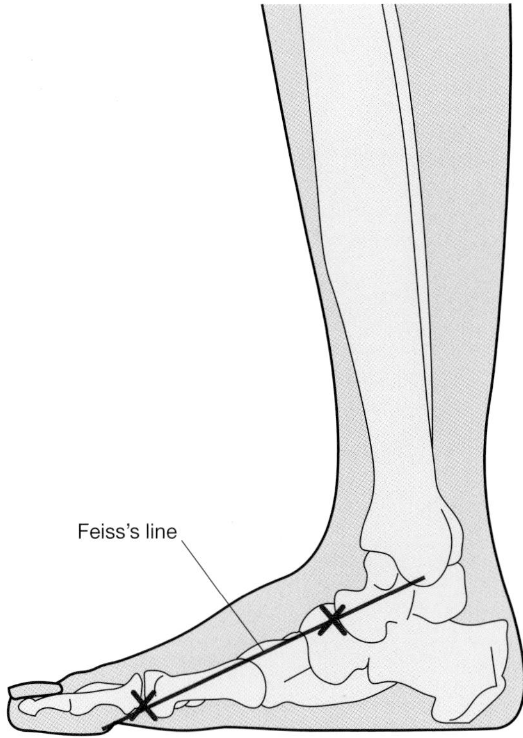

Figure 2.19 Normal medial longitudinal arch.

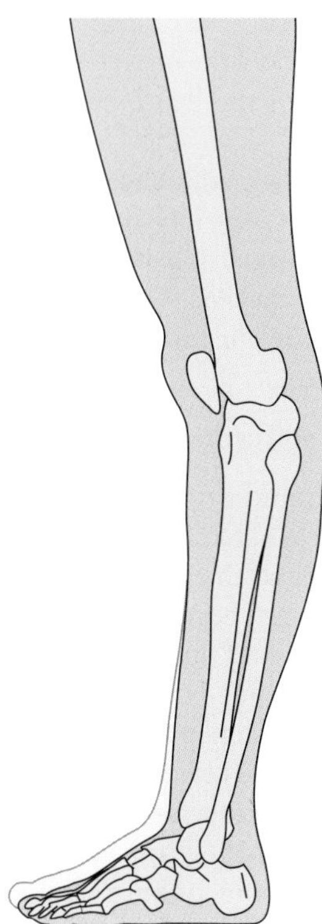

Figure 2.20 Genu recurvatum deformity.

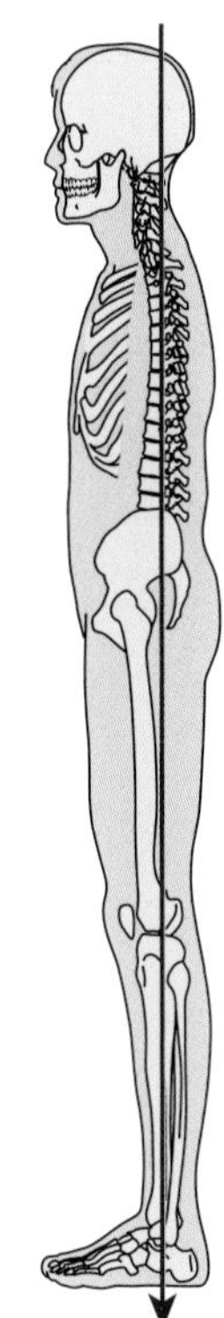

Figure 2.21 Flat back deformity.

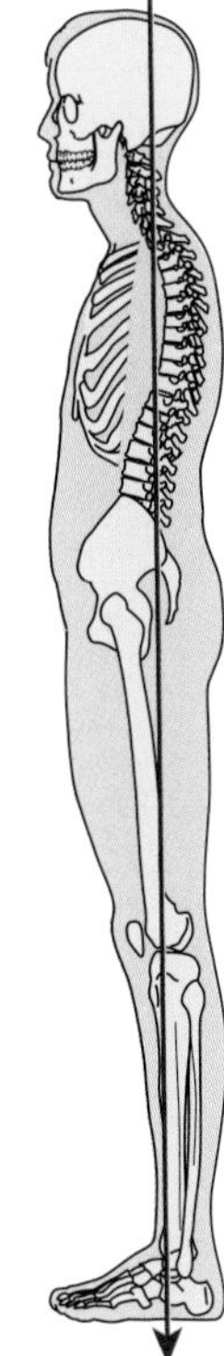

Figure 2.22 Sway back deformity.

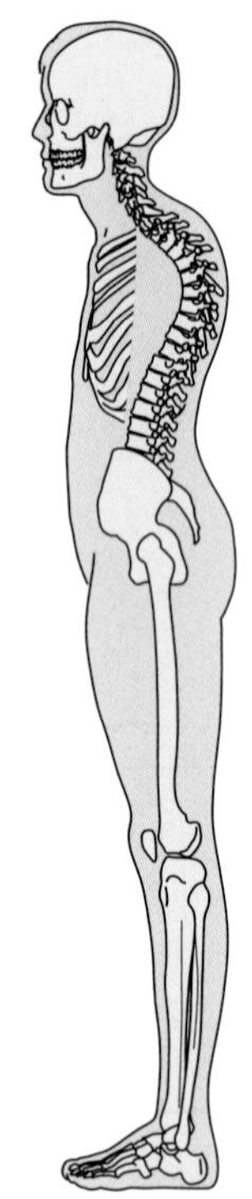

Figure 2.23 Dowager's hump deformity.

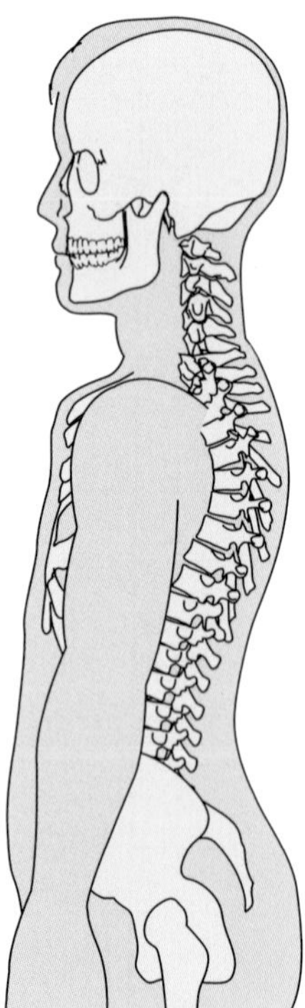

Figure 2.24 Rounded shoulders.

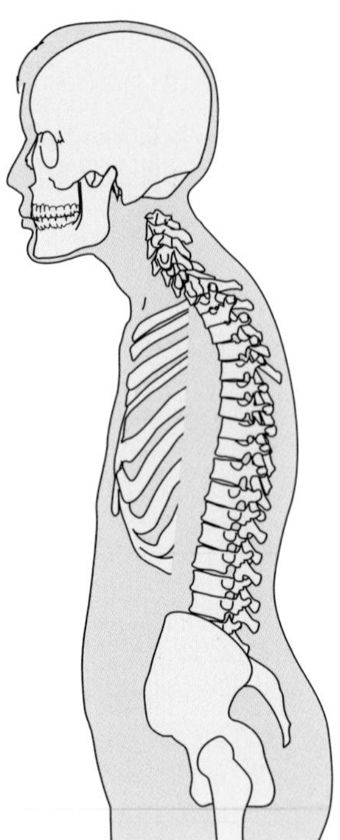

Figure 2.25 Forward head posture.

Sitting Posture

Observe the patient in the sitting position while you are standing behind him or her. Note the differences in the alignment of the head, neck, trunk, and pelvis from the posterior view. These differences can be due to the removal of the influence of the lower extremities. Some patients may have considerably better posture in the sitting position by eliminating deviations in the lower extremities, which create functional leg length discrepancies or muscle imbalances.

Active Movement Testing

The examiner should proceed by directing the patient to move through all available ranges of motion. It is beneficial to have the patient move independently before the clinician begins the palpatory examination, as the degree of movement may be adversely affected if the patient's pain level is increased. Active movement testing will provide the clinician with information regarding the status of both contractile (i.e., muscle, tendon) and noncontractile (ligaments, bones) structures of the joint (Cyriax, 1982). These tests can be used to assess the quantity and the quality of movement. The clinician should observe the degree of movement, the ease with which the patient moves, the willingness of the patient to move, and the rhythm,

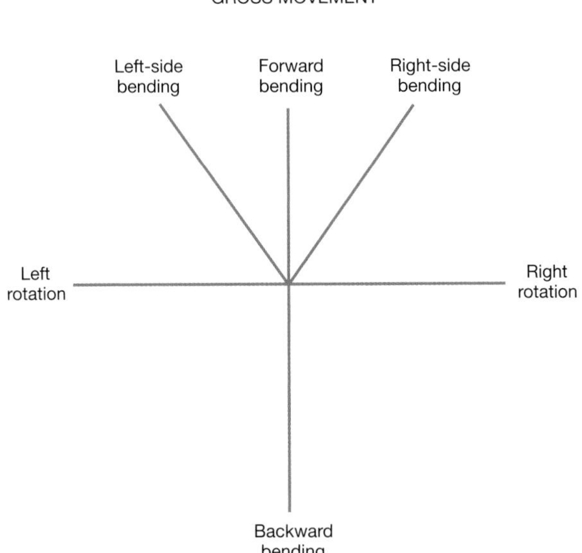

Figure 2.26 Movement diagram.

symmetry, and rate of movement (Cyriax, 1982). This will provide the clinician with information regarding the degree of the patient's flexibility, mobility, and strength.

If on active movement the patient obtains full pain-free active range of motion with an overpressure, the clinician can continue with the resisted testing portion of the examination. If the patient's range of motion is limited, the clinician should utilize passive movement testing to gain a better understanding of the structures causing the restriction.

Objective measurement of movement in the spine can be recorded utilizing a movement diagram (Figure 2.26). This very simple method allows the clinician to document the percentage or actual degrees of movement relative to the total normal anatomical range of motion in all directions. Deviations from the midline and the point of the onset of pain can also be noted. The diagram allows the clinician to quickly ascertain symmetry of movement.

Formal measurement of range of motion can also be documented with a standard goniometer using either the 180- or 360-degree scale. The specifics of appropriately placing and utilizing the goniometer are more thoroughly addressed in a textbook on goniometry. In addition, bubble goniometers, flexible rulers, inclinometers, and tape measures have all been documented in the literature as appropriate measurement tools. More specific information concerning range-of-motion measurements is included in the individual chapters devoted to the joints.

Passive Movement Testing

Passive testing of the physiological movements (cardinal plane, gross joint movement) is used to provide information regarding the state of the noncontractile (inert) elements (Cyriax, 1982). Cyriax defined inert structures as those tissues that lack the inherent ability to contract. These structures (ligaments, joint capsule, fascia, bursa, dura mater, and nerve root) are stretched or stressed when the joint is taken to the end of the available range. It is important, however, to note that even though the muscles are not called on to contract during passive movement, they do exert an influence on the degree of motion. If the muscle is maintained in a shortened state, it will prevent the joint from achieving its full anatomical range.

When performing passive movement testing, it is necessary to have the patient relax and place him or her in a secure and comfortable position. This will allow movement without internal resistance. The movement should be carried out smoothly and gently to allow maximal movement with the least discomfort.

If the patient does not achieve full anatomical range, the end of the available motion is referred to as the pathological limit. The examiner should assess the feel of the limiting tissue at the end of this range. This sensation is referred to as the end feel (end point). The end feel can be hard (bony), abrupt and firm (ligamentous), soft (tissue approximation), or elastic (tendinous). This end feel will help the clinician understand which tissue may be responsible for the loss of motion. Pain can also be a limiting factor. In this case, the clinician will experience the sense that the tissue is not restricting the motion, rather the patient is actively preventing the rest of the movement from occurring. This is referred to as an empty end feel (Cyriax, 1982; Paris, 1991; Kaltenborn, 2011).

If pain is present before a sense of structural resistance is felt, the condition can be considered to be acute. Because of the pain, the patient will prevent the movement well before the anatomical structures limit the range. If resistance is noted before the onset of pain, the condition can be considered to be chronic. The structures being stretched at the end of the range will cause the discomfort (Cyriax, 1982).

Resisted Movement Testing

Resisted movement testing involves an isometric contraction of the muscle that is performed in the neutral (mid) position. The joint must be held still so that the amount of stress placed on the inert (noncontractile) structures is minimized. The patient is instructed to produce a progressive maximal isometric contraction. This is accomplished by the clinician gradually increasing the degree of resistance until a maximal contraction is achieved. Resisted testing will help isolate the musculotendinous unit as the cause of the pain. The clinician should consider the results of the resisted movement tests. It is possible that a muscle that is tested as weak has either a musculoskeletal component, such as a strain or inflammation, or a neurological component, such as a peripheral nerve compression. If the patient has a musculoskeletal dysfunction, the resisted movement will be painful since the damaged structure is stressed. If the test reveals a muscle that is weak and painless, it is possible that the etiology is neurological (Cyriax, 1982).

The clinician must classify the response as strong, weak, painless, or painful. A muscle is considered strong if the patient can maintain a contraction against a moderate degree of resistance. If the muscle is unable to generate enough force to match the applied resistance, it is considered to be weak (Cyriax, 1982). If the patient's pain level remains unchanged despite the examiner's resistance, the response is classified as painless. If the patient's degree of pain increases or changes with the examiner's resistance, the response is classified as painful. This pain–strength relationship will give the clinician better insight into which structures are responsible for the problem. Interpretation using Cyriax's method indicates the following:

1. Strong and painful responses may be indicative of an injury to some part of the muscle or tendon.
2. Weak and painless responses may be indicative of a full rupture of the muscle or may imply an interruption of the nervous innervation of the muscle.
3. Weak and painful responses may be an indication of a gross lesion such as a fracture or metastatic lesion.
4. Strong and painless responses are indicative of normal structures.

Passive Mobility (Accessory) Movement Testing

Accessory movements (joint play) are movements that occur within the joint simultaneously with active or passive physiological movements. A combination of roll, spin, and glide allows the joint to move following the shape of the joint surface. The clinician can also assess the degree of laxity (slack) that is present when separating or gliding the joint surfaces. Laxity is the degree of looseness or "play" that is allowed by the capsule and ligaments in a normal joint while the muscles are relaxed. These movements are not under the volitional control of the patient and are totally independent from muscle contraction. To obtain full, pain-free physiological range of motion, the accessory movements must be present and full. The clinician should compare the findings from the symptomatic side with those obtained from the unaffected side.

Neurological Examination

The neurological examination helps the clinician determine whether the patient's symptomatology stems from the musculoskeletal system, the nervous system, or a combination of both. For example, a patient with complaints of shoulder pain may have a C5 radiculopathy or a subdeltoid bursitis. The clinician cannot differentiate between the two diagnoses without completing a thorough examination of the cervical spine and shoulder. The specifics of these examinations are discussed later in this chapter.

Manual Muscle Testing

If the clinician prefers to obtain specific grades of strength for each individual muscle as opposed to classifying the strength as strong or weak, a formal manual muscle test can be performed. The patient is placed in the appropriate positions with resistance applied to elicit specific muscle contractions. The strength is then evaluated and graded using a system from 0 to 5 or 0 to normal. Generally accepted definitions of the muscle grades are as follows (Kendall *et al.*, 2005):

- Normal (5): The muscle can withstand a strong degree of resistance against gravity.
- Good (4): The muscle can withstand a moderate degree of resistance against gravity.
- Fair (3): The muscle is able to sustain the test position against gravity.
- Poor (2): The muscle is able to complete the range of motion in a plane that is parallel to gravity (gravity eliminated).
- Trace (1): The muscle can perform a palpable contraction but without any visible movement.
- Zero (0): No contraction is present.

Some clinicians may prefer to use plus and minus grades with the above definitions or use a scale from 0 to 10. A discussion related to functional muscle testing is included in each of the chapters on individual joints. Selected manual muscle tests are included in the individual chapters later in this book. However, detailed information regarding the specifics of manual muscle testing is beyond the scope of this book. Some clinicians may want to continue their evaluation with more extensive equipment, such as that required for isokinetic testing.

Deep Tendon (Stretch) Reflexes

It is important to test the deep tendon (stretch or myotatic) reflexes. Comparison of both sides is very important. A patient may present with symmetrically decreased reflexes and be perfectly normal. Normal variations must be taken into account. If the patient presents with hyperreflexia, a correlation can be made with upper motor neuron disease secondary to decreased inhibition by the motor cortex. If the patient presents with hyporeflexia, lower motor neuron disease may be the causative factor secondary to an interruption in the reflex arc. Jendrassik's method of reinforcement, where the patient pulls his or her clasped hands apart, may be needed to determine whether a reflex is present if the patient is very hyporeflexic. Asking the patient to lightly contract the muscle being tested can also enhance a difficult to elicit reflex.

Sensory Testing

The clinician should proceed with the pinprick test to differentiate between sharp and dull sensation and assess the presence or absence of skin sensation. The clinician should correlate the findings with either a dermatomal or peripheral nerve distribution. If the patient appears to have significant neurological deficits, a more detailed sensory examination (including tests for temperature, position, and vibration sensations) would be appropriate. Light touch may also be used as a screening test for sensation.

Nerve Stretch Testing

Nerve stretch tests can be used to determine whether there is compression of a nerve. The most common tests used are the straight-leg raise (SLR) (Laséque's) test and the femoral nerve (prone knee bending) test. An increased dural stretch can be added to the SLR test by flexing the patient's head and neck, adding dorsiflexion of the ankle. This creates additional stretch on the nerve root and increases the positive findings. Butler (1991) adds a slumping maneuver to the SLR and neck flexion in the sitting position, entitling it the "slump test." Peripheral nerves can also be tested by stretching them to provoke or worsen symptoms.

Compression and Distraction

Compression and distraction of the spine can be used to evaluate whether the patient's symptoms are either increased or decreased. Distraction can relieve pressure in an area that is compressed by separating the structures and allowing more space for the nerve root. Pain can also be increased because of increased stretch on the nerve root or if the nerve root is adhered. Compression can increase an already existing pressure by decreasing the space in the nerve root foramen.

Pathological Reflex Testing

Pathological reflexes should also be tested. The clinician should check for the presence of the Babinski or Hoffmann reflex. If either of these is present, a correlation to upper motor neuron disease can be made.

Palpatory Examination

The clinician should start the examination by visually inspecting the skin and subcutaneous tissue over the affected area. Areas of localized swelling, excess fat, abrasion, discoloration, hematoma, and birthmarks should be noted. The clinician should then palpate the area and note areas of increased or decreased moisture and temperature. If warmth, redness, and increased moisture are present, a correlation can be made to an acute lesion. A scratch test can be performed to evaluate the degree of histamine reaction. Skin rolling can determine whether there are any areas of adhesion. In a normal patient, the skin should roll freely.

The clinician should palpate bony landmarks, noting their orientation and areas of tenderness or deformity. When examining the spine, the clinician should pay attention to the alignment of the spinous and transverse processes and note if they are appropriately positioned. The inexperienced clinician may be misled into thinking that a faulty alignment exists when actually a congenital anomaly is present.

The muscles should be palpated and areas of spasm, guarding, knots, and tenderness should be noted. The clinician should be aware that it is easy to be fooled by listening to the patient's complaint without completing the actual physical examination. Very often the area of complaint will not correlate to the area of palpable tenderness or dysfunction. When palpated, trigger points within muscles may radiate pain to a distant location. Ligaments and tendons should also be palpated. Swelling and a sense of bogginess may indicate an acute lesion, whereas stringiness may be found in chronic injuries. Finally, the clinician should palpate the arterial pulses in the area being examined to determine whether any vascular compromise is present.

Correlation

On completion of the examination, the clinician should correlate the information in a logical fashion, so that all the pieces of the puzzle fit together to formulate a diagnosis. If one piece of information does not fit, the clinician should reexamine the patient to guarantee that the finding is accurate. If the information does not fit together, the clinician should consider that the etiology of the problem is coming from another body system and refer the patient accordingly.

CHAPTER 3

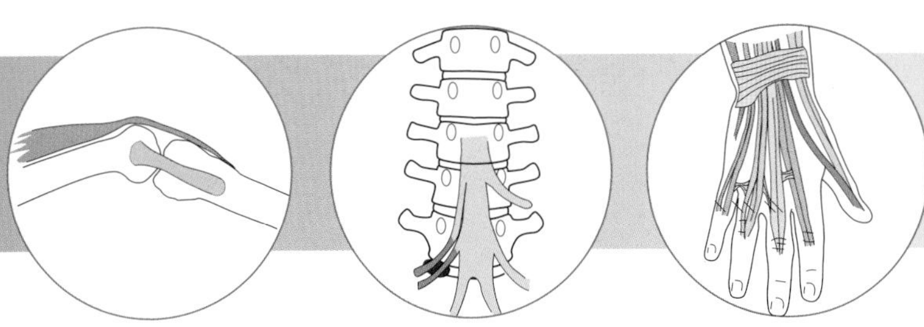

Overview of the Spine and Pelvis

The spine and pelvis represent the central support of the body. The pelvis can be thought of as a trapezoidal structure lying atop two columns (the lower extremities) upon which the spine sits.

The spine is composed of more than 30 segments called vertebrae. The vertebrae permit rotation, lateral bending, and flexion–extension movements. They vary in shape and size, but in general have similar structures (Figure 3.1). Most of the vertebrae have a large central body. Posteriorly, they have a hollow ring through which the spinal cord passes. There are bony projections extending posteriorly from the lateral and posterior aspects of this ring. These bony projections are termed the transverse and spinous processes and serve as points of attachment for spinal ligaments and muscular tissues. Stability of the vertebrae is dependent on soft tissues (intervertebral ligaments and paraspinal muscles) and posterior articulations called the facet joints. The vertebrae can be divided into five subgroups. Each subgroup has a different function; hence, vertebrae, although somewhat similar within a subgroup, vary significantly in their geometry from vertebrae of another subgroup. This change in shape and size reflects the different functions of these subgroups. The different shapes have significant effects on vertebral mobility and stability. The most superior subgroup is termed the cervical spine. There are seven vertebrae within the cervical spine. At the apex is the atlas, or C1 vertebra. It is so named because it carries the "world" (the head) on its shoulders. Its articulation with the base of the skull permits a small amount of front-to-back movement (nodding) and side bending. Beneath the atlas is the axis, or C2 vertebra. Its name comes from the fact that it presents a vertical structure (odontoid), much like that of a gatepost to the atlas, about which the atlas can rotate. This bony odontoid shares space with the spinal cord within the central hollow ring of the atlas (Figures 3.2 and 3.3). As such, any instability, whether traumatic or secondary to another etiology (rheumatoid inflammation), can cause anterior translation of the atlas on the axis. This can result in compression of the odontoid onto the spinal cord within the spinal canal, with life-threatening consequences. Beneath the axis, the remaining five cervical vertebrae are similar in shape and function. They accommodate flexion–extension, lateral (side) bending, and lateral rotation. Below C2, the point of maximum flexion–extension movement is at the C4–C5 and C5–C6 levels. Hence, it is at these sites that osteoarthritic degeneration is most commonly seen. The consequence of this frequency of osteoarthritic degeneration is that radicular symptomatology secondary to cervical osteoarthritis most commonly affects the C4, C5, and C6 nerve roots. This is due to foraminal and disc space narrowing (stenosis) caused by degenerative changes and osteophyte formation at these levels. One additional anatomical curiosity of the cervical spine involves the vertebral artery becoming entombed within the vertebral processes of C2, C3, C4, and C5 as it travels proximal toward the skull. This tethering of the vertebral artery within the bony vertebrae can create a stress point to the vessel with extreme movement of the cervical spine.

The 12 thoracic vertebrae are stabilized by the rib cage into a relatively immobile segment. There are

Musculoskeletal Examination, Fourth Edition. Jeffrey M. Gross, Joseph Fetto and Elaine Rosen.

Companion website: www.wiley.com/go/musculoskeletalexam

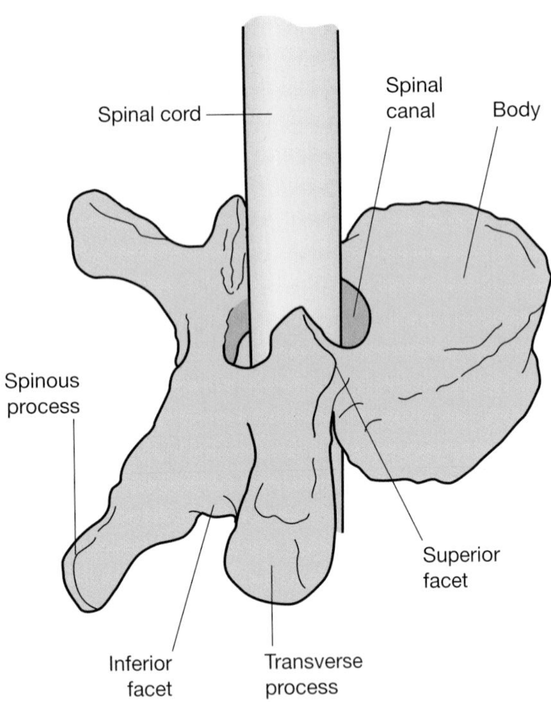

Figure 3.1 A generalized vertebral segment is composed of a large, solid cylindrical body. Posteriorly, there is a bony ring through which the spinal cord and its coverings pass. Transverse and spinous processes project from the ring.

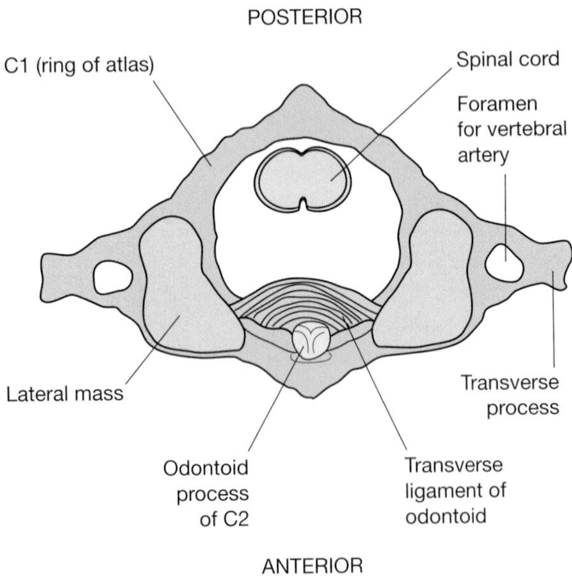

Figure 3.2 A transverse view through the ring of C1 (atlas) shows the spinal canal to be divided into thirds. The anterior third is occupied by the bony odontoid process of C2; the posterior third is filled by the spinal cord; the transverse ligament prevents migration of C1 on C2, not allowing the odontoid to invade the empty central third of the spinal canal.

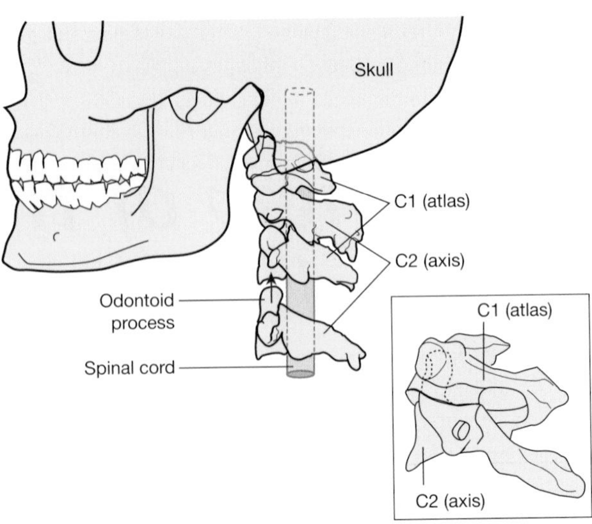

Figure 3.3 The skull rests on the atlas (C1); the head rotates about the odontoid process as if it were a gatepost.

four localized points of significant stress created at the proximal and distal ends of the thoracic spine, at the cervicothoracic and thoracolumbar junctions. This is due to the abrupt change in stiffness at these points.

The five segments of the lumbar spine are very large versions of those found in the cervical spine. This is consistent with the increased load to which they are subjected and the fact that their purpose is to permit motion in all three planes between the rigid pelvis below and the semirigid thorax above. Like the cervical spine, the lumbar spine is a common site of degenerative change. It has been said that the human lumbar spine has not yet sufficiently evolved to accommodate the erect bipedal stance. This is certainly borne out by the fact that back pain is almost a universal ailment among humans at some point during their lives. Of particular importance are the L4–L5 and L5–S1 articulations. A forward-facing convexity called lordosis is quite pronounced at these levels. This lordosis accounts for the slight "hollow" one normally perceives at the region of the low back when lying on the floor with the lower extremities fully extended. This lordosis creates a tremendous forward pressure on the vertically oriented facet joints, which serve to stabilize the lower lumbar segments against forward translation. This constant forward pressure may explain the high frequency of degenerative change seen within these particular facet articulations.

The lumbar, thoracic, and cervical spinal segments rest on a large triangular structure called the sacrum. The sacrum is formed by the fusion of five vertebral segments into one large triangular bone. Similar to the keystone at the top of the arch, the sacrum is keystoned into the pelvic ring between the ilia (innominates). It is held in place by a combination of extremely strong ligaments and a synchondrosis with each iliac wing.

Beneath the sacrum are the vertebral segments of the coccyx. Seen on lateral x-ray films, the coccyx has the appearance of a short tail. It actually represents the vestigial remnants of the tails that existed on our ancestors. Occasionally, an infant will be born with accessory coccygeal segments or an actual tail, which will require surgical removal. The coccyx serves to protect the structures of the lower pelvis and acts as an attachment for some of the lower pelvic musculature and ligaments.

CHAPTER 4

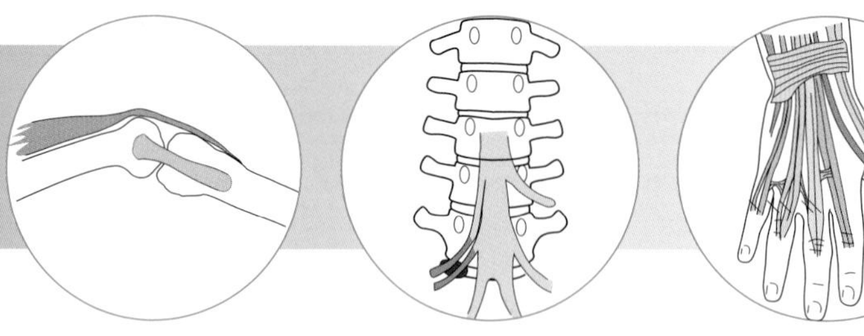

The Cervical Spine and Thoracic Spine

FURTHER INFORMATION

Please refer to Chapter 2 for an overview of the sequence of a physical examination. For purposes of length and to avoid having to repeat anatomy more than once, the palpation section appears directly after the section on subjective examination and before any section on testing, rather than at the end of each chapter. The order in which the examination is performed should be based on your experience and personal preference as well as the presentation of the patient.

Observation

The cervical spine is a flexible column that supports the weight of the head and provides a protected pathway for the spinal cord as it descends. It protects the vertebral arteries, the internal jugular veins, and the sympathetic chain of the autonomic nervous system. It is imperative that special care be taken to monitor these structures during the examination. The distinctive arrangement of the articulations of the upper cervical spine continuing with the facet joints of the lower cervical spine allows for the head to move through space. The muscles and ligaments create a great deal of stability as they counteract the inertia of the head. There is also a unique interaction with the shoulder girdle because of the many mutual muscle attachments. In contrast, the thoracic spine is quite rigid because of its attachment to the rib cage. Active motion is therefore much more restricted (see Figures 4.1, 4.2, 4.3, and 4.4).

Note the manner in which the patient is sitting in the waiting room. Notice how the patient is posturing the head, neck, and upper extremity. Is the patient's head forward or laterally bent? Is the patient supporting their head with their hands or is he or she wearing a cervical collar? Is the arm relaxed at the side or is it being cradled for protection? How willing is the patient to turn the head or look up at you as you approach? Will the patient use the upper extremity? Will he or she extend the arm to you to shake your hand? Pain may be altered by changes in position, so watch the patient's facial expression for indications as to their pain level.

Observe the patient as he or she assumes the standing position and note their posture. Pay particular attention to the position of the head, cervical spine, and thoracic kyphosis. Note the height of the shoulders and their relative positions. Once the patient starts to ambulate, observe whether he or she is willing to swing their arms. Arm swing can be limited

Musculoskeletal Examination, Fourth Edition. Jeffrey M. Gross, Joseph Fetto and Elaine Rosen.

Companion website: www.wiley.com/go/musculoskeletalexam

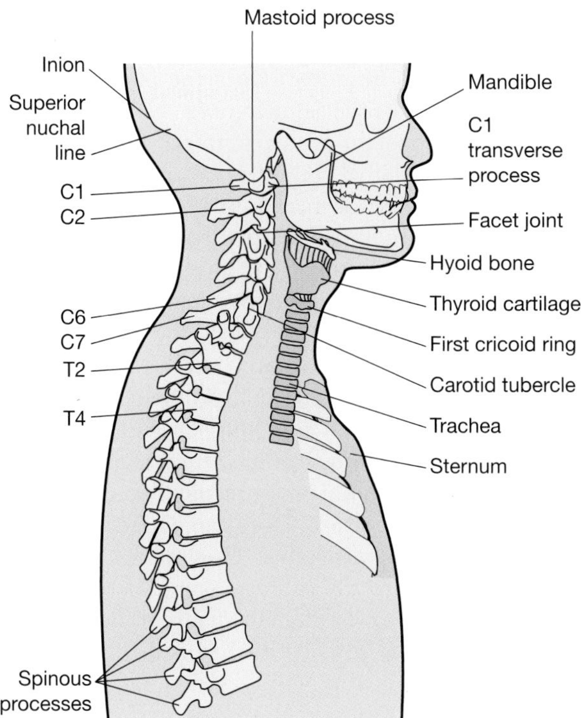

Figure 4.1 Overview of the neck with anterior–posterior relationships.

by pain or loss of motion. Once the patient is in the examination room, ask him or her to disrobe. Observe his or her willingness to bend the head to allow for removal of the shirt. Note the ease with which upper extremities are used and the rhythm of the movements. Observe the posture of the head, neck, and upper back. Observe for symmetry of bony structures. Observe the clavicles and the sternum. An uneven

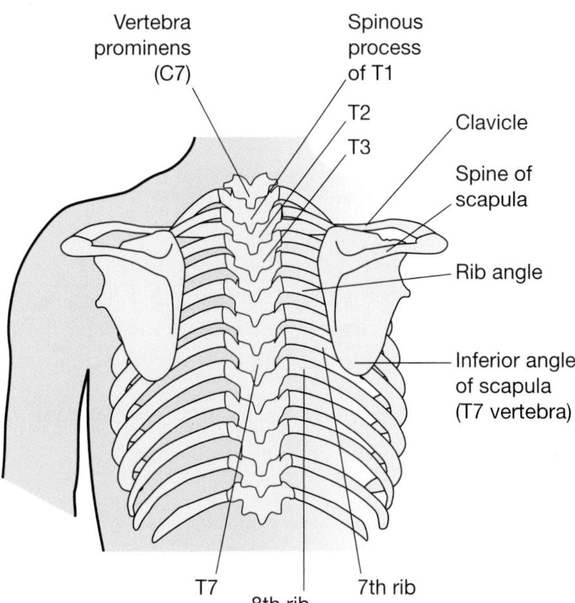

Figure 4.2 Overview of the posterior thorax.

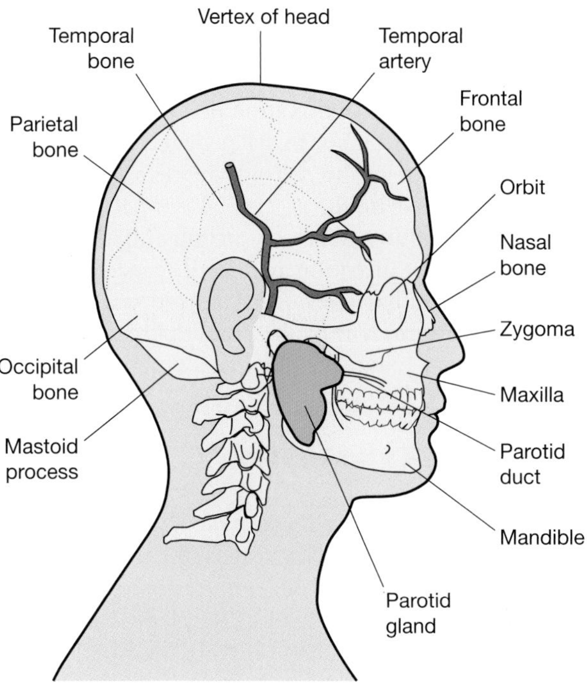

Figure 4.3 Overview of the skull.

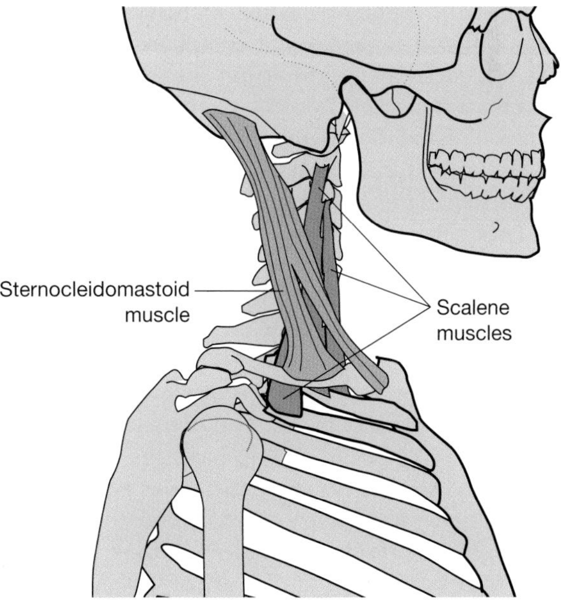

Figure 4.4 The sternocleidomastoid muscle acts both as a cervical flexor and lateral rotator of the cervical spine. The scaleni muscles act to bend the cervical spine laterally and also assist in flexion.

contour may be present secondary to a healed fracture. Observe the scapulae and determine whether they are equidistant from the spine and are lying flat on the rib cage. Is a subluxation present at the glenohumeral joint and if so, to what degree? Notice the size and contour of the deltoid muscle and compare to the opposite deltoid.

Observe for any areas of atrophy in the upper extremities. Pay attention to the rib cage. Does the patient have a barrel chest? Observe the patient's breathing pattern. Is he or she a mouth breather? Note the degree and symmetry of expansion bilaterally.

Subjective Examination

Since the cervical spine is quite flexible, it is an area very commonly affected by osteoarthritis, inflammation, and trauma. You should inquire about the nature and location of the patient's complaints and their duration and intensity. Note if the pain travels up to the patient's head or distally to below the elbow. The behavior of the pain during the day and night should also be addressed. Is the patient able to sleep or is he or she awakened during the night? What position does the patient sleep in? How many pillows do they use? What type of pillow is used?

You should determine the patient's functional limitations. Can the patient independently support the head upright? Is he or she able to read, drive, or lift heavy objects? If the patient complains of radicular pain, ask questions regarding use of the upper extremity. Is the patient able to comb their hair, fasten a bra, bring their hand to their mouth to eat, or remove their jacket? Is the radicular pain associated with numbness or tingling in the arm or hand? Does the patient regularly participate in any vigorous sports or work-related activity that would stress the neck and upper back? What is the patient's occupation? Working at a computer or constant use of the telephone can influence the patient's symptoms.

If the patient reports a history of trauma, it is important to note the mechanism of injury. The direction of force, the position of the head and neck during impact, and the activity the patient was participating in at the time of the injury all contribute to an understanding of the resulting problem and help to better direct the examination. If the patient was involved in a motor vehicle accident, it is important to determine whether he or she was the driver or the passenger. Did the patient strike their head during the accident? Did the patient suffer a loss of consciousness and if so, for how long? Was the patient wearing a seatbelt and if so, what type? The degree of pain, swelling, and disability at the time of the trauma and within the next 24 hours should be noted. Does the patient have a previous history of the same injury?

Is the pain constant or intermittent? The answer to this question will give you information as to whether the pain is chemical or mechanical in nature. Can the pain be altered by position? If the pain is altered by position, one can assume that there is a mechanical basis. Consider the factors that make the patient's complaints increase or ease. Does the pain increase when the patient takes a deep breath? This may be secondary to a musculoskeletal problem or a space-occupying lesion. Does coughing, sneezing, or bearing down increase the symptoms? Increased pain with greater intra-abdominal pressure may be secondary to a space-occupying lesion. Does the patient complain of gastrointestinal problems? Pain may be referred from the viscera to the thoracic spine. If the patient has a central nervous system disorder including a compression of the spinal cord, he or she may present with the following complaints: headaches, dizziness, seizures, nausea, blurred vision, or nystagmus. The patient may notice difficulty swallowing secondary to an anterior disc bulge or a change in the quality of his or her voice. The patient may experience difficulty with the lower extremities and gait disorders. How easily is the patient's condition irritated and how quickly can the symptoms be relieved? The examination may need to be modified if the patient reacts adversely with very little activity and requires a long time for relief.

The patient's disorder may be related to age, gender, ethnic background, body type, static and dynamic posture, occupation, leisure activities, hobbies, and general activity level. It is important to inquire about any change in daily routine and any unusual activities that the patient has participated in.

You should inquire about the nature, location, duration, and intensity of the complaints. The location of the symptoms may provide some insight into the etiology of the complaints. For example, pain that is located over the lateral aspect of the shoulder may actually be referred to C5.

(Please refer to Box 2.1, Chapter 2, p. 15 for typical questions for the subjective examination.)

Gentle Palpation

The palpatory examination is started with the patient in the standing position. This allows you to see the influence of the lower extremities on the trunk and the lumbar spine in the weight-bearing position. If the patient has difficulty standing, he or she may sit on a stool with the back toward you. The patient must be sufficiently disrobed so that the thoracic spine and neck are exposed. You should first search for areas of localized effusion, discoloration, birthmarks, open sinuses or drainage, incisional areas, bony contours and alignment, muscle girth, symmetry, and skinfolds. A *café au lait* spot or a "faun's" beard most commonly found in the lumbar spine might be indicative of a spina bifida occulta. Remember to use the dominant eye (see p. 15) (Isaacs and Bookhout, 2002) when checking for alignment or symmetry. Failure to do this can alter the findings. You should not have to use deep pressure to determine areas of tenderness or malalignment. It is important to use firm but gentle pressure, which will enhance your palpatory skills. By having a sound basis of cross-sectional anatomy, you should not have to physically penetrate through several layers of tissue to have a good sense of the underlying structures. Remember, if the patient's pain is increased at this point in the examination, the patient will be very reluctant to allow you to continue, or may become more limited in his or her ability to move.

Palpation is most easily performed with the patient in a relaxed position. Although the initial palpation may be performed with the patient standing or sitting, the supine, side-lying, or prone positions allow for easier access to the bony and soft-tissue structures.

Posterior Aspect

The easiest position for palpation of the posterior structures is with the patient supine and the examiner sitting behind the patient's head. You can rest your forearms on the table, which enables you to relax your hands during palpation.

Bony Structures

Inion (External Occipital Protuberance)
Place your fingers on the middle of the base of the skull and move slightly superiorly into the hairline and you will feel a rounded prominence, which is the inion (Figure 4.5). This is often referred to as the "bump of knowledge."

Superior Nuchal Line
Place your fingers on the inion and move laterally and inferiorly diagonally toward the mastoid process. You will feel the ridge of the superior nuchal line under your fingers (Figure 4.6).

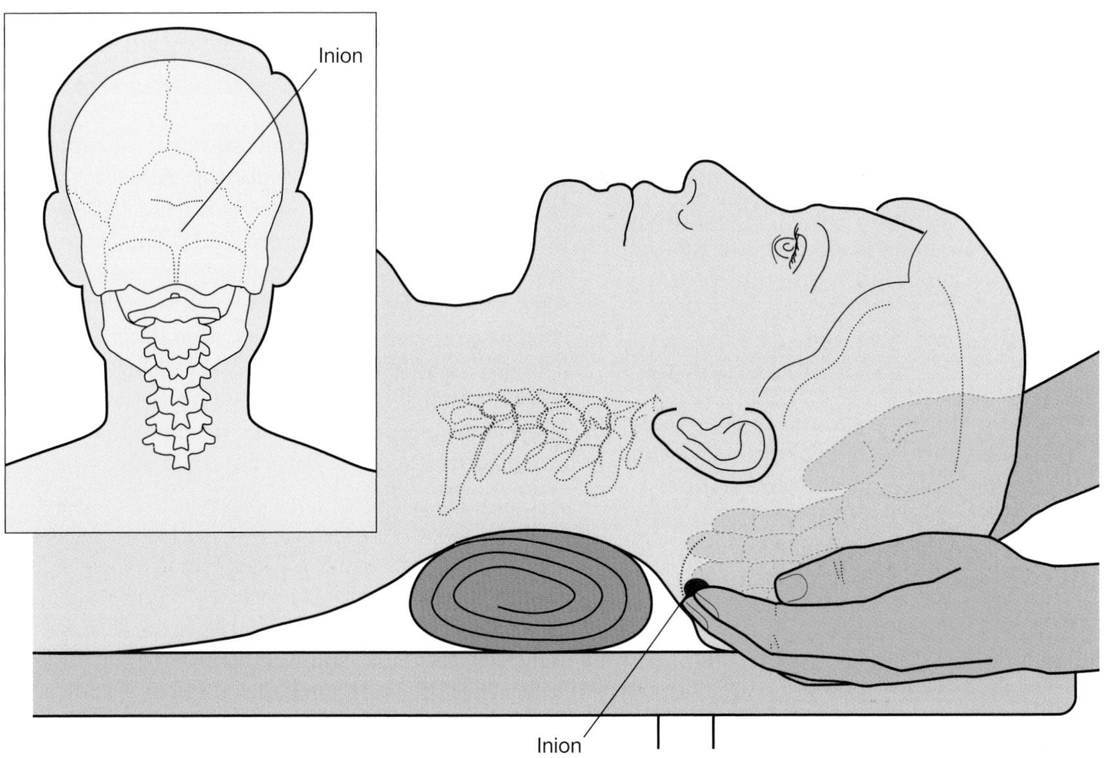

Figure 4.5 Palpation of the inion.

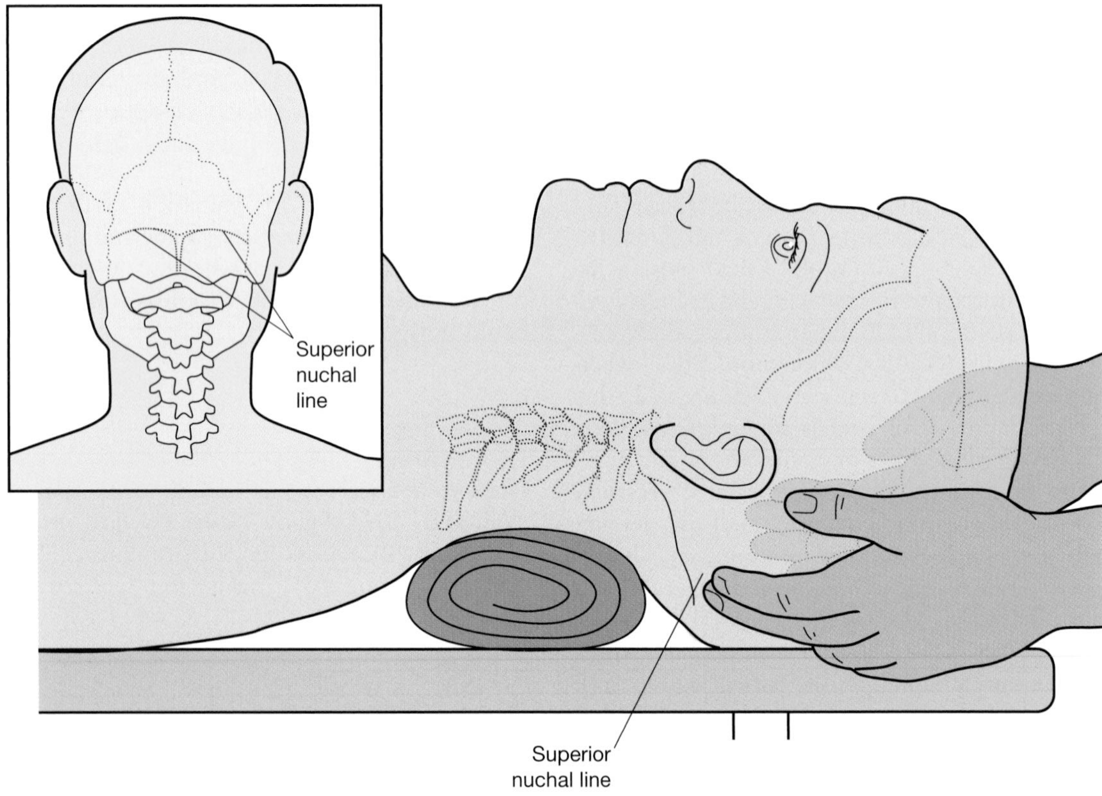

Figure 4.6 Palpation of the superior nuchal line.

Occiput

Place your hands under the base of the patient's head and allow your fingertips to rest on the most inferior aspect. This area is the occiput (Figure 4.7).

Mastoid Processes

Place your fingers directly under the patient's earlobes and you will feel a rounded prominence on each side under your fingers. These are the mastoid processes (Figure 4.8).

Transverse Processes of C1

Place your fingers anterior to the mastoid processes and in the space between the mastoid processes and the angle of the mandible, you will find the projection of the transverse processes of C1 (Figure 4.9). Although they can be deep, be careful not to press too firmly since they are often tender to palpation even in the normal patient.

Spinous Process of C2

Place your finger on the inion and move inferiorly into an indentation (posterior arch of C1). As you continue to move inferiorly, the rounded prominence that you feel is the spinous process of C2 (Figure 4.10).

Spinous Processes

Place your middle fingers in the upper portion of the midline of the posterior aspect of the neck. You will feel blunt prominences under your fingers. These are the spinous processes (Figure 4.11). The spinous processes are often bifurcated, which you may be able to sense as you palpate them. You can start counting the spinous processes from C2 (location described above) caudally. You will notice the cervical lordosis as you palpate. Notice that the spinous processes of C3, C4, and C5 are deeper and closer together, making them more difficult to differentiate individually.

Spinous Process of C7

The spinous process of C7 is normally the longest of all the cervical spinous processes (Figure 4.12). It is referred to as the prominens. However, it may be the same length as the spinous process of T1. To determine whether you are palpating C7 or T1, locate the spinous process you assume is C7. Place one finger on the spinous process that you presume is C7, and one

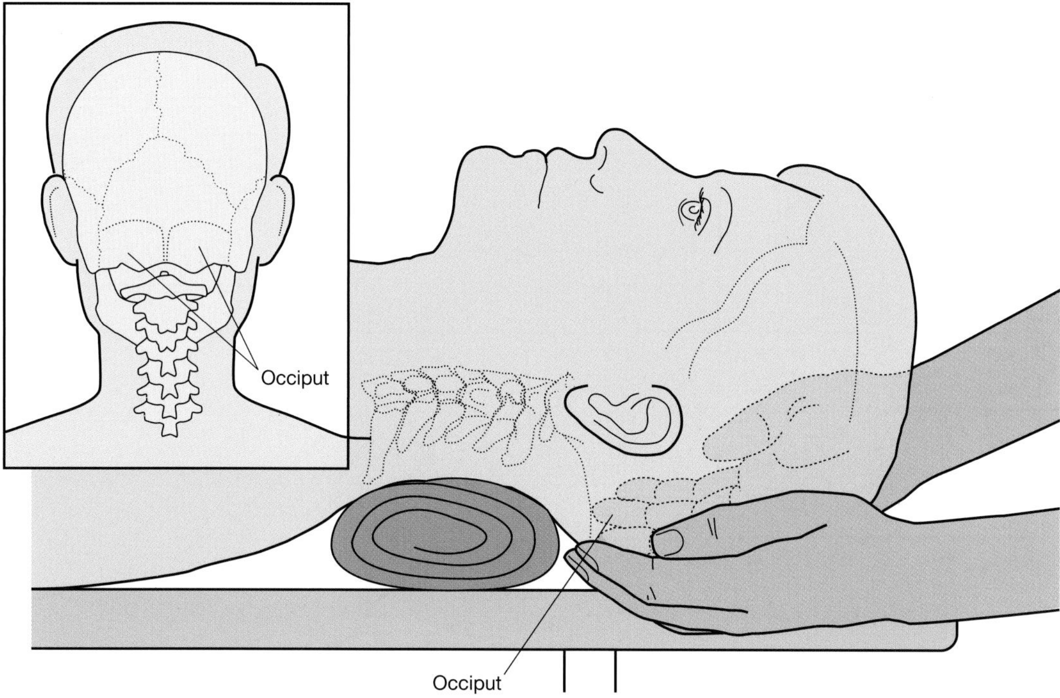

Figure 4.7 Palpation of the occiput.

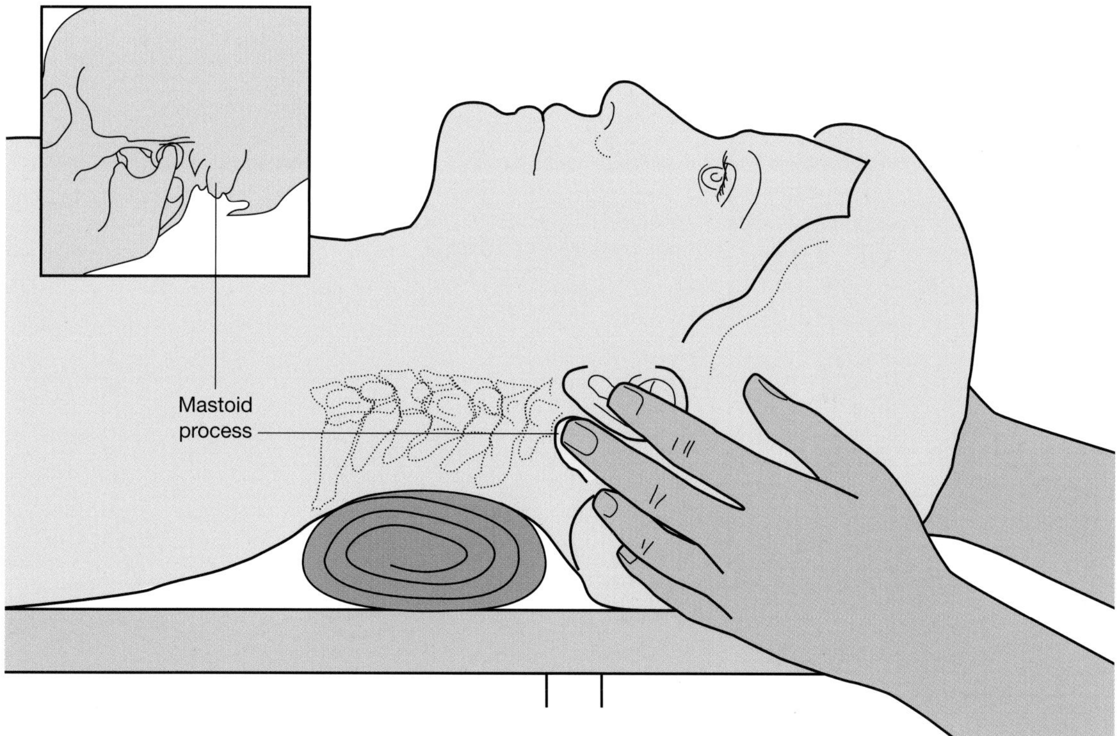

Figure 4.8 Palpation of the mastoid process.

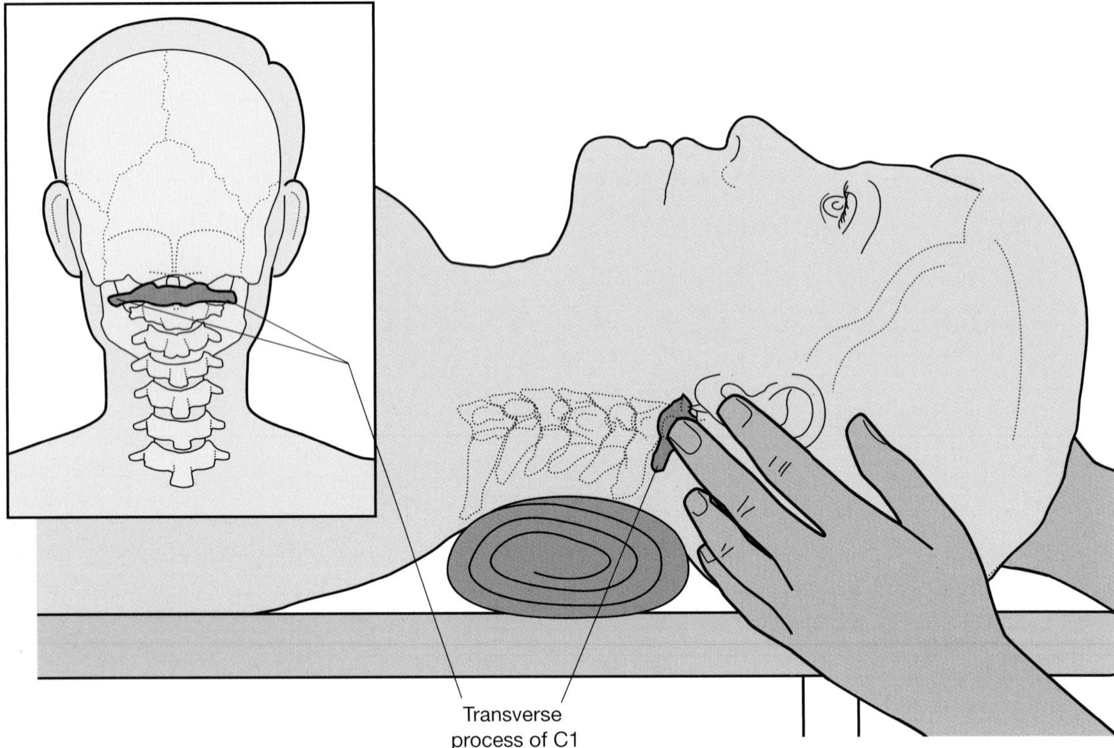

Figure 4.9 Palpation of the transverse process of C1.

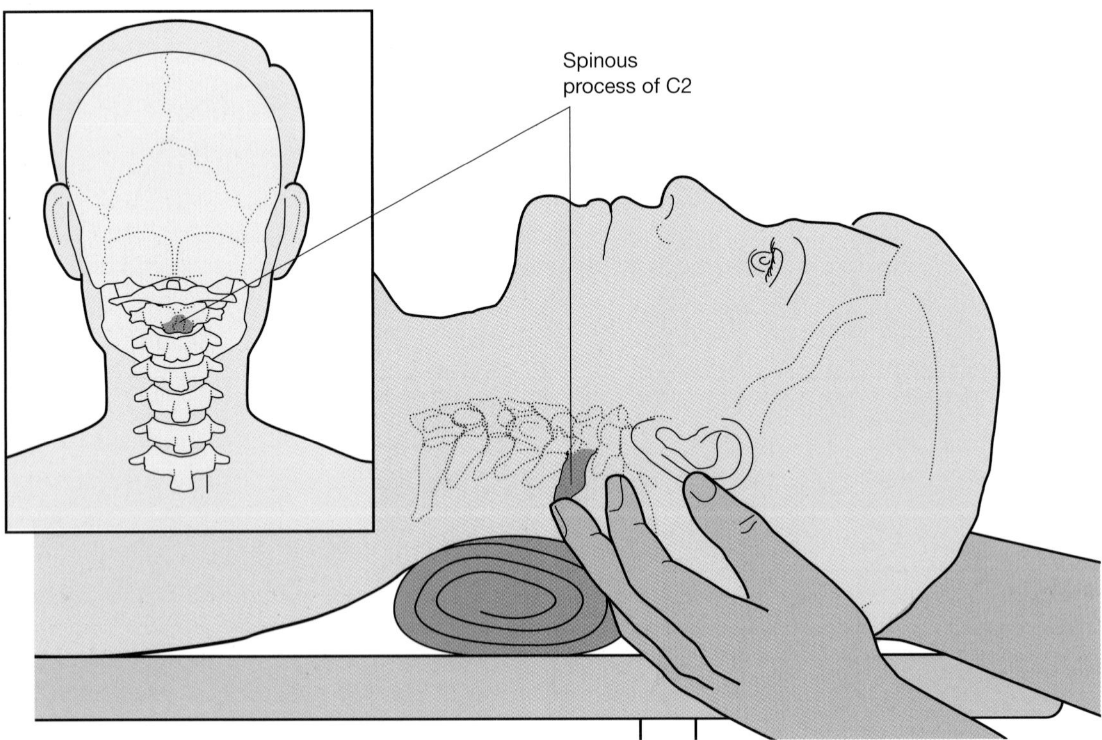

Figure 4.10 Palpation of the spinous process of C2.

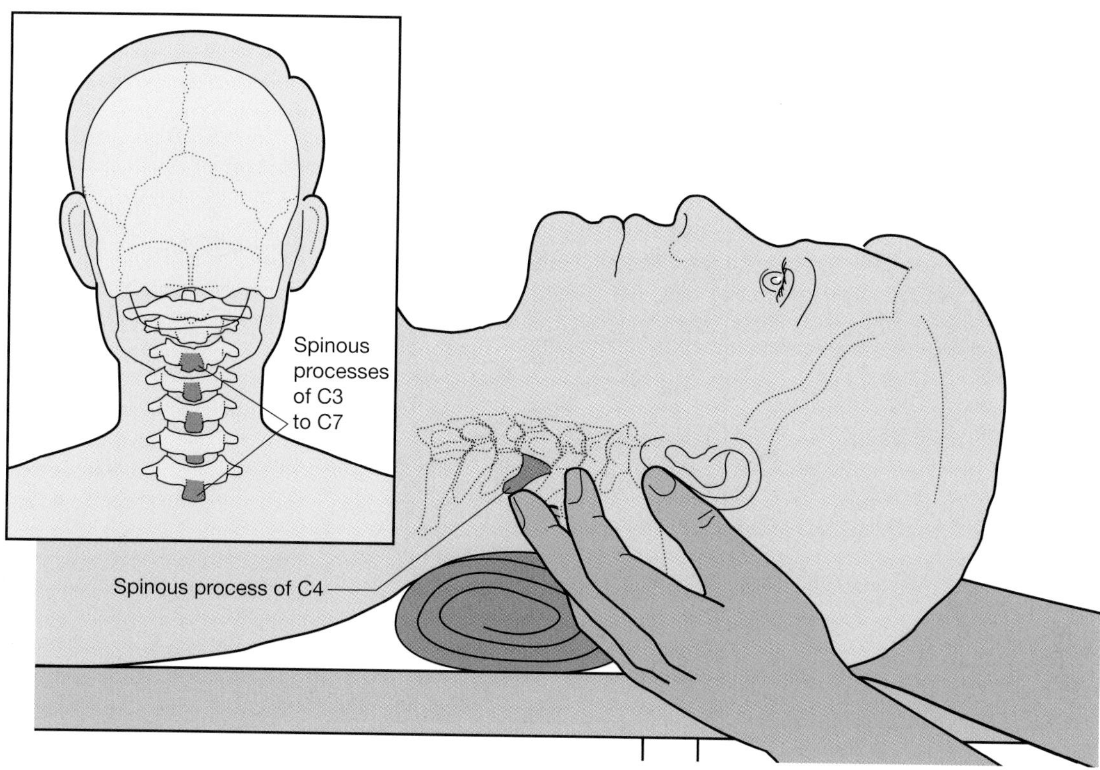

Figure 4.11 Palpation of the spinous processes.

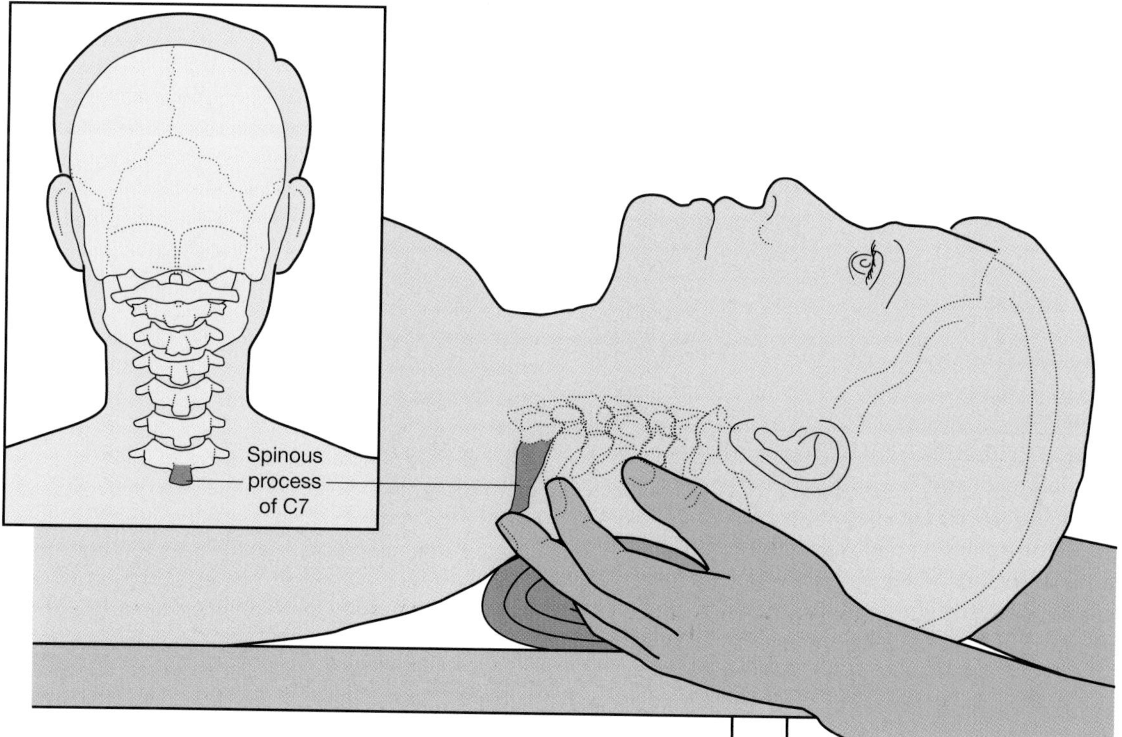

Figure 4.12 Palpation of the spinous process of C7.

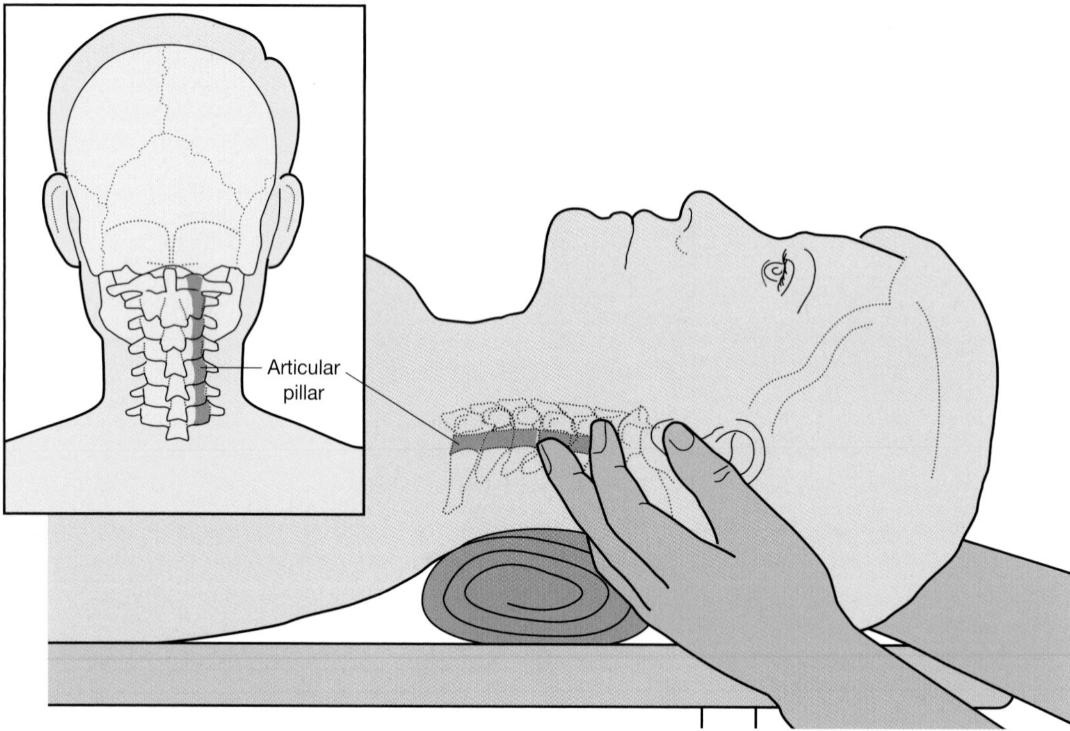

Figure 4.13 Palpation of the articular pillar.

over C6 and T1, and then have the patient extend the head slightly. The C6 vertebra will drop off slightly at the beginning of the movement, followed by C7 with a slight increase in extension, and T1 will not drop off at all. The T1 spinous process is stabilized by the first ribs and therefore does not move.

Articular Pillar (Facet Joints)

Move your fingers laterally approximately 1 in. from the spinous processes, over the erector spinae until you find a depression. You will be on the articular pillar. As you palpate in a caudal direction, you will be able to differentiate the joint lines of the facet joints: they feel like a stick of bamboo (Figure 4.13). If the joints deteriorate secondary to osteoarthritis, they become enlarged and are not as clearly delineated. Note that the facet joints can be tender to palpation even in a normal individual. Facet joints can become locked or dislocated. They will alter the patient's ability to move and limit the available range of motion in a distinctive pattern.

Transverse Processes of the Cervical Spine

Move your fingers to the most lateral aspect of the neck and you will feel a series of blunt prominences. These are the transverse processes (Figure 4.14). The second cervical transverse process can be palpated through the sternocleidomastoid muscle approximately 1 cm inferior to the mastoid process. These processes are normally tender to palpation.

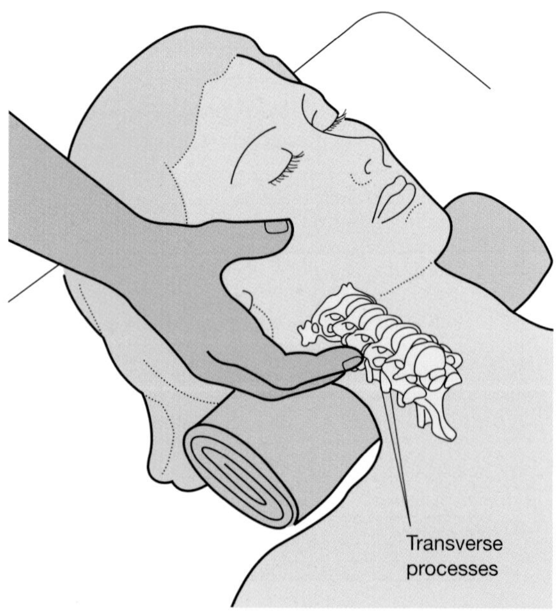

Figure 4.14 Palpation of the transverse processes of the cervical spine.

The following palpations are more easily accomplished with the patient in either the prone or the seated position.

Spinous Processes of the Thoracic Spine

The spinous processes of the thoracic spine are longer and more slender than those of the cervical spine. Since the direction of the spinous processes changes throughout the thoracic spine, a method for relating the location of the spinous process to the transverse process was developed. This is referred to as the "rule of 3's." T1–T3 vertebrae have spinous processes that are posteriorly directed as in the cervical spine. Therefore, the spinous process is at the same level as its own transverse process. T4–T6 vertebrae have spinous processes that are angled in a slightly downward direction. Therefore, the tip of the spinous process is located at a point halfway between the transverse process at the same level and the vertebra below. T7–T9 vertebrae have spinous processes that are angled moderately downward. Therefore, the spinous process is located at the same level as the transverse process of the vertebra below. T10–T12 vertebrae have spinous processes that slowly resume the horizontal direction as in the lumbar spine, where the spinous process is at the same level as the transverse process (Isaacs and Bookhout, 2002) (Figure 4.15).

Transverse Processes of the Thoracic Spine

In T1–T3 vertebrae the transverse processes are at the same level as the spinous processes. The transverse processes of T4–T6 vertebrae are halfway between each vertebra's own spinous process and the one above. The transverse processes of T7–T9 vertebrae are at the level of the spinous process of the vertebra above. The transverse processes of T10–T12 vertebrae are the reverse of those in the previous three groups (T10 process resembles T7–T9 processes, T11 resembles T4–T6, and T12 resembles T1–T3) as the spinous processes become more horizontal (Figure 4.16).

Spine of the Scapula

Palpate the posterior aspect of the acromion and follow medially along the ridge of the spine of the scapula as it tapers and ends at the level of the spinous process of the third thoracic vertebra (Figure 4.17).

Medial (Vertebral) Border of the Scapula

Move superiorly from the medial aspect of the spine of the scapula until you palpate the superior angle, which is located at the level of the second thoracic vertebra. This area serves as the attachment of the levator scapulae and is often tender to palpation. It

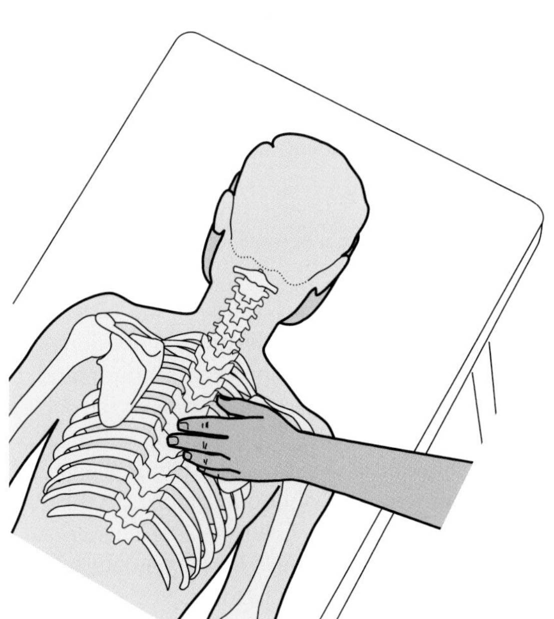

Figure 4.15 Palpation of the spinous processes of the thoracic spine.

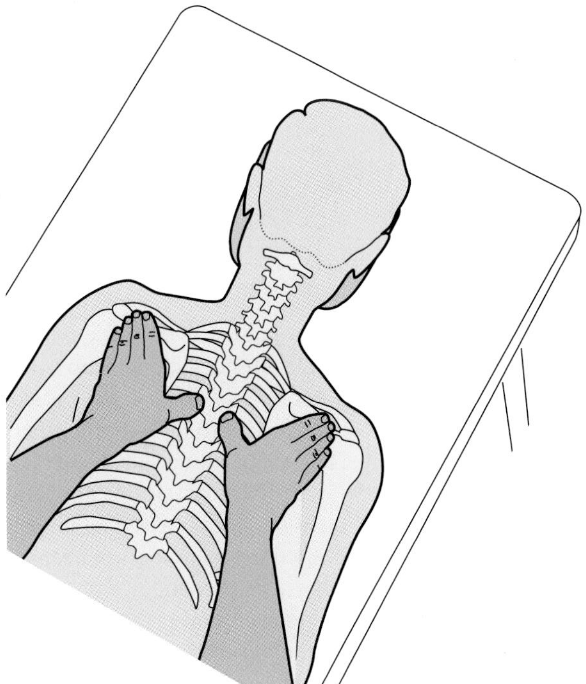

Figure 4.16 Palpation of the transverse processes of the thoracic spine.

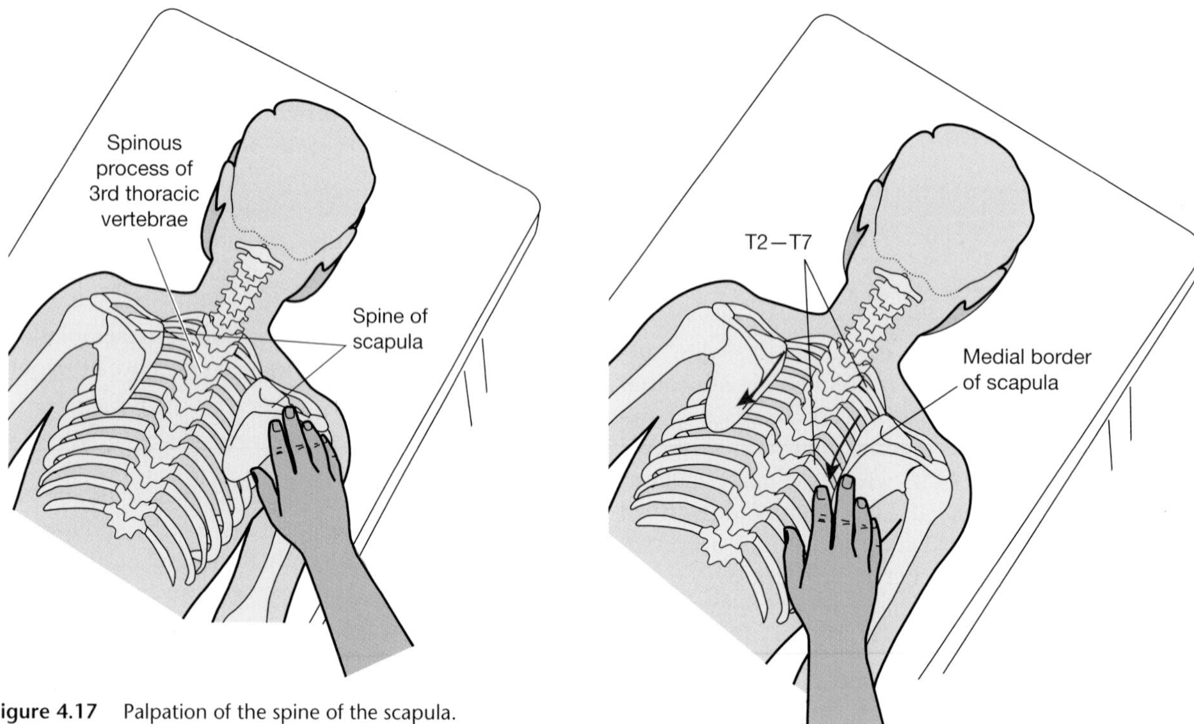

Figure 4.17 Palpation of the spine of the scapula.

Figure 4.18 Palpation of the medial border of the scapula.

is frequently an area of referred pain from the cervical spine. Continue inferiorly along the medial border and note if it lies flat along the rib cage. If the border wings away from the rib cage, it may be indicative of a long thoracic nerve injury. Notice the attachment of the rhomboid major along the length of the medial border from the spine to the inferior angle. The inferior angle is located at the level of the seventh thoracic vertebra (Figure 4.18).

Soft-Tissue Structures

Trapezius Muscle

Stand behind the seated patient or observe the patient in the prone position. Differences in contour and expanse can be easily noted as you observe the patient prior to palpation. To enable you to palpate the fibers of the upper trapezius, allow your fingers to travel laterally and inferiorly from the external occipital protuberance to the lateral third of the clavicle. The muscle is a flat sheet but feels like a cordlike structure because of the rotation of the fibers. It is frequently tender to palpation and often very tight secondary to tension or trauma. You can palpate the muscle using your thumb on the posterior aspect and your index and middle fingers anteriorly. The fibers of the lower trapezius can be traced as they attach from the medial aspect of the spine of the scapula, running medially and inferiorly to the spinous processes of the lower thoracic vertebrae. The fibers become more prominent by asking the patient to depress the scapula. The fibers of the middle trapezius can be palpated from the acromion to the spinous processes of the seventh cervical and upper thoracic vertebrae. The muscle becomes more prominent by asking the patient to adduct the scapulae (Figure 4.19).

Suboccipital Muscles

The suboccipital muscles consist of the rectus capitis posterior major and minor and the obliquus capitis superior and inferior. The rectus minor and the obliquus superior attach from the atlas to the occiput. The rectus major and the obliquus inferior have their distal attachment on the axis. The rectus then travels to the occiput while the obliquus attaches to the transverse processes of atlas (Figure 4.20). This group of muscles is designed to allow for independent function of the suboccipital unit. They can be palpated by placing your fingertips at the base of the occiput while the patient is in the supine position. It is important to recognize that they are very deep structures and that you

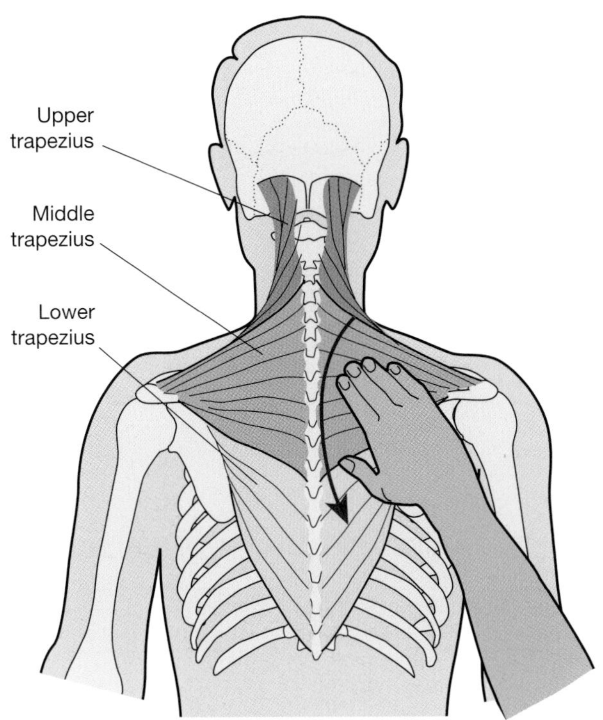

Figure 4.19 Palpation of the trapezius muscle.

are actually palpating the fascia and superficial muscles simultaneously (Porterfield and DeRosa, 1995).

These muscles are often in spasm and become tender to palpation.

Semispinalis Cervicis and Capitis

The semispinalis cervicis has its attachments to the transverse processes of the upper thoracic spine and the spinous process of C2. It functions as a stabilizer of the second cervical vertebra.

The semispinalis capitis has its attachments to the transverse processes of the upper thoracic and lower cervical vertebrae and to the occiput between the superior and inferior nuchal line.

The semispinalis capitis is superficial to the semispinalis cervicis. The two muscles form a cordlike structure. Place your finger over the spinous processes from C2–C7 and move laterally until you feel the rounded cordlike structure (see Figure 4.53).

Greater Occipital Nerves

The greater occipital nerves pierce the upper trapezius near its attachment to the occiput. Locate the proximal attachment of the trapezius and palpate the base of the skull on either side of the external occipital protuberance (see Figure 4.20). The nerves are only

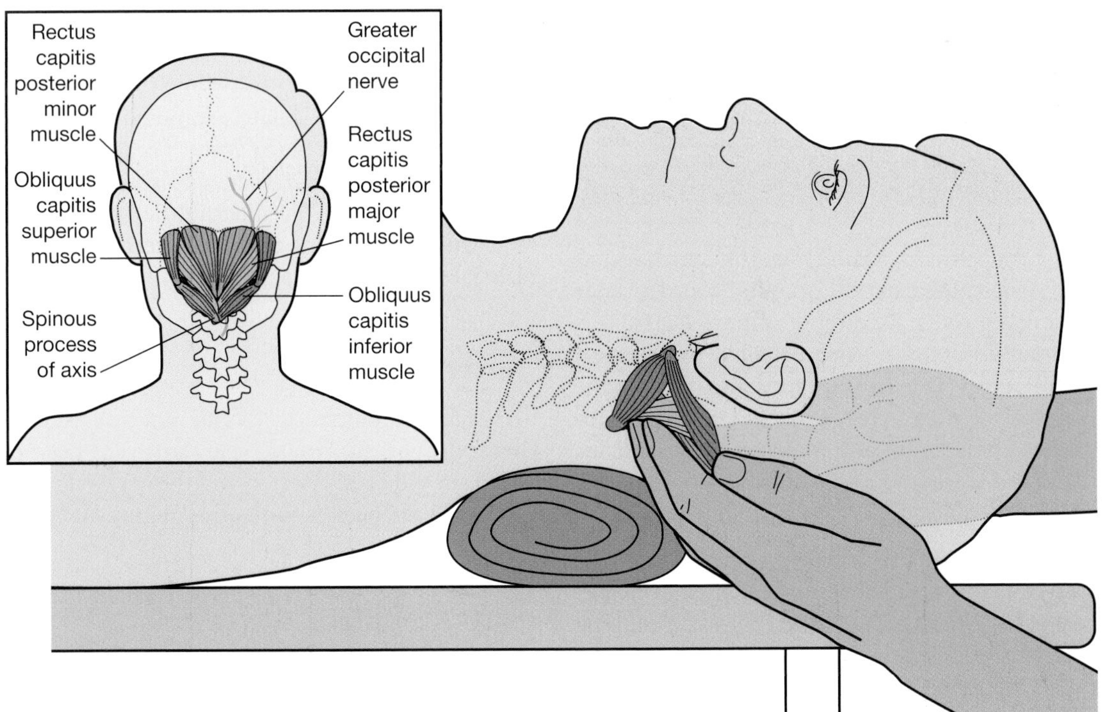

Figure 4.20 Palpation of the suboccipital muscles and the greater occipital nerves.

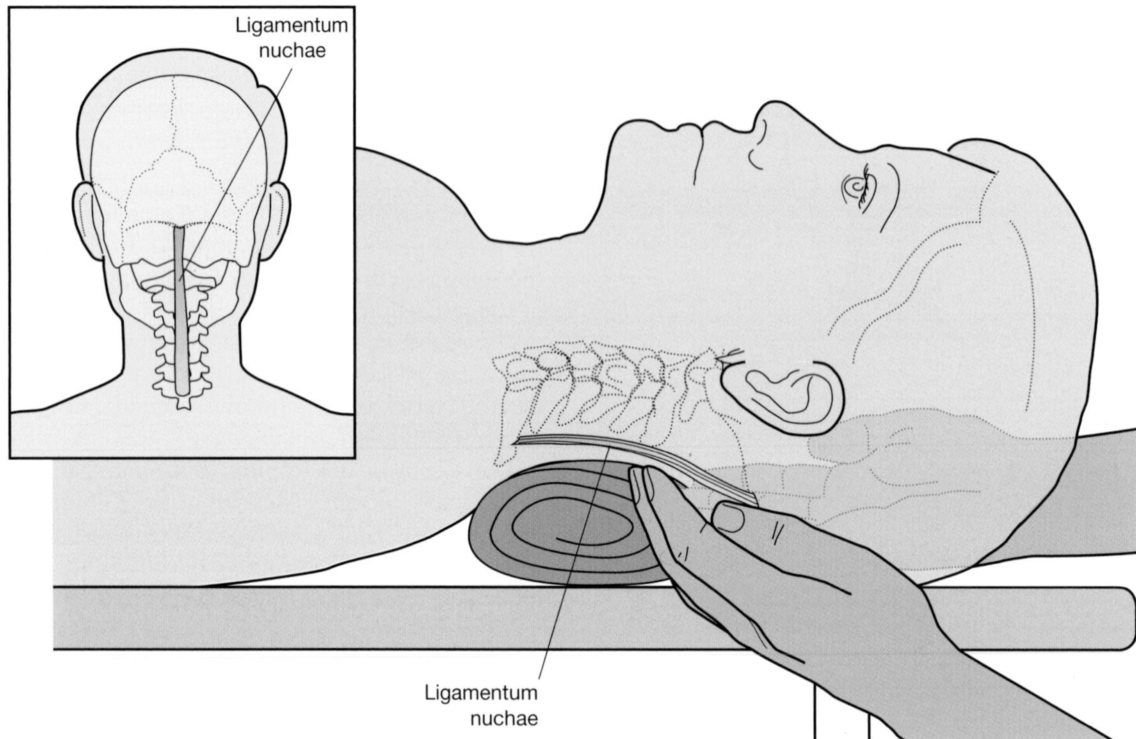

Figure 4.21 Palpation of the ligamentum nuchae.

palpable if they are inflamed. The nerves pierce the semispinalis muscle. An entrapment syndrome with pain, numbness, or burning in the scalp may occur when the semispinalis capitis muscle is hyperirritable (Porterfield and DeRosa, 1995). They may also be the source of headaches in patients with acute cervical strain.

Ligamentum Nuchae

The superficial part of the ligamentum nuchae has its attachment on the external occipital protuberance and the seventh cervical vertebra (Figure 4.21). It is easily palpated on top of and between the cervical spinous processes. It becomes more apparent as the patient flexes the neck. This ligament continues caudally as the supraspinous and interspinous ligaments.

Levator Scapulae

The levator scapulae are attached to the transverse processes of C1–C4 and the superior medial aspect of the scapula. The muscle can function as a scapula elevator and also as a lateral flexor of the neck. However, it also functions as a dynamic check to the anterior pull of the cervical lordosis. It is therefore often obligated to maintain a state of constant contraction. Tenderness can be palpated over its distal attachment on the superior medial border of the scapula. You can palpate the muscle with the patient in either the prone or the seated position (see Figure 8.71). You can facilitate the palpation by asking the patient to rotate away from the side being examined. This will allow for greater tension in the levator scapulae by moving the transverse processes anteriorly while creating laxity in the trapezius by moving the spinous processes toward the side being tested (Porterfield and DeRosa, 1995).

Anterior Aspect

To facilitate palpation of the anterior aspect of the neck, the patient should be in the supine position. The head should be supported and the neck relaxed. Make sure that the neck is in neutral alignment.

Bony Structures

Hyoid Bone

The hyoid bone is located at the anterior aspect of the C3–C4 vertebral bodies. It is useful as a landmark for locating the spinous processes, as you can easily

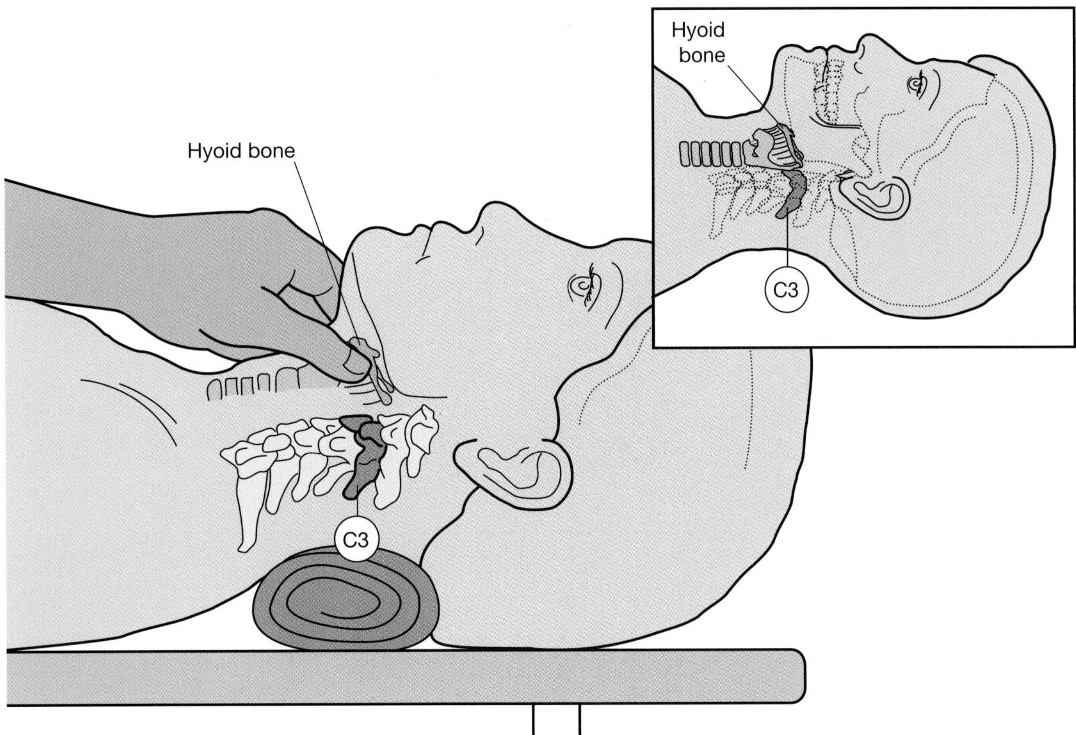

Figure 4.22 Palpation of the hyoid bone.

palpate the anterior surface and then wrap your fingers posteriorly at the same level. The hyoid is a horseshoe-shaped bone. With your thumb and index finger, surround the most superior aspects of the structure and move it from side to side. It is not easy to palpate because it is tucked under the mandible and is suspended by many of the anterior neck muscles. When the patient swallows, movement of the hyoid becomes apparent (Figure 4.22). You may notice crepitus while moving the hyoid laterally, which indicates a roughened cartilage surface.

Thyroid Cartilage

The thyroid cartilage (commonly referred to as Adam's apple) is located at the anterior aspect of the C4–C5 vertebral bodies. Continuing inferiorly from the hyoid bone, you will feel the rounded dome of the thyroid cartilage (Figure 4.23). If the neck is fully extended, the upper part of the thyroid cartilage can be located at the mid position between the chin and the sternum. The thyroid cartilage is partially covered by the thyroid gland. If there is a swollen area noted over the anterior inferior aspect of the cartilage, it might be an enlargement of the thyroid gland known as goiter.

First Cricoid Ring

As you continue to palpate inferiorly along the anterior part of the neck, you reach a tissue that is softer than the thyroid cartilage at the level of the C6 vertebral body. This is the first cricoid ring (Figure 4.24). Palpation of this area creates a very unpleasant sensation for the patient. This is an area commonly used for tracheostomy incisions because of the easy and safe access into the trachea.

Carotid Tubercle

The carotid tubercle is located on the anterior aspect of the transverse process of C6 (Figure 4.25). The common carotid artery is located superficially next to the tubercle. The artery can be easily compressed when palpating the tubercle. Care must be taken not to palpate both carotid tubercles simultaneously because of the possible consequences of decreased blood flow in the carotid arteries. The carotid tubercle is a useful landmark to orient you and confirm your location while examining the anterior cervical spine.

Suprasternal Notch

Stand facing the patient and use your middle or index finger to locate the triangular notch between the two clavicles. This is the suprasternal notch (Figure 4.26).

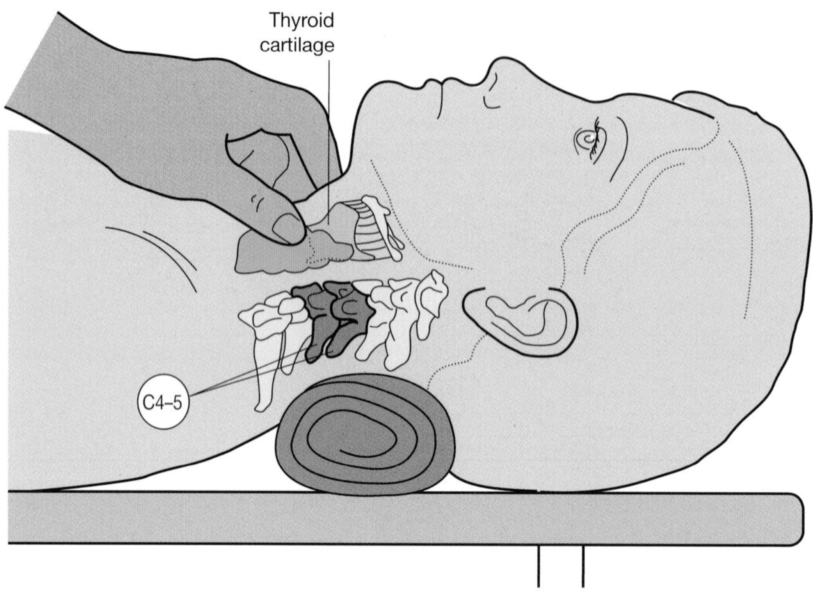

Figure 4.23 Palpation of the thyroid cartilage and gland.

Sternal Angle (Angle of Louis)

You can locate the sternal angle by finding the suprasternal notch and moving inferiorly approximately 5 cm (Bates, 2012, p. 126) until you locate a transverse ridge where the manubrium joins the body of the sternum. If you move your hand laterally, you will find the attachment of the second rib (Figure 4.27).

Sternoclavicular Joint

Move your fingers slightly superiorly and laterally from the center of the suprasternal notch until you feel the joint line between the sternum and the clavicle. The joints should be examined simultaneously to allow for comparison of heights and location. You can get a better sense of the exact location of the sternoclavicular joint by having the patient shrug his or

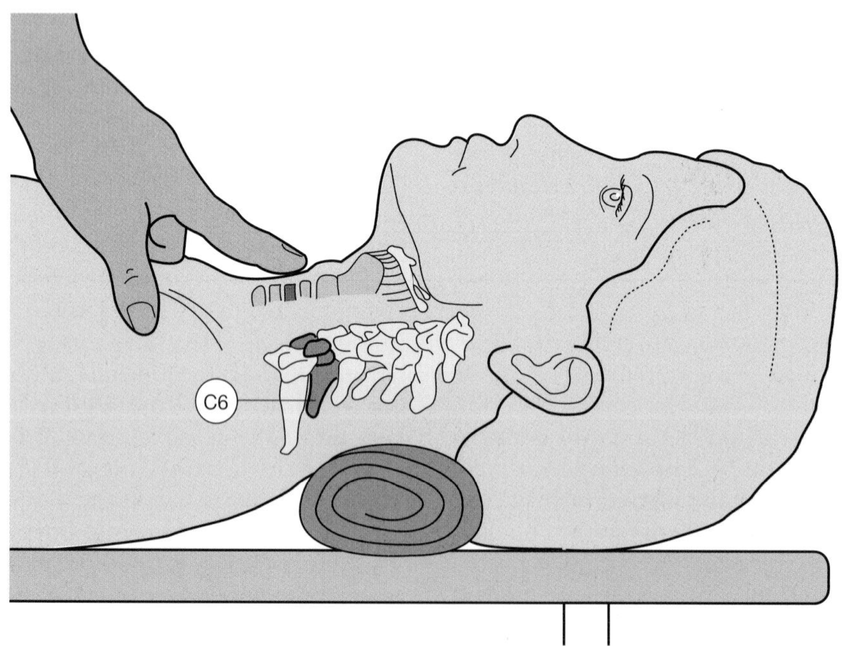

Figure 4.24 Palpation of the first cricoid ring.

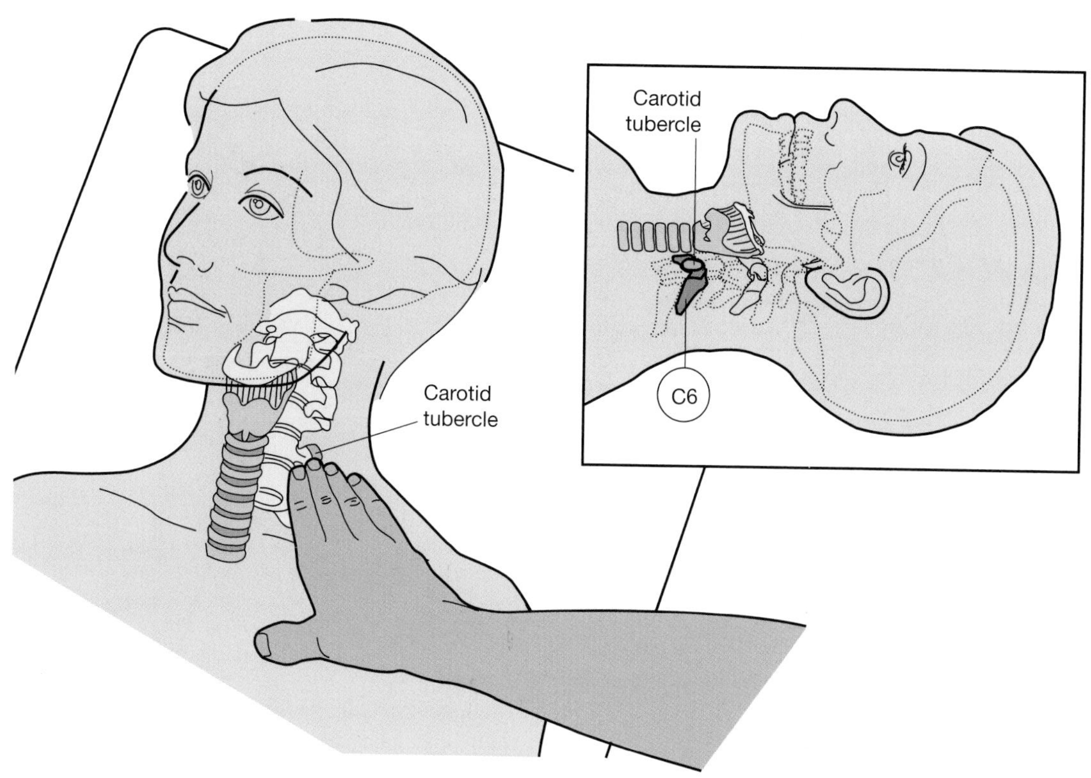

Figure 4.25 Palpation of the carotid tubercle.

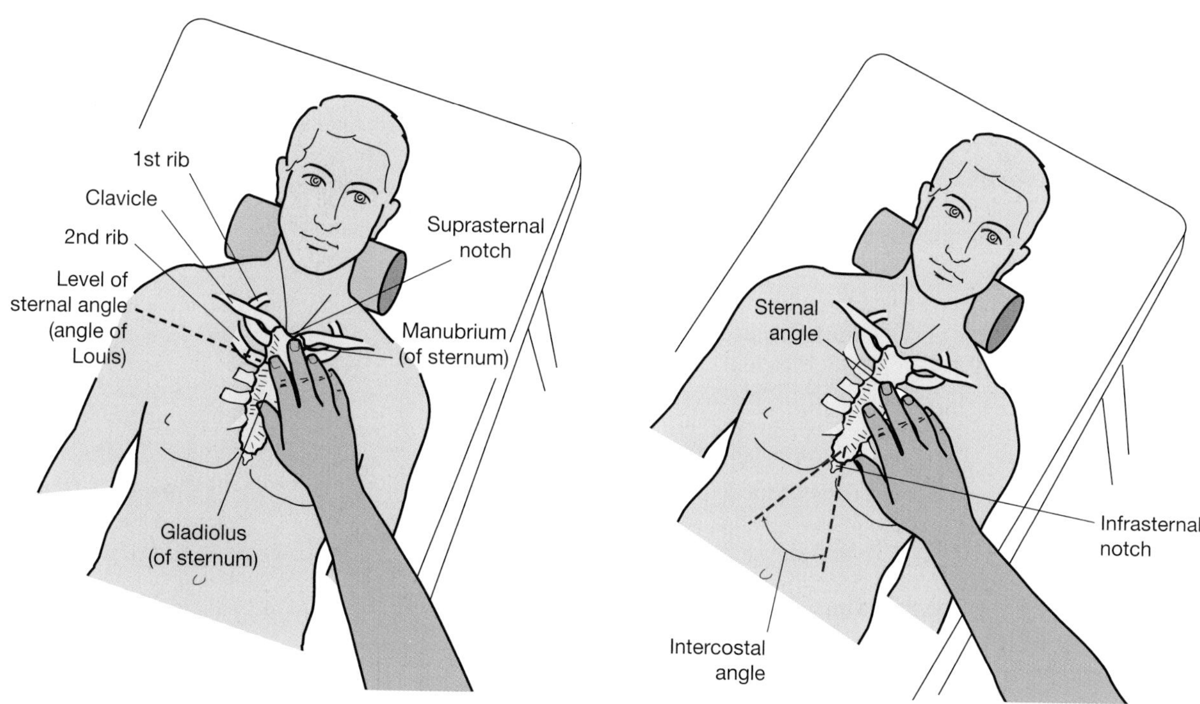

Figure 4.26 Palpation of the suprasternal notch.

Figure 4.27 Palpation of the sternal angle.

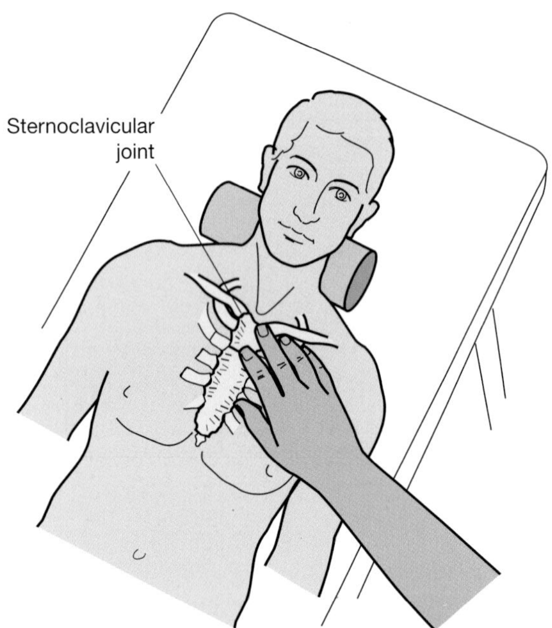

Figure 4.28 Palpation of the sternoclavicular joint.

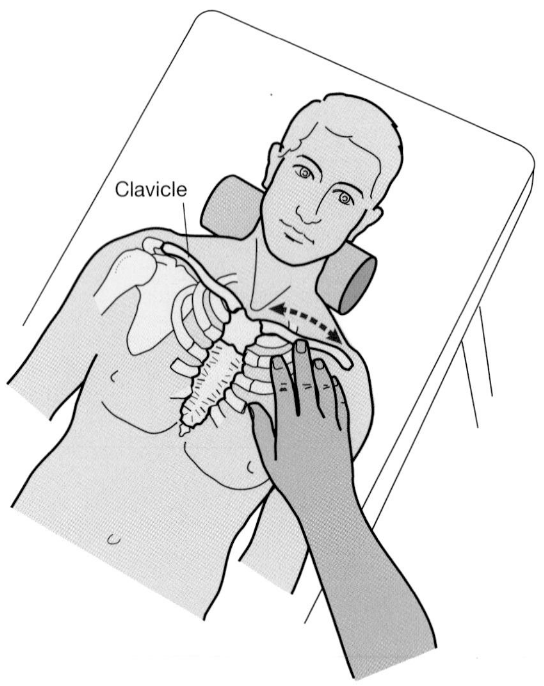

Figure 4.29 Palpation of the clavicle.

her shoulders while you palpate the movement of the joint and the upward motion of the clavicles. A superior and medial displacement of the clavicle may be indicative of dislocation of the sternoclavicular joint (Figure 4.28).

Clavicle and Surrounding Area

Continue to move laterally from the sternoclavicular joint along the superior and anterior curved bony surface of the clavicle. The bony surface should be smooth and continuous. Any area of increased prominence, pain, or sense of motion or crepitus in the bony shaft may be indicative of a fracture. The platysma muscle passes over the clavicle as it courses up the neck and can be palpated by having the patient strongly pull the corners of the mouth in a downward direction (Figure 4.29). The supraclavicular lymph nodes are found on the superior surface of the clavicle, lateral to the sternocleidomastoid in the supraclavicular fossa. If you notice any enlargement or tenderness, a malignancy or infection should be suspected. You can also palpate for the first rib in this space.

First Rib

The first rib is a little tricky to find since it is located behind the clavicle. If you elevate the clavicle and move your fingers posterior and inferior from the middle one-third of the clavicle, you will locate the first rib just anterior to the trapezius muscle (Figure 4.30). This rib is often confused by examiners as being a muscle spasm of the trapezius. It is normally tender to palpation.

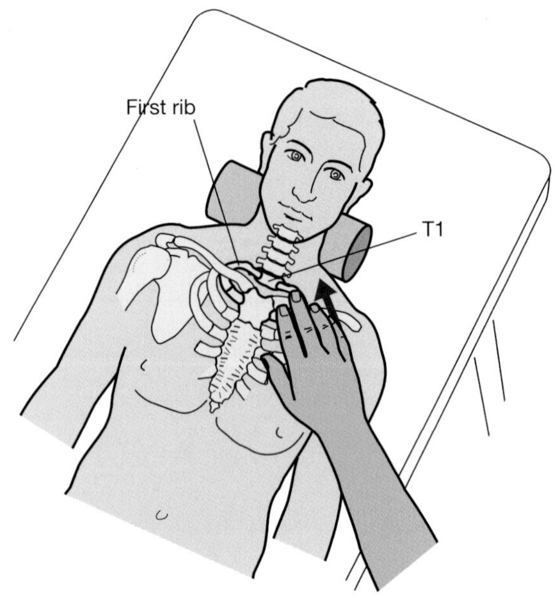

Figure 4.30 Palpation of the first rib.

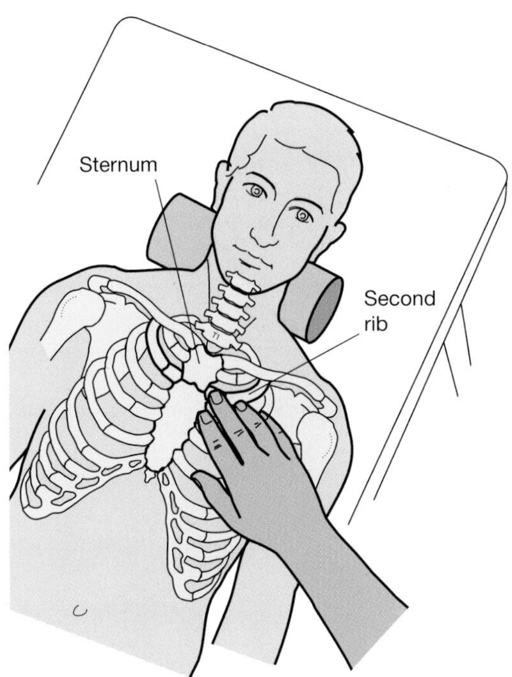

Figure 4.31 Palpation of the ribs.

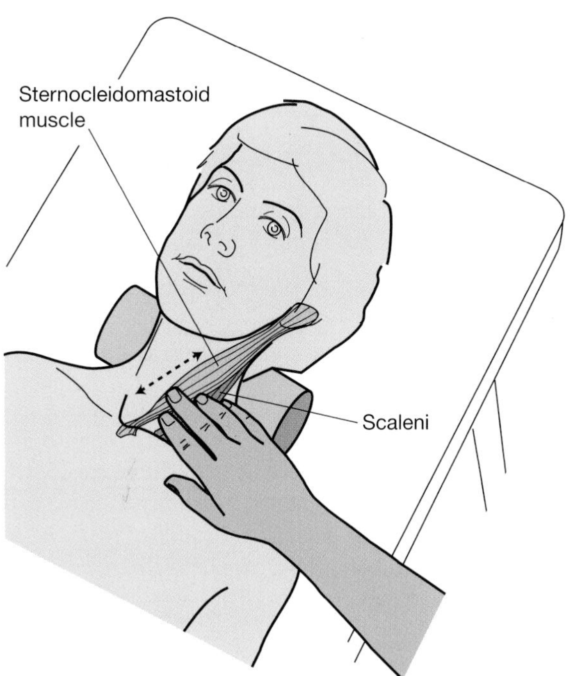

Figure 4.32 Palpation of the sternocleidomastoid muscle and the scaleni muscles.

Ribs

The second rib is the most superior rib that is easily palpable on the anterior part of the chest. Locate the sternal angle (described previously) and move laterally until you locate the second rib. You can then proceed inferiorly and count the ribs by placing your fingers in the intercostal spaces. The fifth rib is located at the xiphisternal joint. Note the symmetry of alignment and movement. Check the rib angles posteriorly along the insertion of the iliocostalis muscle approximately 1 in. lateral to the spinous processes. Observe for both the pump-handle elevation and the bucket-handle lateral expansion movements. The 11th and 12th ribs are found just above the iliac crests.

They are most easily palpated on the lateral aspect along their free ends (Figure 4.31).

Soft-Tissue Structures

Sternocleidomastoid Muscle

To facilitate palpating the sternocleidomastoid muscle, have the patient bend the neck toward the side you are palpating and then simultaneously rotate away. This movement allows the muscle to become more prominent and therefore easier to locate. Palpate the distal attachments on the manubrium of the sternum and the medial aspect of the clavicle and follow the muscle superiorly and laterally until it attaches to the mastoid process. The upper trapezius and sternocleidomastoid meet at their attachment at the skull at the superior nuchal line. Move just medial to the attachment and you will feel the occipital artery (Moore and Dalley, 1999). The sternocleidomastoid is the anterior border of the anterior triangle of the neck; the upper trapezius is the posterior border, and the clavicle the inferior border. It is a useful landmark for palpating enlarged lymph nodes (Figure 4.32).

Scalene Muscles

The scalenus anterior attaches proximally to the anterior tubercles of the transverse processes of all the cervical vertebrae. The scalenus medius attaches proximally to the posterior tubercles of the transverse processes of all the cervical vertebrae. They both have their distal attachment to the first rib. The scalenus anterior is clinically significant because of its relationship to the subclavian artery and the brachial plexus. Compression of these structures may lead to thoracic outlet syndrome. Both the scalenus anterior and medius can assist in elevating the first rib. The scalenus posterior attaches from the posterior tubercles of the transverse processes from C4–C6 into the second rib. The scalenus anterior muscles can work bilaterally to flex the neck. Unilaterally, the group can laterally flex the neck. These muscles work together as stabilizers of the neck in the sagittal plane. They can be injured in acceleration-type accidents. This occurs when the individual is sitting at a standstill and hit from behind. Place your fingers over the lateral aspect of the neck in the posterior triangle and ask the patient to laterally flex away from you. This places the muscles on stretch and facilitates palpation (see Figure 4.32). Inhalation will also make the muscles more distinct.

Lymph Node Chain

Multiple lymph nodes are located in the head and neck. There is a long lymph node chain with the majority of the nodes located deep to the sternocleidomastoid muscle. These are not normally accessible to palpation. If they are enlarged secondary to an infection or a malignancy, they can be palpated by surrounding the sternocleidomastoid with your thumb and finger (Figure 4.33).

Carotid Pulse

The carotid pulse may be visible by inspection. Locate the sternocleidomastoid muscle in the area of the carotid tubercle (see description, p. 51). Place your index and middle fingers medial to the midsection of the muscle belly and press toward the transverse processes of the cervical spine. Ask the patient to rotate the head toward the side you are palpating. This relaxes the muscle and makes the pulse more accessible (Figure 4.34). Remember not to press too hard or the pulse will be obliterated.

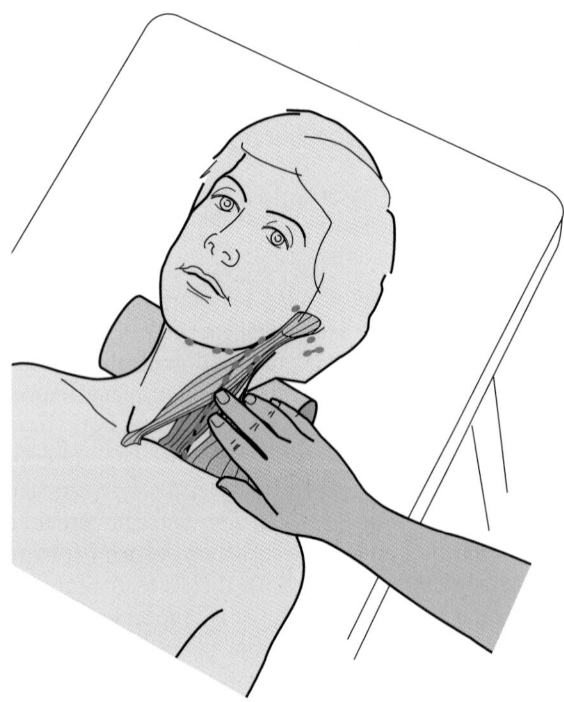

Figure 4.33 Palpation of the lymph node chain.

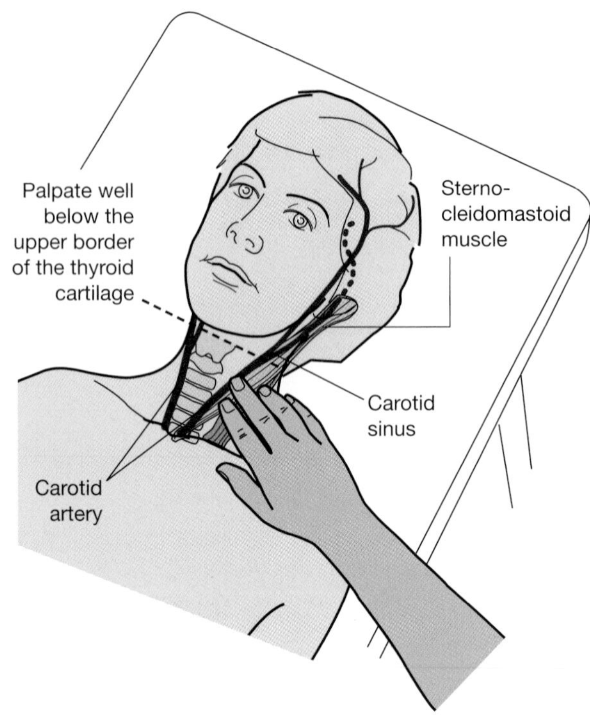

Figure 4.34 Palpation of the carotid pulse.

Parotid Gland

The parotid gland is the largest of the three salivary glands. It is not normally palpable. If it is enlarged, it can be found in the space between the sternocleidomastoid, the anterior mastoid process, and the ramus of the mandible (Figure 4.35). It is enlarged when the patient has the mumps or a ductal stone. The contour of the mandibular angle will appear more rounded.

Trigger Points of the Cervical Spine

The trapezius muscle contains numerous trigger points. Five common trigger points are illustrated in Figures 4.36, 4.37, and 4.38. The sternocleidomastoid muscle contains trigger points that frequently cause symptoms such as nasal congestion, watery eyes, and headaches (Figure 4.39). The scalene muscles may refer pain down as far as the hand (Figure 4.40).

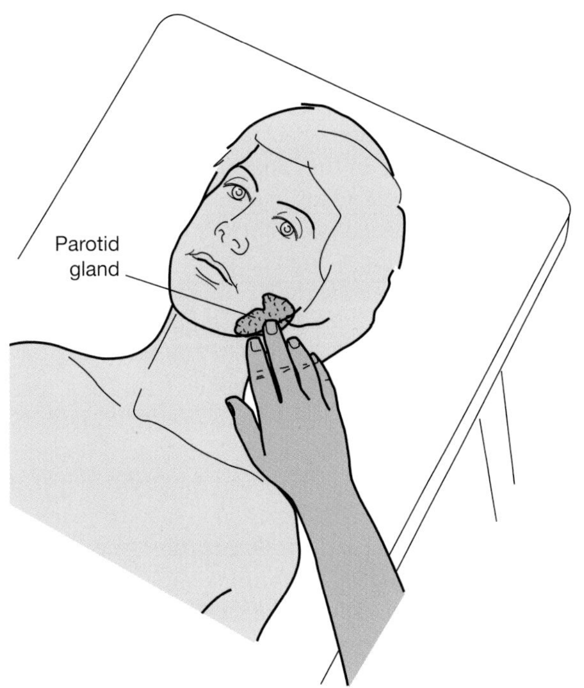

Figure 4.35 Palpation of the parotid gland.

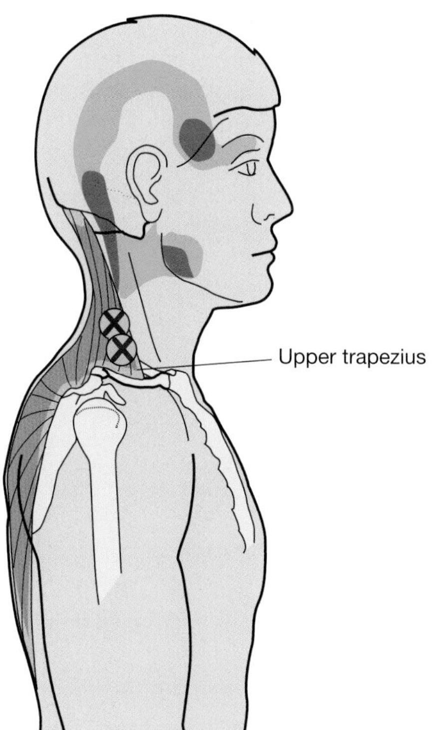

Figure 4.36 A trigger point in the upper trapezius muscle may cause headaches. (Adapted with permission from Travell and Rinzler, 1952.)

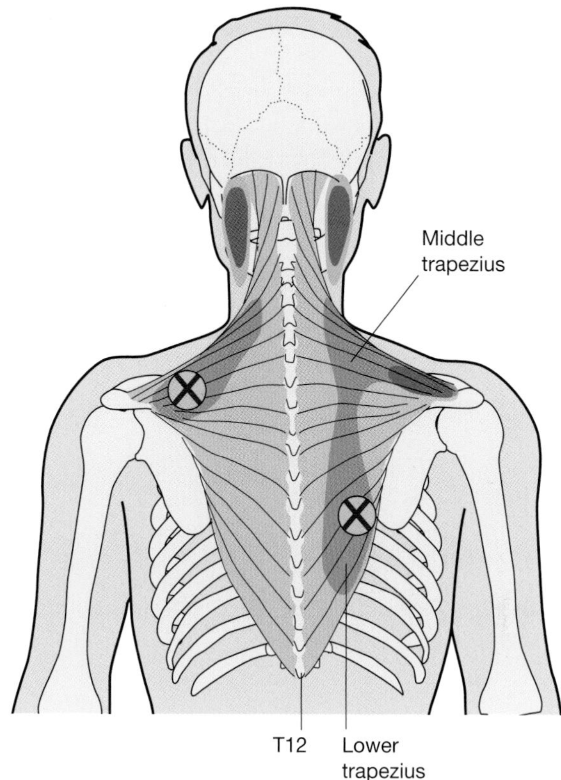

Figure 4.37 Trigger points in the middle and lower trapezius may cause pain in the occipital region and along the paraspinal region. (Adapted with permission from Travell and Rinzler, 1952.)

Trigger points of the splenius capitis and suboccipital muscles also commonly cause headaches (Figures 4.41 and 4.42).

Active Movement Testing

Have the patient sit on a stool or on the examination table with their feet supported in a well-lit area of the examination room. Shadows from poor lighting will affect your perception of the movement. The patient should be appropriately disrobed so that you can observe the neck and upper thoracic spine. You should watch the patient's movements from the anterior, posterior, and both lateral aspects. While observing the patient move, pay particular attention to his or her willingness to move, the quality of the motion, and the available range. Lines in the floor may serve as visual guides to the patient and alter the movement patterns. It may be helpful to ask the patient to repeat movements with the eyes closed.

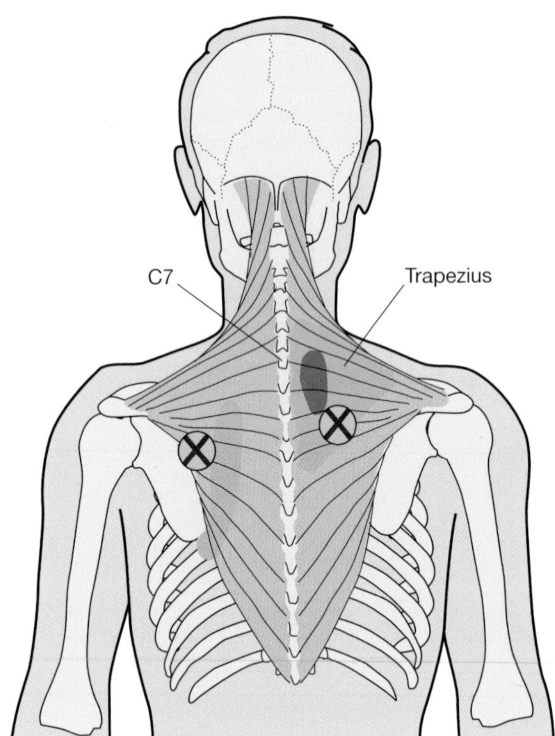

Figure 4.38 Additional trigger points in the left lower and right middle trapezius are shown with their referred pain patterns. (Adapted with permission from Travell and Rinzler, 1952.)

Before your examination of the cervical spine, you should have the patient perform a quick test to clear the joints of the upper extremities. Ask the patient to fully elevate the upper extremities; stress a combination of shoulder internal rotation, adduction, and extension at the end of the range; and passively stress the elbow and wrist. This will check the range of motion of the entire upper extremity. If the movements are painless, these joints are not implicated and you should proceed with the examination of the cervical spine.

You should then have the patient perform the following movements: bending the head forward and backward, lateral (side) bending to the right and left, and rotation to the right and left. You should observe the alignment and symmetry of the spinal curves. You may note a flattening in a particular area as the patient bends to the side or a deviation to one side during forward bending. These deviations should alert you to more carefully examine the involved area. If the motion is pain free at the end of the range, you can add an additional overpressure to "clear" the joint (Cyriax, 1982). You can also ask the patient to sustain the position for 15 seconds to determine whether the symptoms can be reproduced. Sustained movements can also be combined to increase the degree of nerve root compression symptoms. If the patient experiences pain in any of these movements, you should note the position that increases or alleviates the symptoms.

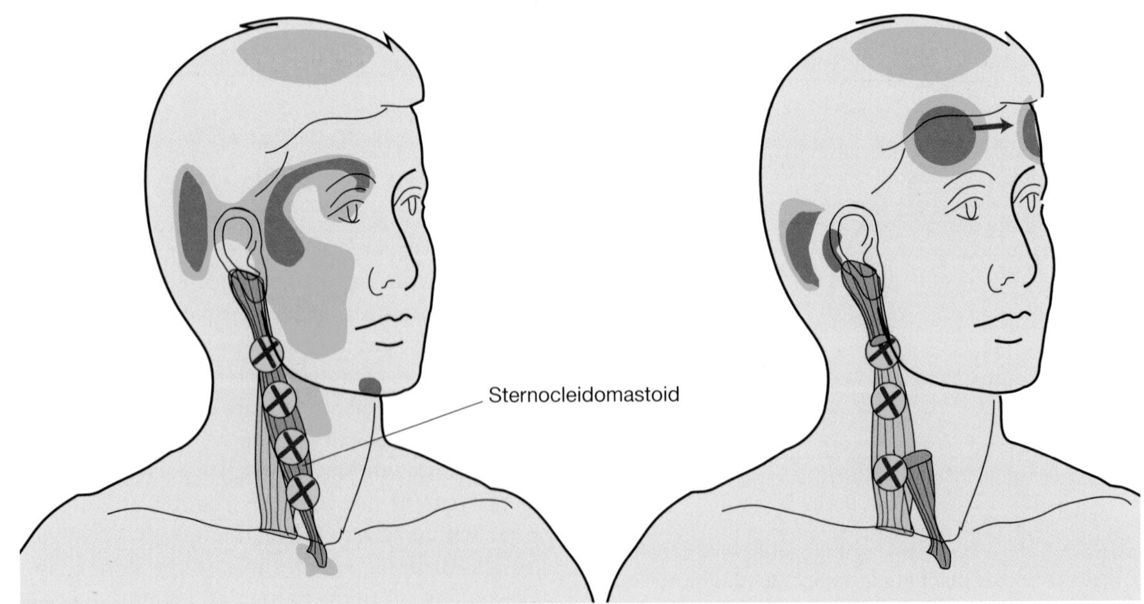

Figure 4.39 Trigger points in the sternocleidomastoid muscle may cause referred pain in the face and head and also symptoms of watery eyes and runny nose. (Adapted with permission from Travell and Rinzler, 1952.)

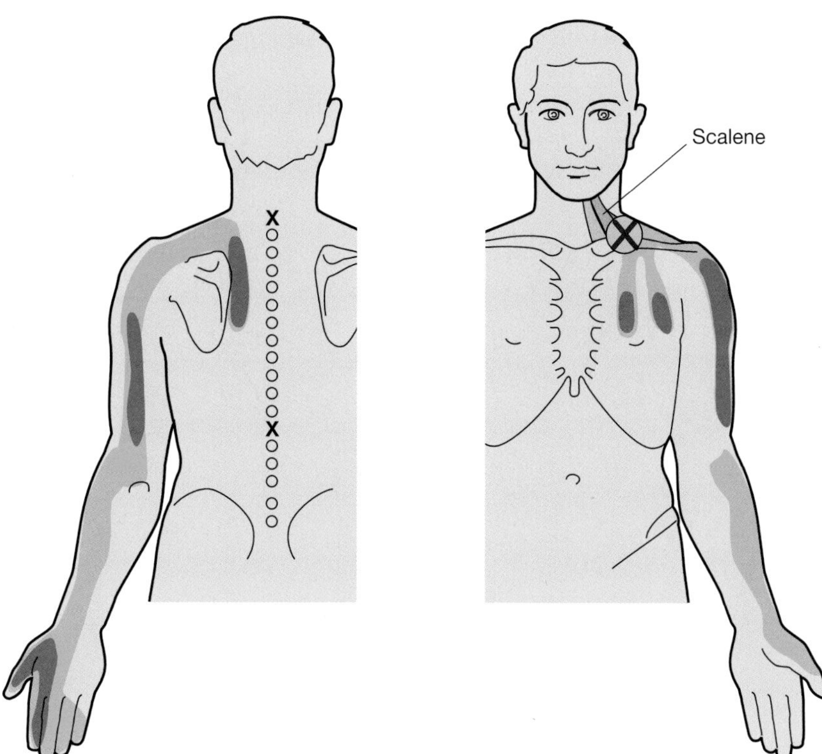

Figure 4.40 Trigger points within the scalene muscles may refer pain all the way to the hand. (Adapted with permission from Travell and Rinzler, 1952.)

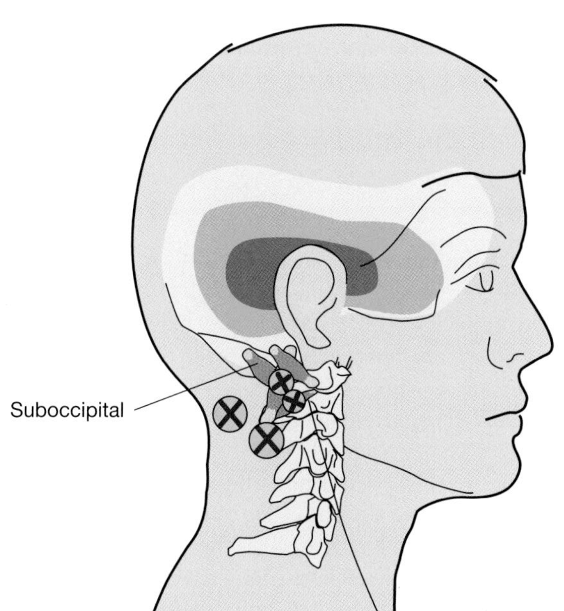

Figure 4.41 Trigger points in the suboccipital muscles radiate pain in the region of the greater occipital nerve. (Adapted with permission from Travell and Rinzler, 1952.)

Forward Bending

Instruct the patient to sit on a stool with the feet firmly on the ground approximately 6 in. apart. Stand behind the patient to observe them from the back during the movement. Note the patient's normal resting posture, as changes in the normal thoracic and lumbar curves can influence the resting position and mobility of the cervical spine. It is also helpful to observe the patient from the side to obtain a better view of the cervical lordosis. Instruct the patient to sit in an erect posture before you begin your examination. Ask the patient to drop the head forward with the chin toward the chest (Figure 4.43a). Observe the degree of range of motion and any deviation to the right or left. Note the smoothness with which each intervertebral level opens as the cervical lordosis reverses. Note whether the range is limited by pain or the patient's anticipation of pain. The patient achieves full flexion when the chin, with mouth closed, touches the chest. It is accepted as normal if there is a two-finger space between the chin and chest. The normal range of motion of flexion is 80–90 degrees (Magee, 2008).

The amount of movement can be recorded on a movement diagram. Deviations to the side and the

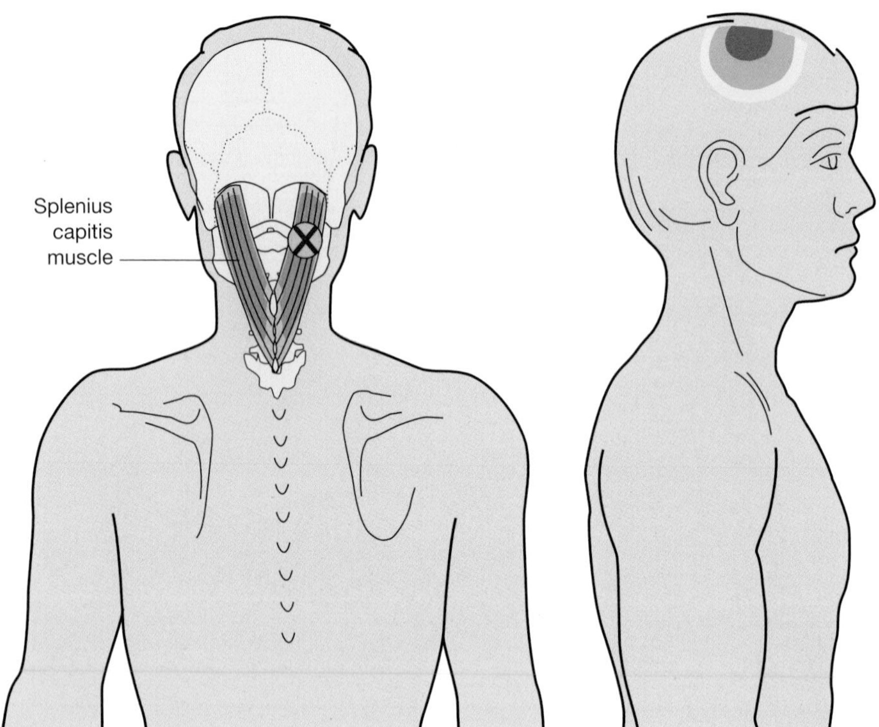

Figure 4.42 A trigger point in the splenius capitis muscle may cause referred pain on the top of the head. (Adapted with permission from Travell and Rinzler, 1952.)

onset of symptoms can also be recorded. A more objective method of measuring the range can be accomplished in one of the few ways. One method is to use a ruler to measure the distance from the patient's chin to the sternal notch. Another is by using a standard goniometer or a gravity-assisted bubble goniometer (inclinometer) specifically designed for the cervical spine, or a cervical range of motion device (CROM) to give you the actual degrees of movement.

Backward Bending

Instruct the patient to sit on a stool or on the examination table with their feet firmly on the ground approximately 6 in. apart. Stand behind the patient to observe the movement. Instruct the patient to sit in an erect posture before you begin your examination. Ask the patient to raise the chin and look toward the ceiling (Figure 4.43b). Normal range is achieved when the patient's forehead and nose are on a horizontal plane. Note the smoothness with which each intervertebral level closes. Note whether the range is limited by pain or the patient's anticipation of pain.

Range of motion is most easily recorded on a movement diagram. Another method of recording is to use a ruler to measure the distance from the patient's chin to the sternal notch as the neck is extended. A standard goniometer or one specifically designed for the cervical spine can be used to give you the actual degrees of movement. Normal range of motion is 70 degrees (Magee, 2008).

Lateral (Side) Bending

Instruct the patient to sit on a stool or on the examination table with their feet firmly on the ground approximately 6 in. apart. Stand behind the patient to observe the movement. Instruct the patient to sit in an erect posture before you begin your examination. Ask the patient to allow their ear to approach the shoulder on the side to which he or she is moving (Figure 4.43c). Do not allow the patient to substitute by raising the shoulder to meet the ear. Lateral bending should be repeated on the right and left sides. Compare the degree and quality of movement from side to side. Note any breaks in the continuity of the curve. An angulation of the curve may indicate an area of hypermobility or hypomobility. Note the smoothness with which each intervertebral level opens. Note

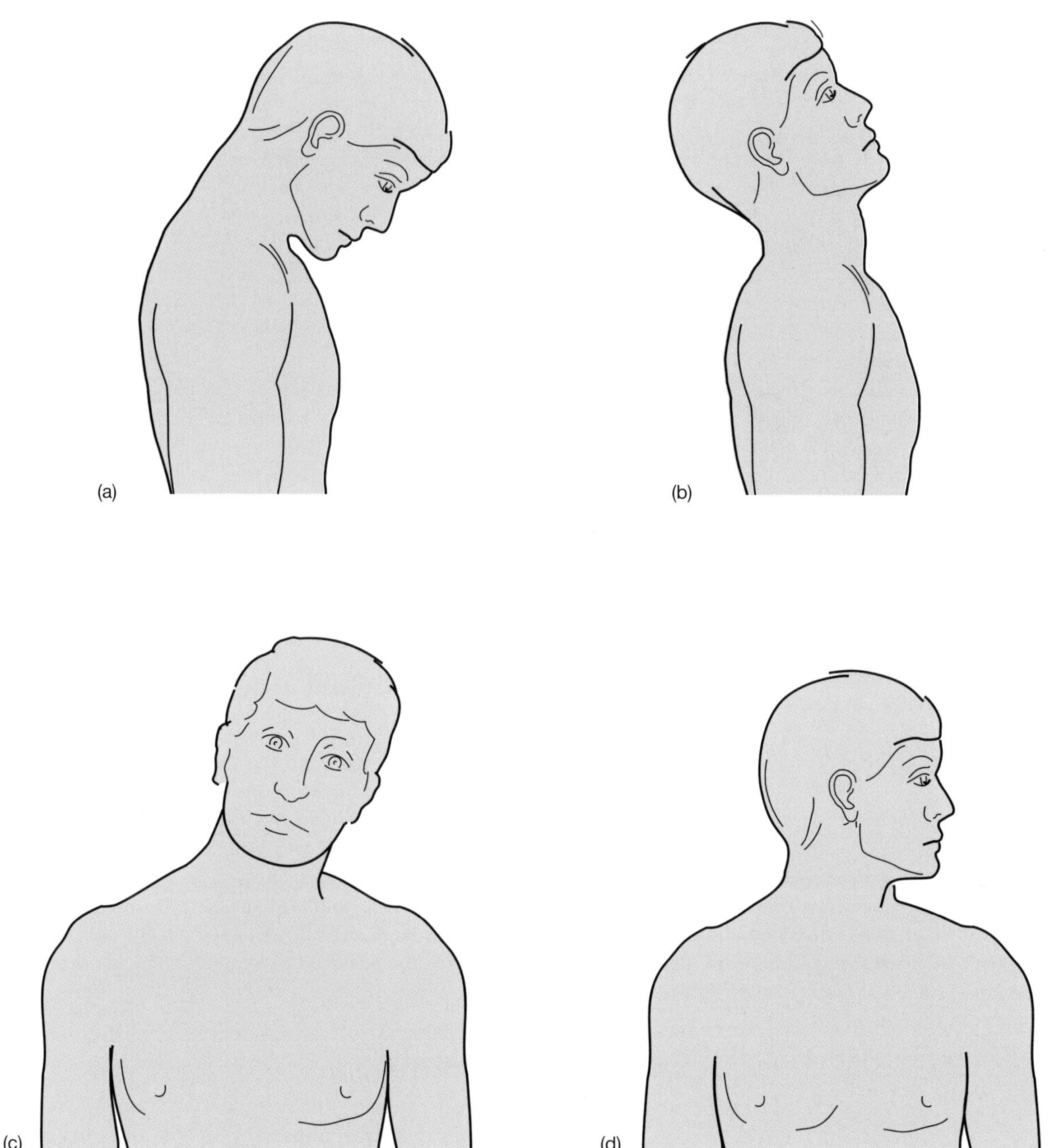

Figure 4.43 Active movement testing. (a) Cervical forward bending. (b) Cervical backward bending. (c) Cervical sidebending. (d) Cervical rotation.

whether pain or the patient's anticipation of pain limits the range.

Range of motion is most easily recorded on a movement diagram. You can also use a ruler to measure the distance from the mastoid process to the tip of the acromion process and compare one side to the other. A standard goniometer or one specifically designed for the cervical spine can be used to give you the actual degrees of movement. Normal range of motion is 20–45 degrees (Magee, 2008).

Rotation

Instruct the patient to sit on a stool or on the examination table with their feet firmly on the ground approximately 6 in. apart. Stand behind the patient to observe the movement. Instruct the patient to sit in an erect posture before you begin your examination. Ask the patient to turn the head in the horizontal plane so that the chin moves toward the shoulder (Figure 4.43d). The patient may try to substitute by rotating the trunk. Rotation should be repeated on the right and left sides. Compare the degree and quality of movement from side to side. Note any discontinuity of the curve. Note the smoothness with which each intervertebral level opens. Note whether the range is limited by pain or the patient's anticipation of pain.

Range of motion is most easily recorded on a movement diagram. You can use a ruler to measure the distance from the chin to the acromion process and compare one side to the other. A standard goniometer or one specifically designed for the cervical spine can be used to give you the actual degrees of movement. Normal range of motion is 70–90 degrees (Magee, 2008).

Upper Cervical Spine

Tucking the chin in will produce flexion of the upper cervical spine and extension of the lower cervical spine. Jutting the chin produces extension of the upper cervical spine and flexion of the lower cervical spine.

Thoracic Motion

Active motion of the upper thoracic spine can be evaluated as an extension of the cervical spine. After the patient takes up all the motion in each direction of the cervical spine, instruct him or her to continue the flexion, extension, lateral bending, and rotation movements to a greater degree until you can sense movement in the middle thoracic vertebrae. The lower thoracic spine can be evaluated as an extension of the lumbar spine. Recognize that the thoracic spine is the most restricted area of the spine because of the costal attachments.

Passive Movement Testing

Passive movement testing can be divided into two categories: physiological movements (cardinal plane), which are the same as the active movements, and mobility testing of the accessory (joint play, component) movements. Using these tests helps to differentiate the contractile from the noncontractile (inert) elements. These elements (ligaments, joint capsule, fascia, bursa, dura mater, and nerve root) (Cyriax, 1982) are stretched or stressed when the joint is taken to the end of the available range. At the end of each passive physiological movement, you should sense the end feel and determine whether it is normal or pathological. Assess the limitation of movement and see if it fits into a capsular pattern. The capsular pattern of the cervical spine is equally limited lateral bending and rotation, followed by extension that is less limited (Magee, 2008). This pattern is only clearly noticeable when multiple segments are involved. Paris described a capsular pattern for the cervical spine secondary to a facet lesion. With the facet lesion on the right, lateral bending is limited to the left, rotation is limited to the left, and forward bending deviates to the right (Paris, 1991).

Since the structures of the cervical and thoracic spine can be easily injured, it is imperative that you take a history and are aware of the radiological findings before you initiate the passive movement portion of the examination. Patients may have fractures, subluxations, or dislocations that are not easily diagnosed on the initial clinical evaluation. If these injuries exist, the patient's well-being may be jeopardized during the examination process.

Passive Physiological Movements

Passive testing of the physiological movements is most easily performed with the patient in the sitting position. You should place one hand over the top of the patient's head and rest your fingers on the anterior aspect of the skull and your palm over the patient's forehead. Your other hand should grasp the patient's occiput. This hold will allow you to support the patient's head and allow him or her to relax while you perform the passive movements.

Mobility Testing of Accessory Movements

Mobility testing of accessory movements will give you information about the degree of laxity present in the joint and the end feel. The patient must be totally relaxed and comfortable to allow you to move the joint and obtain the most accurate information. Before beginning the mobility testing portion of the examination, you must be sure that the vertebral artery is not compromised and that the cervical spine is stable.

Intervertebral Mobility of the Cervical Spine

Flexion Intervertebral Mobility Testing

Place the patient in the sitting position either on a stool or on a low table with their feet supported, with

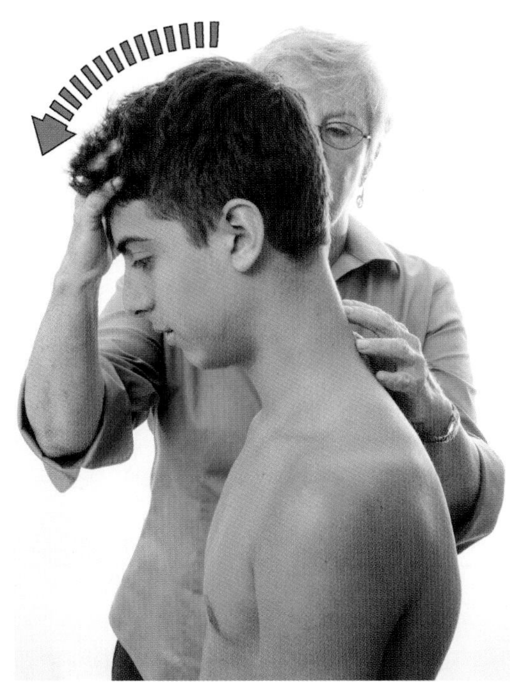

Figure 4.44 Mobility testing of cervical spine flexion.

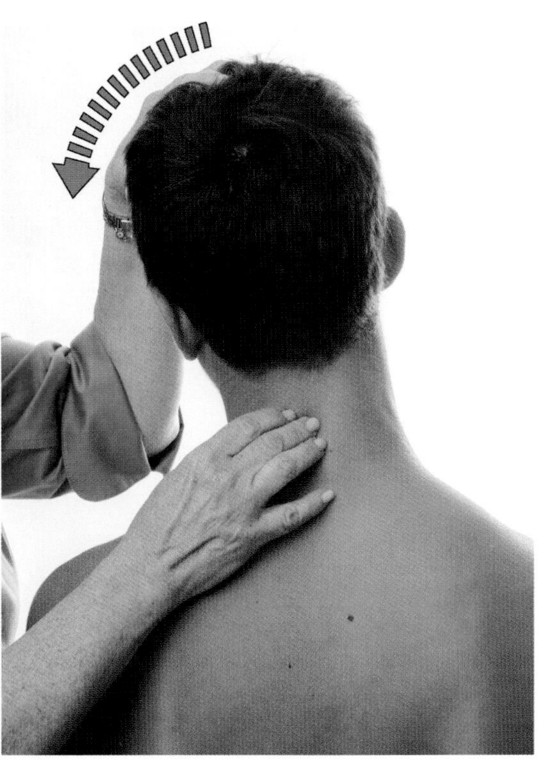

Figure 4.45 Mobility testing of cervical spine lateral (side) bending.

the head and neck in neutral alignment. Stand beside the patient to observe the movement occurring posteriorly. Support the patient's head by placing your hand over his or her forehead onto the skull. Place the middle finger of your other hand in the interspace between the spinous processes of C2 and C3. Flex the patient's head and neck until you feel movement at the segment you are palpating. Note the opening of the intervertebral space. You can slightly extend the neck to get a better sense of opening and closing. Slightly increase the degree of flexion to palpate the next intervertebral segment and continue in a caudal direction (Figure 4.44). You can also palpate over the facet joints during passive flexion. The test should be repeated bilaterally to evaluate all of the joints (http://www.youtube.com/watch?v=_3NSw2SqzJI).

Extension Intervertebral Mobility Testing

Cervical extension is evaluated in the same manner as described above for flexion except that you should be feeling a closing between the spinous processes as you extend the neck.

Lateral Bending Intervertebral Mobility Testing

Place the patient in the sitting position either on a stool or on a low table with their feet supported, with the head and neck in neutral alignment. Stand beside the patient to observe the movement occurring posteriorly. Support the patient's head by placing your hand over the top of the skull. Place the middle finger of your other hand over the facet joint on the side that you are testing. Start by placing your middle finger over the facet joint between C2 and C3. Bend the patient's head and neck toward the side you are evaluating until you feel movement at the segment being palpated. Note the closing of the facet joint. You can laterally bend the head and neck slightly in the opposite direction to get a better sense of opening and closing. Slightly increase the degree of sidebending to palpate the next intervertebral segment and continue in a caudal direction (Figure 4.45). This movement can also be palpated over the facet joints on the opposite side of the movement and you will palpate an opening of the facet joint. The test should be repeated on both sides to evaluate all of the joints (http://www.youtube.com/watch?v=H_GQp-f6rQc).

Rotation Intervertebral Mobility Testing

Place the patient in the sitting position either on a stool or on a low table with their feet supported, with the head and neck in neutral alignment. Stand beside the patient to observe the movement occurring posteriorly. Support the patient's head by placing your hand over the forehead onto the skull. Place the middle finger of your other hand on the lateral aspect of the

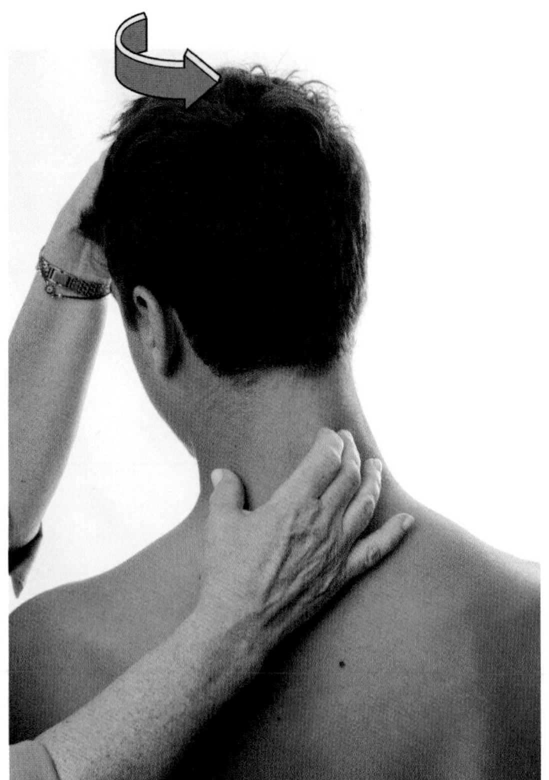

Figure 4.46 Mobility testing of cervical spine rotation.

spinous process of C2. Rotate the patient's head and neck away from the side on which you have placed your finger until you feel the spinous process pressing into your finger at the segment you are palpating. Slightly increase the degree of rotation to palpate the next intervertebral segment and continue in a caudal direction (Figure 4.46). You can also palpate by rotating the head toward your palpating finger. You will then feel the spinous process moving away from you. The test should be repeated on both sides to evaluate all the joints (http://www.youtube.com/watch?v=DwfzoyUxry4).

Thoracic Spine Movements

Passive motion of the upper thoracic spine can be evaluated as a continuation of the cervical spine. After you evaluate all the motions in each direction, continue the flexion, extension, lateral bending, and rotation movements to a greater degree until you can sense movement down to the middle thoracic vertebrae. The middle thoracic spine can be evaluated with the patient in the sitting position. Hold the patient by placing your arm around the patient's crossed upper extremities and grasping the opposite shoulder. Your hand placements and the method of palpation are the same as described above for the cervical spine. The lower thoracic spine can be evaluated as a continuation of the lumbar spine. When evaluating the lumbar spine, you should move the pelvis and lower extremities with a greater amount of range in a cranial direction until you can sense mobility in the lower thoracic vertebrae.

Cervical Traction

Place the patient in the supine position. Stand behind the patient's head. Place your hands so that your fingertips grasp under the occiput. Use your body weight and lean back, away from the patient, to create the traction force (Figure 4.47) (http://www.youtube.com/watch?v=_wEEEhIkZrg).

Accessory Movements of the Cervical Spine

Posteroanterior Central Pressure (Ventral Glide) on the Spinous Process

Place the patient in the prone position with the neck in neutral rotation midway between flexion and extension. Stand on the side of the patient so that your dominant eye is centered over the spine, with your body turned so that you are facing the patient's head. Place your overlapping thumbs onto the spinous process. Press directly over the process in an anterior direction until all the slack has been taken up (Figures 4.48a and 4.48b).

Posteroanterior Unilateral Pressure on the Articular Pillar

Place the patient in the prone position with the neck in neutral rotation midway between flexion and extension. Stand on the side of the patient so that your dominant eye is centered over the spine, with your body turned so that you are facing the patient's head. Place your overlapping thumbs onto the articular pillar on the side closest to you. Press directly over the pillar in an anterior direction until all the slack has been taken up. This will cause a rotation of the vertebral body away from the side that you are contacting (Figures 4.49a and 4.49b).

Transverse Pressure on the Spinous Process

Place the patient in the prone position with the neck in neutral rotation midway between flexion and extension. Stand on the side of the patient so that your dominant eye is centered over the spine, with your body turned so that you are facing the side of the patient.

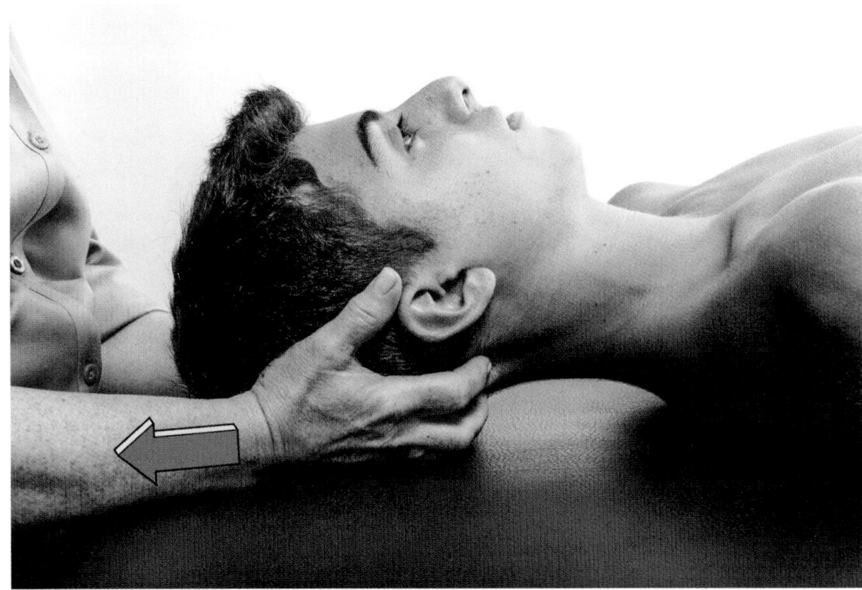

Figure 4.47 Cervical spine traction.

Place your thumbs on the lateral aspect of the spinous process. Push the process away from you until you have taken up all the slack. This will cause rotation of the vertebral body toward the direction that you are contacting (Figures 4.50a and 4.50b).

First Rib Ventral–Caudal Glide

Place the patient in the sitting position either on a stool or on a low table with their feet supported, with the head and neck rotated to the right. Stand behind the patient. Support the patient by placing your left hand over the patient's head and rest your elbow on the shoulder. Place the lateral aspect of your index finger of the right hand over the superior dorsal aspect of the right first rib. Press in a ventral and caudal direction until all the slack is taken up (Figure 4.51). This should then be repeated with rotation to the left to palpate the left first rib.

Resistive Testing

Movements of the head and neck are flexion, extension, rotation, and lateral bending. Testing the

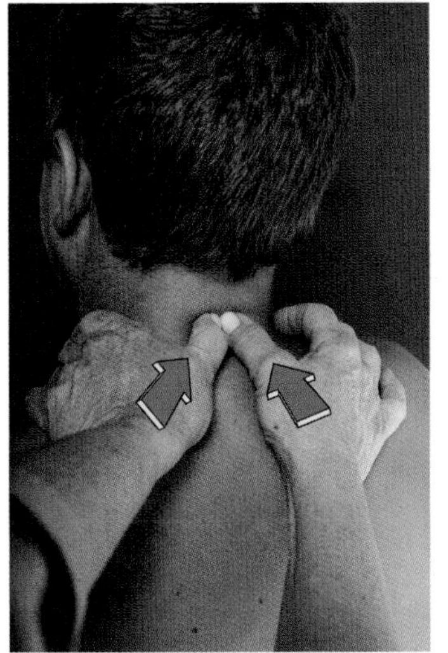

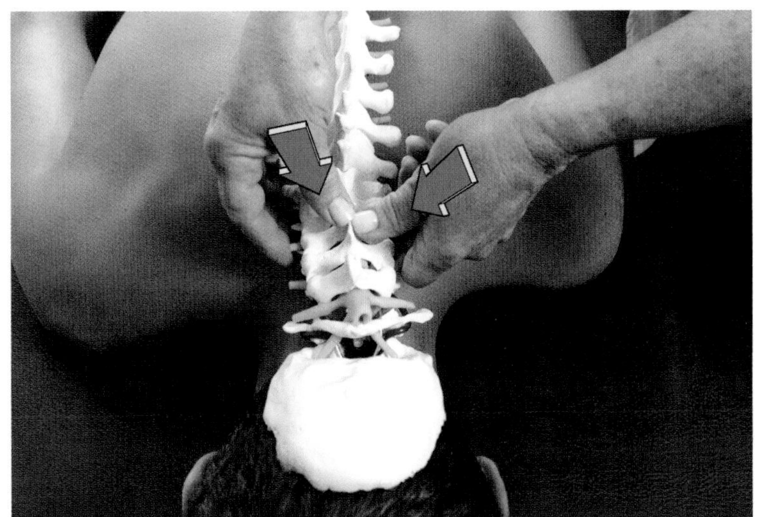

(a) (b)

Figure 4.48 (a, b) Mobility testing of central posteroanterior pressure on the spinous processes.

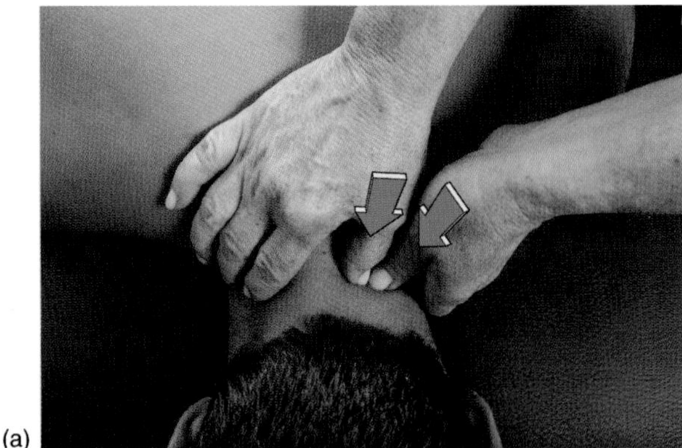

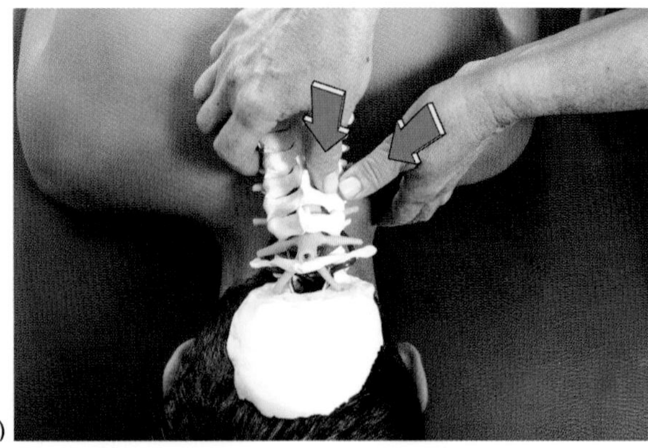

Figure 4.49 (a, b) Mobility testing of the posteroanterior pressure on the articular pillar.

strength of the cervical muscles is best performed with the patient in the seated position. Testing the cervical muscles with gravity eliminated is performed with the patient lying supine. Significant weakness of cervical muscles may be found in neuromuscular diseases such as myasthenia gravis and polymyositis.

Cervical Flexion

The sternocleidomastoid muscle is the primary cervical flexor. The scalenus anterior, medius, and posterior, as well as the intrinsic neck muscles (see Figure 4.4) assist it.

- Position of the patient: Seated.
- Resisted test (Figure 4.52): Place one of your hands on the patient's sternum to prevent substitution of neck flexion by flexion of the thorax. Place the palm of your other hand on the patient's forehead and ask the patient to bring the head downward so as to look at the floor. Resist this movement with your hand as he or she pushes against you.

Cervical Extension

The primary extensors of the cervical spine are the trapezius (superior fibers), the semispinalis capitis, splenius capitis, and splenius cervicis (Figure 4.53).

These muscles are assisted by the levator scapulae and the intrinsic neck muscles.

Position of patient: Seated. Stand behind the patient.

Resisted test (Figure 4.54): Place one hand on the patient's shoulder over the scapula for stabilization. Place your other hand over the occiput and vertex of the patient's skull and ask the patient to bring the head backward against your resistance as he or she tries to look to the ceiling. The patient may attempt to lean backward and you should resist this movement with your stabilizing hand.

Rotation

The sternocleidomastoid muscle is the prime rotator of the cervical spine (see Figure 4.55). The left

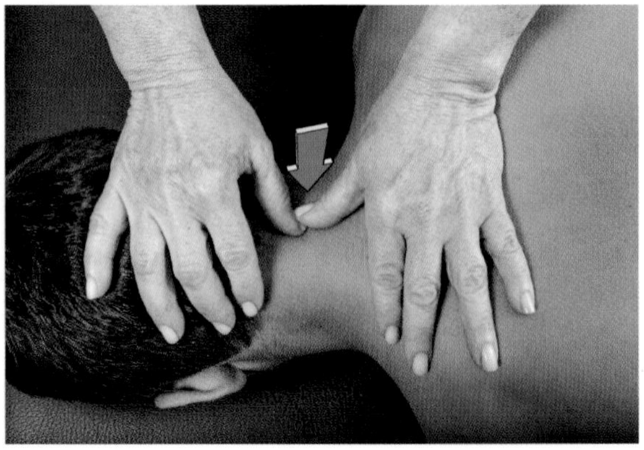

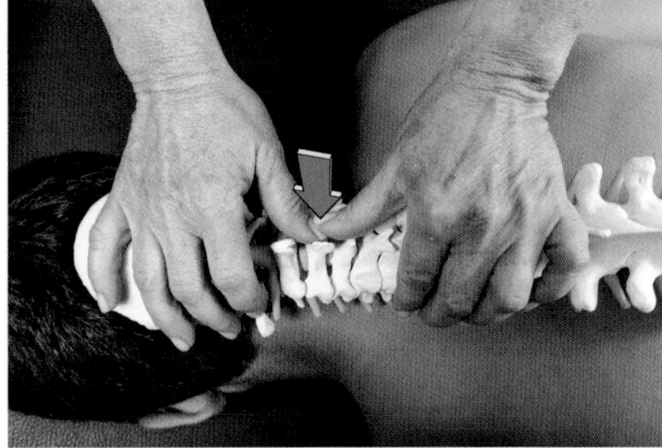

Figure 4.50 (a, b) Mobility testing of transverse pressure on the spinous process.

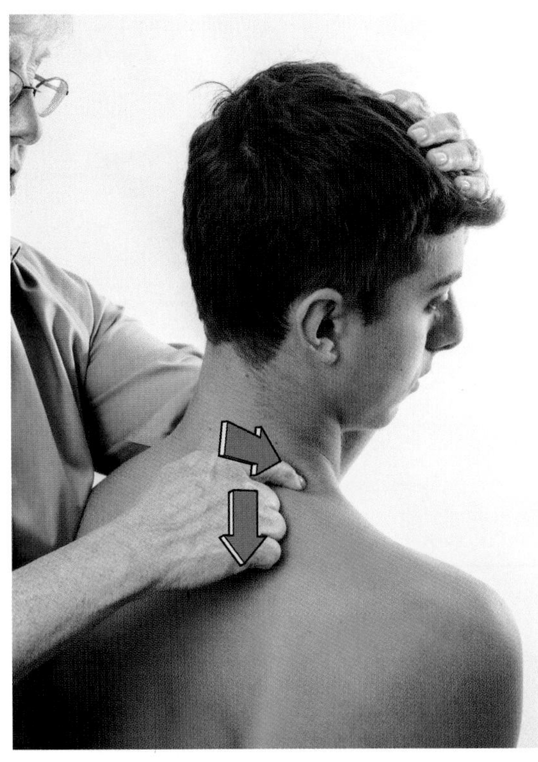

Figure 4.51 Mobility testing of first rib ventral–caudal glide.

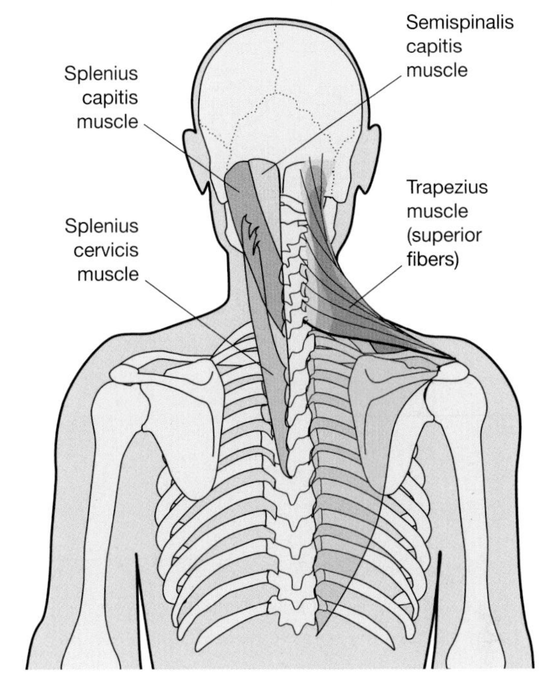

Figure 4.53 The cervical extensors.

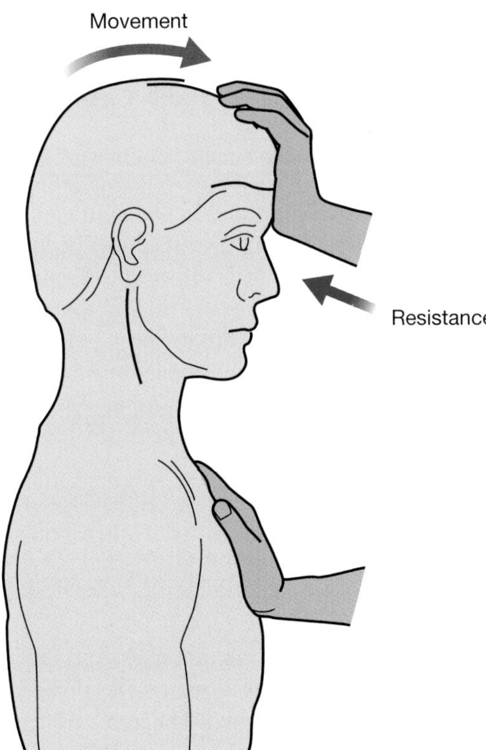

Figure 4.52 Testing cervical flexion.

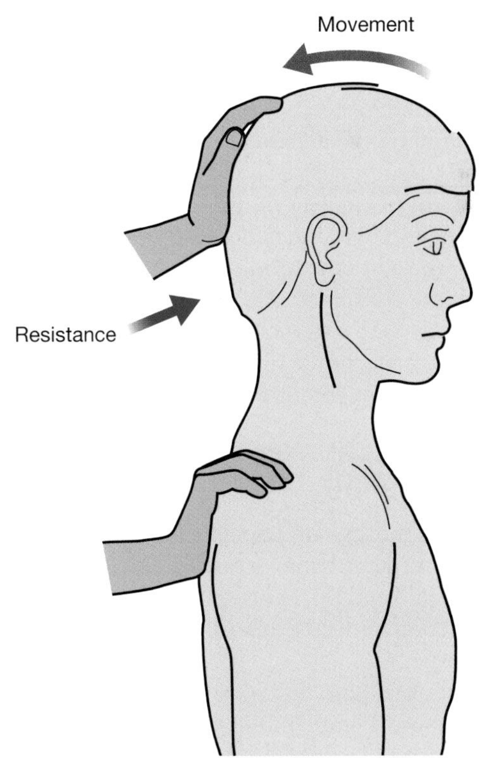

Figure 4.54 Testing cervical extension.

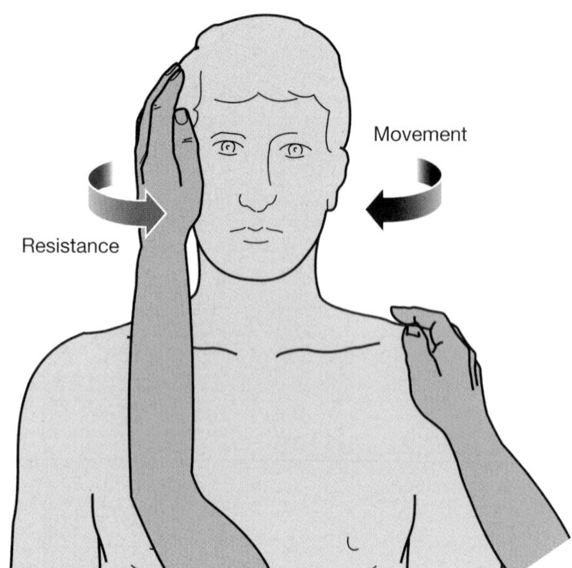

Figure 4.55 Testing lateral rotation. Resisting rotation of the head to the left tests the right sternocleidomastoid muscle.

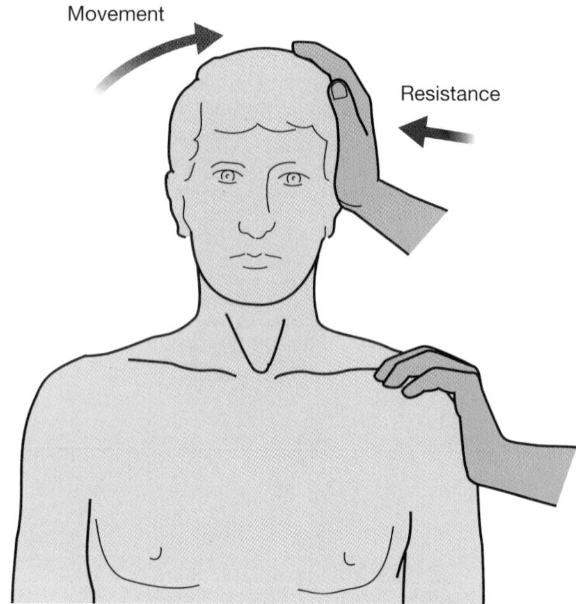

Figure 4.56 Testing lateral bending.

sternocleidomastoid rotates the head to the right (Figure 4.4). It also side bends the head to the left.

- Position of patient: Seated, with you in front of the patient.
- Resisted test (Figure 4.55): To test the left sternocleidomastoid muscle, you should resist right rotation of the head as follows. Place your right hand on the patient's left shoulder to stabilize the torso. Cup your left hand and place it so that the patient's chin is in the palm of your hand and your fingers cover the patient's cheek. Ask the patient to rotate the head in a horizontal plane against the resistance of your left hand.

Weakness of the sternocleidomastoid muscle may be due to damage to the spinal accessory nerve. Compare left and right rotation.

Lateral Bending

The primary muscles of lateral bending are the scaleni muscles, and the intrinsic muscles of the neck assist them. Lateral bending is not a pure motion and occurs in conjunction with rotation of the cervical spine (see Figure 4.4).

- Position of patient: Seated, with you at the side.
- Resisted test (Figure 4.56): Test left lateral bending by placing your left hand on the patient's left shoulder to stabilize the torso. Place your right hand over the temporal aspect of the skull above the ear and ask the patient to tilt the ear toward the shoulder as you resist this motion. Compare your findings with those of the opposite side.

Neurological Examination of the Cervical Spine and Upper Extremity

The Brachial Plexus

The brachial plexus (Figure 4.57) is composed of the C5, C6, C7, C8, and T1 nerve roots. In some individuals, C4 is included, and this is referred to as a prefixed brachial plexus. In others, T2 is included, and this is called a postfixed brachial plexus.

During embryogenesis, the upper limb bud rotates so that the upper nerve roots, C5 and C6, become lateral in the arm, and the lower nerve roots, C8 and T1, become medial in the arm.

The five nerve roots that form the plexus join to form three trunks. C5 and C6 form the upper trunk, C7 forms the middle trunk, and C8 and T1 join to form the lower trunk. The trunks are located at the level of the clavicle.

Each trunk splits into an anterior and posterior division. The posterior divisions of the three trunks join to form the posterior cord. The anterior divisions of the upper and middle trunks form the lateral cord, and the anterior division of the lower trunk continues on as the medial cord. The names posterior, lateral,

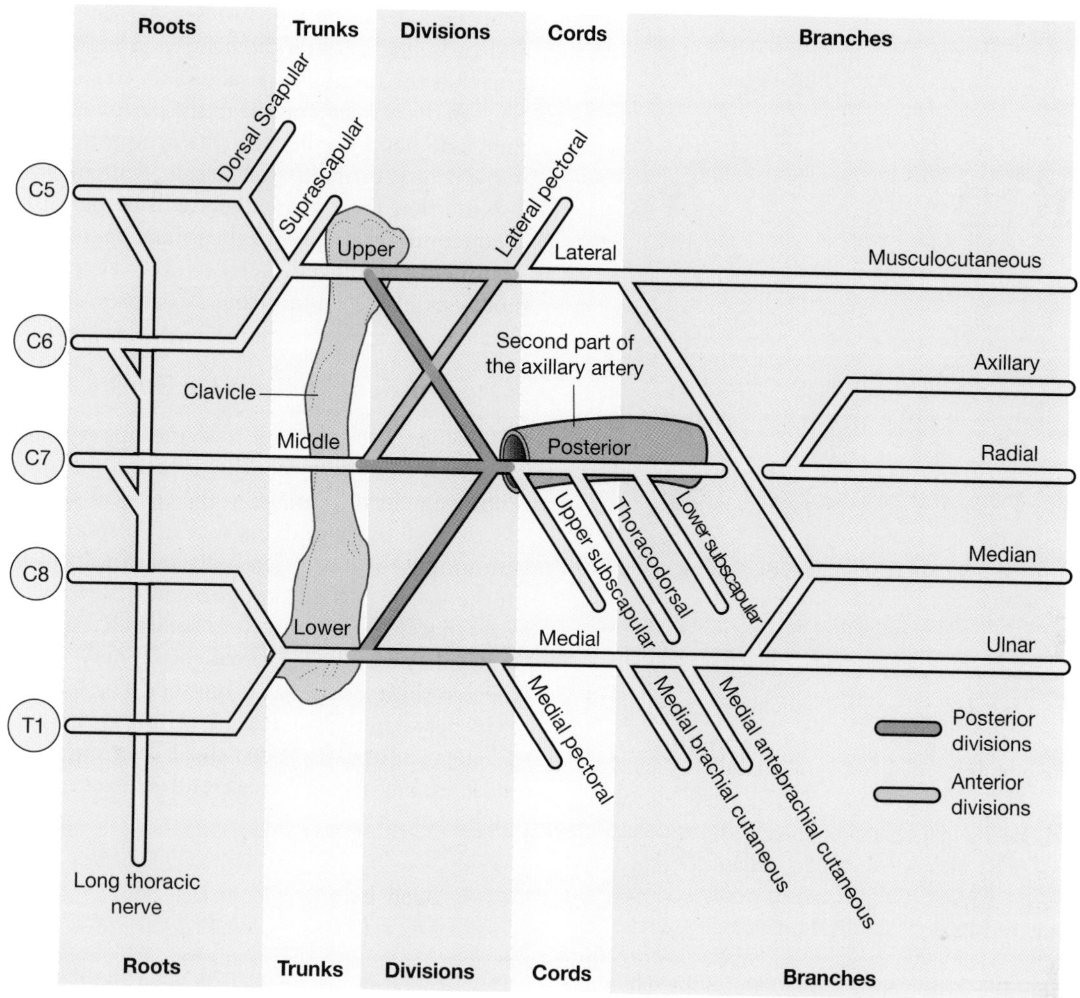

Figure 4.57 The brachial plexus. The anterior divisions of the upper and middle trunks form the lateral cord and the anterior division of the lower trunk forms the medial cord. The three posterior divisions of the trunk form the posterior cord.

and medial cords are based on their relationship to the second part of the axillary artery and the axilla.

Portions of the lateral and medial cords join to form the median nerve. The lateral cord continues on as the musculocutaneous nerve, and the medial cord continues on as the ulnar nerve. The posterior cord branches into the axillary and radial nerves.

Upper Limb Tension Test (Brachial Plexus Tension Test, Elvey's Test)

Performing a mobility test can test the component nerves of the brachial plexus.

Median Nerve

The patient is supine with the scapula unobstructed. Depress the shoulder and maintain the position. Extend the elbow and externally rotate the upper extremity. Then extend the wrist, fingers, and thumb. If nerve root irritation is present, local palpation of the nerve will increase the symptoms (Butler, 1991) (Figure 4.58) (http://www.youtube.com/watch?v=g3DSgCOXpWc).

Radial Nerve

The patient is supine with the scapula unobstructed. Depress the shoulder and maintain the position. Extend the elbow and internally rotate the upper extremity. Then flex the wrist. Adding ulnar deviation and flexion of the thumb can enhance the position. If nerve root irritation is present, local palpation of the nerve will increase the symptoms (Butler, 1991) (Figure 4.59) (http://www.youtube.com/watch?v=x3ivtuDwCDI).

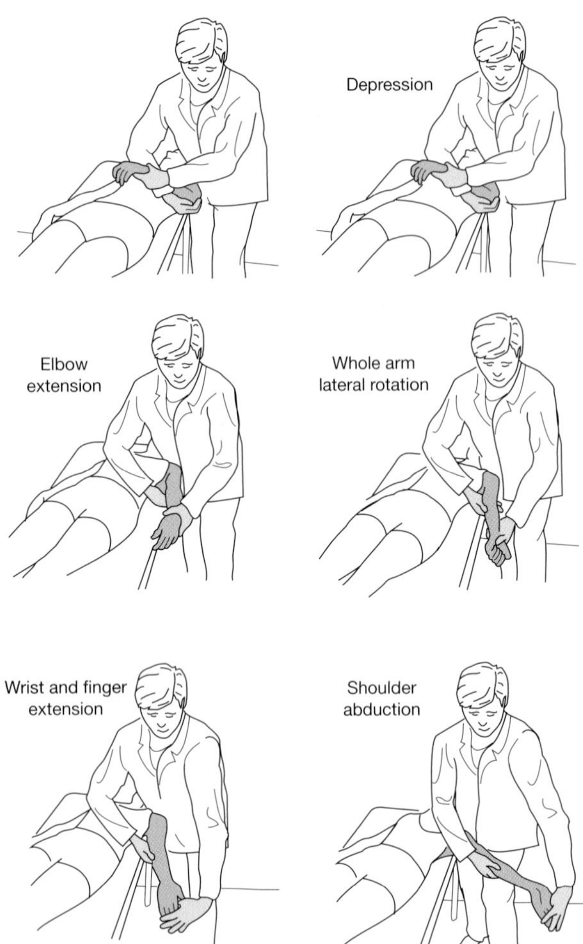

Figure 4.58 The median nerve stretch test. (Adapted from Butler, 1991.)

Adding cervical lateral bending away from the side being tested and some adduction or extension of the shoulder can enhance both tests.

Ulnar Nerve

The starting position is the same as for the median nerve. Extend the patient's wrist and supinate the forearm. Then fully flex the elbow and depress the shoulder. Add external rotation and abduct the shoulder. The neck can be placed in lateral bending (Figure 4.60) (http://www.youtube.com/watch?v=g3DSgCOXpWc).

The patient will likely complain of numbness or pain in the thumb, index, and middle fingers. This is a normal response. In 70% of normal patients, lateral bending away from the test side will exacerbate the symptoms (Kenneally *et al.*, 1988). The test is abnormal if the patient notes symptoms in the ring and little finger while the head is in neutral. To confirm that the findings are secondary to root irritation, slacken the position of one of the peripheral joints and then side bend the neck. If the symptoms return, the nerve root is probably the source (Kaltenborn, 2012).

Note that these maneuvers will be painful if there is concomitant disease of the joints, ligaments, or tendons being mobilized. Refer to other chapters for specific tests of these important structures.

Neurological Testing by Root Level

Neurological examination of the upper extremity is required to determine the location of nerve root impingement or damage in the cervical spine, as may be caused by spondylosis or a herniated disc. By examining the motor strength, sensation, and reflexes in the upper extremities, you can determine the root level that is functioning abnormally. Recall that in the cervical spine, the C1 through C7 nerves exit above the vertebrae of the same number. The C8 nerve root exits between the C7 and T1 vertebral bodies, and the T1 nerve root exits below the T1 vertebral body. Key muscles, key sensory areas, and reflexes are tested for each root level.

The C5 Root Level

Motor

The biceps muscle, which flexes the elbow, is innervated by the musculocutaneous nerve and represents the C5 root level (Figure 4.61). Many authors also consider the deltoid muscle, innervated by the axillary nerve, to be a key C5 muscle. The patient flexes the elbow with the forearm fully supinated. Resist this movement with your hand placed on the anterior aspect of the mid forearm (see pp. 218–219, Figure 9.33 for further information).

Sensation

The key sensory area for C5 is the lateral antecubital fossa.

Reflex

The biceps reflex is tested by placing your thumb on the biceps tendon as the patient rests his or her forearm on yours. Take the reflex hammer and tap your thumb briskly and observe for contraction of the biceps and flexion of the elbow (see pp. 223–224, Figures 9.43, 9.45 for further information).

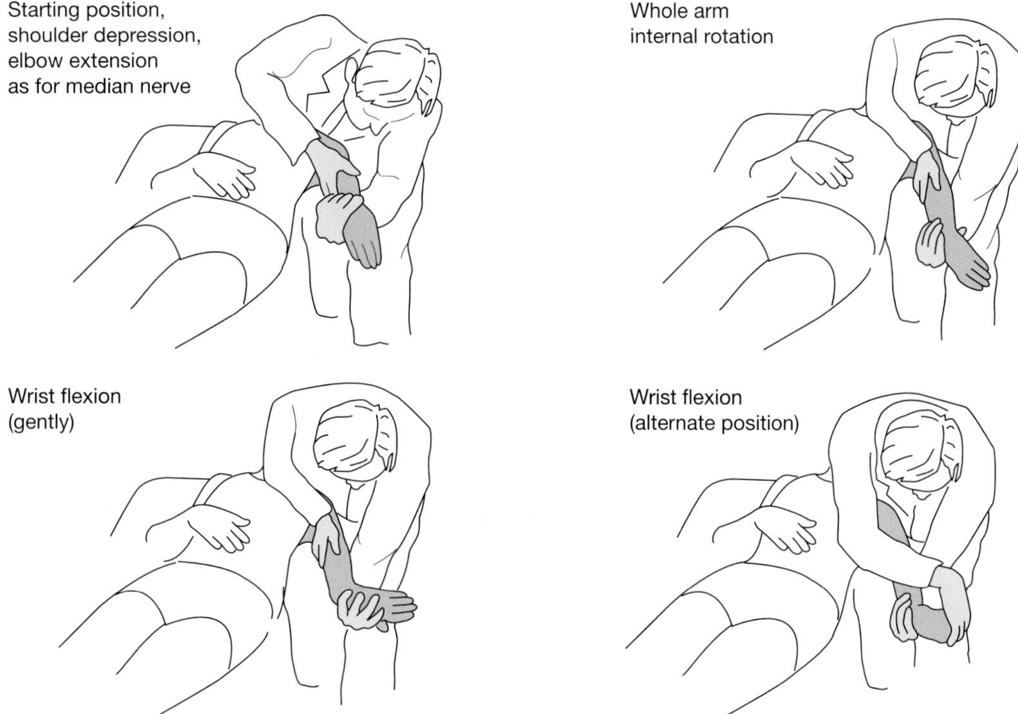

Figure 4.59 The radial nerve stretch test.

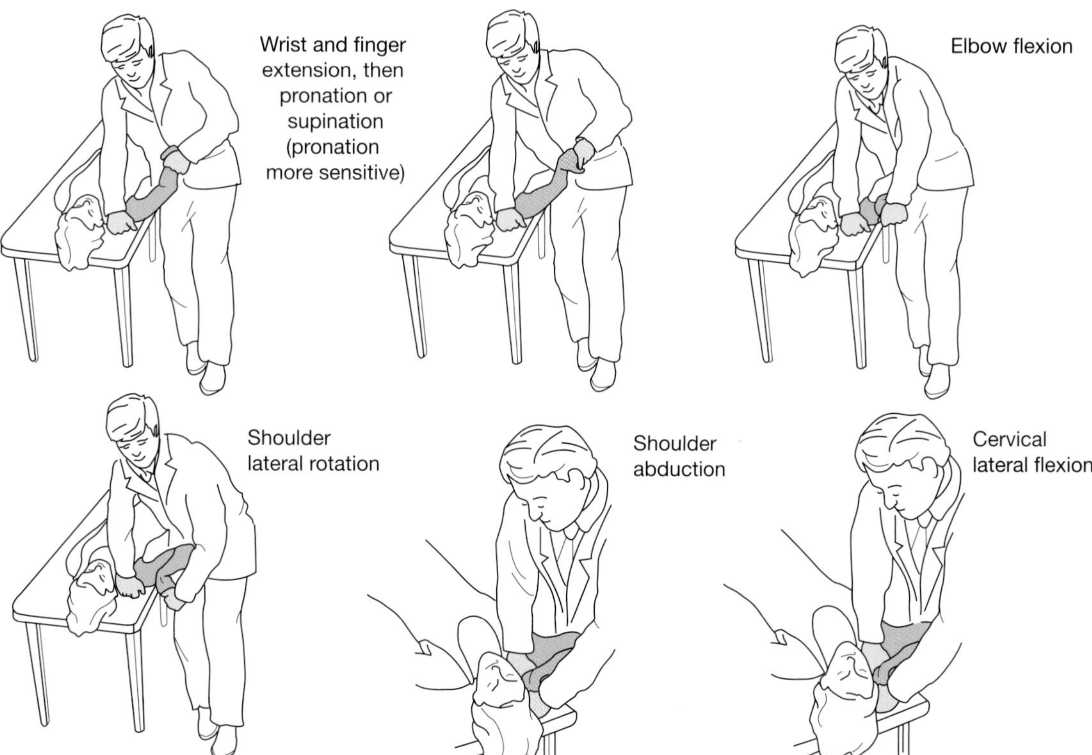

Figure 4.60 The ulnar nerve stretch test. (Adapted from Butler, 1991.)

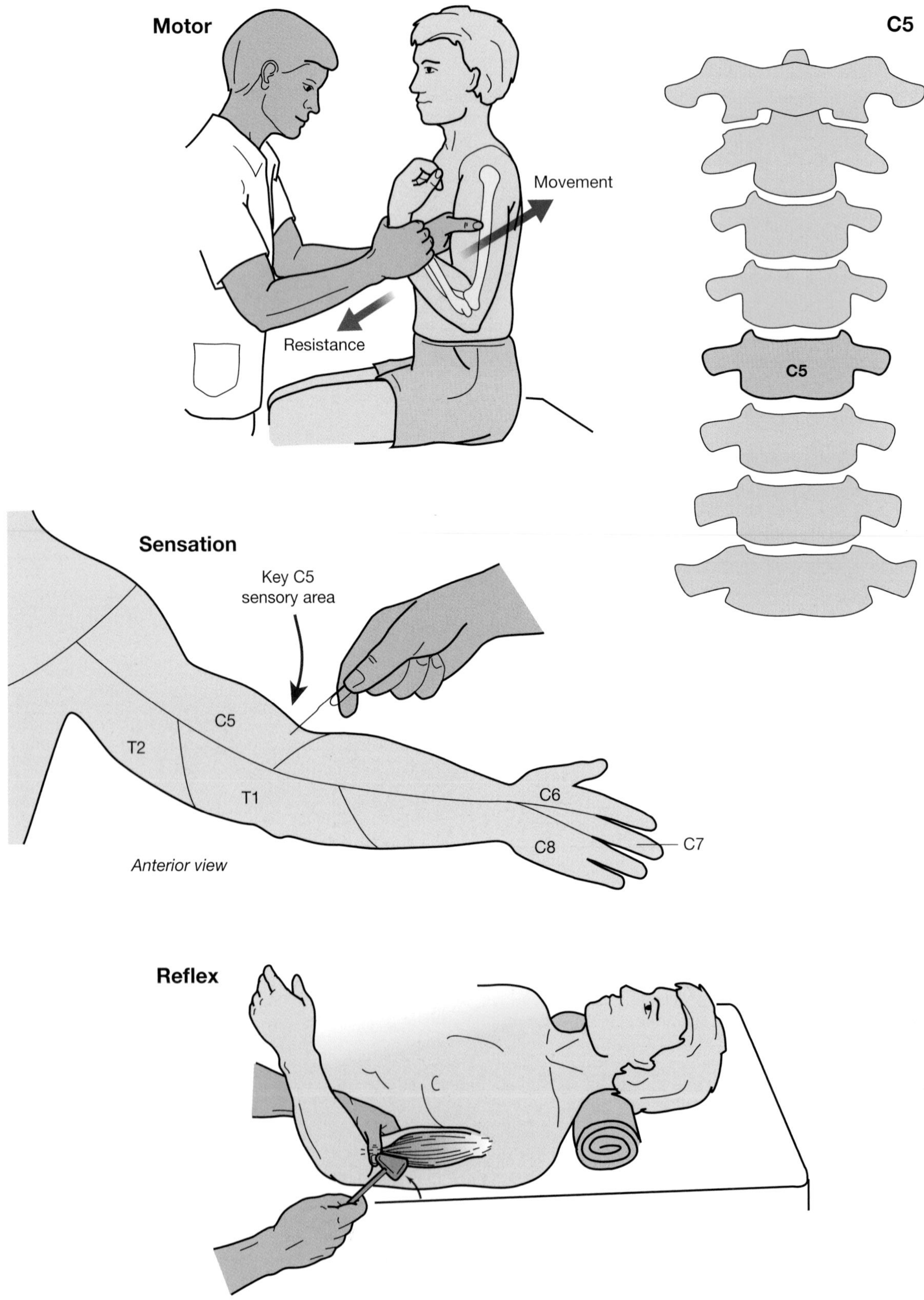

Figure 4.61 The C5 root level.

The C6 Root Level

Motor

The wrist extensors (extensor carpi radialis longus and brevis) are innervated by the radial nerve and represent the C6 root level (Figure 4.62). Test wrist extension by having the patient pronate the forearm and raise his or her hand, as if to say "stop." Resist this motion with your hand against the posterior aspect of the metacarpals (see pp. 264, 266, Figure 10.55 for further information).

Sensation

The key sensory area for C6 is the anterior distal aspect of the thumb.

Reflex

The brachioradialis reflex is used to test the C6 nerve root level. To test this reflex, have the patient rest the forearm over yours, with the elbow in slight flexion. Use the flat end of the reflex hammer to tap the distal part of the radius. The test result is positive when the brachioradialis muscle contracts and the forearm jumps up slightly (see pp. 223–224, Figure 9.45 for further information). The biceps reflex can also be tested to evaluate the C6 root level because both the C5 and C6 roots innervate the biceps nerve roots.

The C7 Root Level

Motor

Elbow extension (triceps brachii) is examined to test the C7 root level (Figure 4.63). The triceps is innervated by the radial nerve. Testing elbow extension is performed by having the patient lie supine with the shoulder flexed to 90 degrees and the elbow flexed. Stabilize the arm with one hand placed just proximal to the elbow and apply a downward flexing resistive force with your other hand placed on the forearm just proximal to the wrist. Ask the patient to extend the hand upward against your resistance (see pp. 219–220, Figure 9.36 for further information).

Sensation

The key sensory area for C7 is located on the anterior distal aspect of the long finger.

Reflex

The triceps reflex tests the C7 nerve root level. This test is performed by having the patient's forearm resting over yours. Hold the patient's arm proximal to the elbow joint with your hand, to stabilize the upper arm. Ask the patient to relax. Tap the triceps tendon with the reflex hammer just proximal to the olecranon process. The test result is positive when a contraction of the triceps muscle is visualized (see pp. 223–225, Figure 9.46 for further information).

The C8 Root Level

Motor

The long flexors of the fingers (flexor digitorum profundus), which are innervated by the median and ulnar nerves, are tested to evaluate the C8 root level (Figure 4.64). Finger flexion is tested by asking the patient to curl the second through fifth fingers toward the palm as you place your fingers against the patient's palmar finger pads to prevent him or her from forming a fist (see p. 267, Figure 10.58 for further information).

Sensation

The key sensory area for C8 is located over the anterior distal aspect of the fifth finger.

Reflex

The finger flexor jerk is not often tested. The reader is referred to neurological textbooks for further information regarding this reflex.

The T1 Root Level

Motor

The small and index finger abductors (abductor digiti quinti, first dorsal interosseous) are tested to evaluate the T1 root level (Figure 4.65). These muscles are innervated by the ulnar nerve. The patient is examined with the forearm pronated. Ask the patient to spread the fingers apart as you apply resistance to this movement against the outer aspects of the proximal phalanges of the index and little fingers (see pp. 269–272, Figures 10.66, 10.67, 10.70 for further information).

Sensation

The key sensory area for T1 is located on the medial aspect of the arm just proximal to the antecubital fossa.

Reflex

None.

T2 Through T12 Root Levels

The thoracic root levels are tested primarily by sensation, and the key sensory areas are located just to the side of the midline on the trunk as illustrated in Figure 4.66. The only exception to this is the T2 key sensory area, which is located in the anteromedial aspect of the distal axilla.

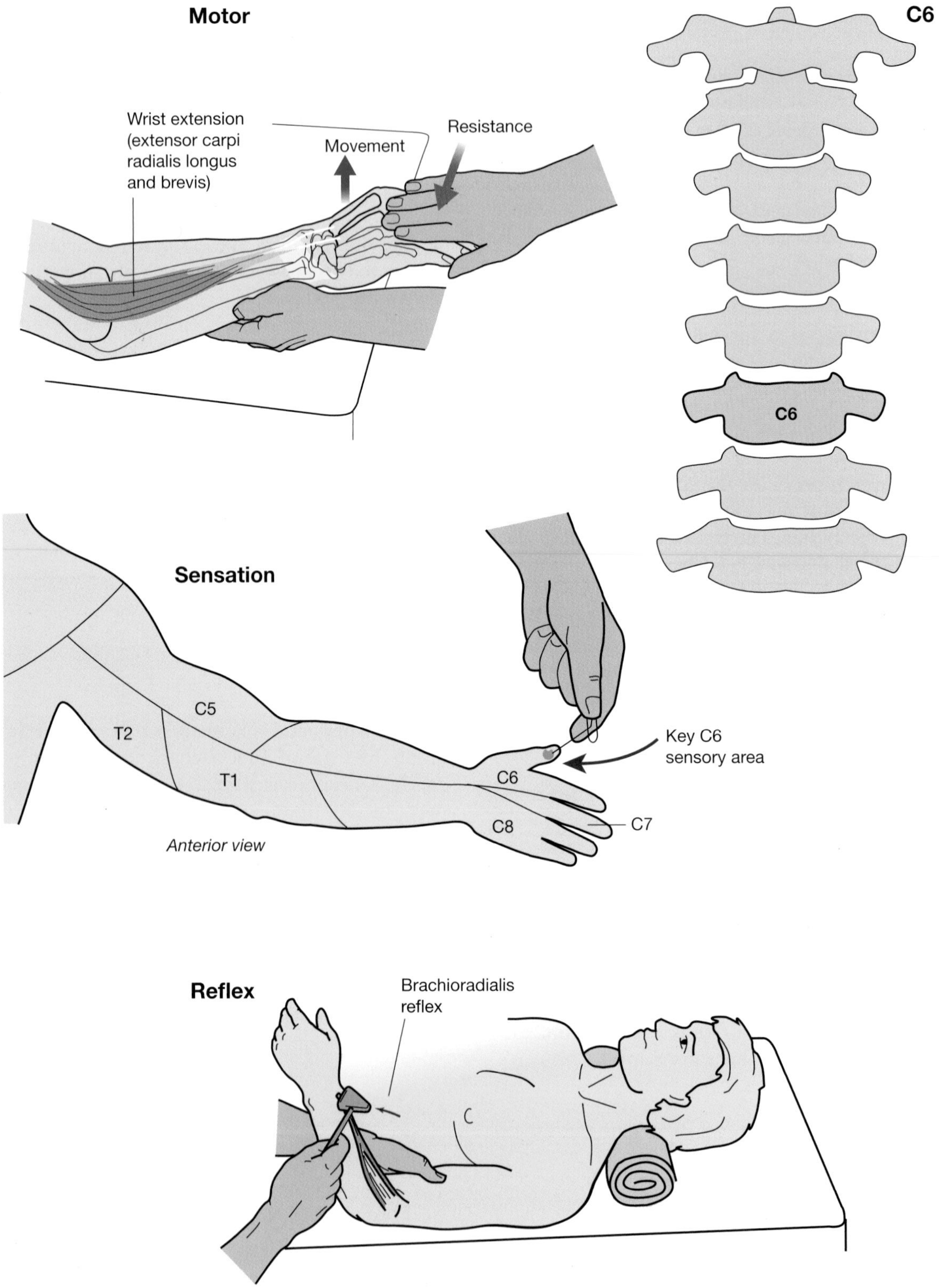

Motor
C6
Wrist extension (extensor carpi radialis longus and brevis)
Movement
Resistance
C6
Sensation
C5
T2
T1
C6
C8
C7
Key C6 sensory area
Anterior view
Reflex
Brachioradialis reflex

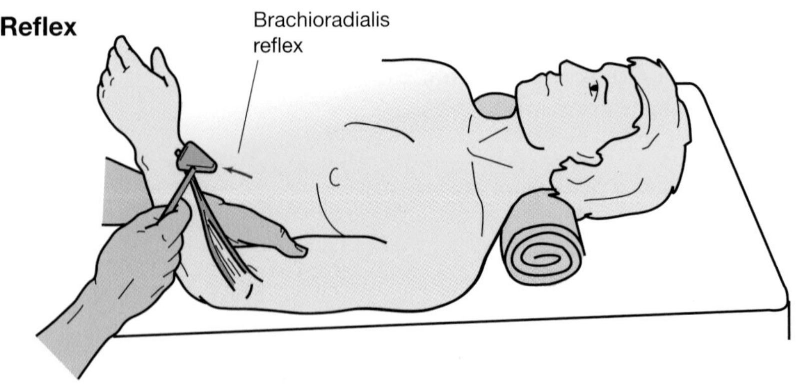

Figure 4.62 The C6 root level.

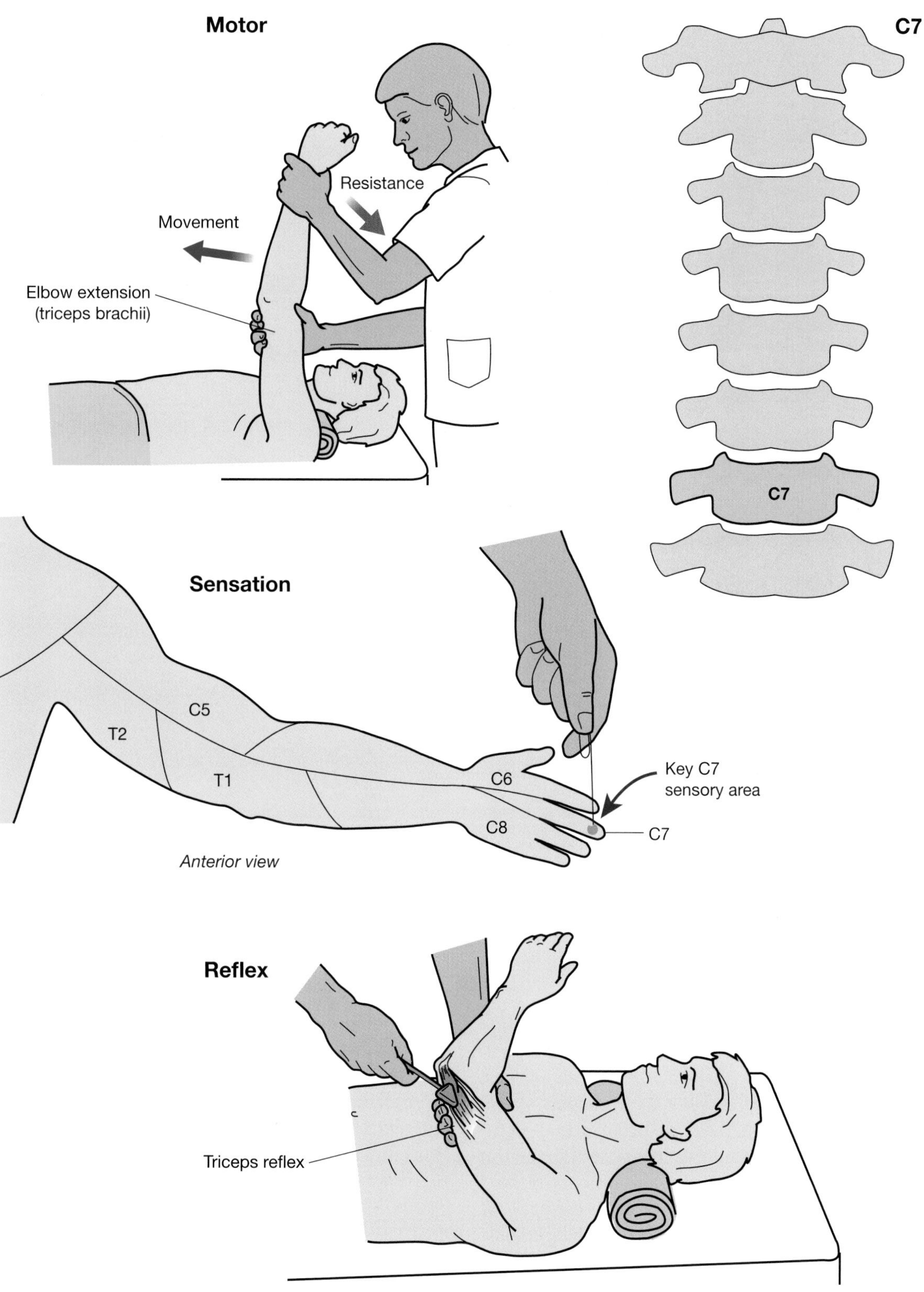

Figure 4.63 The C7 root level.

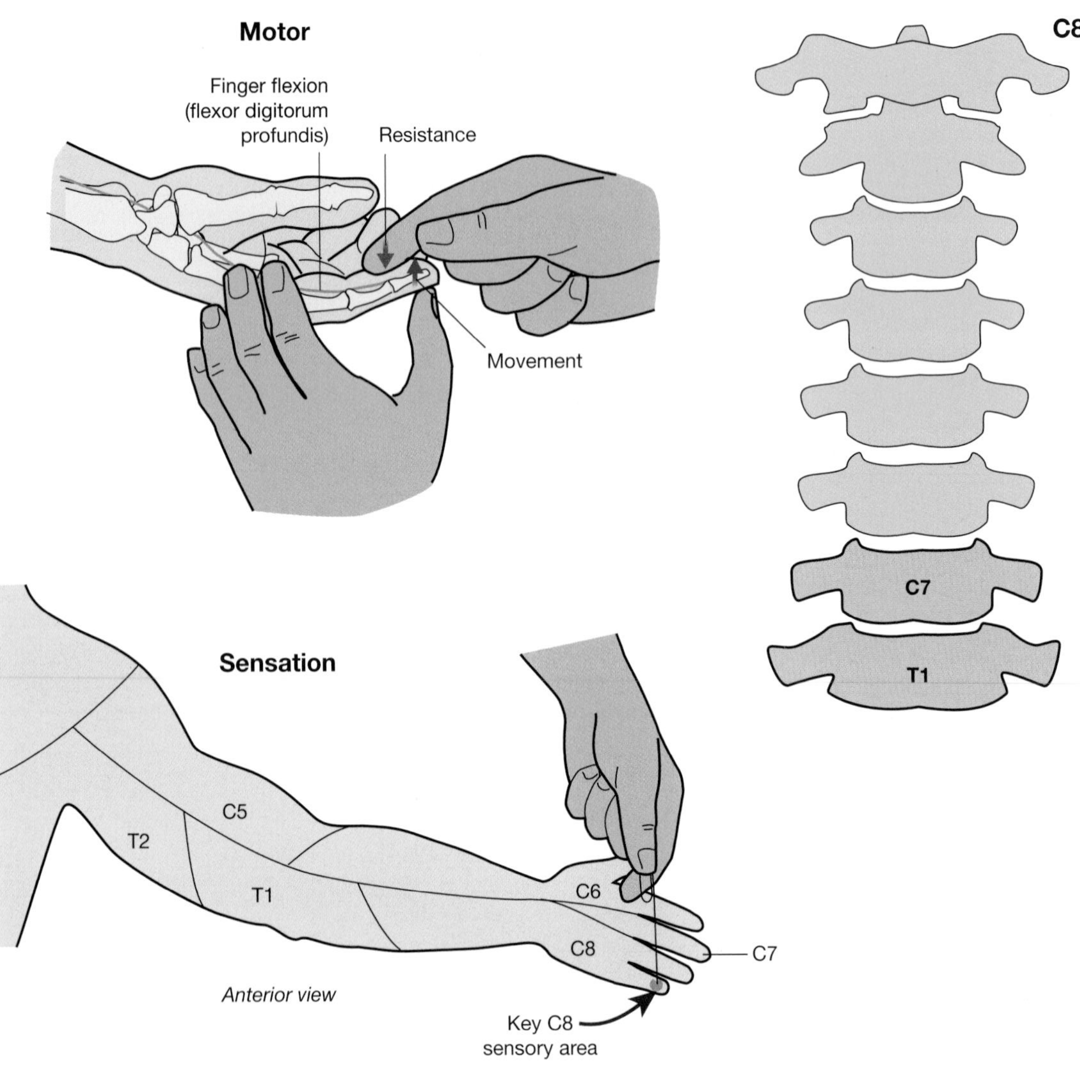

Figure 4.64 The C8 root level.

Special Tests

Compression of the cervical spine from above is performed to reproduce or amplify the radicular symptoms of pain or paresthesias that occur due to compression of the cervical nerve roots in the neural foramina. The neural foramina become narrowed when the patient extends the neck, rotates the neck, or laterally bends the head toward the side to be tested.

Spurling Test

The Spurling test (Figure 4.67) is performed with the patient's neck in lateral flexion or ipsilateral rotation. The patient is sitting. Place your hand on top of the patient's head and press down firmly or bang the back of your hand with your fist. If the patient complains of an increase in radicular symptoms in the extremity, the test finding is positive. The distribution of the pain and abnormal sensation is useful in determining which root level may be involved (http://www.youtube.com/watch?v=h8GxF73P6GQ).

Distraction Test

The distraction test (Figure 4.68) is performed in an effort to reduce the patient's symptoms by opening

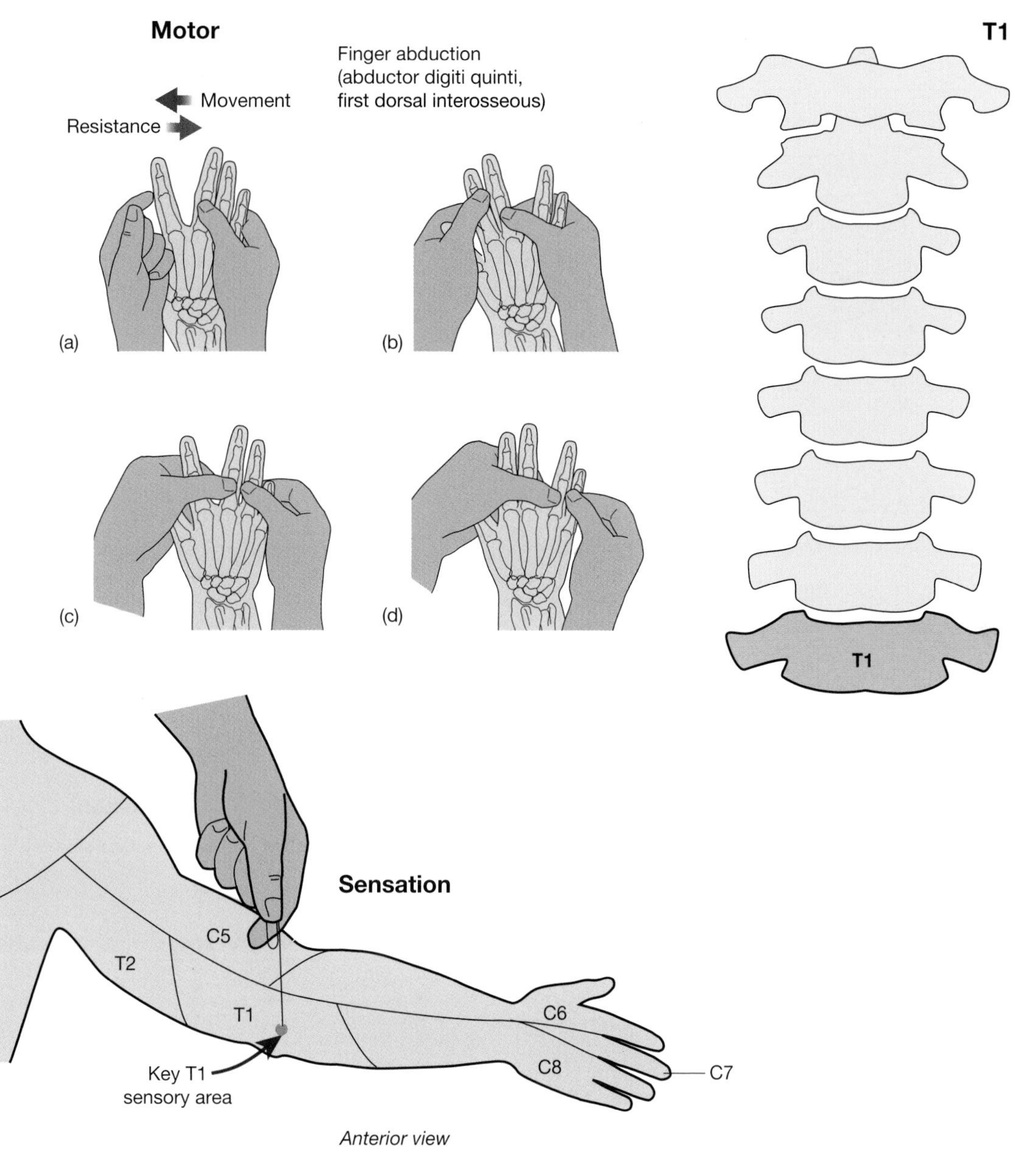

Figure 4.65 The T1 root level.

the neural foramina. The patient is sitting. Place both of your hands under the patient's occipital bones, supporting the weight of the head. Lift the patient's head slowly to distract the cervical spine. If the patient notes relief or diminished pain, the test finding is positive for nerve root damage. Be careful to protect the temporomandibular joint when pulling up on the chin (http://www.youtube.com/watch?v=v_zoQI_HLt8).

Upper Cervical Instability Testing

Sharp-Purser Test

The patient is placed in the sitting position. Ask the patient to flex their head. Extreme caution should be exercised with upper cervical stability testing since it is possible to compromise the spinal cord. The initial positive finding is the reproduction of the

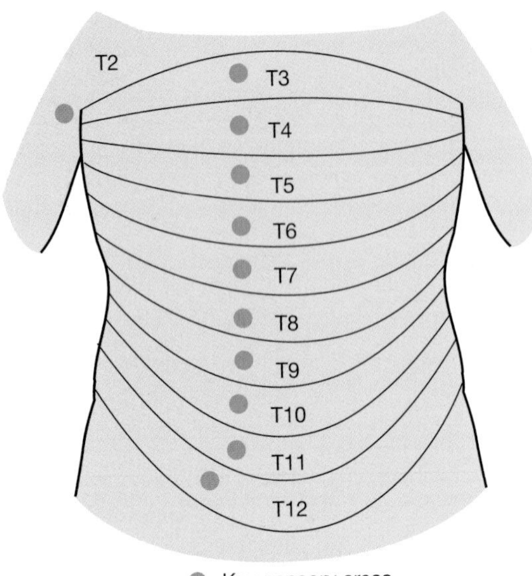

Figure 4.66 The thoracic dermatomes and their key sensory areas.

patient's complaints. The therapist can postulate that the symptoms are caused by incompetency of the transverse ligament allowing for forward translation of C1 on C2. The therapist then stabilizes the spinous processes of C2 using their thumb and index finger and simultaneously translates the patient's head posteriorly with their forearm anterior to the patient's forehead. The positive finding is the reduction of the patient's symptoms. The assumption is that the unstable upper cervical spine has been reduced, thus

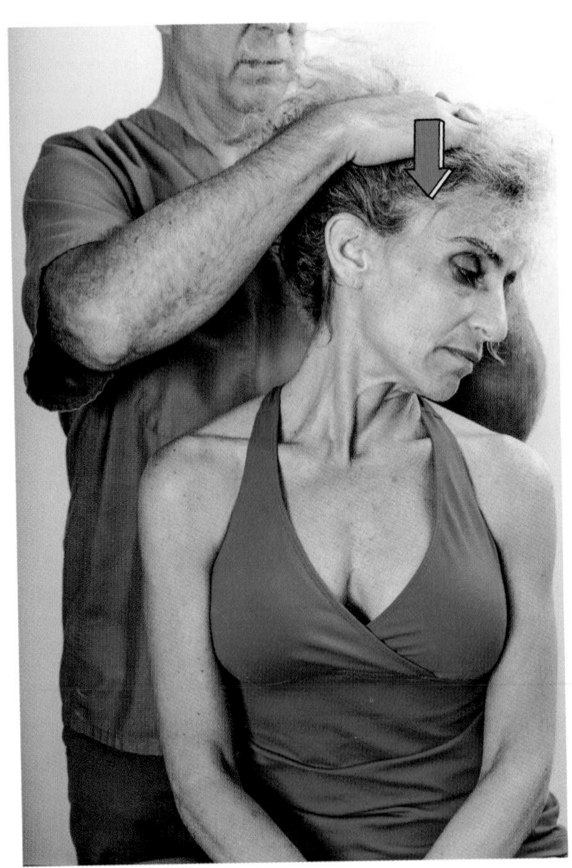

Figure 4.67 The Spurling test. The patient's head is flexed laterally. Compression causes the neural foramina on the same side to narrow in diameter.

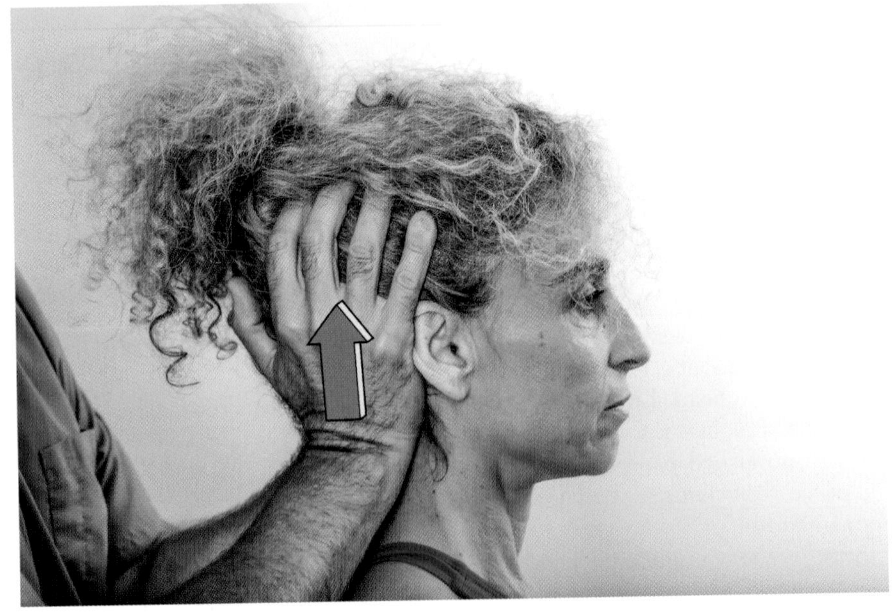

Figure 4.68 The distraction test. Distracting the cervical spine increases the diameter of the neural foramina.

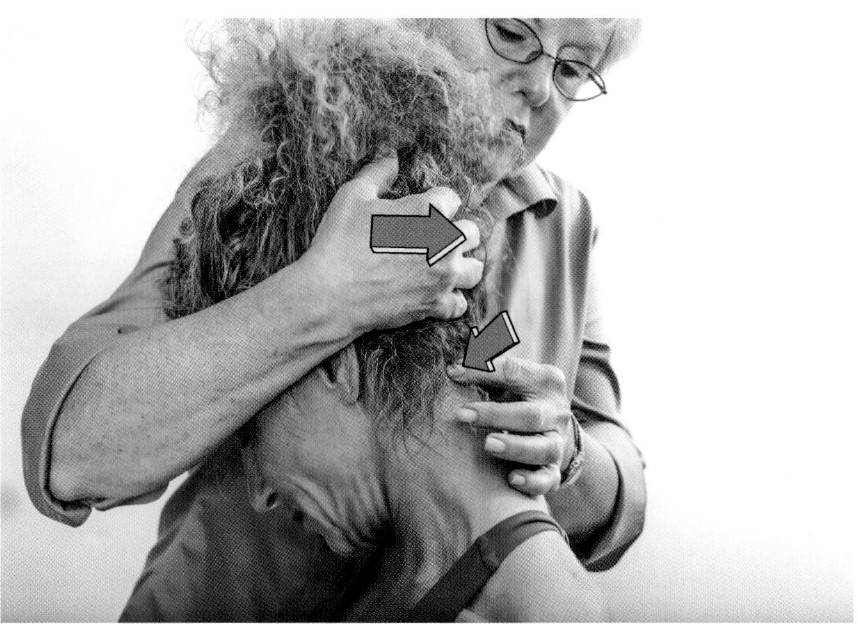

Figure 4.69 Sharp-Purser test. Stabilize at C2 and translate the head posteriorly.

relieving the compression on the spinal cord (Figure 4.69) (Aspinall, 1990) (http://www.youtube.com/watch?v=ZxYCFei_LQw).

Aspinall's Transverse Ligament Test

If the Sharp-Purser test is negative and you have suspicions that the patient has an upper cervical instability of the transverse ligament, you can perform this additional test. This test can compromise the spinal cord, therefore extreme caution should be used. The patient is placed in the supine position stabilizing the occiput in flexion. Apply a gradually increasing pressure over the posterior aspect of C1. Your direction of force is from posterior to anterior. The patient may perceive a feeling of a "lump" in their throat which can increase during testing. This sensation or movement between the atlas and the occiput are considered to be positive findings. Check for any vertebral artery symptoms (Figure 4.70) (Aspinall, 1990) (http://www.youtube.com/watch?v=Ljkd_q-apbU).

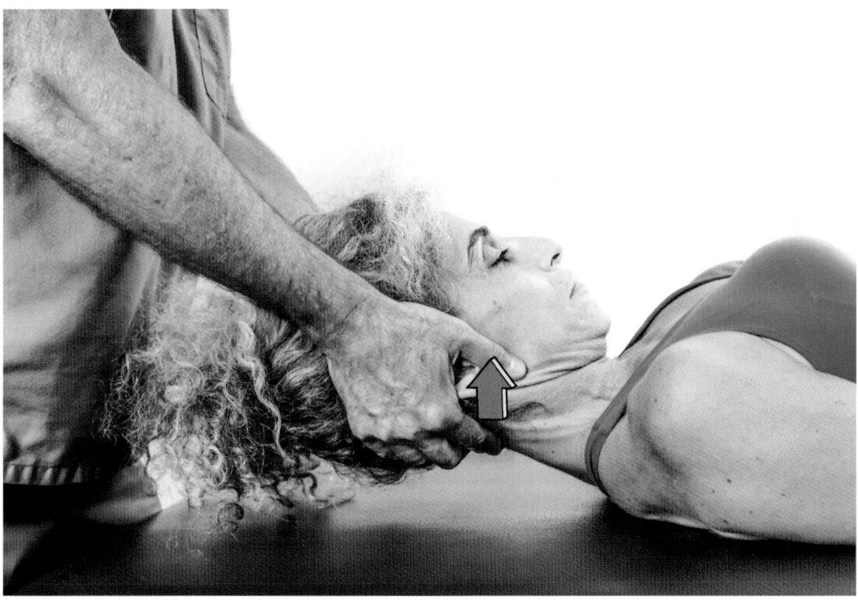

Figure 4.70 Aspinall's transverse ligament test. Direct force gradually from posterior to anterior.

Alar Ligament Stress Tests

Lateral Flexion Alar Ligament Stress Test

The patient is in the supine or sitting position. Use one hand to stabilize the spinous process of C2 and then passively side bend the patient's neck in the neutral position, followed by sidebending in both flexion and extension. The positive finding is movement between the head and neck. If the alar ligament is intact, only a minimal amount of movement should be present (Figure 4.71) (Aspinall, 1990) (http://www.youtube.com/watch?v=FYgBiQNQ06g).

Rotational Alar Ligament Stress Test

The patient is in the supine or sitting position. Use one hand to stabilize the spinous process of C2 and then passively rotate the patient's head in both directions, starting with the asymptomatic side. Normally, only 20–30 degrees of rotation can occur if the ligament is stable. If excessive movement is present, the test is considered positive for increased laxity of the contralateral alar ligament (Figure 4.72) (Magee, 2008).

Lhermitte's Sign

Lhermitte's sign (Figure 4.73) is used to diagnose meningeal irritation and may also be seen in multiple sclerosis. The patient is sitting. Passively flex the patient's head forward so that the chin approaches the chest. If the patient complains of pain or paresthesias down the spine, the test result is positive. The patient may also complain of radiating pain into the upper or lower extremities. Flexion of the hips can also be performed simultaneously with head flexion (i.e., with the patient in the long sitting position) (http://www.youtube.com/watch?v=-YJepJhe9IU).

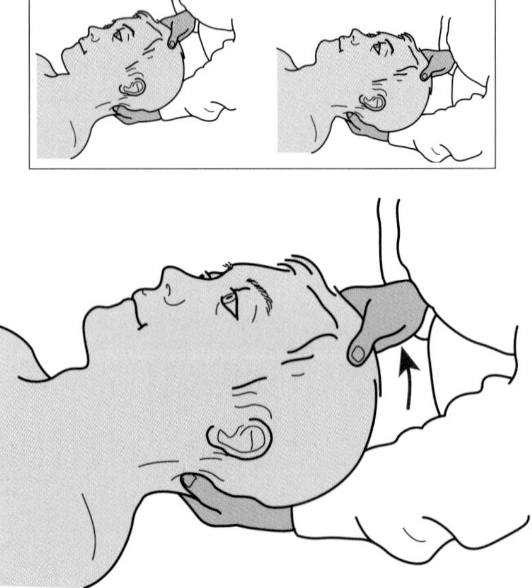

Figure 4.71 Lateral flexion alar ligament stress test. Attempt passive sidebending of the head in neutral, flexion, and extension.

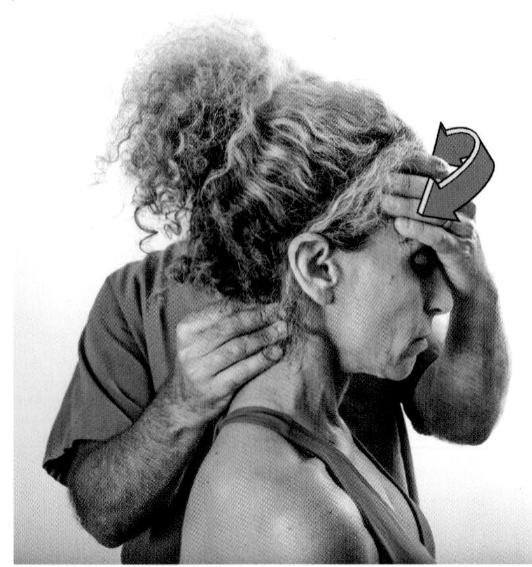

Figure 4.72 Rotational alar ligament stress test. Stabilize at C2. Passively rotate the head, first to the asymptomatic side and then to the other side.

Vertebral Artery Test

Movement of the cervical spine affects the vertebral arteries because they course through the foramina of the cervical vertebrae. These foramina may be stenotic and extension of the cervical spine may cause symptoms such as dizziness, lightheadedness, or nystagmus. The vertebral artery test is performed prior to manipulation or passive motion to the end of the range of the cervical spine, to test the patency of the vertebral arteries. The patient is most easily tested in a supine position. Place the patient's head and neck in the following positions passively for at least 30 seconds, and observe for symptoms or signs as previously described: head and neck extension, head and neck rotation to the right and left, and head and neck rotation to the right and left with the neck in extension (with or without lateral bending to the opposite side). Take time between each position to allow the patient to re-equilibrate. In general, turning the head to the right will affect the left vertebral artery more and

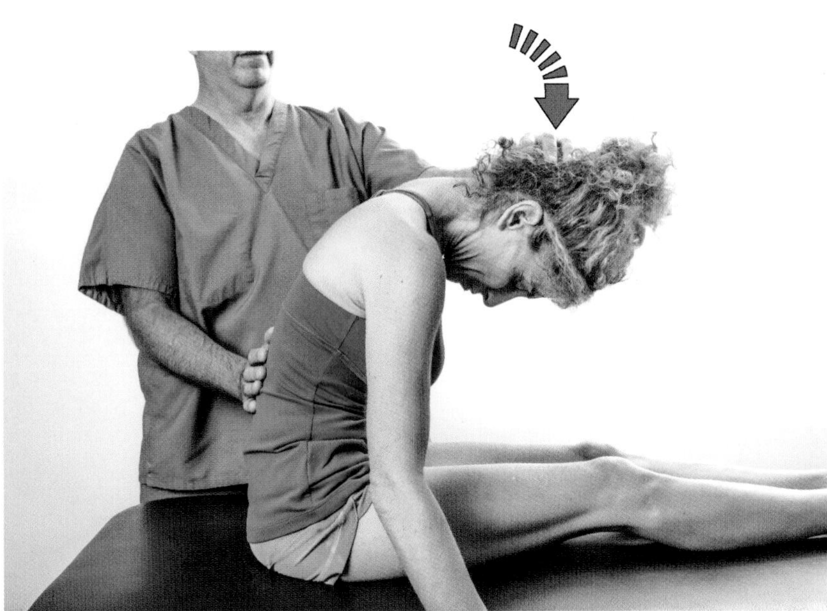

Figure 4.73 Lhermitte's sign. Do not apply any pressure with your right hand. Gently bend the head forward to stretch the dura.

vice versa (Figure 4.74) (http://www.youtube.com/watch?v=74l7mdVHvss).

Shoulder Abduction (Relief) Test (Bakody's Sign)

The patient is in either the sitting or supine position. Ask the patient to abduct their symptomatic arm and bring their hand to the top of their head. The positive finding is the relief of the symptoms by shortening the length of the neural tissues and therefore decreasing pressure on the nerve roots. This is usually associated with cervical radiculopathy from a C4 to C5 or C5 to C6 disc herniation. The test is usually negative if the complaints are caused by spondylosis (Figure 4.75) (Magee, 2008) (http://www.youtube.com/watch?v=4xHsrhd86LM).

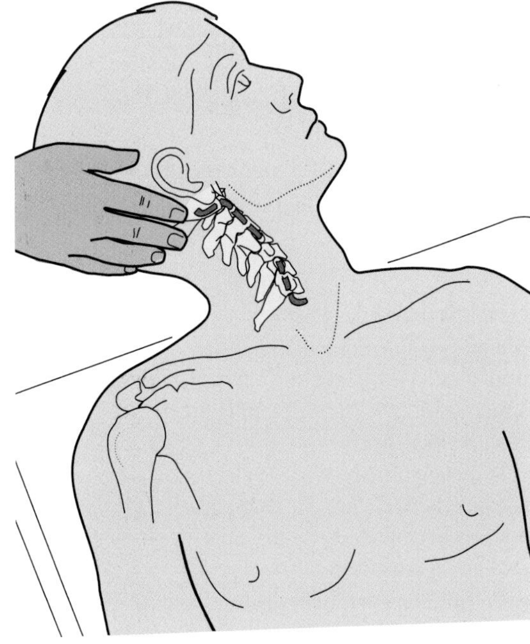

Figure 4.74 Vertebral artery test. This test should be performed if cervical manipulation is being contemplated.

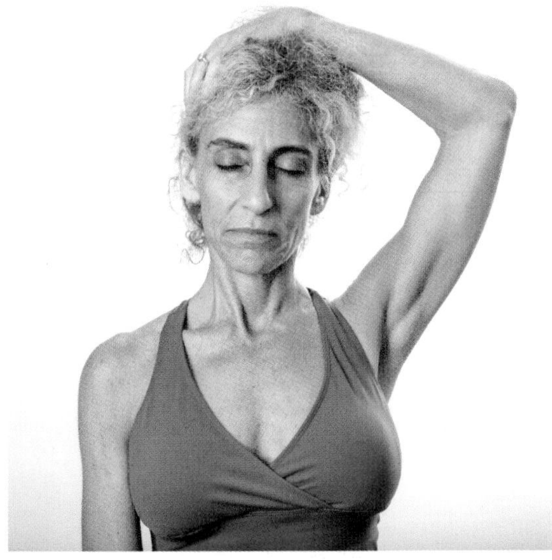

Figure 4.75 Shoulder abduction (relief) test (Bakody's sign). Radicular pain is relieved by this position.

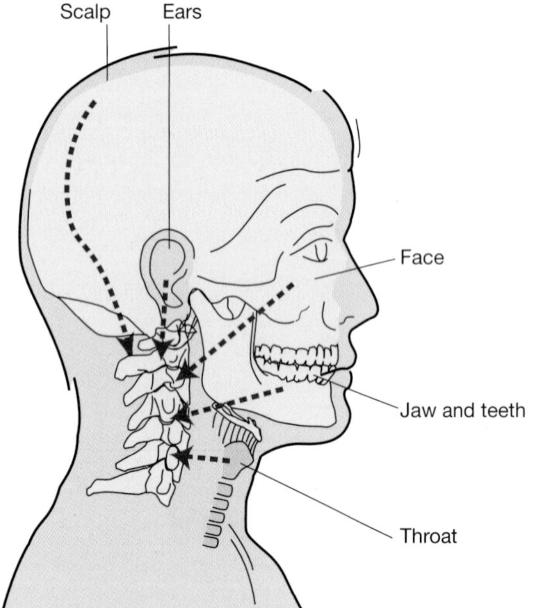

Figure 4.76 The scalp, ears, face, jaw, teeth, and throat may all refer pain to the cervical spine.

Valsalva Maneuver

The patient can be in any position. The Valsalva maneuver occurs when the patient exhales with considerable force and maintains their mouth in a closed position. This maneuver increases the intrathoracic pressure. The positive finding is increased symptoms in the upper extremities if the patient has any type of space-occupying lesion (tumor, disc) creating increased pressure on the spinal cord.

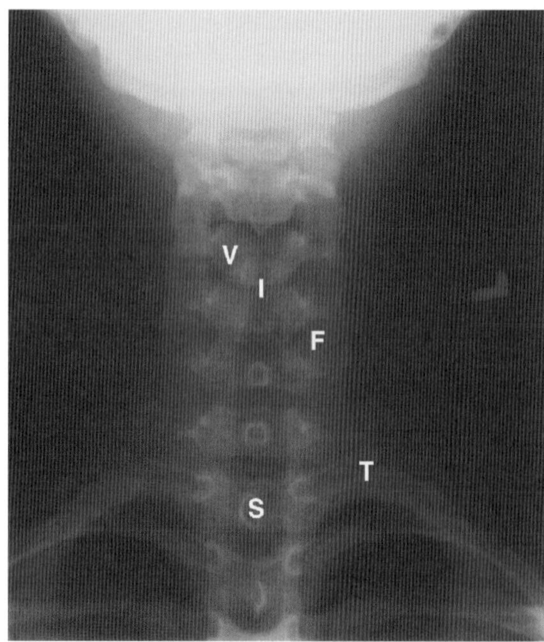

Figure 4.77 Anteroposterior view of the cervical spine.

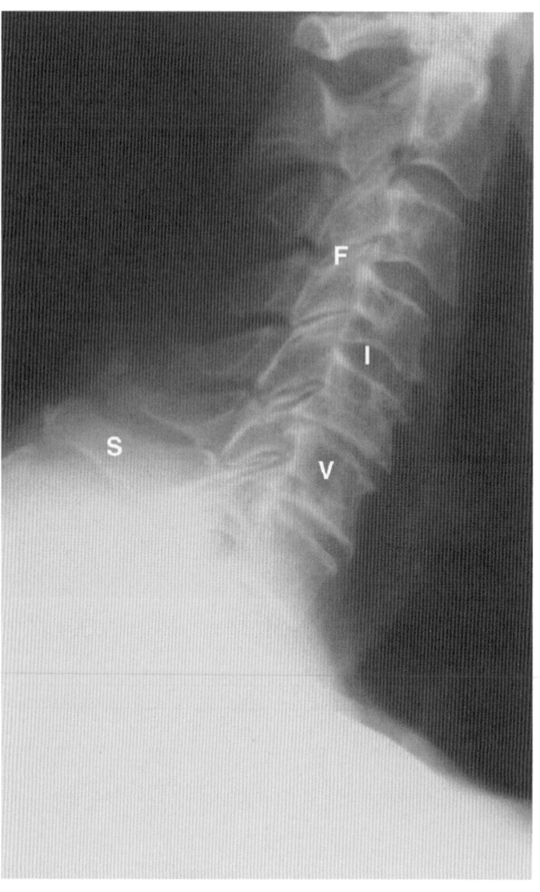

Figure 4.78 Lateral view of the cervical spine.

Referred Pain Patterns

Pain in the cervical spine may result from disease or infection in the throat, ears, face, scalp, jaw, or teeth (Figure 4.76).

Radiological Views

Radiological views of the cervical spine are provided in Figures 4.77, 4.78, 4.79, and 4.80.

V = Vertebral body
D = Intervertebral disc
Sc = Spinal cord
S = Spinous process
N = Neural foramen
P = Pedicle of vertebral arch
I = Intervertebral disc space
F = Facet joints
T = T1 transverse process

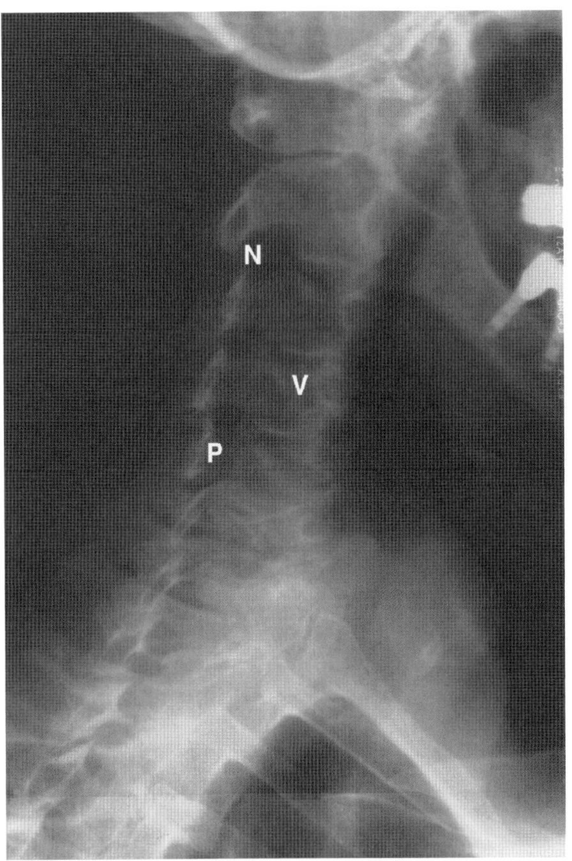

Figure 4.79 Oblique view of the cervical spine.

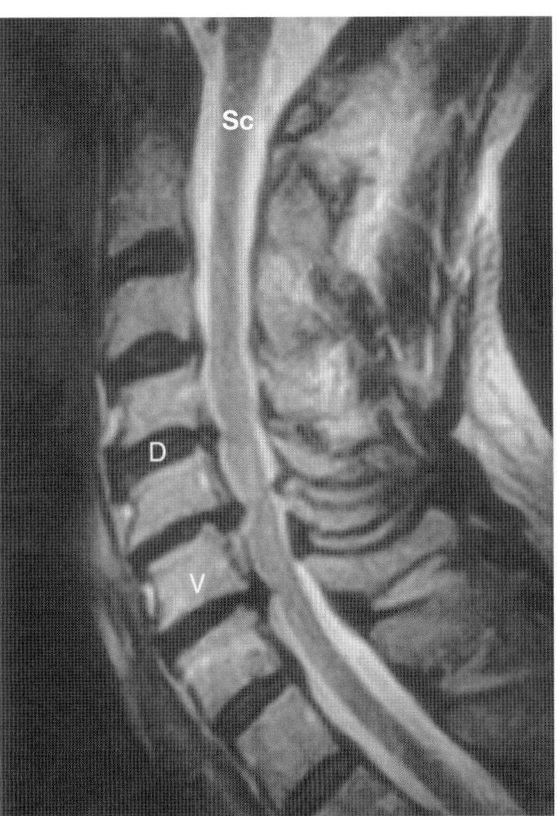

Figure 4.80 Magnetic resonance image of the cervical spine, sagittal view.

SAMPLE EXAMINATION

History: 45-year-old patient who presents with pain at the superomedial border of the right scapula, aggravated with rotation of the head to the right. The patient gives a history of being evaluated after a motor vehicle accident in which he was the driver of a car struck from behind, airbags deployed. He recalls looking in the rear view mirror just as the car was struck. There was no loss of consciousness reported. He was evaluated and released from his local emergency room, where x-rays were reported to show no fractures or dislocation, but noted "straightening of the cervical lordosis." The patient has no prior history related to his neck.

Physical Examination: 45-year-old male, ambulatory, wearing a soft collar, sweater, and tied shoes. There was no increase in symptoms on vertical compression or distraction of the cervical spine. There was limitation of 50% of the range of motion of the cervical spine in all planes due to pain. Resistive testing of the upper extremities was within normal limits. Sensation was intact in both upper extremities. Deep tendon reflexes were brisk and symmetrical.

There was no evidence of bowel and bladder dysfunction. Cervical mobility testing was not restricted. Flexibility testing was restricted in the right trapezius. The left trapezius and bilateral sternocleidomastoids revealed normal flexibility testing. He had tenderness to palpation over the right paracervical and trapezius muscles with trigger points. Vascular testing was negative.

Presumptive Diagnosis: Acute paracervical/trapezial strain.

Physical Examination Clues: (1) The patient was ambulatory, indicating no gross myelopathy. (2) He was dressed with a sweater and tied shoes, and all neurological testing was negative indicating no compromise of movement or motor function in the upper extremities. (3) He had well-localized tenderness, identifying injury to specific anatomic structures. (4) He had negative findings with vertical compression and distraction and intact mobility testing of the cervical spine, indicating no irritation of intervertebral joints or cervical roots exiting from the spinal foramina. (5) He had negative neurologic and vascular signs in the upper extremities, indicating a less serious degree of injury.

PARADIGM FOR A HERNIATED CERVICAL DISC

A 45-year-old male presents 2 days after the car he was driving was struck from behind. At the time of the accident, he had immediate pain in the posterior aspect of his neck which radiated down the entire right upper extremity into the small finger of his right hand. He noted weakness in his grip and loss of dexterity in fine motor movements of the digits of his right hand. There was also a sensation of "pins and needles" in the ring and small fingers. He gave no history of complaints relative to his head or neck existing prior to the accident.

On physical examination, the patient is able to ambulate independently without support. He holds his neck in a rigid posture and resists neck rotation in any direction. He has full active movement of his upper extremities, but has weakness in the grip of his right hand. Biceps and triceps reflexes appear to be equal bilaterally. However, there is diminished light touch on the ulnar aspect of the hand. Pain is produced on vertical compression of the cervical spine and with passive cervical spine extension. The patient can actively forward flex his neck 20 degrees without causing himself distress. His lower extremity examination is unremarkable. X-rays demonstrate loss of cervical lordosis and narrowing of the C6–C7 disc space without fracture or displacement of the bony structures. There are signs of mild early osteoarthritis of the facet joints at the mid cervical levels.

This is a paradigm for an acute herniated cervical disc because of:

A history of acute trauma
No prior history of symptoms
Immediate onset of pain and neurological symptoms at the time of injury
Inability to extend the cervical spine
Limited painless active flexion of the cervical spine
Pain with vertical compression
Motor and sensory deficits in a specific distribution

CHAPTER 5

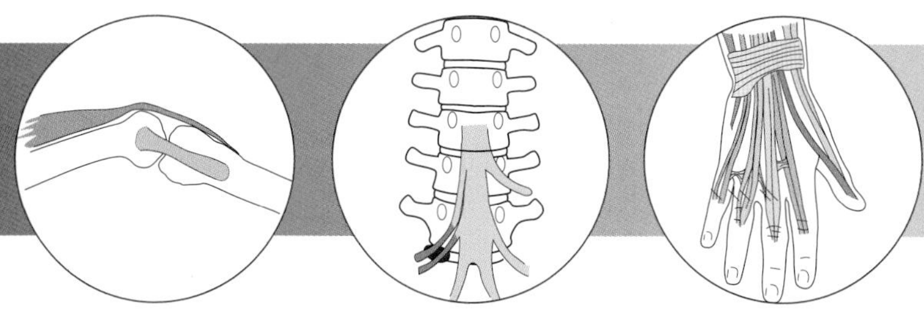

The Temporomandibular Joint

FURTHER INFORMATION

Please refer to Chapter 2 for an overview of the sequence of a physical examination. For purposes of length and to avoid having to repeat anatomy more than once, the palpation section appears directly after the section on subjective examination and before any section on testing, rather than at the end of each chapter. The order in which the examination is performed should be based on your experience and personal preference as well as the presentation of the patient.

Functional Anatomy of the Temporomandibular Joint

The temporomandibular joint (TMJ) is a synovial articulation. It is formed by the domed head of the mandible resting in the shallow mandibular fossa at the inferolateral aspect of the skull beneath the middle cranial fossa. Similar to the acromioclavicular joint of the shoulder, the articular surfaces of the TMJ are separated by a fibrous articular disc. The surface area of the mandibular head is similar in size to that of the tip of the small finger, yet it is subjected to many hundreds of pounds of compressive load with each bite of an apple or chew of a piece of meat.

Downward movement of the jaw is accomplished by a combination of gravity and muscular effort. The masseter and temporalis muscles perform closing of the mouth. The temporalis muscle inserts on the coronoid process. As such it functions very much like the flexors of the elbow. The masseter is attached to the lateral surface of the mandible along its posterior inferior angle. The mandible is stabilized against the infratemporal surface of the skull by contraction of the pterygoid muscles. The lateral pterygoid is attached directly onto the medial aspect of the articular disc.

There are numerous neurological structures about the TMJ. Branches of the auricular temporal nerve provide sensation to the region. The last four cranial nerves (IX, X, XI, and XII) lie deep and in close proximity to the medial surface of the TMJ.

Given the great magnitude of repetitive forces traversing the relatively small articular surfaces of the TMJ, it is remarkable that it normally functions as well as it does over many years of use. It is equally understandable why when the anatomy of the TMJ has been altered this articulation may become an extremely painful and challenging problem.

Trauma to the face and jaw may cause subluxation or dislocation of the TMJ. Untreated compromise of ligamentous stability will result, just as in the knee, in the rapid development of premature degenerative arthritis of the joint.

Instability of the TMJ may also be the result of exuberant synovitis secondary to inflammatory disease, such as rheumatoid arthritis, stretching capsular ligaments. The resultant instability causes further inflammation, swelling, pain, and compromise of joint function.

Musculoskeletal Examination, Fourth Edition. Jeffrey M. Gross, Joseph Fetto and Elaine Rosen.

Companion website: www.wiley.com/go/musculoskeletalexam

Damage to the articular disc either by direct trauma, inflammation, or simple senescence exposes the articular surfaces of the TMJ to excessive loads. This is yet another pathway leading to the premature and rapid onset of a painful osteoarthritic joint.

Given the density of neurological structures in close proximity to the TMJ, pain referred from the TMJ may be perceived about the face, scalp, neck, and shoulder. Complaints in these areas resulting from TMJ pathology are often difficult to analyze. This situation often leads to incomplete or inaccurate diagnoses and inappropriate treatment plans. As with other pathological articular conditions, a greater likelihood of success with treatment requires a thorough knowledge of local anatomy together with an accurate history and a meticulous physical examination of the patient.

The TMJ is a synovial joint, lined with fibrocartilage and divided in half by an articular disc. The TMJs must be examined together along with the teeth and the cervical spine.

Observation

Note the manner in which the patient is sitting in the waiting room. Notice how the patient is posturing the head, neck, and upper extremities. Refer to Chapter 4 (see pp. 34–36) for additional questions relating to the cervical spine. Is there facial symmetry? Is the jaw in the normal resting position (mouth slightly open but lips in contact)? How is the chin lined up with the nose in the resting position and in full opening? (Iglarsh and Snyder-Mackler, 1994) Is the patient supporting his or her jaw? Are they having difficulty talking and opening their mouth? Are the teeth in contact or slightly apart? Is there a crossbite, underbite, overbite, or malocclusion? Patients with a crossbite present with their mandibular teeth laterally displaced to their maxillary teeth. Patients with an underbite present with their mandibular teeth anteriorly displaced to their maxillary teeth. Patients with an overbite present with their maxillary teeth extending below the mandibular teeth. Is hypertrophy of the masseters present? Is there normal movement of the tongue? The patient should be able to move the tongue up to the palate, protrude, and click it. Observe the tongue. Is there scalloping on the edges or does the patient bite the tongue? This may indicate that the tongue is too wide or rests between the teeth (Iglarsh and Snyder-Mackler, 1994).

What is the resting position of the tongue and where is it when the patient swallows? The normal resting position of the tongue should be on the hard palate. Are all the patient's teeth intact? Do you notice any swelling or bleeding around gums?

Observe the patient as he or she assumes the standing position and note their posture. Pay particular attention to the position of the head, cervical, and thoracic spine. Additional information relating to posture of the spine can be found in Chapters 2 and 4 (see pp. 16–26 and pp. 34–36). Pain may be altered by changes in position so watch the patient's facial expression for indications as to their pain level.

Subjective Examination

The TMJs are extremely well utilized and are opened approximately 1800 times during the day (Harrison, 1997). These joints are essential in our ability to eat, yawn, brush our teeth, and talk. They are intimately related to the head and cervical spine and should be included in their examination. Approximately 12.1% of Americans experience head and neck pain (Iglarsh and Snyder-Mackler, 1994). Unfortunately, however, these problems are frequently overlooked in the examination process.

You should inquire about the nature and location of the patient's complaints and their duration and intensity. Note if the pain travels up to the patient's head or distally to below the elbow. The behavior of the pain during the day and night should also be addressed. Is the patient able to sleep or is he or she awakened during the night? What position does the patient sleep in? How many pillows do they use? What type of pillow is used? Additional subjective questions relating to the cervical spine can be found in Chapter 4 (p. 36) and in Box 2.1 (p. 15) for typical questions of subjective examination.

Does the patient report trauma to the TMJ? Was the patient hit in the jaw or did he or she fall on their face? Did he or she bite down on something hard? Was the mouth held open excessively for a prolonged period of time (at the dentist's office)? Did the patient overuse the joint by talking for a prolonged period of time or chewing on a tough piece of meat? Was traction applied to the neck, compressing the jaw with part of the harness?

Does the patient experience pain on opening or closing of the mouth? Pain in the fully opened position may be from an extra-articular problem, while pain with biting may be an intra-articular problem

(Magee, 2008). Does the patient complain of clicking with movement? Crepitus may be indicative of degenerative joint disease. Has the patient ever experienced locking of the jaw? This may be due to displacement of the disc. If the jaw locks in the open position, the TMJ might have dislocated (Magee, 2008). Is there limited opening of the mouth? Does the patient have pain with yawning, swallowing, speaking, and shouting? Is there pain while eating? Does the patient chew equally on both sides of their mouth? Has the patient had previous dental interventions? Teeth may have been pulled or ground down. Does the patient clench or grind (bruxism) his or her teeth? If the front teeth are in contact and the back teeth are not, there is a malocclusion. Has the patient worn braces? When and for how long? The braces will have altered the occlusion. Has the patient been wearing a dental appliance? What type of appliance are they using and how long have they been wearing it? Has the appliance been helpful in alleviating the patient's symptoms?

Special Questions

Was the patient breastfed or bottle fed (Iglarsh and Snyder-Mackler, 1994)? Did the patient suck on a pacifier or on their fingers and for how long? Is the patient a mouth breather? This alters the position of the tongue on the palate. Does the patient complain of problems swallowing? This may be due to cranial nerve problems of the CN VII (facial nerve) and CN V (trigeminal nerve). Earaches, dizziness, or headaches may be due to TMJ, inner ear, or upper cervical spine problems.

Consider the factors that make the patient's complaints increase or ease. He or she may present with the following complaints: headaches, dizziness, seizures, nausea, blurred vision, nystagmus, or stuffiness. How easily is the patient's condition irritated and how quickly can the symptoms be relieved? The examination may need to be modified if the patient reacts adversely with very little activity and requires a long time for relief.

The patient's disorder may be related to age, gender, ethnic background, body type, static and dynamic posture, occupation, leisure activities, hobbies, and general activity level. Psychosocial issues, stress level, and coping mechanisms should be addressed. It is important to inquire about any change in daily routine and any unusual activities that the patient has participated in.

Gentle Palpation

The palpatory examination is started with the patient in the sitting position.

You should first search for areas of localized effusion, discoloration, birthmarks, open sinuses or drainage, incisional areas, bony contours and alignment, and muscle girth and symmetry.

Remember to use the dominant eye when checking for alignment or symmetry. Failure to do this can alter the findings. You should not have to use deep pressure to determine areas of tenderness or malalignment. It is important to use firm but gentle pressure, which will enhance your palpatory skills. By having a sound basis of cross-sectional anatomy, you should not have to physically penetrate through several layers of tissue to have a good sense of the underlying structures. Remember, if the patient's pain is increased at this point in the examination, the patient will be very reluctant to allow you to continue, or may become more limited in his or her ability to move.

Palpation is most easily performed with the patient in a relaxed position. Although the initial palpation may be performed with the patient sitting, the supine and prone positions allow for easier access to the bony and soft-tissue structures.

The easiest position for palpation of the posterior structures is with the patient supine and the examiner sitting behind the patient's head. You can rest your forearms on the table, which enables you to relax your hands during palpation.

Posterior Aspect

Bony Structures

Mastoid Processes
Please refer to Chapter 4 (see pp. 38–39, Figure 4.8).

Transverse Processes of C1
Please refer to Chapter 4 (see pp. 38, 40, Figure 4.9).

Soft-Tissue Structures

Trapezius
Please refer to Chapter 4 (see pp. 44–45, Figure 4.19).

Suboccipital Muscles
Please refer to Chapter 4 (see pp. 44–45, Figure 4.20).

Semispinalis Cervicis and Capitis
Please refer to Chapter 4 (see pp. 45, 63, Figure 4.53).

Greater Occipital Nerves
Please refer to Chapter 4 (see pp. 45–46, Figure 4.20).

Ligamentum Nuchae
Please refer to Chapter 4 (see p. 46, Figure 4.21).

Levator Scapulae
Please refer to Chapter 4 (see pp. 46, 173) and Figure 8.71.

Anterior Aspect

To facilitate palpation of the anterior aspect of the neck, the patient should be in the supine position. The head should be supported and the neck relaxed. Make sure that the neck is in neutral alignment.

Bony Structures

Mandible
Run your fingers along the entire bony border of the mandible starting medial and inferior to the ears, move inferiorly to the angle of the mandible and then anteriorly and medially. Palpate both sides simultaneously (Figure 5.1).

Teeth
Wearing gloves, the examiner is able to retract the lips and examine the teeth. Note if any teeth are missing or loose, the type of bite, and any malocclusion.

Hyoid
Please refer to Chapter 4 (see pp. 46–47, Figure 4.22).

Thyroid
Please refer to Chapter 4 (see pp. 47–48, Figure 4.23).

Cervical Spine
Please refer to Chapter 4 (see pp. 36–52) for a full description of palpation of all bony prominences and soft-tissue structures.

Soft-Tissue Structures

Temporalis
Palpate on the lateral aspect of the skull over the temporal fossa. Ask the patient to close their mouth and you will be able to feel the muscle contract. Spasm of the muscle may be a cause of headaches (Figure 5.2).

Lateral and Medial Pterygoid
Place your gloved little or index finger between the cheek and the superior gum. Travel past the molar until you reach the neck of the mandible. Ask the patient to open their jaw and you will note tightness in the muscle. You will not be able to differentiate between the lateral and medial portions of the muscle

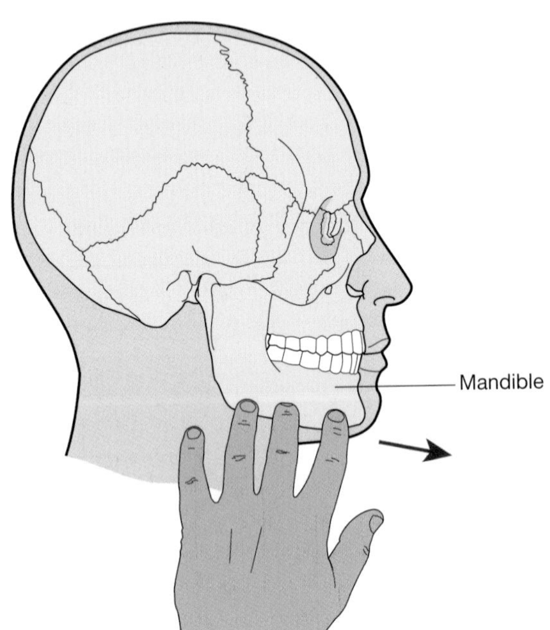

Figure 5.1 Palpation of the mandible.

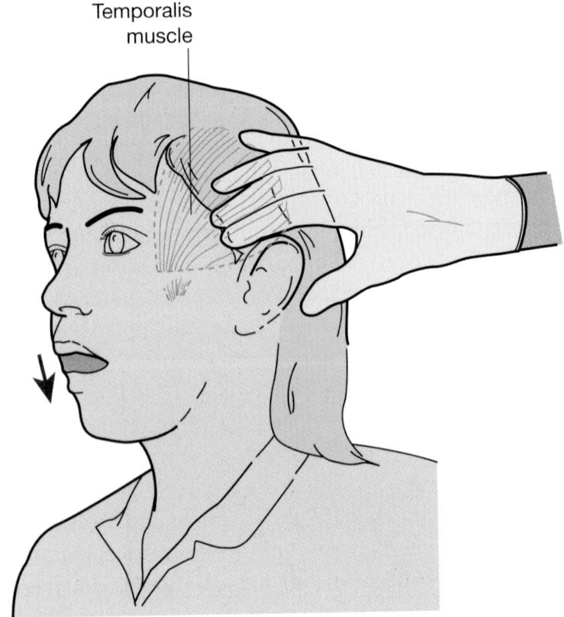

Figure 5.2 Palpation of the temporalis muscle.

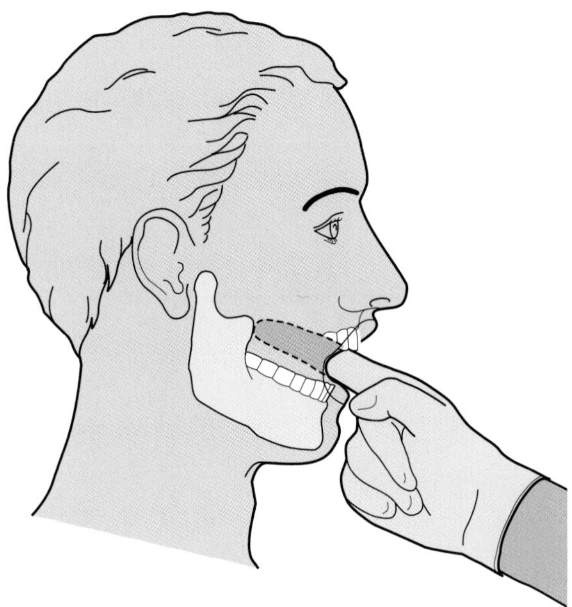

Figure 5.3 Palpation of the pterygoid muscles.

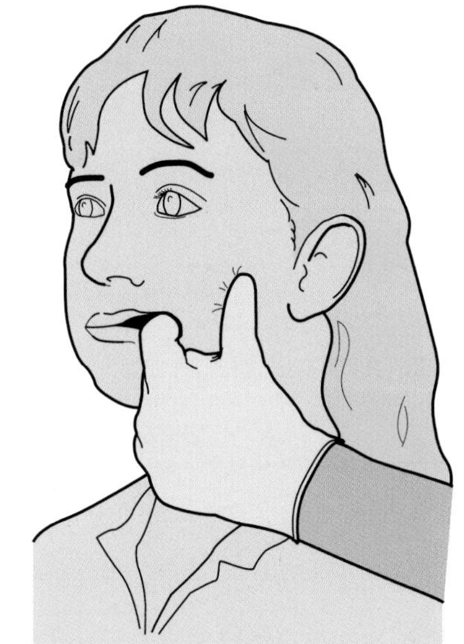

(a)

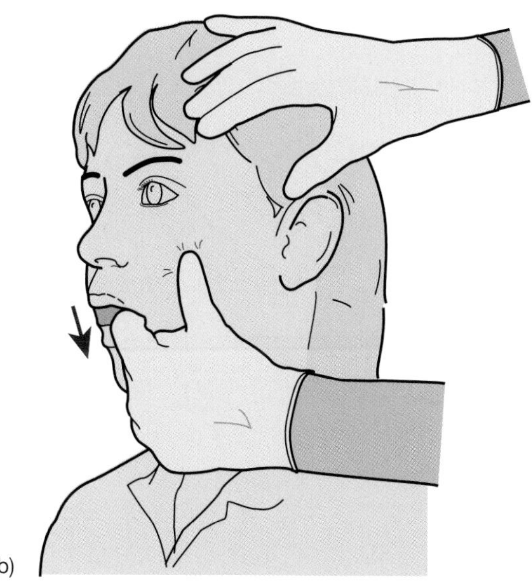

(b)

Figure 5.4 Palpation of the masseter muscle.

(Iglarsh and Snyder-Mackler, 1994). Spasm in the muscle can cause pain in the ear and discomfort while eating (Figure 5.3).

Masseter

Place your gloved index finger in the patient's mouth and slide the finger pad along the inside of the cheek approximately halfway between the zygomatic arch and the mandible. Simultaneously, palpate the external cheek with your index thumb. Ask the patient to close their mouth and you will feel the muscle contract (Figure 5.4).

Sternocleidomastoid Muscle

Please refer to Chapter 4 (see p. 51, Figure 4.32).

Scaleni Muscles

Please refer to Chapter 4 (see pp. 51–52, Figure 4.32).

The Suprahyoid Muscle

The suprahyoid muscle can be palpated externally inferior to the chin, in the arch of the mandible (Rocabado and Iglarsh, 1991). The infrahyoid muscle can be palpated on either side of the thyroid cartilage. A contraction of the muscle is felt if you gently resist cervical flexion at the beginning of the range (Rocabado and Iglarsh, 1991). Spasm in the suprahyoid muscle can elevate the hyoid and create difficulty swallowing. Pain can also be felt in the mouth near the muscles' origin (Figure 5.5).

Trigger Points of the TMJ Region

Myofascial pain of the TMJ region is quite common and can occur due to dental malocclusion, bruxism, excessive gum chewing, prolonged mouth breathing (while wearing diving gear or a surgical mask), and trauma. Activation of these trigger points can cause headaches and can mimic TMJ intrinsic joint disease.

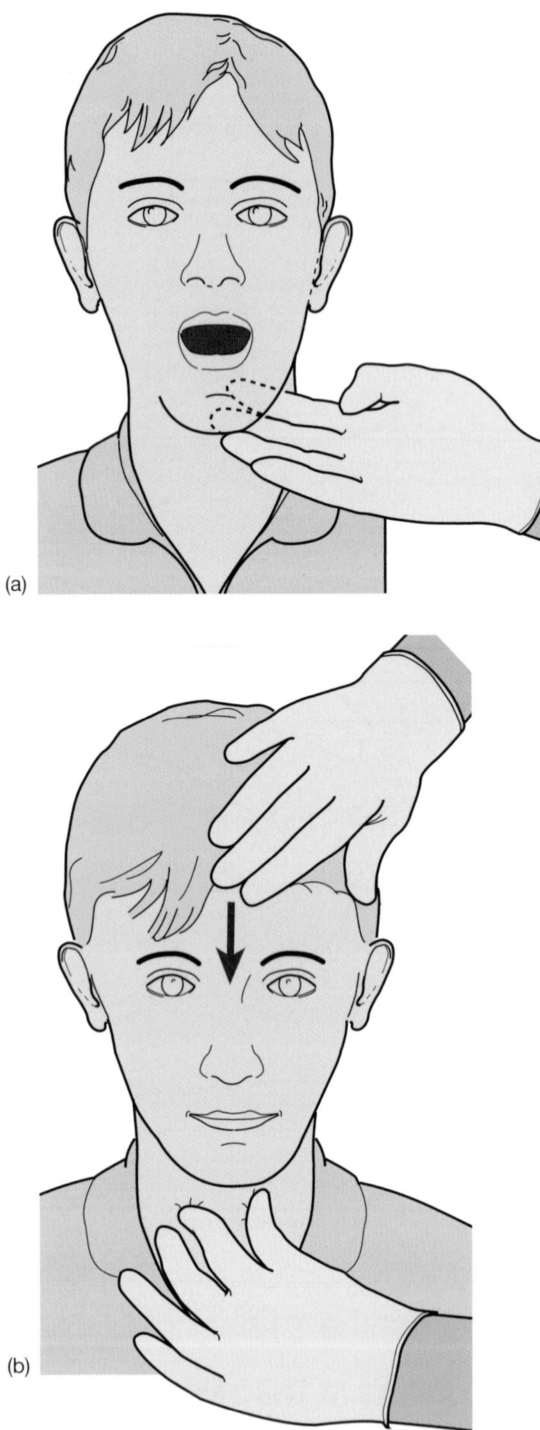

Figure 5.5 Palpation of the suprahyoid (a) and infrahyoid muscles (b).

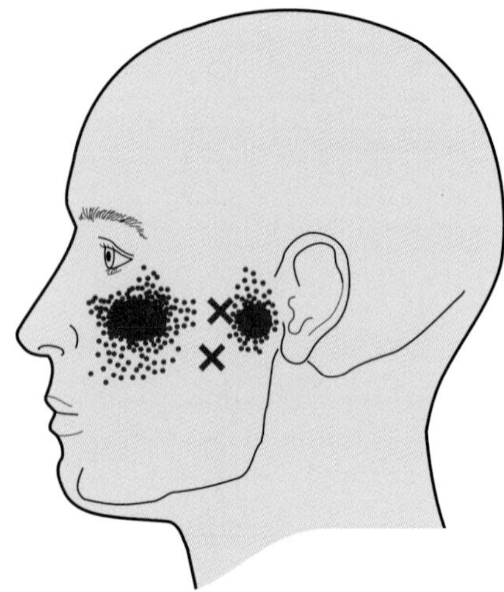

Figure 5.6 Trigger points of the lateral pterygoid, shown with common areas of referred pain.

The masseter and lateral pterygoid are the most commonly affected, followed by the temporalis and medial pterygoid muscles. The location and referred pain zones for trigger points in these muscles are illustrated in Figures 5.6, 5.7, 5.8, and 5.9.

Active Movement Testing

Have the patient sit on a stool in a well-lit area of the examination room. Shadows from poor lighting will affect your perception of the movement. The patient should be appropriately disrobed so that you can observe the neck and upper thoracic spine. You should watch the patient's movements from the anterior, posterior, and both lateral aspects. While observing the patient move, pay particular attention to his or her willingness to move, the quality of the motion, and the available range. Lines in the floor may serve as visual guides to the patient and alter the movement patterns. It may be helpful to ask the patient to repeat movements with the eyes closed. A full assessment of cervical movement should be performed first. (Refer to Chapter 4, pp. 53–58 for a full description.) Note the position of the patient's mouth with all the cervical movements.

Assess the active range of motion of the TMJs. Active movements of the TMJs include: opening of the mouth, closing of the mouth, protrusion, and lateral mandibular deviation to the right and left. While observing the patient move, pay particular attention to his or her willingness to move, the quality of the

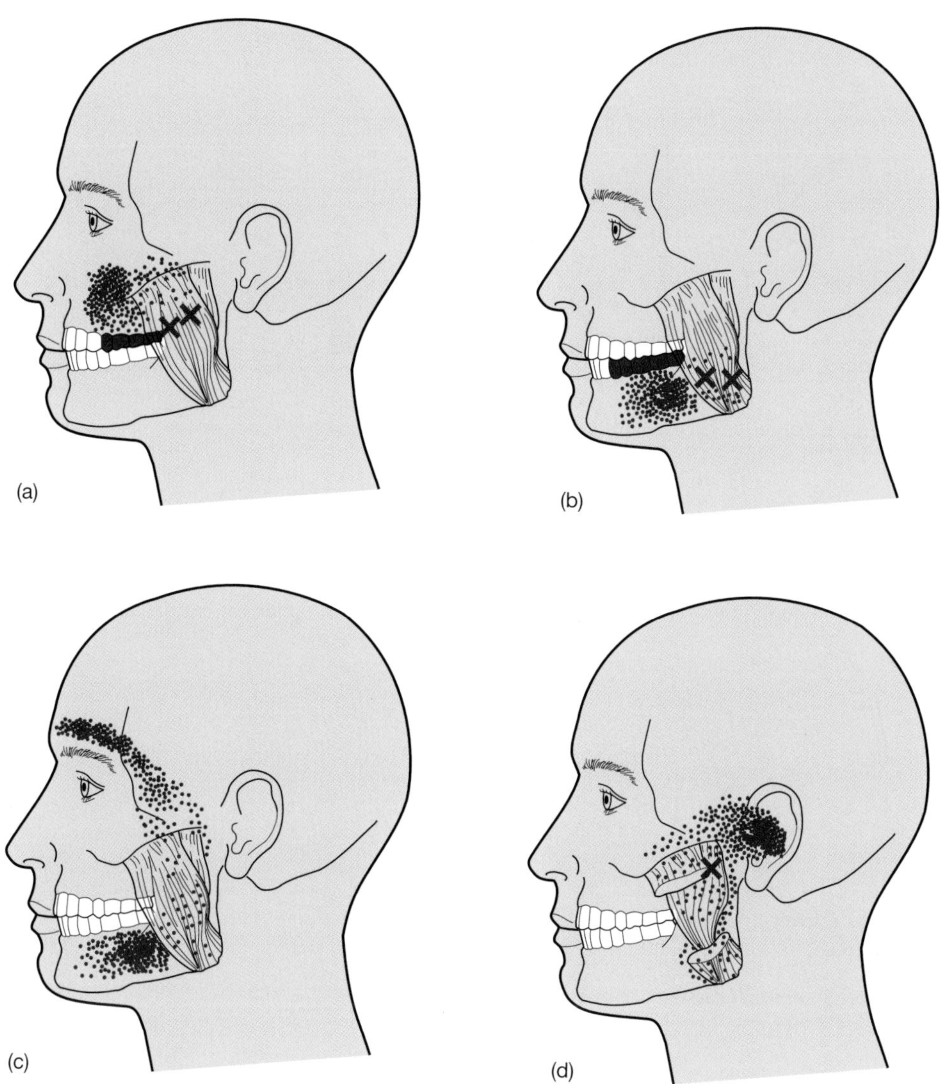

Figure 5.7 Trigger points of the masseter, shown with common areas of referred pain.

motion, the available range, and any deviations that might be present.

Movement can be detected by placing your fourth or fifth fingers with the finger pads facing anteriorly into the patient's ears to allow you to palpate the condyles. The TMJs can also be palpated externally, by placing your index finger anterior to the ear. Note any clicking, popping, or grinding with the movement. Pain or tenderness, especially on closing, is indicative of posterior capsulitis (Magee, 2008). During opening of the jaw, the condyle must move forward. Full opening requires that the condyles rotate and translate equally (Magee, 2008). If this symmetrical movement does not occur, you will note a deviation. Loss of motion can be secondary to rheumatoid arthritis, congenital bone abnormalities, soft tissue or bony ankylosis, osteoarthritis, and muscle spasm (Hoppenfeld, 1976).

The TMJ is intimately related to both the cervical spine and the mouth. To be complete in the evaluative process, cervical active range of motion should be included in the examination of the TMJ. Details of cervical spine testing can be found in Chapter 4 (pp. 53–54, 56–58, Figure 4.43).

Opening of the Mouth

Ask the patient to open their mouth as far as they can. Both TMJs should be working simultaneously and synchronously, allowing the mandible to open

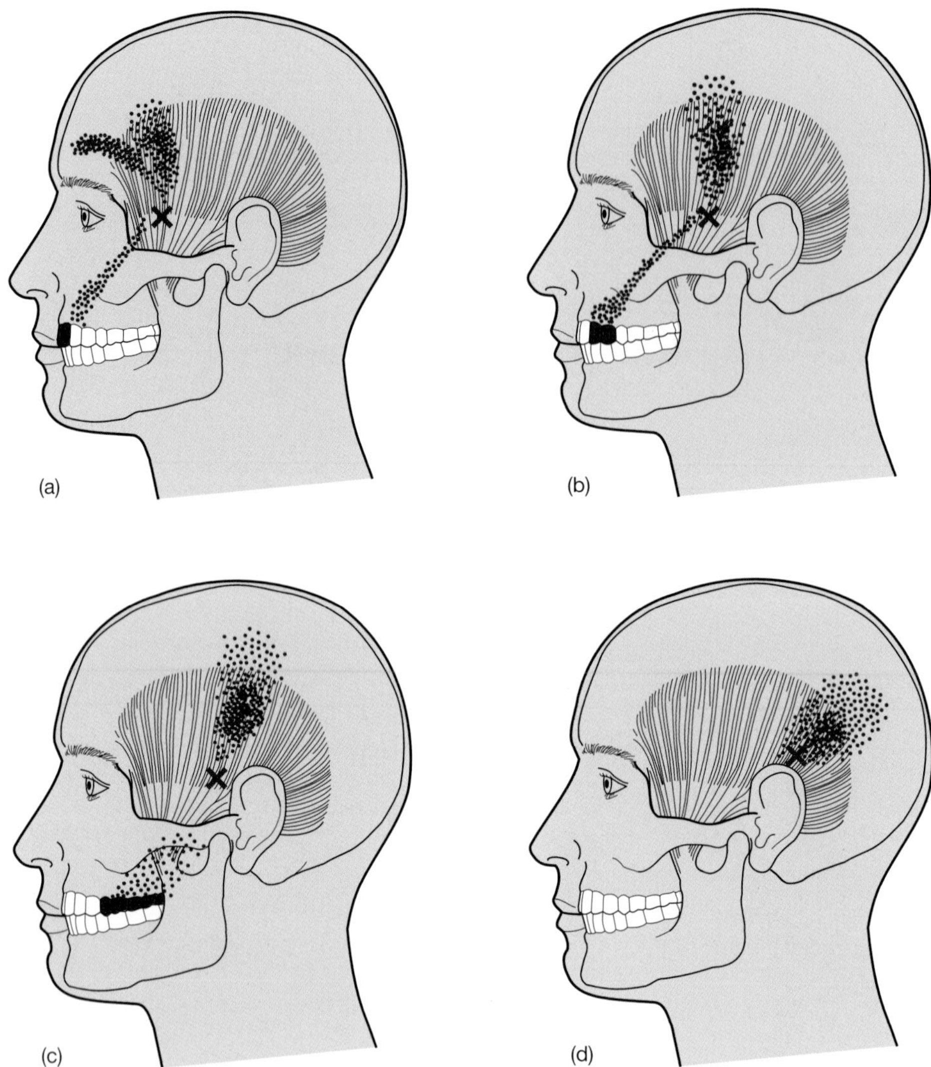

Figure 5.8 Trigger points of the temporalis, shown with common areas of referred pain.

evenly without deviation to one side. The clinician should palpate the opening by placing their fifth fingers into the patient's external auditory meatus with the finger pads facing anteriorly and should feel the condyles move away from their fingers. If one's TMJ is hypomobile, the jaw will deviate to that side. Normal range of motion of opening is between 35 and 55 mm from the rest position to full opening (Magee, 2008). The opening should be measured between the bottom of the maxillary and top of the mandibular incisors. If the jaw opens less than 25–33 mm, it is classified as being hypomobile. If opening is greater than 50 mm, the joint is classified as hypermobile (Iglarsh and Snyder-Mackler, 1994). A quick functional test is performed by asking the patient to place two to three flexed fingers, at their knuckles, between the upper and lower teeth (Figure 5.10).

Closing of the Mouth

The patient is instructed to close their mouth from full opening. The clinician should palpate the opening by placing their fifth fingers into the patient's external auditory meatus with the finger pads facing anteriorly and should feel the condyles move toward their fingers.

Protrusion of the Mandible

The patient should be instructed to jut the jaw anteriorly so that it protrudes out from the upper teeth.

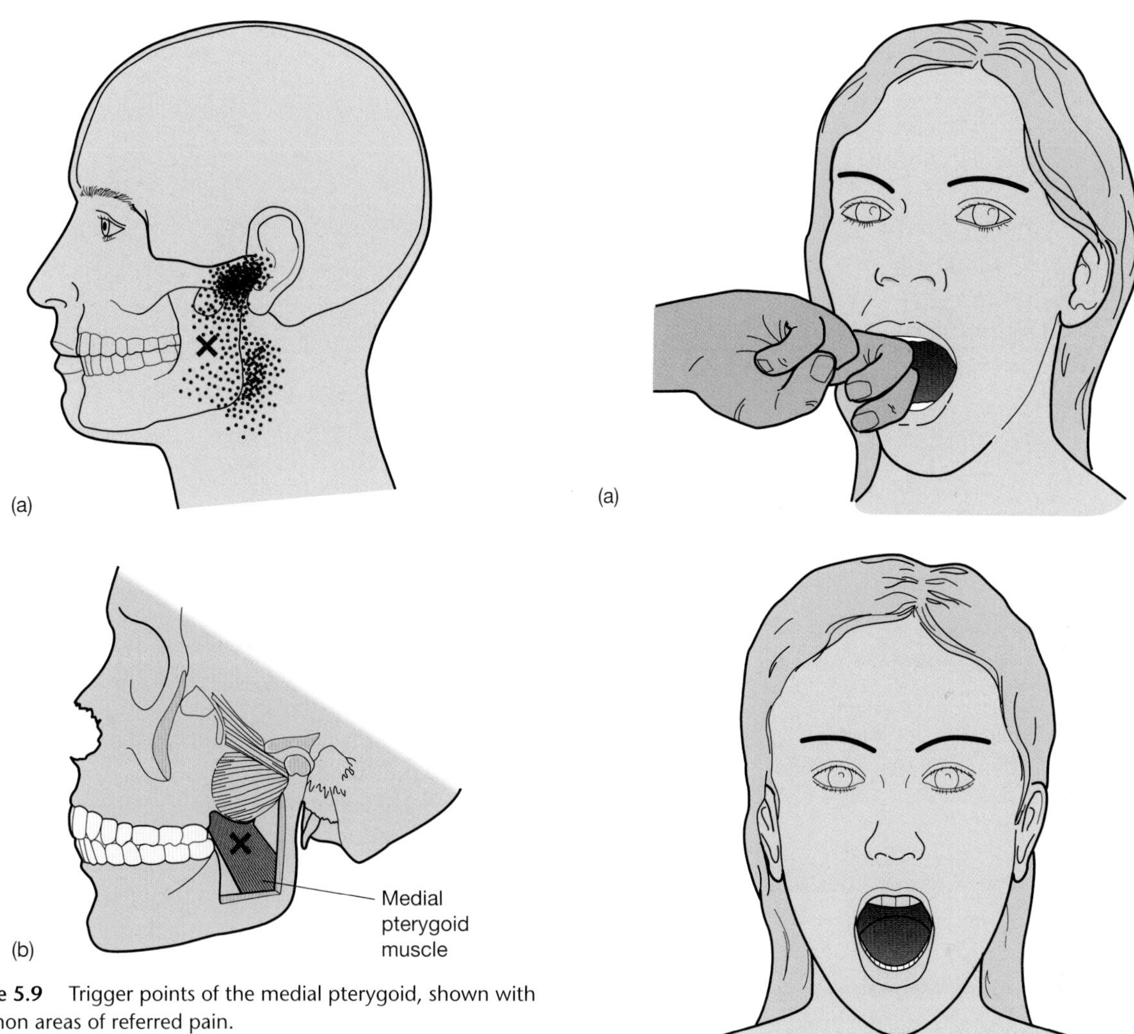

Figure 5.9 Trigger points of the medial pterygoid, shown with common areas of referred pain.

Figure 5.10 Observe as the patient opens their mouth as far as they can. Both TMJs should be working simultaneously and synchronously allowing the mandible to open evenly without deviation to one side. A quick functional test is performed by asking the patient to place two to three flexed fingers, at their knuckles, between the upper and lower teeth.

The movement should not be difficult for the patient to perform. Measure the distance from the superior aspect of the lower teeth as they protrude anteriorly past the upper teeth. Normal range of motion for this movement should be between 3 and 6 mm from the resting position to the protruded position (Iglarsh and Snyder-Mackler, 1994; Magee, 2008) (Figure 5.11).

Lateral Mandibular Deviation

The patient should be instructed to disengage his or her bite and then move the mandible first to one side, back to the midline, and then to the other side. The clinician should pick points on both the upper and lower teeth to be used as markers for measuring the amount of lateral deviation. The normal amount of lateral deviation is 10–15 mm (Magee, 2008), approximately one-fourth of the range of opening (Iglarsh and Snyder-Mackler, 1994). Lateral deviation to one side from the normal resting position or an abnormal degree of deviation may be caused by muscle dysfunction of the masseter, temporalis, or lateral pterygoid, or problems with the disc or lateral ligament on the opposite side from which the jaw deviates (Magee, 2008) (Figure 5.12).

Measurements of TMJ movements can be made by using a ruler marked in millimeters, or a Boley gauge (Iglarsh and Snyder-Mackler, 1994).

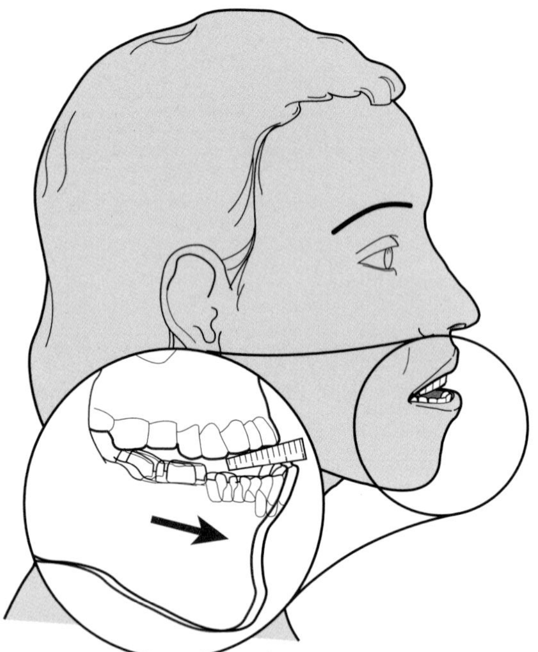

Figure 5.11 Observe as the patient juts the jaw anteriorly so that it protrudes out from the upper teeth.

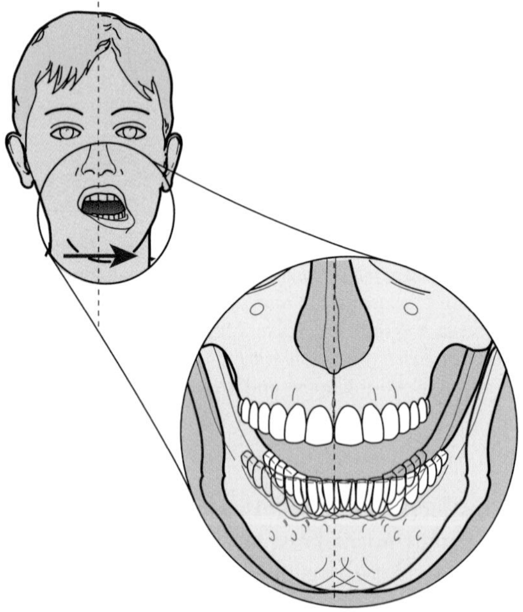

Figure 5.12 Observe as the patient disengages his or her bite and then moves the mandible first to one side, back to the midline, and then to the other side.

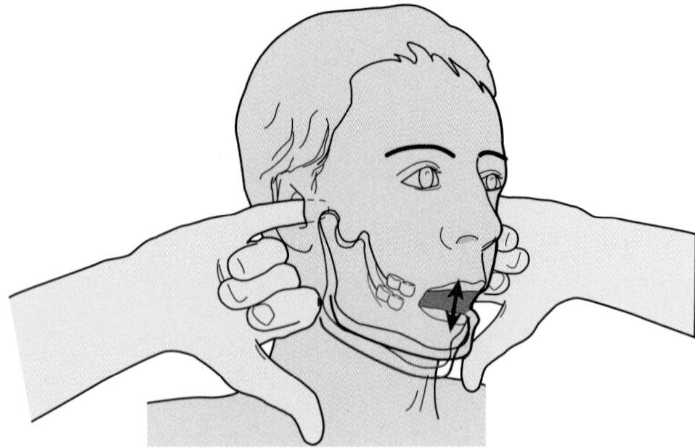

Figure 5.13 The freeway space is the point within the open pack position where the soft tissues of the temporomandibular joints are the most relaxed.

Assessing the Freeway Space

The freeway space is the point within the open pack position where the soft tissues of the TMJs are the most relaxed. The patient can achieve this position by leaving their tongue on their hard palate and leaving the mandible slightly depressed. You can assess the freeway position by placing your fourth finger's pad facing anteriorly into the patient's external auditory meatus as the patient slowly closes their mouth. The freeway space is achieved when you palpate the mandibular heads touching your finger pads (Iglarsh and SnyderMackler, 1994). The normal measurement is 2–4 mm (Harrison, 1997) (Figure 5.13).

Measurement of Overbite

Ask the patient to close their mouth. Mark the point where the maxillary teeth overlap the mandibular teeth. Ask the patient to open their mouth and measure from the top of the mandibular teeth to the line that you marked. This measurement is usually 2–3 mm (Iglarsh and Snyder-Mackler, 1994; Rocabado (unpublished data, 1982) (Figure 5.14).

Measurement of Overjet

Overjet is the distance that the maxillary teeth protrude anteriorly over the mandibular teeth. Ask the patient to close their mouth and measure from underneath the maxillary incisors to the anterior surface of the mandibular incisors. This measurement is usually 2–3 mm (Iglarsh and Snyder-Mackler, 1994; Rocabado (unpublished data, 1982) (Figure 5.14).

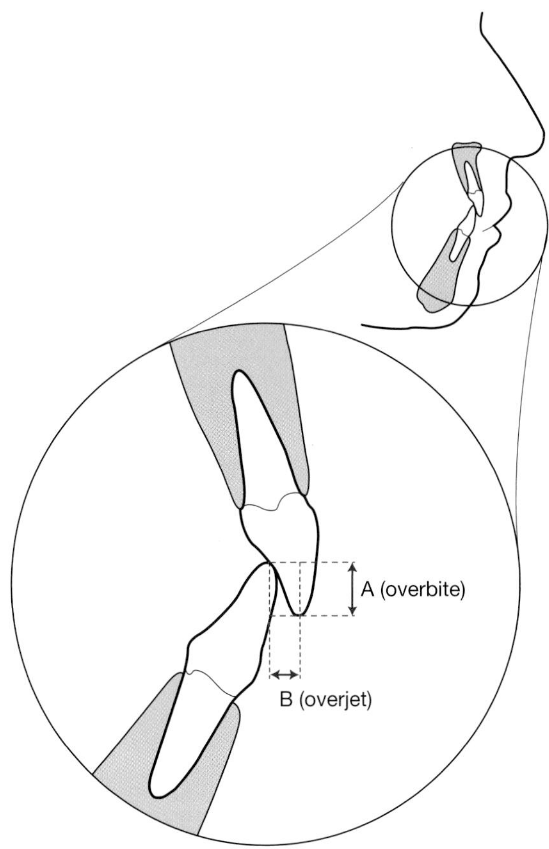

Figure 5.14 Overbite is the point where the maxillary teeth overlap the mandibular teeth. Overjet is the distance that the maxillary teeth protrude anteriorly over the mandibular teeth.

Mandibular Measurement

Measure from the back of the TMJ to the notch of the chin. Compare both sides. If one side is asymmetrical from the other a structural or developmental deformity may be present. Normal measurements should be between 10 and 12 cm (Magee, 2008) (Figure 5.15).

Swallowing and Tongue Position

The patient is instructed to swallow with their tongue in the normal relaxed position. The gloved clinician separates the patient's lips and observes the position of the tongue. The normal position should be at the top of the palate (Figure 5.16).

Passive Movement Testing

Passive movement testing can be divided into two categories: physiological movements (cardinal plane), which are the same as the active movements, and mobility testing of the accessory (joint play, component) movements. Using these tests helps to differentiate the contractile from the noncontractile (inert) elements. These elements (ligaments, joint capsule, fascia, bursa, dura mater, and nerve root) (Cyriax, 1982) are stretched or stressed when the joint is taken to the end of the available range. At the end of each passive physiological movement, you should sense the end feel and determine whether it is normal or pathological.

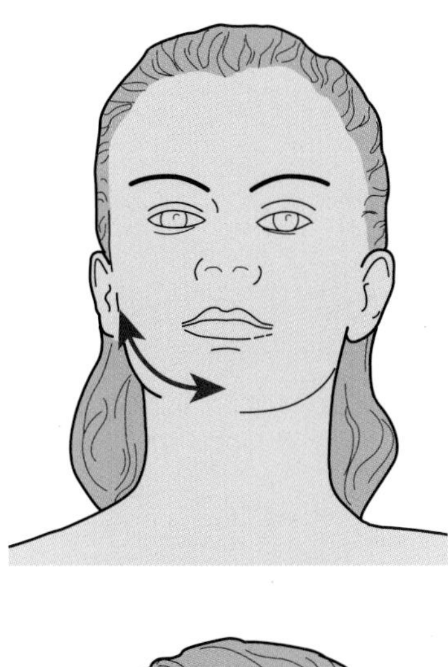

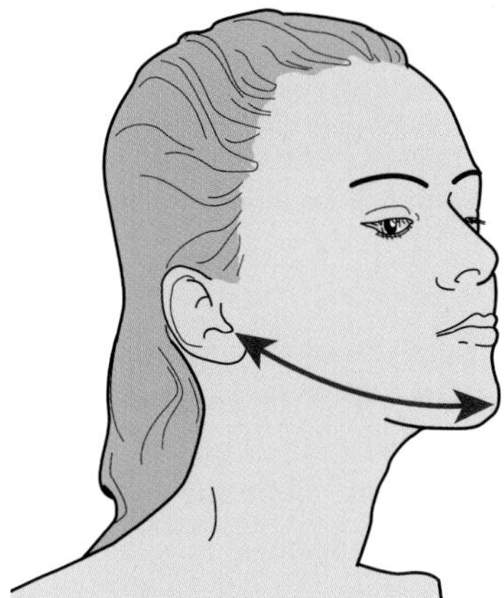

Figure 5.15 Measurement of the mandible is taken from the back of the TMJ to the notch of the chin. Compare the measurement of both sides.

Passive Physiological Movements

Passive testing of the physiological movements is easiest if they are performed with the patient in the sitting position. Testing of the cervical spine movements is described in Chapter 4 on the Cervical Spine

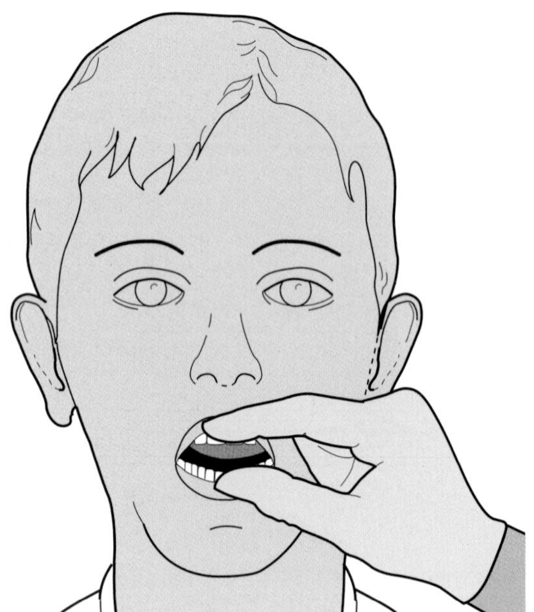

Figure 5.16 The normal position of the tongue is at the top of the palate.

(pp. 58–60). Passive movement testing of the TMJ is rarely performed unless the clinician is examining the end feel of the movement. The end feel of opening is firm and ligamentous, while the end feel of closing is hard, teeth to teeth.

Mobility Testing of Accessory Movements

Mobility testing of accessory movements will give you information about the degree of laxity or hypomobility present in the joint and the end feel. The patient must be totally relaxed and comfortable to allow you to move the joint and obtain the most accurate information.

Distraction of the TMJ

The patient is in the sitting position with the examiner to one side of the patient. The clinician places their gloved thumb into the patient's mouth on the superior aspect of the patient's molars and pushes inferiorly. The examiner's index finger simultaneously rests on the exterior surface of the mandible and pulls inferiorly and anteriorly. The test should be performed unilaterally with one hand testing mobility and the other hand available to stabilize the head. The end feel should be firm and abrupt (Figure 5.17).

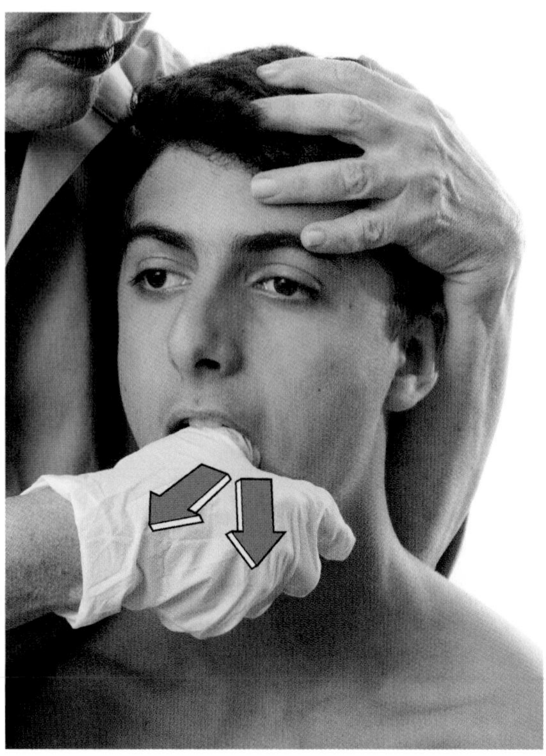

Figure 5.17 Mobility testing of distraction of the temporomandibular joint.

Resistive Testing

Movements of the jaw are complex due to the freedom of movement allowed by the TMJs. The cervical muscles serve to stabilize the head as the muscles of mastication act on the mandible. The temporalis and masseter are the main closing muscles. The inferior portion of the lateral pterygoid functions to open the mouth and protrude the mandible. The superior portion of the lateral pterygoid stabilizes the mandibular condylar process and disc during closure of the mouth. Extreme weakness of these muscles is unusual except in cases of central nervous system or trigeminal nerve damage.

Jaw Opening

The primary mouth opener is the lateral pterygoid (inferior portion) (Figure 5.18). The anterior head of the digastric muscle assists this muscle.

- Position of patient: Sitting, facing you.
- Resisted test: Place the palm of your hand under the patient's chin and ask them to open their mouth from the closed position as you resist their

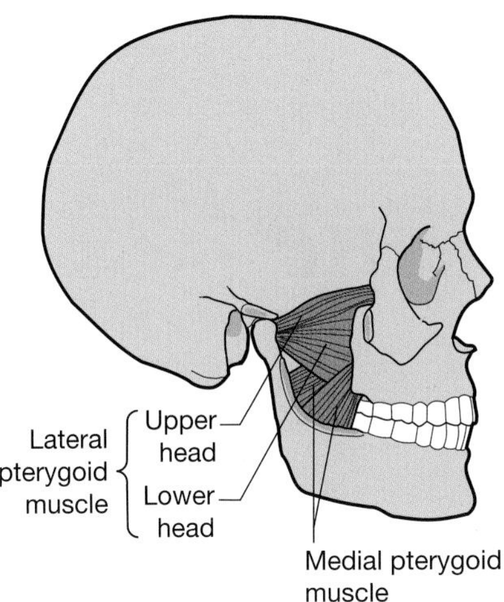

Figure 5.18 Lateral and medial pterygoid muscles.

effort. Normally, the patient will be able to overcome maximal resistance.

Jaw Closing

The masseter (Figure 5.19) and temporalis (Figure 5.20) are the primary muscles that close the mouth.

The medial pterygoid (Figure 5.18) assists them.

- Position of patient: Sitting, facing you.
- Resisted test: Ask the patient to close their mouth tightly and then attempt to open their jaw by pulling down on the mandible.

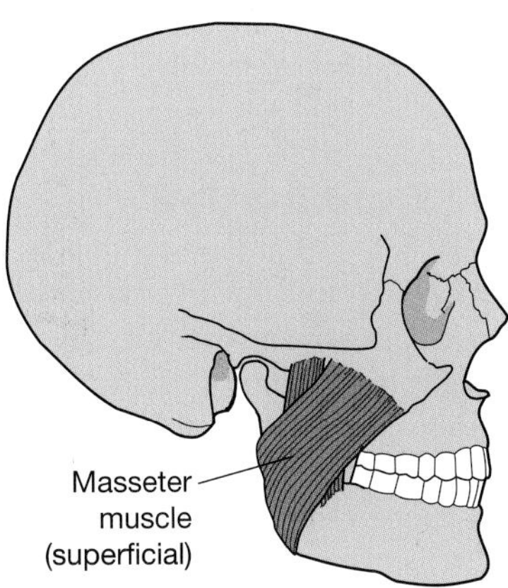

Figure 5.19 Masseter.

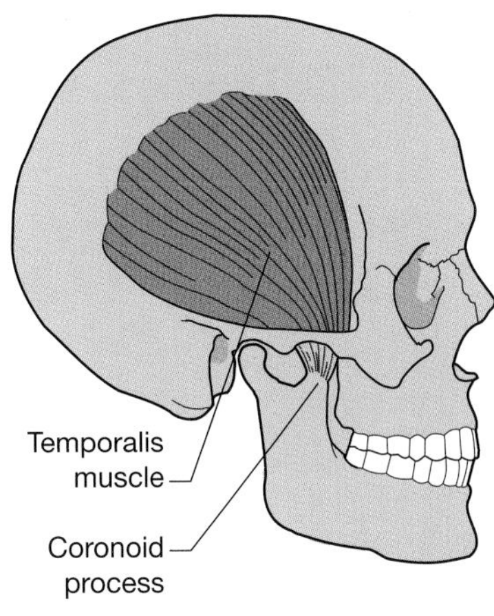

Figure 5.20 Temporalis.

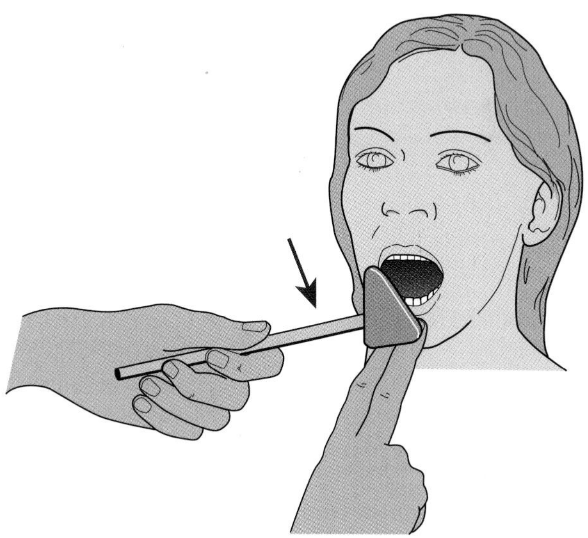

Figure 5.21 Jaw jerk. Make sure the patient is relaxed.

Reflex Testing

Jaw Jerk

The trigeminal (fifth cranial) nerve mediates the jaw reflex. This reflex results from contraction of the masseter and temporalis muscles following a tap on the chin (mandible). To perform the reflex, the patient should relax the jaw in the resting position, with the mouth slightly open. Place your index and long fingers under the lower lip, on the chin, and tap your fingers with the reflex hammer (Figure 5.21). A normal response is closure of the mouth. An exaggerated response indicates an upper motor neuron lesion. A reduced response indicates a trigeminal nerve disorder.

CHAPTER 6

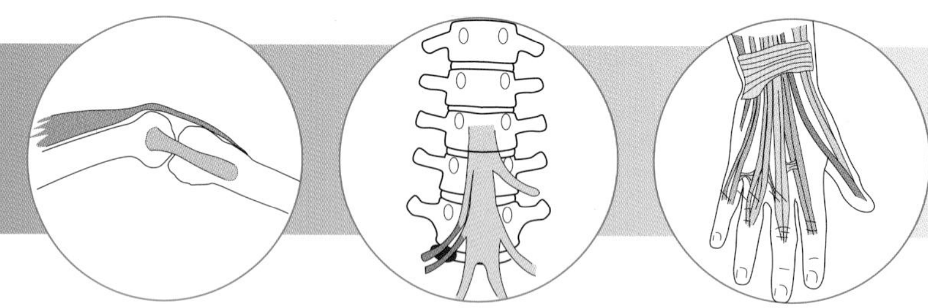

The Lumbosacral Spine

FURTHER INFORMATION

Please refer to Chapter 2 for an overview of the sequence of a physical examination. For purposes of length and to avoid having to repeat anatomy more than once, the palpation section appears directly after the section on subjective examination and before any section on testing, rather than at the end of each chapter. The order in which the examination is performed should be based on your experience and personal preference as well as the presentation of the patient.

Observation

The lumbar spine and sacroiliac joints are intimately related. They function together to support the upper body and transmit weight through the pelvis to the lower extremities. In addition, they receive ground reaction forces through the lower extremities at the time of heel strike and through the stance phase of gait. A disruption of the balance of these forces can inflict an injury to either or both.

Observe the patient in your waiting room. Is the patient able to sit or is he or she pacing because sitting is too uncomfortable? If the patient is sitting, is he or she symmetrical or leaning to one side? This may be due to pain in the ischial tuberosity secondary to bursitis, sacroiliac dysfunction, or radiating pain from the low back. Pain may be altered by changes in position. Watch the patient's facial expression to give you insight into their pain level.

Observe the patient as he or she assumes the standing position. How difficult is it for the patient to go from flexion to extension? Can the patient evenly distribute weight between both lower extremities? Observe the patient's posture. Note any structural deformities such as kyphosis or scoliosis. Are the spinal curves normal, diminished, or exaggerated? Observe the patient's total spinal posture from the head to the sacral base. It is also important to recognize the influence of the lower extremities. Observe any structural deviations in the hips, knees, and feet. Once the patient starts to ambulate, a brief gait analysis should be initiated. Note any gait deviations and whether the patient requires or is using an assistive device. Details and implications of deviations are discussed in Chapter 14.

Subjective Examination

Inquire about the etiology of the patient's symptoms. Was there a traumatic incident or did the pain develop insidiously? Is this the first episode or does the patient have a prior history of low-back pain? Is the patient pregnant or has she recently delivered a baby? Is the patient's symptomatology related to her menstrual cycle? Pregnancy and

Musculoskeletal Examination, Fourth Edition. Jeffrey M. Gross, Joseph Fetto and Elaine Rosen.

Companion website: www.wiley.com/go/musculoskeletalexam

menstruation influence the degree of ligamentous laxity, making the patient more susceptible to injury. Is the pain constant or intermittent? Can the pain be altered by position? What exaggerates or alleviates the patient's complaints? Does coughing, sneezing, or bearing down increase the symptoms? Increased pain with increased intra-abdominal pressure may be secondary to a space-occupying lesion such as a tumor or a herniated disc. How easily is the patient's condition irritated and how quickly can the symptoms be relieved? Your examination may need to be modified if the patient reacts adversely with very little activity and requires a long time for relief.

The patient's disorder may be related to age, gender, ethnic background, body type, static and dynamic posture, occupation, leisure activities, hobbies, and general activity level. It is important to inquire about any change in daily routine and any unusual activities in which the patient may have participated. If an incident occurred, the details of the mechanism of injury are important to help direct your examination.

You should inquire about the nature and location of the complaints as well as the duration and intensity of the symptoms. The course of the pain during the day and night should be addressed. The location of the symptoms may give you some insight into the etiology of the complaints. Pain, numbness, or tingling that is located over the anterior and lateral part of the thigh may be referred from L3 or L4. Pain into the knee may be referred from L4 or L5 or from the hip joint. The patient may complain about pain over the lateral or posterior aspect of the greater trochanter, which may be indicative of trochanteric bursitis or piriformis syndrome. Note any pain or numbness in the saddle (perineal) area. This may be indicative of radiation from S2 and S3. Inquire about any changes in bowel, bladder, and sexual function. Alteration of these functions may be indicative of sacral plexus problems. (Please refer to Box 2.1, see p. 15 for typical questions for the subjective examination.)

Gentle Palpation

The palpatory examination starts with the patient standing. This allows you to see the influence of the lower extremities on the trunk in the weight-bearing position. If the patient has difficulty standing, he or she may sit on a stool with their back toward you. The patient must be sufficiently disrobed so that the entire back is exposed. You should first search for areas of localized effusion, discoloration, birthmarks, open sinuses or drainage, and incisional areas. Note the bony contours and alignment, muscle girth and symmetry, and skinfolds. A *cafe au lait* spot or a "faun's" beard may be indicative of spina bifida occulta or neurofibromatosis. Remember to use your dominant eye when checking for alignment or symmetry. Failure to do this can alter your findings. You should not have to use deep pressure to determine areas of tenderness or malalignment. It is important to use a firm but gentle pressure, which will enhance your palpatory skills. If you have a sound basis of cross-sectional anatomy, it should not be necessary to physically penetrate through several layers of tissue to have a good sense of the underlying structures. Remember that if you increase the patient's pain at this point in the examination, the patient will be very reluctant to allow you to continue, or may become more limited in his or her ability to move.

Palpation is most easily performed with the patient in a relaxed position. Although the initial palpation can be performed with the patient standing or sitting, the supine, side-lying, and prone positions may also be used to allow for easier access to the bony and soft-tissue structures.

Posterior Aspect

Bony Structures

Iliac Crest

The iliac crest is very prominent since it is so superficial and is therefore easy to palpate. Place your extended hands so that the index fingers are at the waist. Allow your hands to press medially and rest on the superior aspect of the ridge of the crests. Then place your thumbs on the lumbar spine in line with the fingers on the crests. The L4–L5 vertebral interspace is located at this level. This is a useful starting landmark when palpating the lumbar spinous processes (Figure 6.1).

Iliac crests that are uneven in height may occur secondary to a leg-length difference, a pelvic obliquity, scoliosis, or a sacroiliac dysfunction.

Spinous Processes

The spinous processes of the lumbar spine are quadrangular in shape and are positioned in a horizontal fashion just posterior to the vertebral body. Locate the posterior superior iliac spine (PSIS) and allow your finger to drop off in the medial and superior direction at a 30-degree angle. You will locate the spinous process of L5. Another consistent method to locate

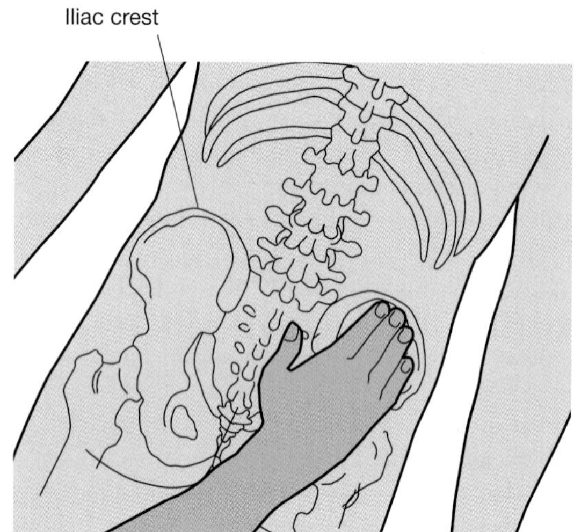

Figure 6.1 Palpation of the iliac crest.

the vertebra is by placing your hands on the iliac crest and moving medially where you will find the vertebral interspace of L4–L5. You can count up the spinous processes from either of these starting points. You can locate the spinous process of L1 by locating the 12th rib and moving your hand medially and down one level. If you choose this method, locate the remaining spinous processes by counting down to L5 (Figure 6.2).

Tenderness or a palpable depression from one level to another may indicate the absence of the spinous process or a spondylolisthesis.

Transverse Processes

The transverse processes of the lumbar spine are long and thin and are positioned in a horizontal fashion. They vary in length, with L3 being the longest and L1 and L5 the shortest. The L5 transverse process is most easily located by palpating the PSIS and moving medially and superiorly at a 30–45-degree angle. The transverse processes are more difficult to palpate in the lumbar spine because of the thickness of the overlying tissue. They are most easily identified in the trough located between the spinalis and the longissimus muscles (Figure 6.3).

Posterior Superior Iliac Spines

The PSISs can be found by placing your extended hands over the superior aspect of the iliac crests and allowing your thumbs to reach diagonally in an inferior medial direction until they contact the bony prominence. Have your thumbs roll so that they are under the PSISs and are directed cranially to more

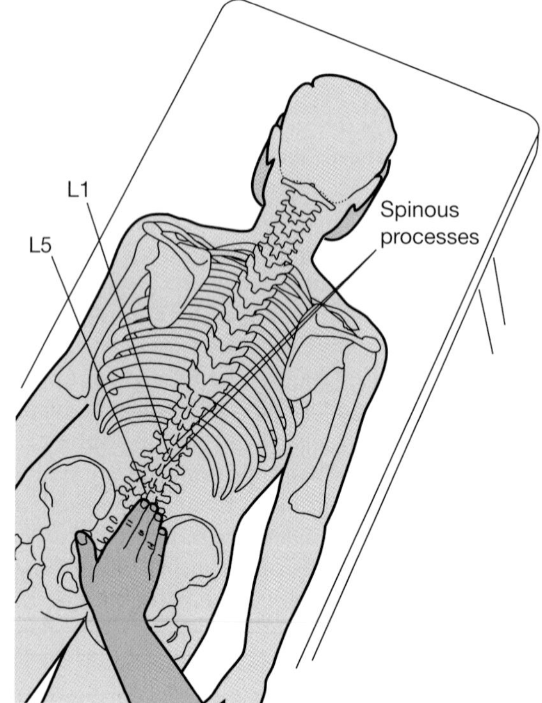

Figure 6.2 Palpation of the spinous processes.

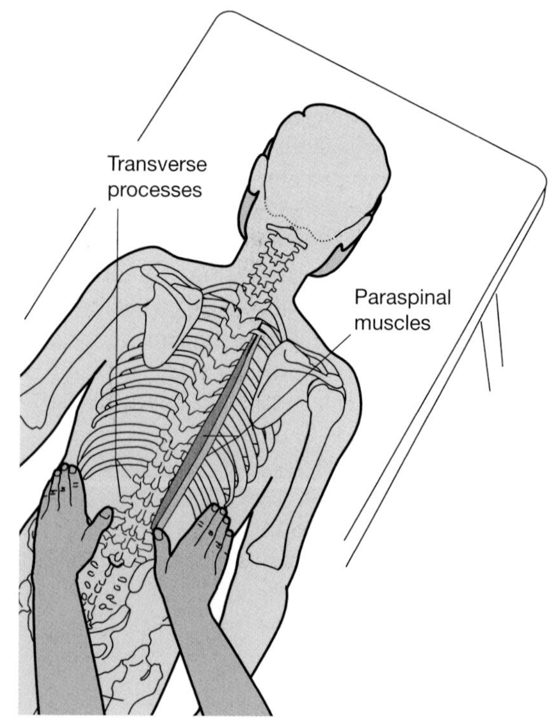

Figure 6.3 Palpation of the transverse processes.

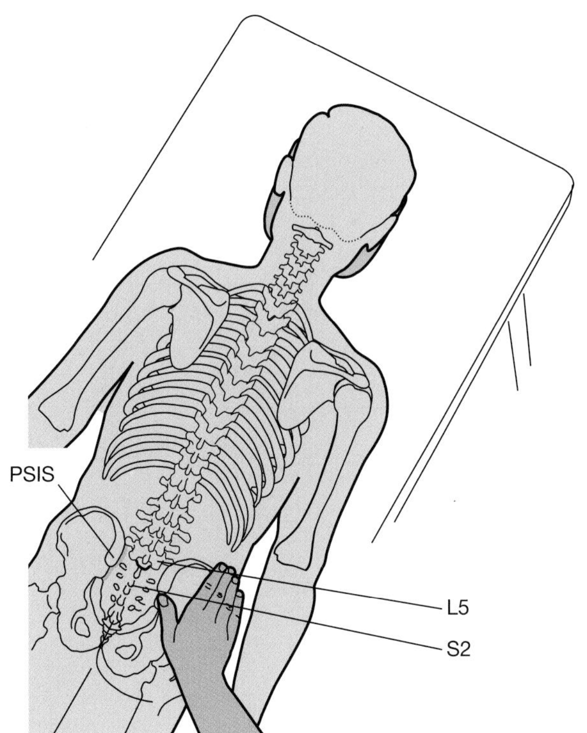

Figure 6.4 Palpation of the posterior superior iliac spine (PSIS).

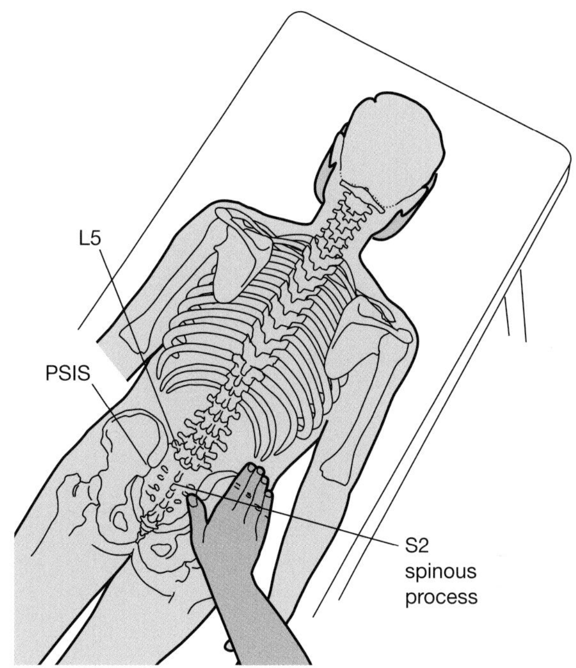

Figure 6.5 Palpation of the sacroiliac joint.

accurately determine their position. Many individuals have dimpling that makes the location more obvious. However, you should be careful because dimpling is not present in all individuals, and if it is present, it may not coincide with the PSISs. If you move your thumbs in a medial and superior angle of approximately 30 degrees, you will come in contact with the posterior arch of L5. If you move your thumbs at a caudal and inferior angle of approximately 30 degrees, you will come in contact with the base of the sacrum. If you are having difficulty, you may also locate the PSISs by following the iliac crests posteriorly and then inferiorly until you arrive at the spines (Figure 6.4).

Sacroiliac Joint

The actual joint line of the sacroiliac joint is not palpable because it is covered by the posterior aspect of the innominate bone. You can get a sense of its location by allowing your thumb to drop off medially from the PSIS. The sacroiliac joint is located deep to this overhang at approximately the second sacral level (Figure 6.5).

Sacral Base

Locate the PSISs on both sides (described above). Allow your thumbs to drop off medially and then move anteriorly until you contact the sacral base. The dropoff between the PSIS and sacral base is referred to as the sacral sulcus (Figure 6.6). Palpation of the sacral base is useful in determining the position of the sacrum.

Inferior Lateral Angle

Place your fingers on the inferior midline of the posterior aspect of the sacrum and locate a small vertical depression, this is the sacral hiatus. Move your fingers laterally approximately 3/4 in. and you will be on the inferior lateral angle (Figure 6.7).

Ischial Tuberosity

You can place you thumbs under the middle portion of the gluteal folds at approximately the level of the greater trochanters. Allow your thumb to face superiorly and gently probe through the gluteus maximus until the thumb is resting on the ischial tuberosity. Some people find it easier to perform this palpation with the patient lying on the side with the hip flexed, allowing the ischial tuberosity to be more accessible since the gluteus maximus is pulled up, reducing the muscular cover (Figure 6.8). If this area is tender to palpation, it may be indicative of an inflammation of the ischial bursa or an ischiorectal abscess.

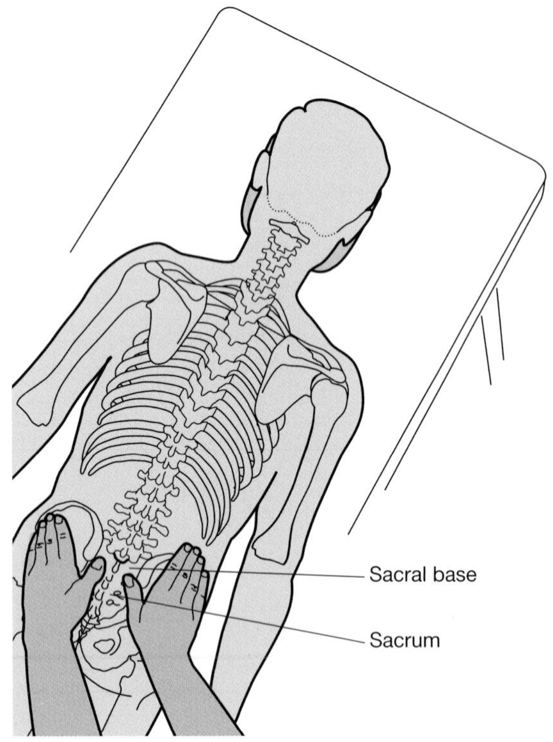

Figure 6.6 Palpation of the sacral base.

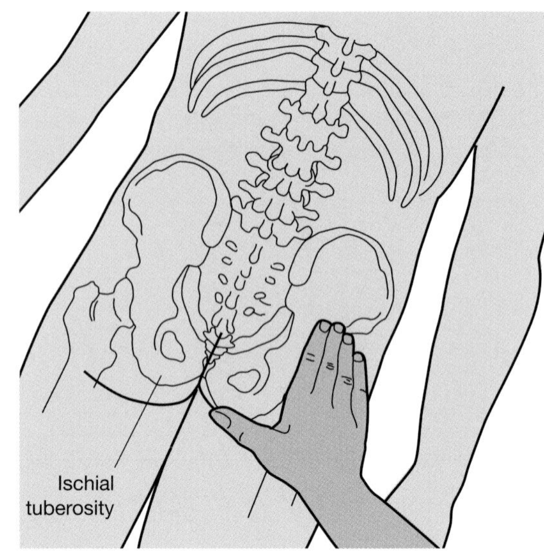

Figure 6.8 Palpation of the ischial tuberosity.

Coccyx

The tip of the coccyx can be found in the gluteal cleft. To palpate the anterior aspect, which is essential to determine the position, a rectal examination must be performed (Figure 6.9). Pain in the coccyx is referred to as coccydynia and is usually secondary to direct trauma to the area.

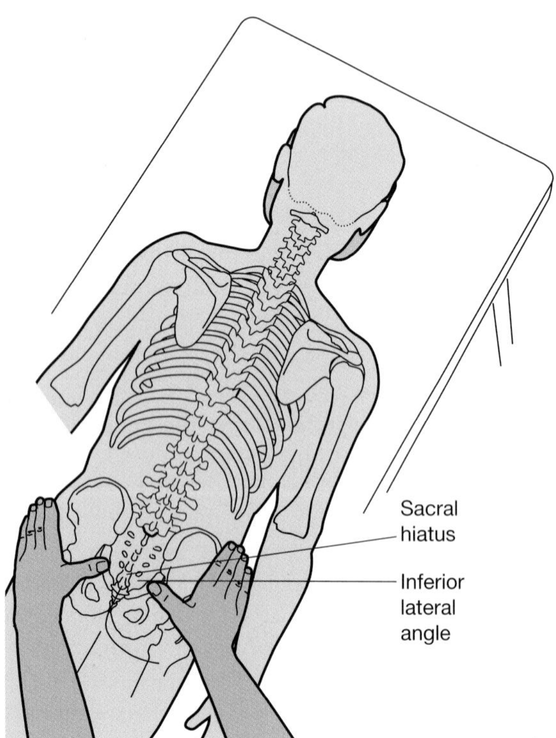

Figure 6.7 Palpation of the inferior lateral angle.

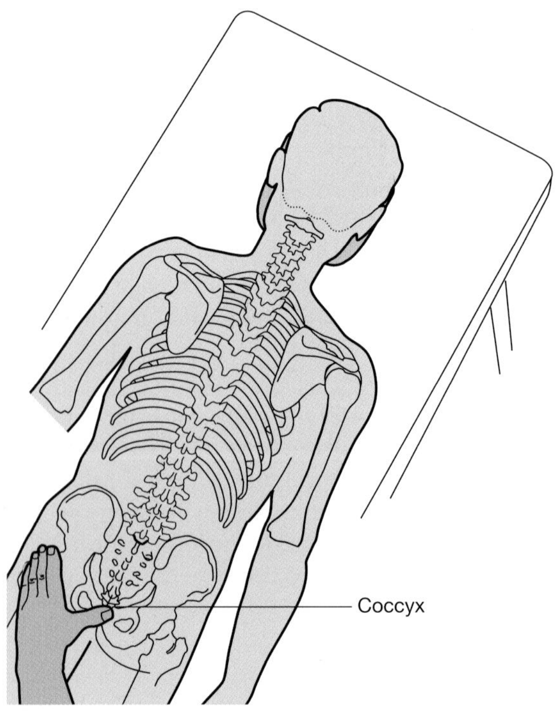

Figure 6.9 Palpation of the coccyx.

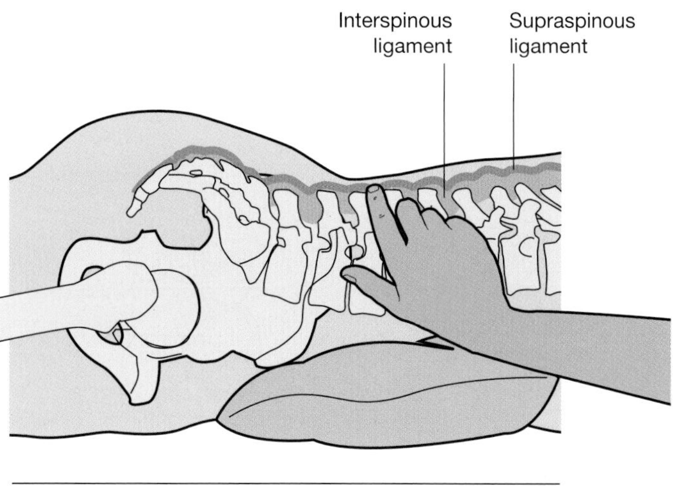

Figure 6.10 Palpation of the supraspinous ligament.

Soft-Tissue Structures

Supraspinous Ligament

The supraspinous ligament joins the tips of the spinous processes from C7 to the sacrum. This powerful fibrous cord that is blended with the fascia is denser and wider in the lumbar than in the cervical and thoracic spines. The ligament can be palpated by placing your fingertip between the spinous processes. The tension of the ligament is more easily noted if the patient is in a slight degree of flexion (Figure 6.10).

Erector Spinae (Sacrospinalis) Muscles

The erector spinae muscles form a thick fleshy mass in the lumbar spine. The intermediate muscles of the group are the spinalis (most medial), longissimus, and iliocostalis (most lateral) muscles. They are easily palpated just lateral to the spinous processes. Their lateral border appears to be a groove (Figure 6.11). These muscles are often tender and in spasm in patients with an acute low-back pain.

Quadratus Lumborum Muscle

Place your hands over the posterior aspect of the iliac crest. Press medially in the space below the rib cage and you will feel the tension of the quadratus lumborum as it attaches to the iliolumbar ligament and the iliac crest (Figure 6.12). The muscle can be made more distinct by asking the patient to lift the pelvis toward the thorax. The quadratus lumborum is important in the evaluation of the lumbar spine. It can adversely affect alignment and muscle balance because of its attachment to the iliolumbar ligament. It can also play a role in changing pelvic alignment because of its intimate relationship to the iliac crest.

Sacrotuberous Ligament

Place the patient in the prone position and locate the ischial tuberosities as described above. Allow your thumbs to slide off in a medial and superior direction.

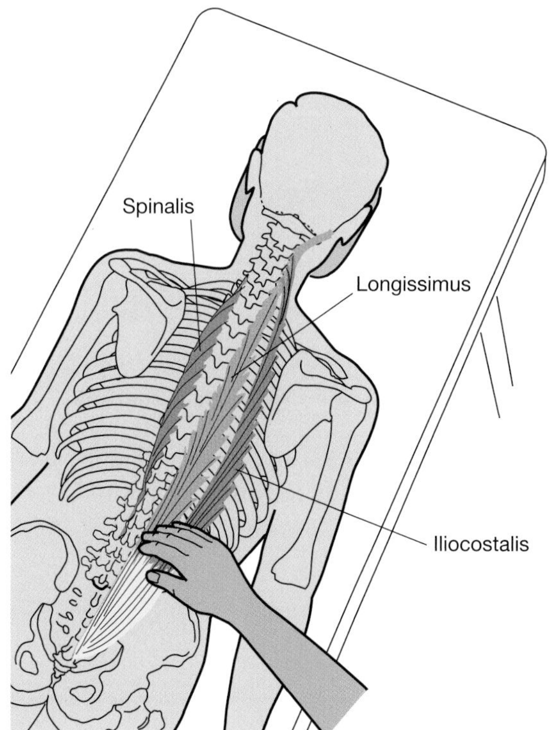

Figure 6.11 Palpation of the erector spinae muscles.

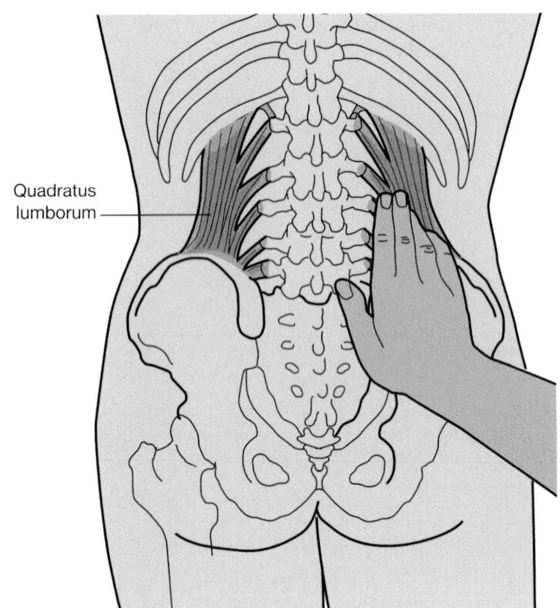

Figure 6.12 Palpation of the quadratus lumborum muscle.

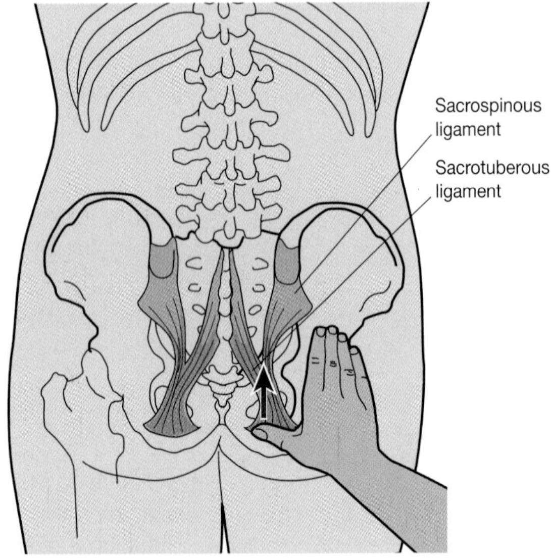

Figure 6.13 Palpation of the sacrotuberous ligament.

You will feel a resistance against your thumbs, which is the attachment of the sacrotuberous ligament (Figure 6.13).

Side-Lying Position

Soft-Tissue Structures

Piriformis Muscle

The piriformis muscle is located between the anterior inferior aspect of the sacrum and the greater

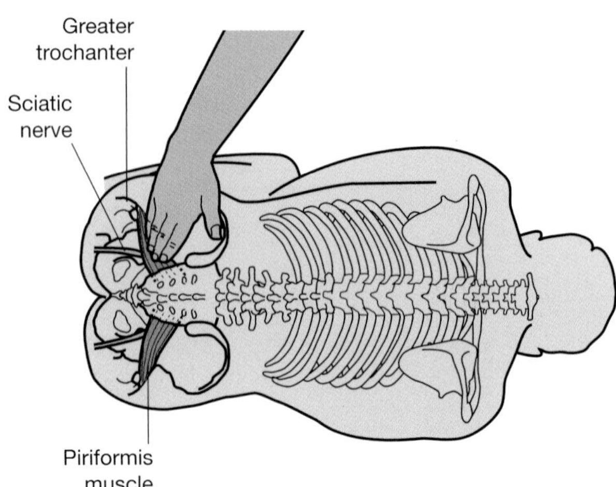

Figure 6.14 Palpation of the piriformis muscle.

trochanter. This muscle is very deep and is normally not palpable. However, if the muscle is in spasm, a cordlike structure can be detected under your fingers as you palpate the length of the muscle (Figure 6.14). Because of its attachment to the sacrum, the piriformis is able to influence the alignment of the sacrum by pulling it anteriorly. The sciatic nerve runs either under, over, or through the muscle belly. Compression or irritation of the nerve can occur when the muscle is in spasm.

Sciatic Nerve

The sciatic nerve is most easily accessed while the patient is lying on the side, which allows the nerve to have less muscle cover since the gluteus maximus is flattened. Locate the mid position between the ischial tuberosity and greater trochanter. The nerve usually travels under the piriformis muscle, but in some patients it pierces the muscle. You may be able to roll the nerve under your fingers if you take up the soft-tissue slack. Tenderness in this area can be due to an irritation of the sciatic nerve secondary to lumbar disc disease or a piriformis spasm (Figure 6.15).

Anterior Aspect

Bony Structures

Anterior Superior Iliac Spine

Place your hands on the iliac crests and allow your thumbs to reach anteriorly and inferiorly, on a diagonal, toward the pubic ramus. The most prominent protuberance is the anterior superior iliac spine (ASIS). To determine their position most accurately,

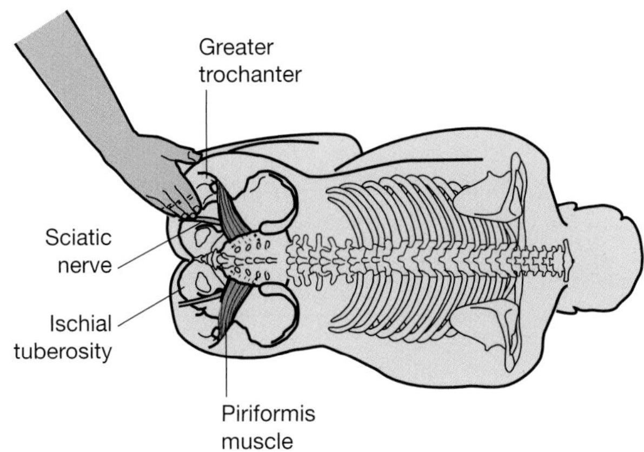

Figure 6.15 Palpation of the sciatic nerve.

roll the pads of your thumbs in a cranial direction so that they can rest under the ASISs. This area is normally superficial but can be obscured in an obese patient. Differences in height from one side to the other may be due to an iliac rotation or shear (Figure 6.16).

Pubic Tubercles

The patient should be in the supine position. Stand so that you face the patient and start the palpation

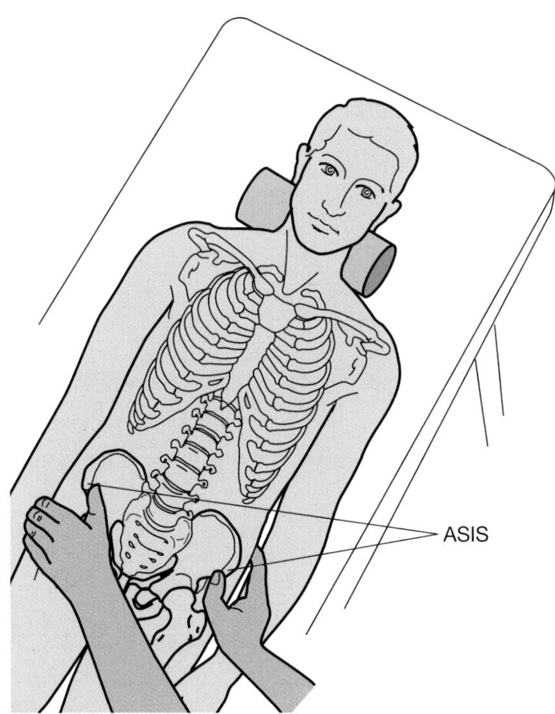

Figure 6.16 Palpation of the anterior superior iliac spine (ASIS).

superior to the pubic ramus. Place your hands so that your middle fingers are on the umbilicus and allow your palms to rest over the abdomen. The heel of your hand will be in contact with the superior aspect of the pubic tubercles. Then move your finger pads directly over the tubercles to determine their relative position. They are located medial to the greater trochanters and the inguinal crease. Make sure that your dominant eye is in the midline. The tubercles are normally tender to palpation. If they are asymmetrical either in height or in an anterior–posterior dimension, there may be a subluxation or dislocation or a sacroiliac dysfunction (Figure 6.17).

Soft-Tissue Structures

Abdominal Muscles

The abdominal muscles play a major role in supporting the trunk. They also play a role in influencing the position of the pubic symphysis and sacroiliac alignment. The group consists of the rectus abdominis, obliquus externus abdominis, and the obliquus internus abdominis. The rectus abdominis covers the anterior aspect of the trunk and attaches from the fifth through seventh ribs to the crest of the pubis. The muscles are segmentally innervated. The muscle belly of the rectus abdominis can be made more distinct by asking the patient to place the arms behind the head and perform a curl-up. Note for symmetry in the muscle and observe for any deficits (Figure 6.18).

Psoas Muscle

The psoas muscle is extremely important in patients with a low-back condition because of its attachment to the lumbar transverse processes and the lateral aspects of the vertebral bodies of T12 and L1–L5. The muscle can be palpated at its insertion on the lesser trochanter and medial and deep to the ASIS on the medial aspect of the sartorius (Figure 6.19). The belly is made more distinct by resisting hip flexion.

Trigger Points of the Lumbosacral Region

Trigger points and myofascial pain are frequently noted in the abdominal muscles and in the intrinsic and extrinsic lumbar spinal muscles. Trigger points in the abdominal muscles may radiate pain posteriorly, and trigger points in the lumbar spinal muscles may radiate pain anteriorly. Occasionally, trigger points in the lumbosacral spine will mimic the symptoms of a herniated disc. Characteristic locations of referred

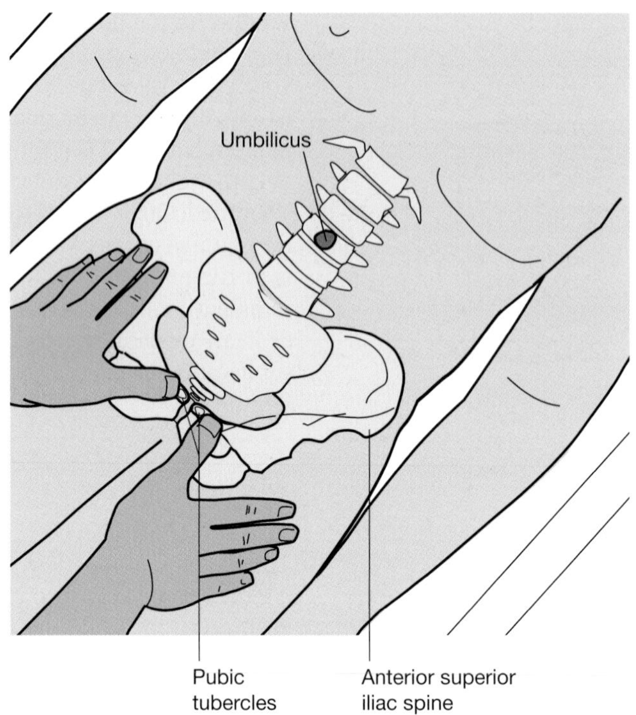

Figure 6.17 Palpation of the pubic tubercles.

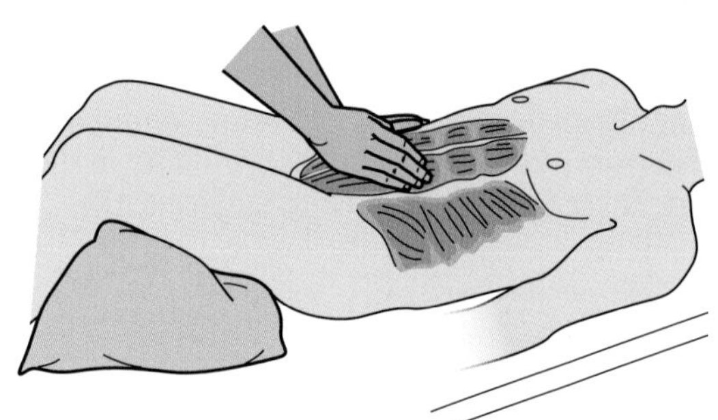

Figure 6.18 Palpation of the abdominal muscles.

pain patterns of trigger points in the abdominal and lumbosacral spinal muscles are illustrated in Figures 6.20, 6.21, 6.22, 6.23, 6.24, and 6.25.

Active Movement Testing

The patient should be appropriately disrobed so that you can observe the entire back. Have the patient stand without shoes in a well-lit area of the examination room. Shadows from poor lighting will affect

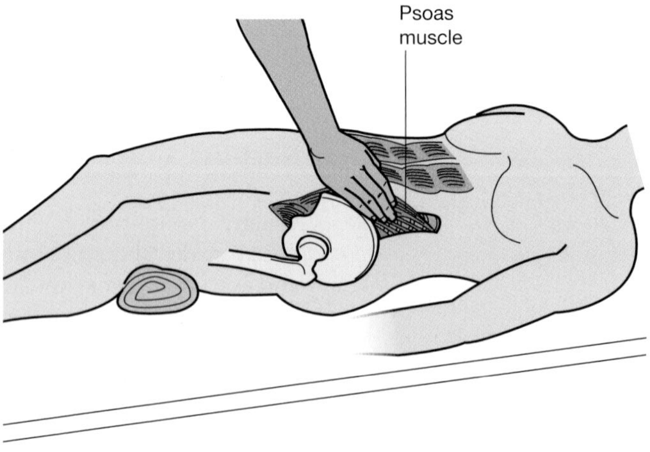

Figure 6.19 Palpation of the psoas muscle.

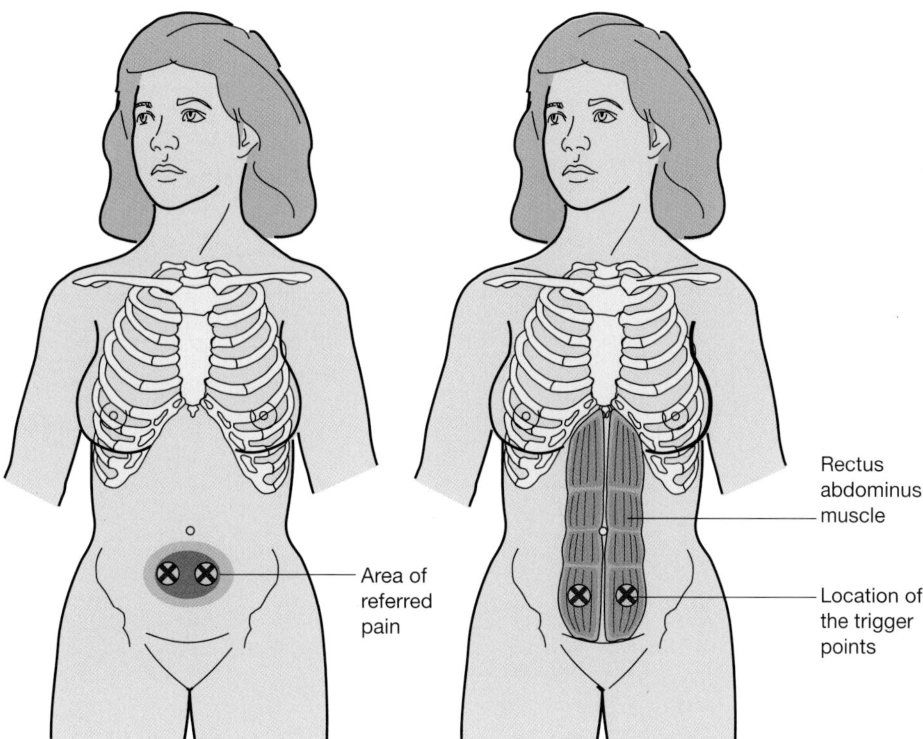

Figure 6.20 Trigger points in the rectus abdominis may simulate the pain of dysmenorrhea. (Adapted with permission from Travell and Rinzler, 1952.)

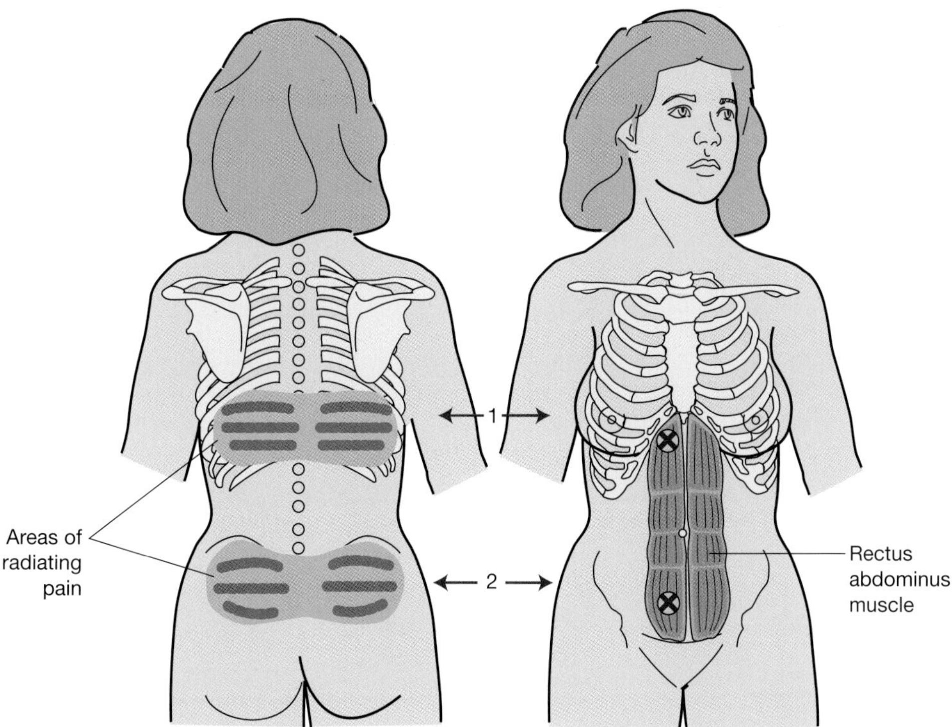

Figure 6.21 Trigger points in the rectus abdominis may also radiate pain into the posterior lower part of the thorax and lower back. (Adapted with permission from Travell and Rinzler, 1952.)

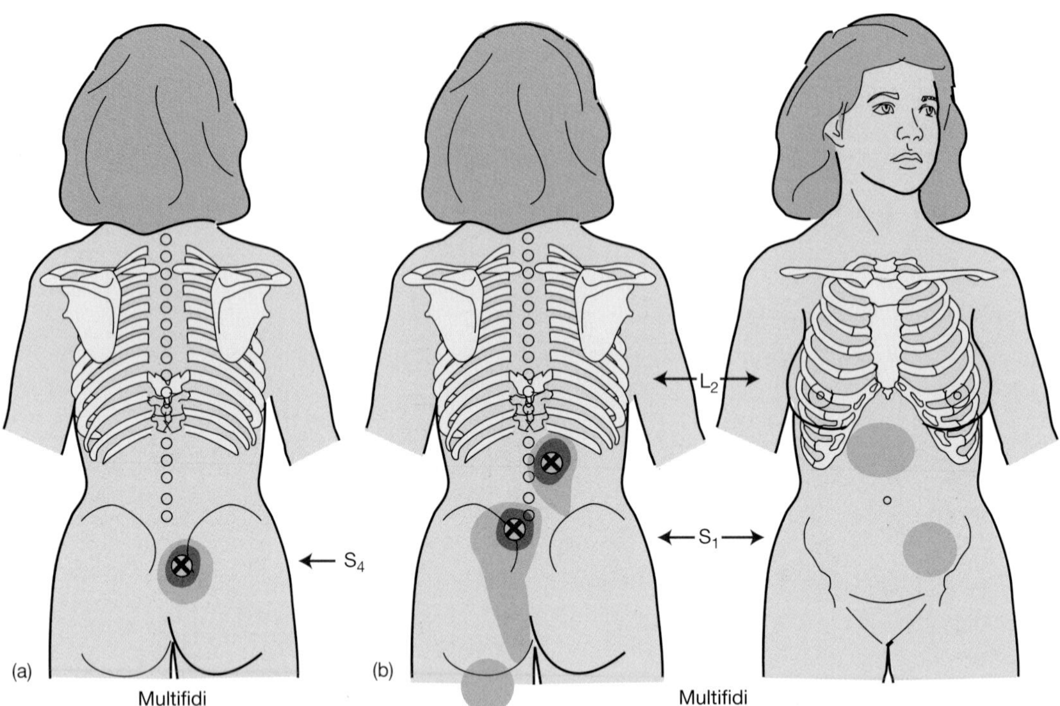

Figure 6.22 Trigger points within the multifidi muscles may cause referred pain in the paraspinal region. Pain may also radiate anteriorly or inferiorly. (Adapted with permission from Travell and Rinzler, 1952.)

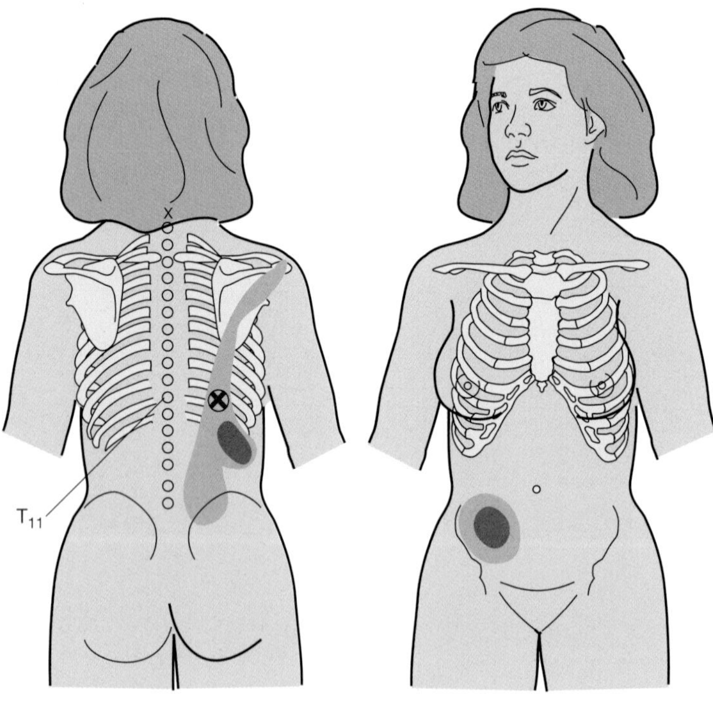

Figure 6.23 Trigger points in the iliocostalis thoracis muscle may radiate pain superiorly and inferiorly as well as anteriorly. (Adapted with permission from Travell and Rinzler, 1952.)

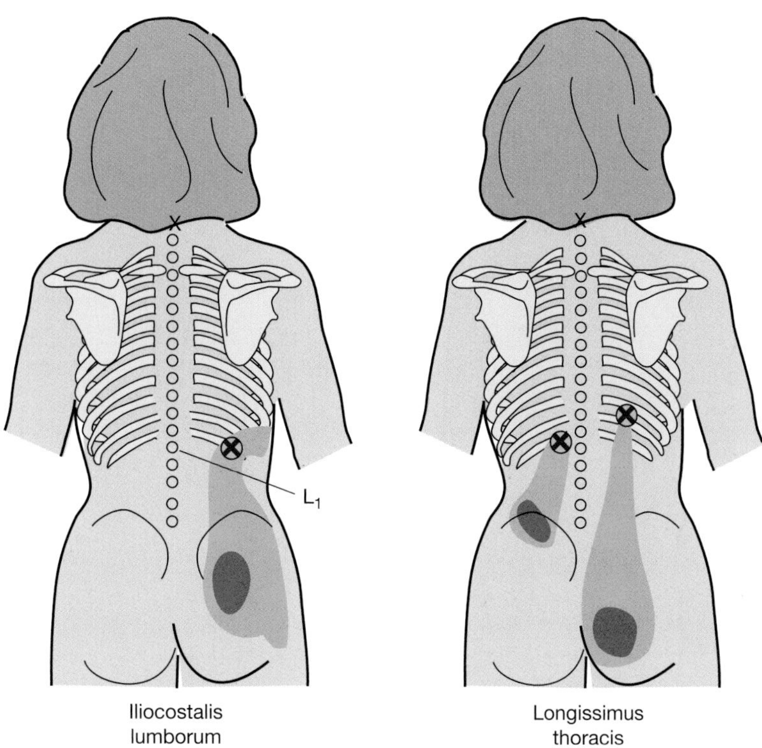

Figure 6.24 Trigger points in the iliocostalis lumborum and longissimus thoracis muscles radiate pain inferiorly. (Adapted with permission from Travell and Rinzler, 1952.)

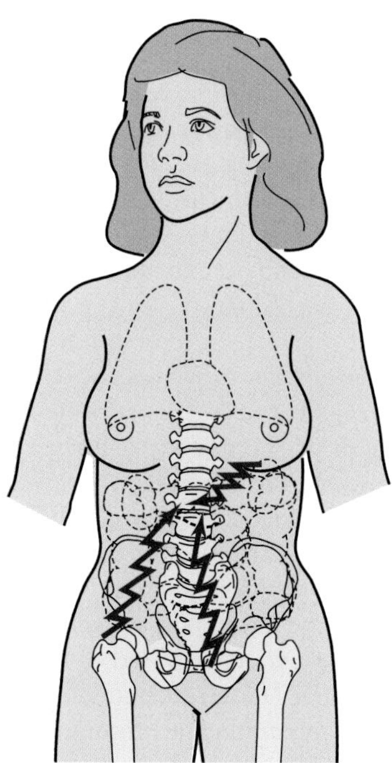

Figure 6.25 Pelvic, abdominal, and retroperitoneal organs may radiate pain to the lumbar spine. The hip may also cause low-back pain.

your perception of the movement. You should observe the patient's active movements from the anterior, posterior, and both lateral aspects. While observing the patient move, pay particular attention to his or her willingness to move, the quality of the motion, and the available range. Lines in the floor may serve as visual guides to the patient and alter his or her movement patterns. It may be helpful to ask the patient to repeat movements with the eyes closed.

Before your examination of the lumbar spine movements, you should have the patient perform a quick test to clear the joints of the lower extremities, by asking the patient to perform a full flat-footed squat. This will check the range of motion (ROM) of the hip, knee, ankle, and foot. If the movement is full and painless, the joints can be cleared.

You should then have the patient perform the following movements: forward and backward bending, lateral bending to the right and left, and rotation to the right and left. You should observe for the amount of available range, smoothness of movement, the willingness of the patient to move, and the alignment and symmetry of the spinal curves. You may note a flattening in a particular area as the patient bends to the side or a deviation to one side during forward

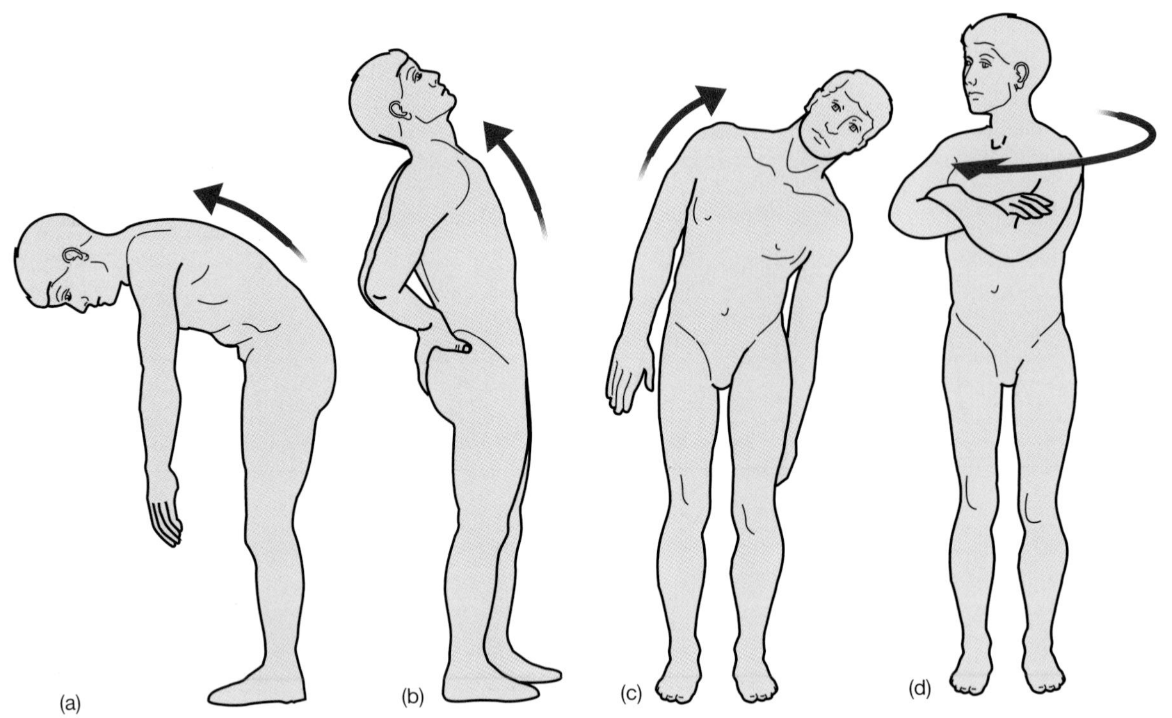

Figure 6.26 Active movement testing. (a) Lumbar forward bending. (b) Lumbar backward bending. (c) Lumbar side bending. (d) Lumbar rotation.

bending. These deviations should alert you to examine the involved area more carefully. The patient may demonstrate a pattern of limitation referred to as the *capsular pattern* (see section on Passive Movement Testing). If the motion is pain free at the end of the range, you can add an additional overpressure to clear the joint (Cyriax, 1982). You can also ask the patient to sustain the position for 15 seconds to determine whether the symptoms can be reproduced. Sustained movements of lateral bending and rotation can also be combined with flexion and extension to increase the degree of compression. If the patient experiences pain during any of these movements, you should note the position that increases the symptoms and whether any position alleviates the symptoms.

Forward Bending

Instruct the patient to stand with the feet approximately 6 in. apart. Stand behind the patient to observe the back during the movement. In addition, observe the patient from the side, to have a better view of the lumbosacral curve contour. To initiate the movement, ask the patient to bend the head forward by tucking the chin toward the chest, then drop the arms, and allow the trunk to roll forward with the fingertips reaching downward. Have the patient go as far as he or she can (Figure 6.26a). Observe the available range and deviation to either side if one occurs. If you feel that the patient is able to compensate for the deviation by using visual cues, have the patient close their eyes during the movement. Observe how much movement is actually coming from the lumbar spine and not by substitution from the hip joint and the normal lumbar–pelvic rhythm (Cailliet, 1995). To separate the movements, you can stabilize the pelvis with your arm to limit the degree of hip flexion. Patients also try to substitute by allowing knee flexion. Note the smoothness of the movement as each intervertebral level opens. At the end range, note if the range is limited by pain or the patient's anticipation of pain. The normal ROM of flexion is 80 degrees (American Academy of Orthopedic Surgeons, 1965).

McKenzie (1981) also has the patient perform flexion in the supine position, asking the patient to bring the knees up to the chest. The movement is therefore initiated from below, as opposed to above when the patient is standing. Therefore, pain noted at the beginning of the movement may be originating from L5–S1.

The amount of movement can be recorded on a movement diagram. Deviations to the side and the onset of symptoms can also be recorded. Objective methods of measuring the ROM in flexion are as follows: (1) Use a ruler to measure the distance from the patient's middle fingertip to the floor. (2) Measure the distance from T12 to the S1 spinous processes while the patient is in neutral position. Then have the patient complete a forward bend and measure from the same landmarks. The normal excursion observed should be 7–8 cm. To perform the Schober test, measure the point midway between the PSISs, which is approximately the level of the second sacral vertebra. Mark 5 cm below and 10 cm above. Measure the distance between the outer landmarks, first in neutral and then in flexion (Magee, 2008). Record the difference in the distance measured. A gravity-assisted bubble goniometer (inclinometer) can be placed on the patient to give you the actual degrees of movement.

Backward Bending

Instruct the patient to stand with the feet approximately 6 in. apart. Stand behind the patient to observe the back during the movement. Ask the patient to place his or her hands behind the back so that the palms contact the buttocks. Instruct the patient to allow the neck to extend, but not hyperextend, and then slowly allow the trunk to move backward toward their hands (Figure 6.26b). Patients will often substitute by flexing their knees when they have limited back extension. Observe the smoothness with which each intervertebral level closes. Note whether the range is limited by pain or the patient's anticipation of pain.

As an alternative method of performing back extension, Isaacs and Bookhout (2002) and Greenman (2003) prefer to have the patient bend backward by allowing him or her to prop up on the elbows and support the chin on the hands (sphinx position) while in a prone position. This allows for easier palpation of the bony position since the patient's muscles are relaxed. McKenzie (1981) prefers to have the patient perform a full push-up with the arms fully extended and the pelvis sagging to the table. This allows the patient to passively extend the back by using the upper-extremity muscles (McKenzie, 1981).

ROM should be recorded on a movement diagram. Normal ROM is 30 degrees (American Academy of Orthopedic Surgeons, 1965).

Lateral Bending

Instruct the patient to stand with the feet approximately 6 in. apart. Stand behind the patient to observe the back during the movement. Instruct the patient to allow their ear to approach the shoulder on the side to which he or she is moving. Then ask the patient to slide the hand down the lateral aspect of the lower extremity as he or she bends the trunk to that side (Figure 6.26c). This movement should be repeated to the right and left and comparison of the degree and quality of movement should be noted. Patients may try to increase the motion by lifting their lower extremity off the floor and hiking their hip. This can be minimized by stabilizing the pelvis with your arm as the patient performs the movement testing. Note any discontinuity of the curve. An angulation of the curve may indicate an area of hypermobility or hypomobility. Note the smoothness with which each intervertebral level contributes to the overall movement. Note whether the range is limited by pain or the patient's anticipation of pain. ROM is most easily recorded on a movement diagram. You can measure the distance from the tip of the middle finger to the floor and compare one side to the other. Normal ROM is 35 degrees (American Academy of Orthopedic Surgeons, 1965).

McKenzie (1981) prefers to have the patient perform a side-gliding movement while standing instead of side bending. This movement is accomplished by instructing the patient to move the pelvis and trunk to the opposite direction while maintaining the shoulders level in the horizontal plane. This movement combines rotation and side bending simultaneously.

If the patient experiences increased symptoms as he or she bends toward the side with the pain, the problem may be caused by an intra-articular dysfunction or a disc protrusion lateral to the nerve root. If the patient experiences increased symptoms as he or she bends away from the side with the pain, the problem may be caused by a muscular or ligamentous lesion, which will cause tightening of the muscle or ligament. The patient may have a disc protrusion medial to the nerve root. A detailed neurological examination will help differentiate between the diagnoses.

Rotation

Instruct the patient to stand with the feet approximately 6 in. apart. Stand behind the patient to observe the back during the movement. Instruct the patient to start by turning the head in the direction in which he or she is going to move and allowing the trunk to continue to turn (Figure 6.26d). Patients tend to compensate for limitation of rotation by turning the entire body. This can be minimized by stabilizing the pelvis with your arm or having the patient perform the test while sitting. This movement should be repeated toward the right and left. Compare the degree and quality of movement from side to side. Note any discontinuity of the curve. Note the smoothness with which each intervertebral level contributes. Note whether the range is limited by pain or the patient's anticipation of pain. ROM can be recorded on a movement diagram. Normal ROM is 45 degrees (American Academy of Orthopedic Surgeons, 1965).

Passive Movement Testing

Passive movement testing can be divided into two categories: physiological movements (cardinal plane), which are the same as the active movements, and mobility testing of the accessory (joint play, component) movements. You can determine whether the noncontractile (inert) elements can be incriminated by using these tests. These elements (ligaments, joint capsule, fascia, bursa, dura mater, and nerve root) (Cyriax, 1982) are stretched or stressed when the joint is taken to the end of the available range. At the end of each passive physiological movement, you should sense the end feel and determine whether it is normal or pathological. Assess the limitation of movement and determine whether it fits into a capsular pattern. The capsular pattern of the lumbar spine is equally limited to lateral bending and rotation followed by extension (Magee, 2008). This pattern is only clearly noticeable when multiple segments are involved. Paris (1991) described a capsular pattern for the lumbar spine secondary to a facet lesion. With the facet lesion on the right, lateral bending is limited to the left, rotation is limited to the right, and forward bending deviates to the right.

Physiological Movements

Passive testing of the gross physiological movements is difficult to accomplish in the lumbar spine because of the size and weight of the trunk. Maneuverability of the trunk is cumbersome and the information that can be obtained is of limited value. You can obtain a greater sense of movement and understanding of the end feel by performing passive intervertebral movement testing.

Mobility Testing

Mobility testing of intervertebral joint movements and accessory movements will give you information about the degree of laxity present in the joint and the end feel. The patient must be totally relaxed and comfortable to allow you to move the joint and obtain the most accurate information.

Intervertebral Mobility of the Lumbar Spine

Flexion

Place the patient in the side-lying position facing you, with the head and neck in neutral alignment. Stand so that you are facing the patient. Be careful not to allow the trunk to rotate or else your findings will be distorted. Place your middle finger in the interspace between the spinous process of L5 and S1. Flex the patient's hips and knees. Support the patient's lower extremities on your hip creating flexion of the lumbar spine to the level that you are palpating by increasing the degree of hip flexion. Note the opening of the intervertebral space. You can slightly extend the spine to get a better sense of opening and closing. Slightly increase the degree of flexion to palpate the next intervertebral segment and continue in a cranial fashion (Figure 6.27) (http://www.youtube.com/watch?v=mHQoY1aw UTU).

Side Bending

Place the patient in the prone position with the neck in neutral rotation. Stand on the side of the patient that is on the side of your dominant eye, with your body turned so that you are facing the patient's head. Place your middle finger in the interspace between the spinous processes of L5 and S1. Hold the patient's lower extremity that is closer to you. Flex the patient's knee to shorten the lever arm and support the lower extremity with your arm. Move the lower extremity into abduction until you feel movement at the interspace that you are palpating. This will create bending to the side on which you are standing and you will feel a narrowing of the interspace. You can also palpate on the opposite side and you will feel opening of the interspace. Slightly increase the degree of side bending by creating additional abduction to palpate the next intervertebral segment and continue in a cranial fashion (Figure 6.28) (http://www.youtube.com/watch?v=GjE2kUyaUjI).

Rotation

Place the patient in the prone position with the neck in neutral rotation. Stand on the side of the patient that is on the side of your dominant eye, with your body turned so that you are facing the

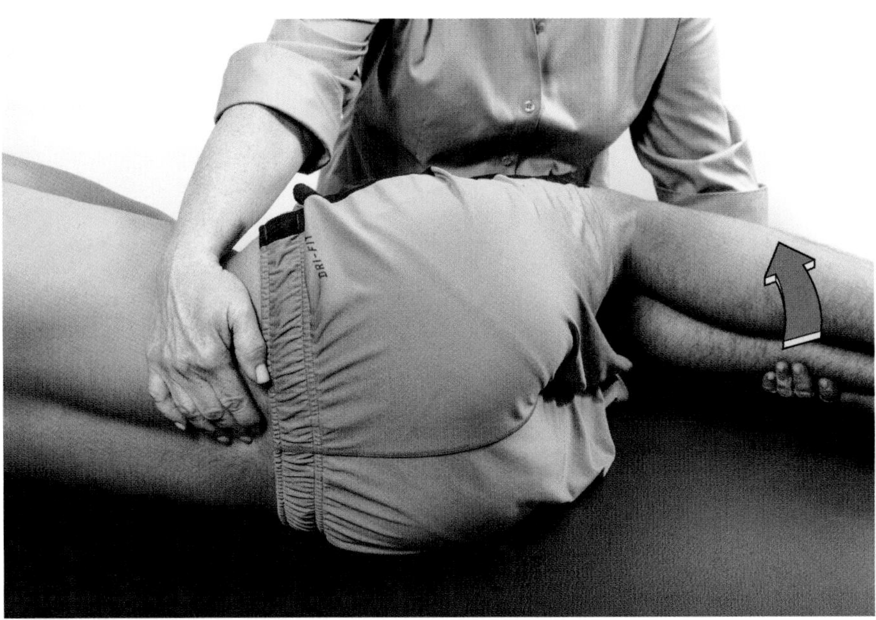

Figure 6.27 Mobility testing of lumbar spine flexion.

patient's head. Place your middle finger on the side of the spinous process of L5 that is closest to you. Hold the patient's innominate bone on the side opposite from which you are standing. Lift the pelvis toward the ceiling. This will create rotation of L5 away from you and you will sense the spinous process moving into your palpating finger (Figure 6.29) (http://www.youtube.com/watch?v=qcb4XYj5f4Y).

Accessory Movements of the Lumbar Spine

Central Posteroanterior Spring on the Spinous Process

Place the patient in the prone position with the neck in neutral rotation. Stand on the side of the patient that is on the side of your dominant eye, with your body turned so that you are facing the patient's head. Place the central portion of your palm (between the thenar and hypothenar eminences) over the spinous

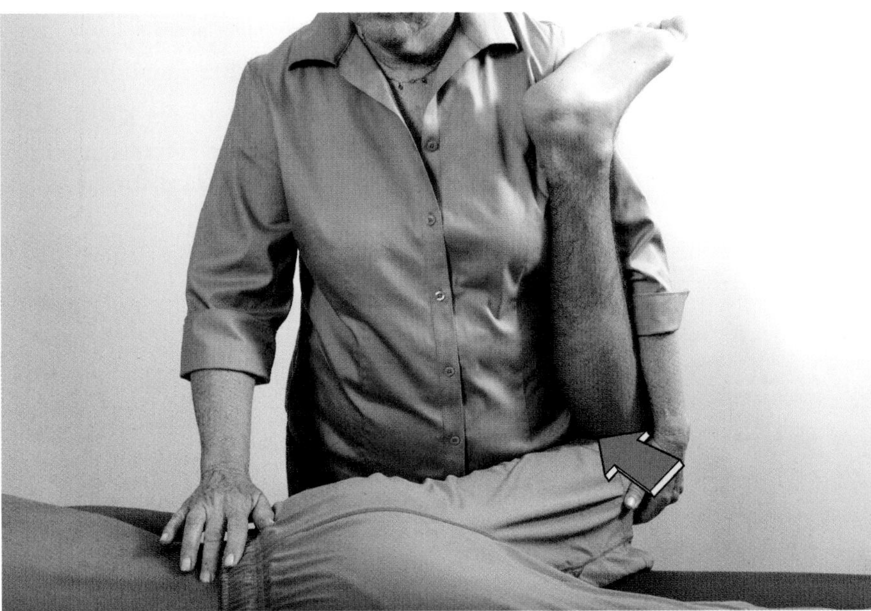

Figure 6.28 Mobility testing of lumbar spine side bending.

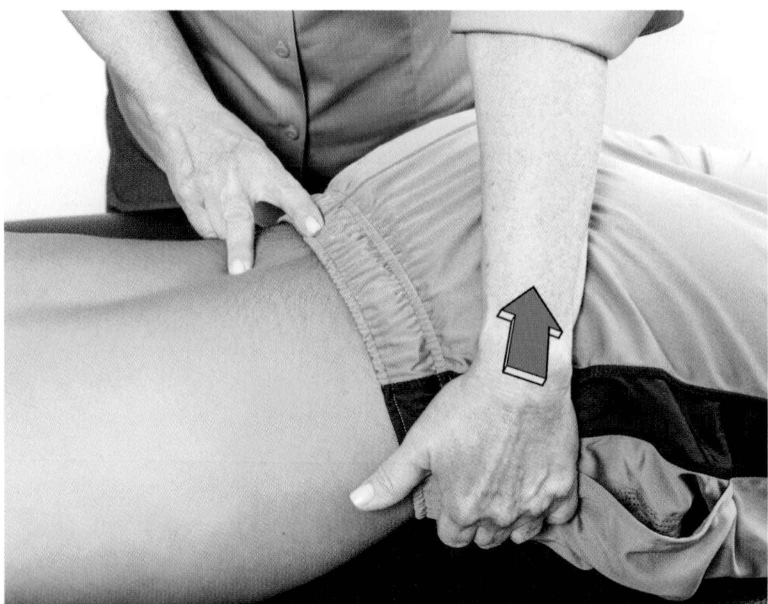

Figure 6.29 Mobility testing of lumbar spine rotation.

process and press directly over the process in an anterior direction until all the slack has been taken up (Figures 6.30a and 6.30b).

Posteroanterior Spring on the Transverse Process

Place the patient in the prone position with the neck in neutral rotation. Stand on the side of the patient that is on the side of your dominant eye, with your body turned so that you are facing the patient's head. Place the hypothenar eminence, just medial to the pisiform, over the transverse process on the side closest to you. Press on the process in an anterior direction until all the slack has been taken up. This will cause a rotation of the vertebral body away from the side that you are contacting (Figures 6.31a and 6.31b).

Transverse Pressure on the Spinous Process

Place the patient in the prone position with the neck in neutral rotation. Stand on the side of the patient that is on the side of your dominant eye, with your body turned so that you are facing the side of the patient. Place your thumbs on the lateral aspect of the spinous process. Push the process away from you until you have taken up all the slack. This will cause rotation of the vertebral body toward you (Figures 6.32a and 6.32b).

Sacroiliac Joint Examination

After concluding the examination of the lumbar intervertebral mobility tests and accessory movements, proceed with the examination of the sacroiliac joint.

(a) 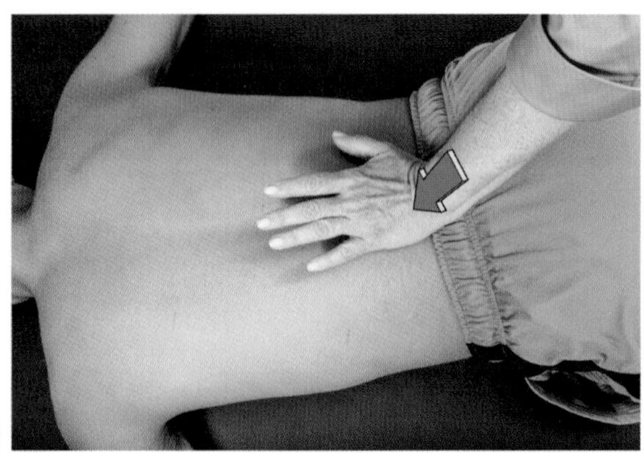

(b) 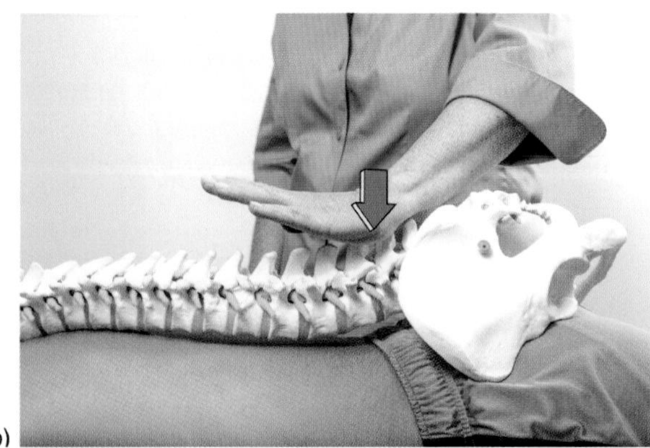

Figure 6.30 (a, b) Mobility testing of central posteroanterior spring on the spinous process.

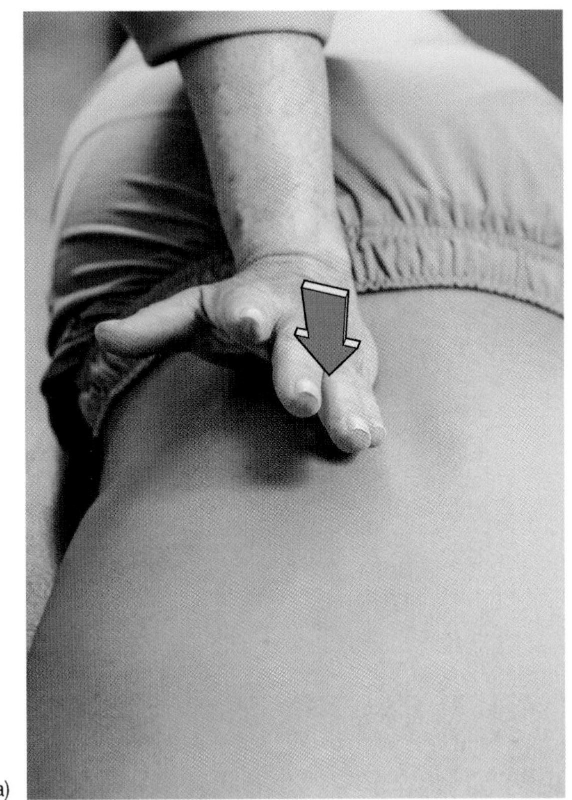

(a)

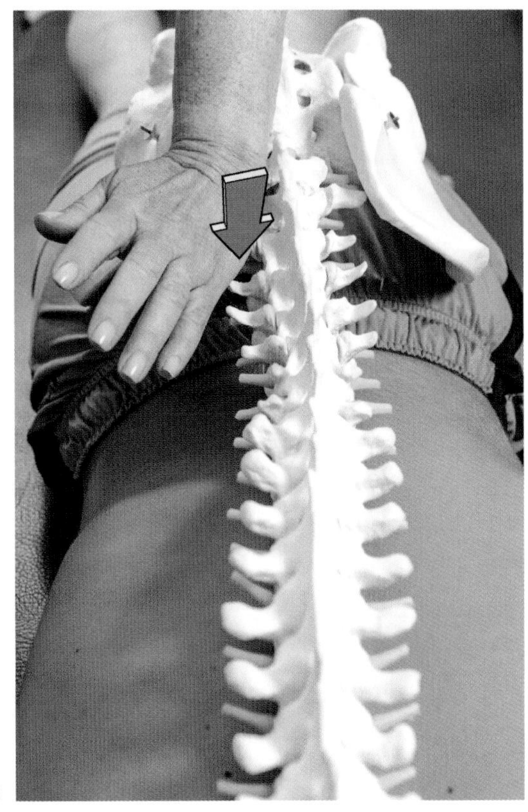

(b)

Figure 6.31 (a, b) Mobility testing of central posteroanterior spring on the transverse process.

Standing Flexion Test

This is a mobility test for the ilium moving on the sacrum. Instruct the patient to stand with the feet approximately 6 in. apart. Stand behind the patient to observe the movement. Remember to use your dominant eye. Locate the PSISs and place your thumbs under them. Maintain contact with the PSISs throughout the movement. Ask the patient to bend as far forward as he or she can. Observe the movement of the PSISs in relation to each other. They should move equally. If there is a restriction, the side that moves first and furthest is considered to be hypomobile (Figure 6.33). If the patient presents with tight hamstrings, a false positive finding can occur (Greenman, 2003; Isaacs *et al.*, 2002) (http://www.youtube.com/watch?v=x6QzLvlnGhs).

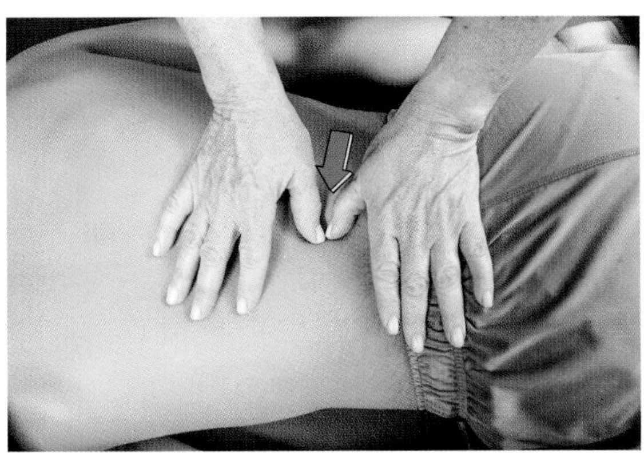

(a)

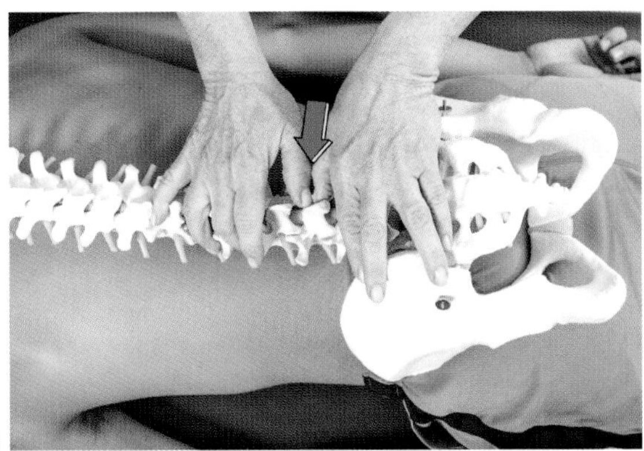

(b)

Figure 6.32 (a, b) Mobility testing of transverse pressure on the spinous process.

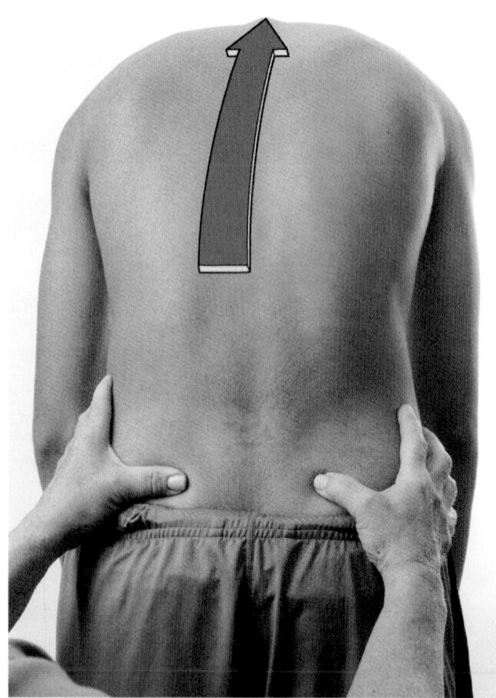

Figure 6.33 Mobility testing of the sacroiliac joint: standing forward-bending test.

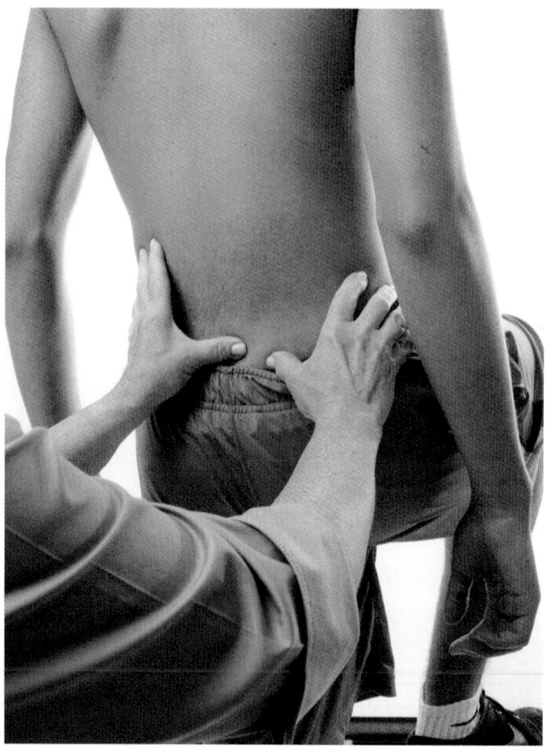

Figure 6.34 Mobility testing of the sacroiliac joint: stork test.

Stork (Gillet, Marching) Test

This is a mobility test for the ilium moving on the sacrum. Instruct the patient to stand with the feet approximately 6 in. apart. Stand behind the patient to observe the movement. Remember to use your dominant eye. Locate the PSIS on the side that you are testing and place one thumb under it. Place your other thumb just medial to the PSIS, on the sacral base. Ask the patient to raise the lower extremity on the side being tested so that the hip and knee are flexed to 90 degrees. Note the movement of the PSIS in relation to the sacrum. This test should be repeated on the contralateral side. Compare the amount of movement from one side to the other. If the PSIS does not drop down into your thumb on one side, the ilium is considered to be hypomobile (Greenman, 2003) (Figure 6.34) (http://www.youtube.com/watch?v=pvsDU6IJoSc).

Backward-Bending Test

Instruct the patient to stand with the feet approximately 6 in. apart. Stand behind the patient to observe the movement. Remember to use your dominant eye. Place your thumbs medial to the PSISs bilaterally on the sacral base. Instruct the patient to bend backward. Observe as your thumbs move in an anterior direction. An inability to move anteriorly demonstrates hypomobility of the sacrum moving on the ilium (Greenman, 2003; Isaacs and Bookhout, 2002) (Figure 6.35).

Seated Flexion Test

This is a mobility test for the sacrum moving on the ilium. This test eliminates the influence of the lower extremities. Instruct the patient to sit on a stool with the feet firmly on the ground for support. Stand behind the patient to observe the movement. Remember to use your dominant eye. Locate the PSISs and place your thumbs under them. Maintain contact with the PSISs throughout the movement. Ask the patient to bend as far forward as he or she can with their arms between their knees. Observe the movement of the PSISs in relation to each other. The side that moves first and furthest is considered to be hypomobile (Greenman, 2003; Isaacs and Bookhout, 2002) (Figure 6.36) (http://www.youtube.com/watch?v=IflCSTcr7cQ).

Posteroanterior Spring of the Sacrum

This is a test for posterior to anterior mobility of the sacrum. Place the patient in the prone position with the neck in neutral rotation. Stand on the side of the

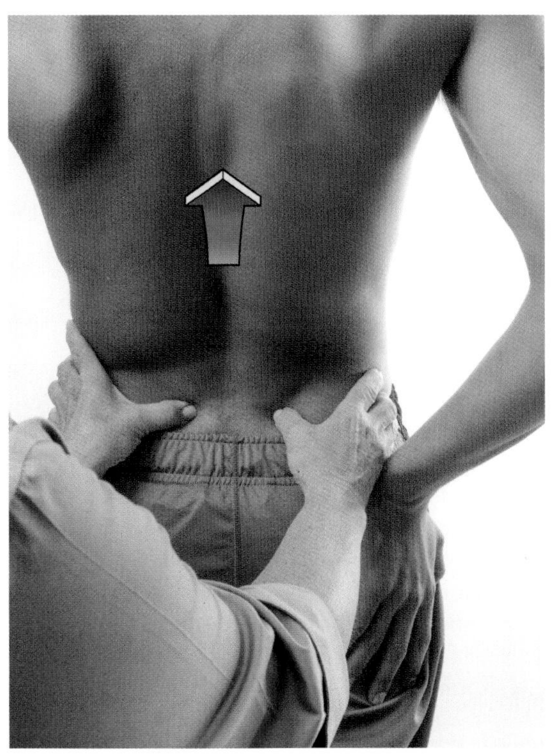

Figure 6.35 Mobility testing of the sacroiliac joint: backward-bending test.

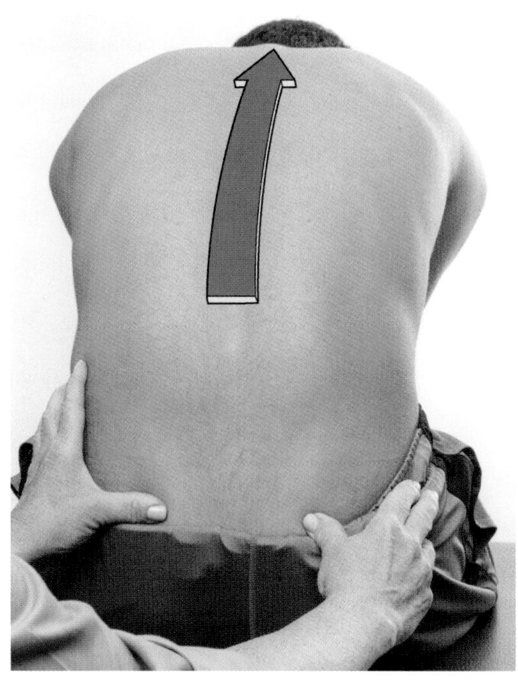

Figure 6.36 Mobility testing of the sacroiliac joint: sitting forward-bending test.

patient that is on the side of your dominant eye, with your body turned so that you are facing the patient's head. Place your hands over the central aspect of the posterior sacrum using the palm as the contact point. Press directly over the sacrum in an anterior direction until all the slack has been taken up (Paris, 1991) (Figures 6.37a and 6.37b).

Resistive Testing

Trunk Flexion

The rectus abdominis is the primary trunk flexor. It is assisted by the obliquus internus and externus muscles (Figure 6.38).

- Position of patient (Figure 6.39): Supine with hands clasped behind the head.

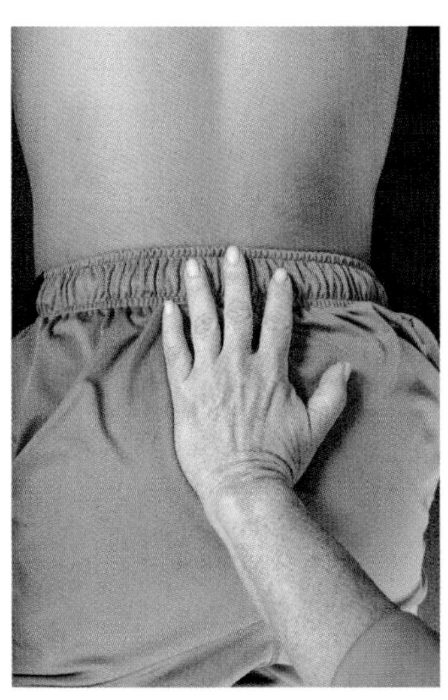

(a)

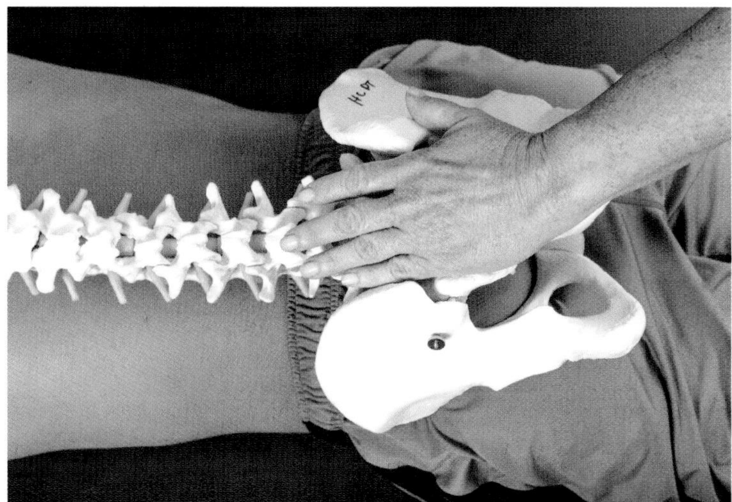

(b)

Figure 6.37 (a, b) Mobility testing of the sacroiliac joint: posteroanterior spring of the sacrum.

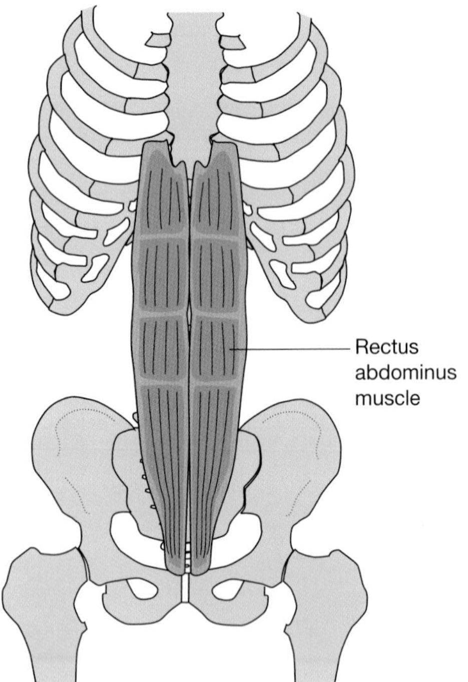

Figure 6.38 The trunk flexors.

- Resisted test: Stabilize the patient's lower extremities by pressing down on the anterior aspect of the thighs and ask the patient to perform a curl-up, lifting the scapulae off the table. Observe the umbilicus for movement cranially or caudally. Movement toward the head indicates stronger contraction of the upper aspect of the muscle, and movement toward the feet indicates stronger contraction of the lower segments of the rectus abdominis. Observe the umbilical region for a bulging of the abdominal contents through the linea alba. This represents an umbilical hernia. Trunk flexion is made easier if the patient attempts the test with the arms relaxed at the side.

Weakness of trunk flexion results in increased risk of lower back pain and may cause difficulty in getting up from a seated position.

Trunk Rotation

The rotators of the trunk are the obliquus internus and externus muscles (Figure 6.40). Accessory muscles include the multifidi, rotatores, rectus abdominis, latissimus dorsi, and semispinalis muscles.

- Position of patient (Figure 6.41): Supine with the hands behind the neck.
- Resisted test: Stabilize the patient's lower extremities by pressing down on the anterior aspect of the thighs and ask the patient to raise the left shoulder blade up and twist the body so as to bring the left elbow toward the right hip. This tests for the left obliquus externus and the right obliquus internus muscles. Now ask the patient to repeat the procedure, bringing the right shoulder and scapula off the table and twisting toward the left to test the right obliquus externus and left obliquus internus muscles.

Weakness of the trunk rotators causes reduced expiratory effort and may result in a functional scoliosis. The risk of lower back pain is also increased.

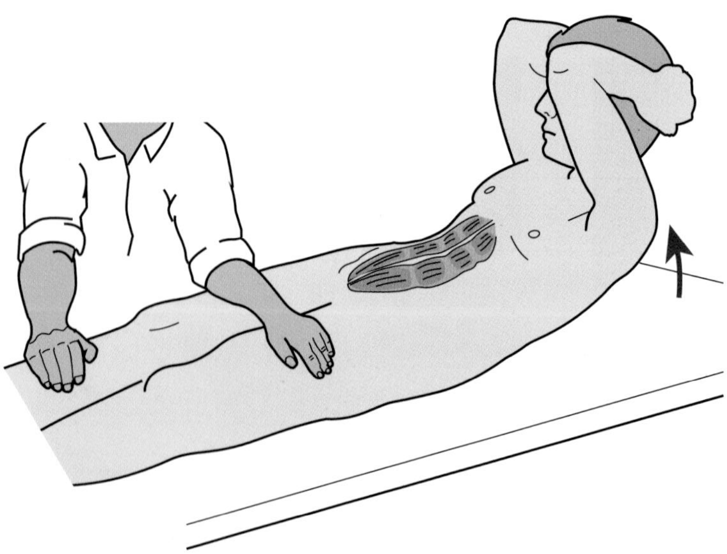

Figure 6.39 Testing trunk flexion.

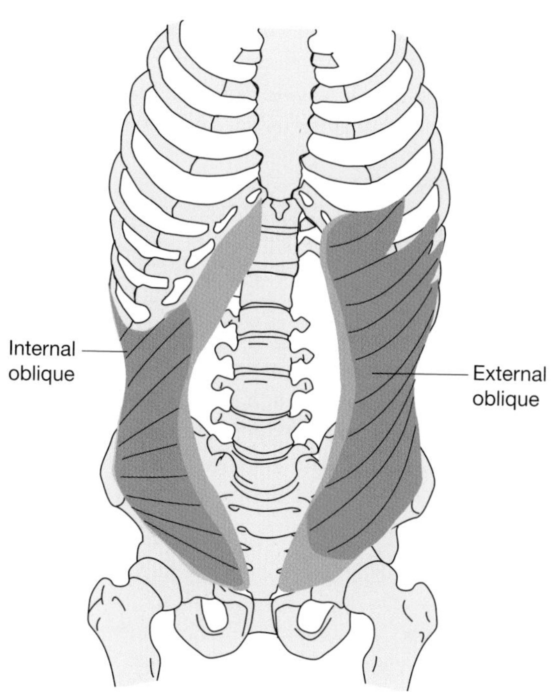

Figure 6.40 The trunk rotators.

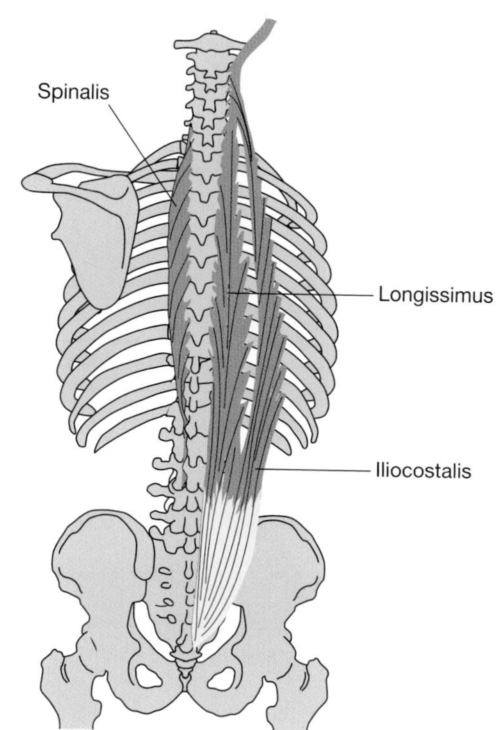

Figure 6.42 The trunk extensors.

Trunk Extension

The extensors of the trunk are the erector spinae, which include the iliocostalis thoracis, longissimus thoracis, spinalis thoracis, and iliocostalis lumborum (Figure 6.42).

- Position of patient (Figure 6.43): Prone with arms at the side. Place a pillow beneath the abdomen for patient comfort and to reverse the lumbar lordosis.
- Resisted test: Stabilize the patient's pelvis with one of your forearms and ask the patient to raise the neck and sternum upward as the patient attempts to raise the trunk against your resistance applied to the middle of the back.

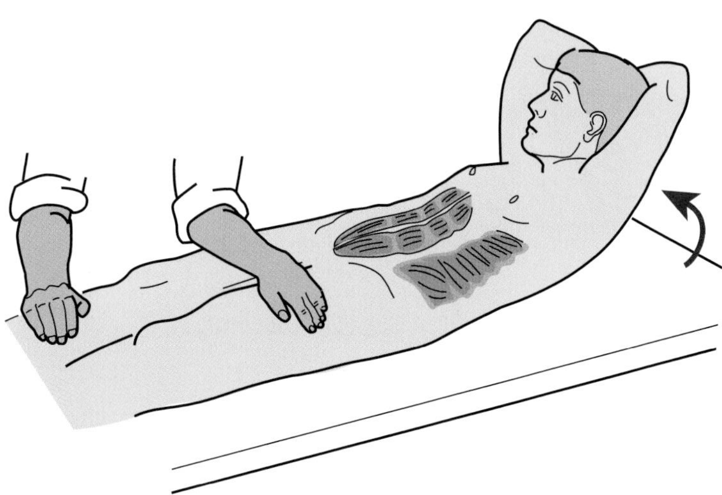

Figure 6.41 Testing trunk rotation.

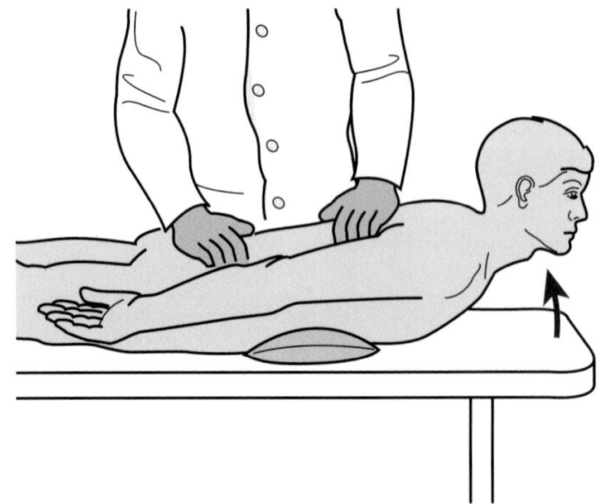

Figure 6.43 Testing trunk extension.

Weakness of the back extensor muscles results in a loss of the lumbar lordosis and an increase in the thoracic kyphosis. Weakness on one side results in lateral curvature with concavity toward the strong side.

Neurological Testing

The Lumbar Plexus

The lumbar plexus is composed of the L1 through L4 nerve roots, with some contribution from T12 (Figure 6.44). The nerve roots branch into anterior and posterior divisions near to the spine. The peripheral nerves that are formed from the anterior divisions innervate the adductor muscles of the hip. The nerves that form

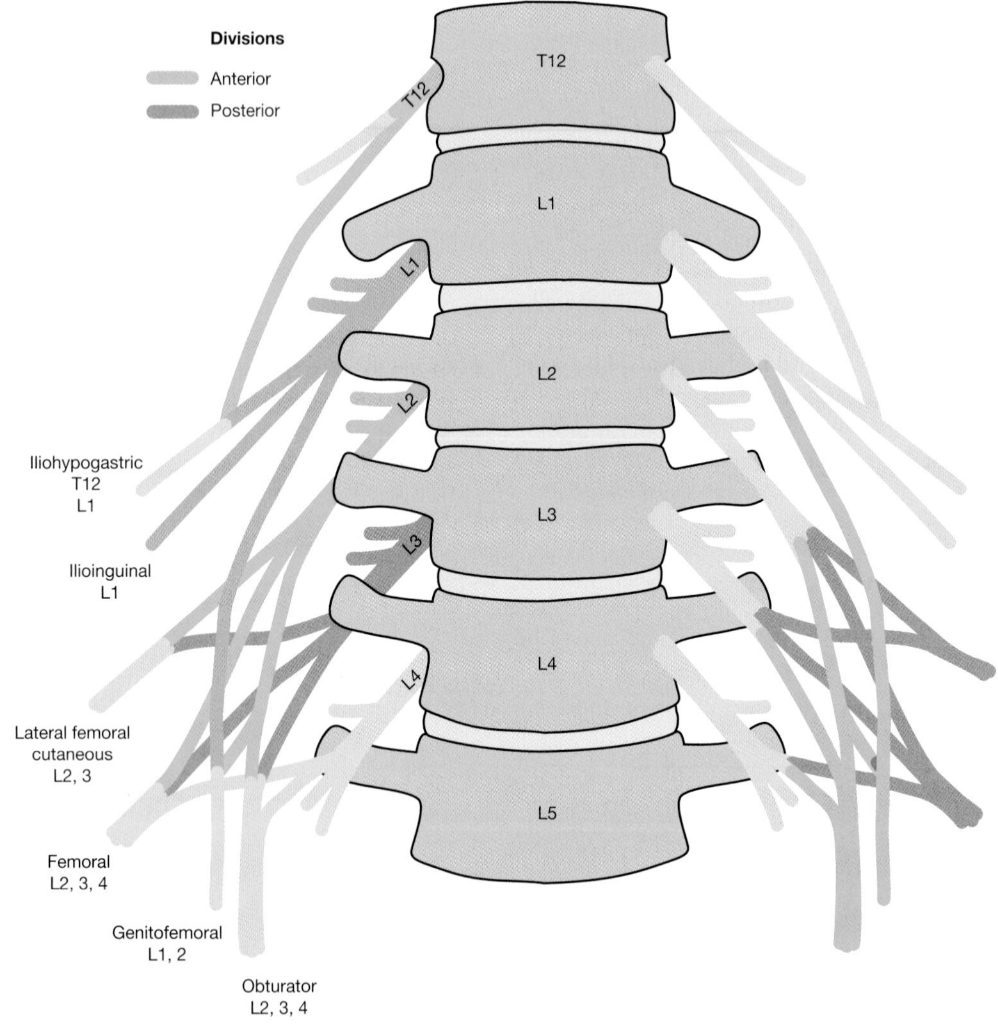

Figure 6.44 The lumbar plexus. The lumbar plexus is formed by the ventral primary rami of L1, L2, L3, and L4 and possibly T12. Note that the peripheral nerves from the anterior divisions innervate the adductor muscles of the hip, and the peripheral nerves from the posterior divisions innervate the hip flexors and knee extensors.

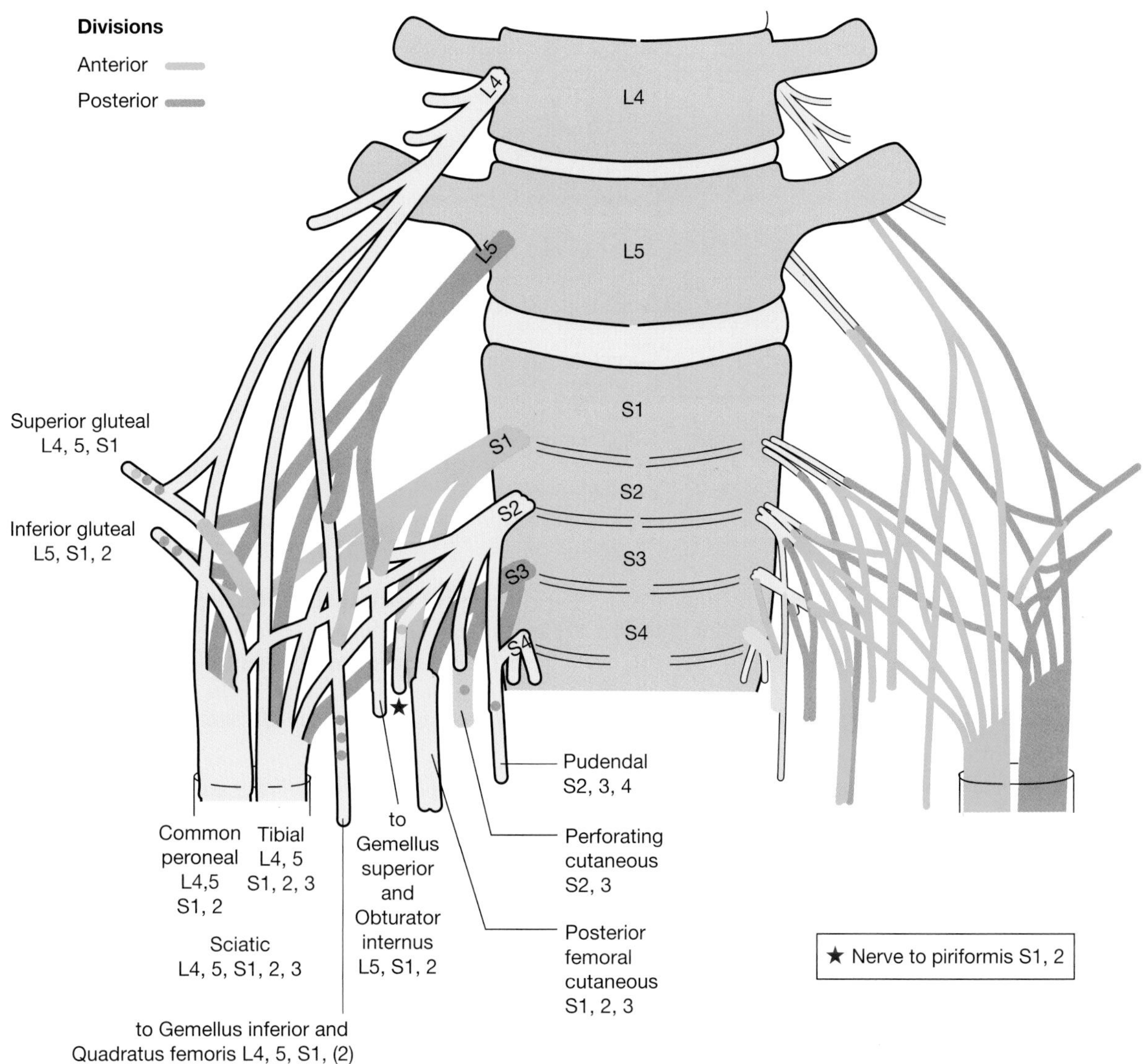

Figure 6.45 The lumbosacral plexus. This plexus is formed by the ventral primary rami of L4, L5, S1, S2, and S3.

from the posterior divisions innervate the hip flexors and knee extensors.

The Lumbosacral Plexus

The lumbosacral plexus is composed of the nerve roots from L4 through S3 (Figure 6.45).

Because of the rotation of the lower limb that occurs during embryogenesis, the anterior divisions and the peripheral nerves that emanate from them innervate the posterior aspect of the lower extremity and the plantar surface of the foot. The posterior divisions of the lumbosacral nerve roots and the peripheral nerves derived from them innervate the lateral abductors and an extensor of the hip, the dorsiflexor muscles of the ankle, and the extensor muscles of the toes.

Testing by Neurological Level

Pathology of the lumbosacral spine is common and neurological testing is necessary to determine where in the lumbosacral spine the pathology exists. The muscles of the lower extremity are usually innervated by specific nerve roots. Muscles that share a common nerve root innervation are in the same myotome (Table 6.1).

Table 6.1 The Lumbosacral Plexus: Muscle Organization

Root Level	Muscle Test	Muscles Innervated at this Level
L1–L2	Hip flexion (adduction)	Psoas, iliacus, sartorius, adductor longus, pectineus, gracilis, adductor brevis
L3	Knee extension (hip adduction)	Quadriceps, adductor magnus, and longus, brevis
L4	Ankle dorsiflexion (knee extension)	Tibialis anterior, quadriceps, adductor magnus, obturator externus, tibialis posterior, tensor fascia latae
L5	Toe extension (hip abduction)	Extensor hallucis longus, extensor digitorum longus, gluteus medius and minimus, obturator internus, peroneus tertius, semimembranosus, semitendinosus, popliteus
S1	Ankle plantar flexion Hip extension Knee flexion Ankle eversion	Gastrocnemius, soleus, gluteus maximus, biceps femoris, semitendinosus, obturator internus, piriformis, peroneus longus and brevis, extensor digitorum brevis
S2	Knee flexion	Biceps femoris, piriformis, flexor digitorum longus, flexor hallucis longus, gastrocnemius, soleus, intrinsic foot muscles

The skin of the lower extremity is innervated by peripheral nerves that emanate from specific nerve roots. Skin that shares innervation from a particular nerve root shares a common dermatome (Figure 6.46).

Knowledge of the myotomes, dermatomes, and peripheral nerve innervations (Figure 6.47) of the skin and muscles will assist you in the diagnosis of neurological pathology. Remember that there is significant variability from patient to patient with respect to patterns of innervation. With this in mind, the neurological examination is organized by root levels.

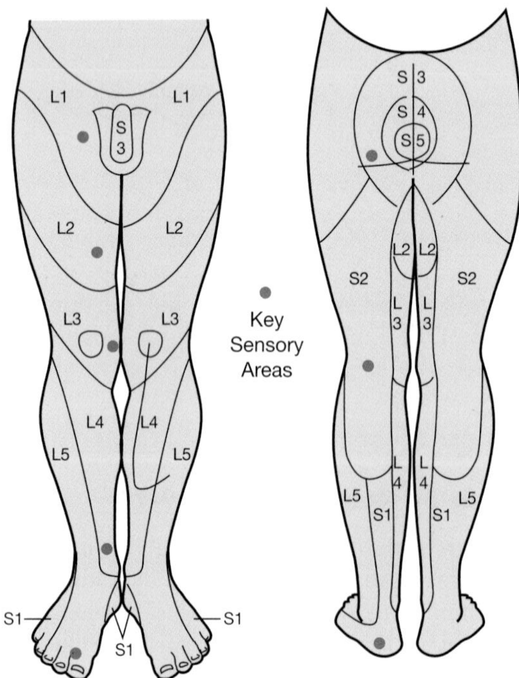

Figure 6.46 The dermatomes and key sensory areas of the lower extremity.

The L1 and L2 Levels

Muscle Testing

The L1 and L2 nerve roots (Figure 6.48) innervate the iliopsoas muscle, which is a hip flexor. Test hip flexion by having the patient sit at the edge of the table with the knees bent to 90 degrees. Ask the patient to raise the knee upward as you apply resistance to the anterior mid aspect of the thigh (see pp. 313–314 for more information).

Sensation Testing

The L1 dermatome is located over the inguinal ligament. The key sensory area is located over the medial third of the ligament. The L2 dermatome is located over the proximal anteromedial aspect of the thigh. The key sensory area is located approximately midway from the groin to the knee in the medial aspect of the thigh.

Reflex Testing

There is no specific reflex for the L1 and L2 levels.

The L3 Level

Muscle Testing

The L3 root level (Figure 6.49) is best tested by examining the quadriceps muscle, which extends the knee.

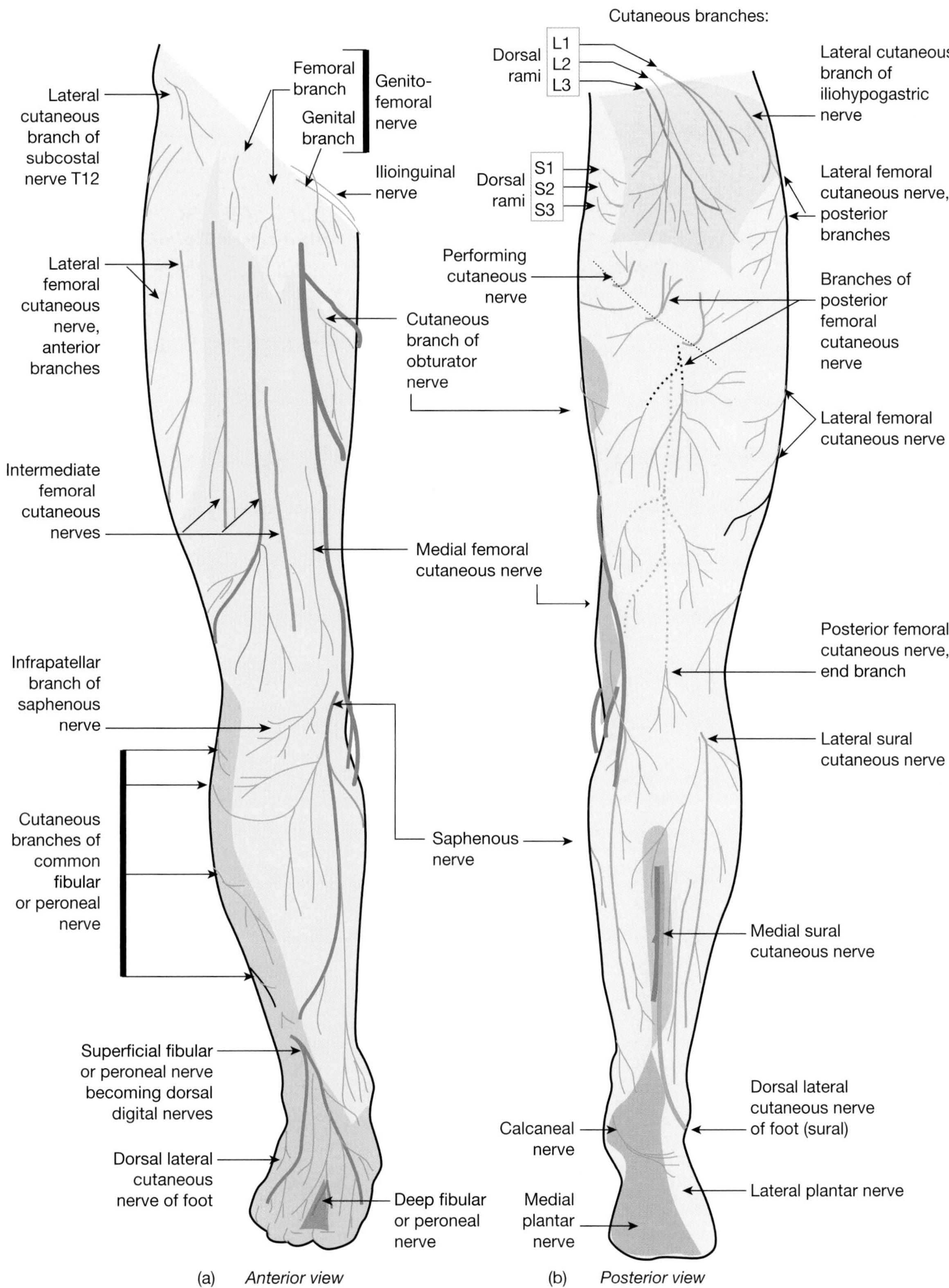

Figure 6.47 The cutaneous innervation of a lower limb.

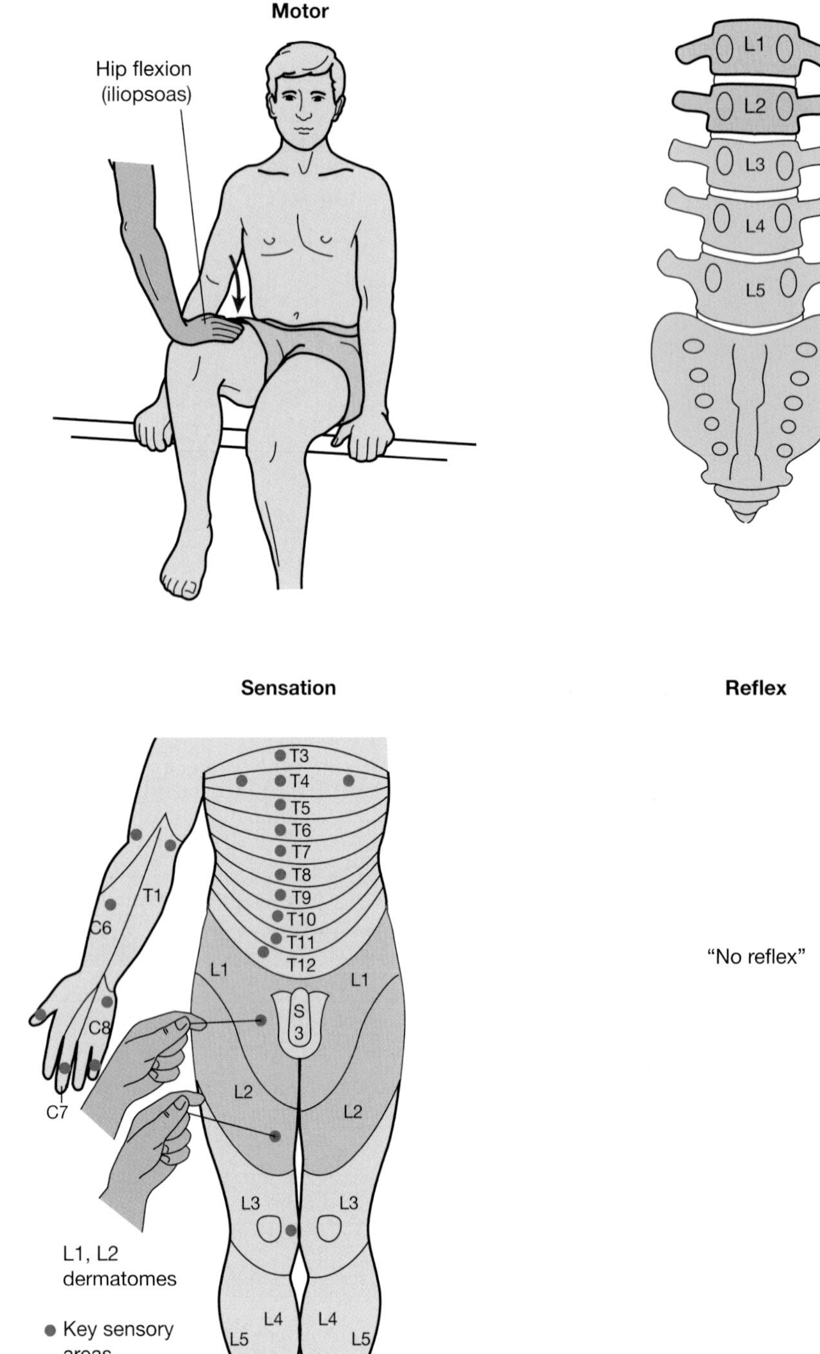

Figure 6.48 The L1 and L2 root levels.

This is performed by having the patient sit on the edge of the examining table with the knees bent to 90 degrees. Ask the patient to extend the knee as you apply resistance to the anterior aspect of the lower leg (see pp. 361–362, Figure 12.57 for further information).

Sensation Testing

The L3 dermatome is located on the anteromedial aspect of the thigh. It extends just below the medial aspect of the knee. The key sensory area for L3 is located just medial to the patella.

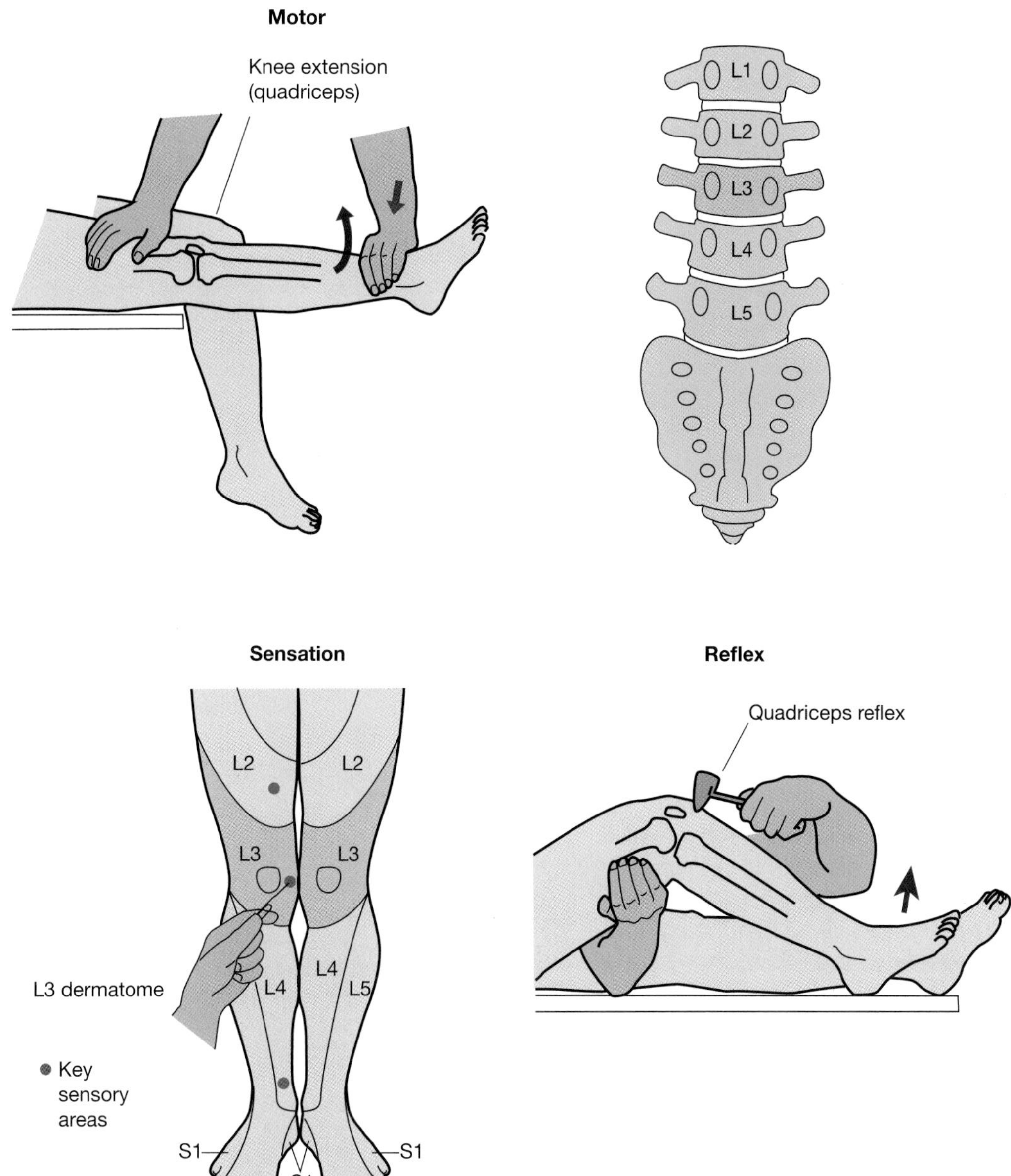

Figure 6.49 The L3 root level.

Reflex Testing

There is no specific reflex for the L3 level. The L3 nerve root does contribute to the quadriceps reflex at the knee (see L4 level below).

The L4 Level

Muscle Testing

The L4 nerve root (Figure 6.50) is best examined by testing dorsiflexion, which is performed by the tibialis anterior muscle. The patient is in a sitting position or supine. Ask the patient to bring the foot upward and inward, bending at the ankle, while you apply resistance to the dorsum of the foot (see p. 410, Figure 13.69 for further information).

Sensation Testing

The L4 dermatome is located over the medial aspect of the leg and extends beyond the medial malleolus. The key sensory area of L4 is located just proximal to the medial malleolus.

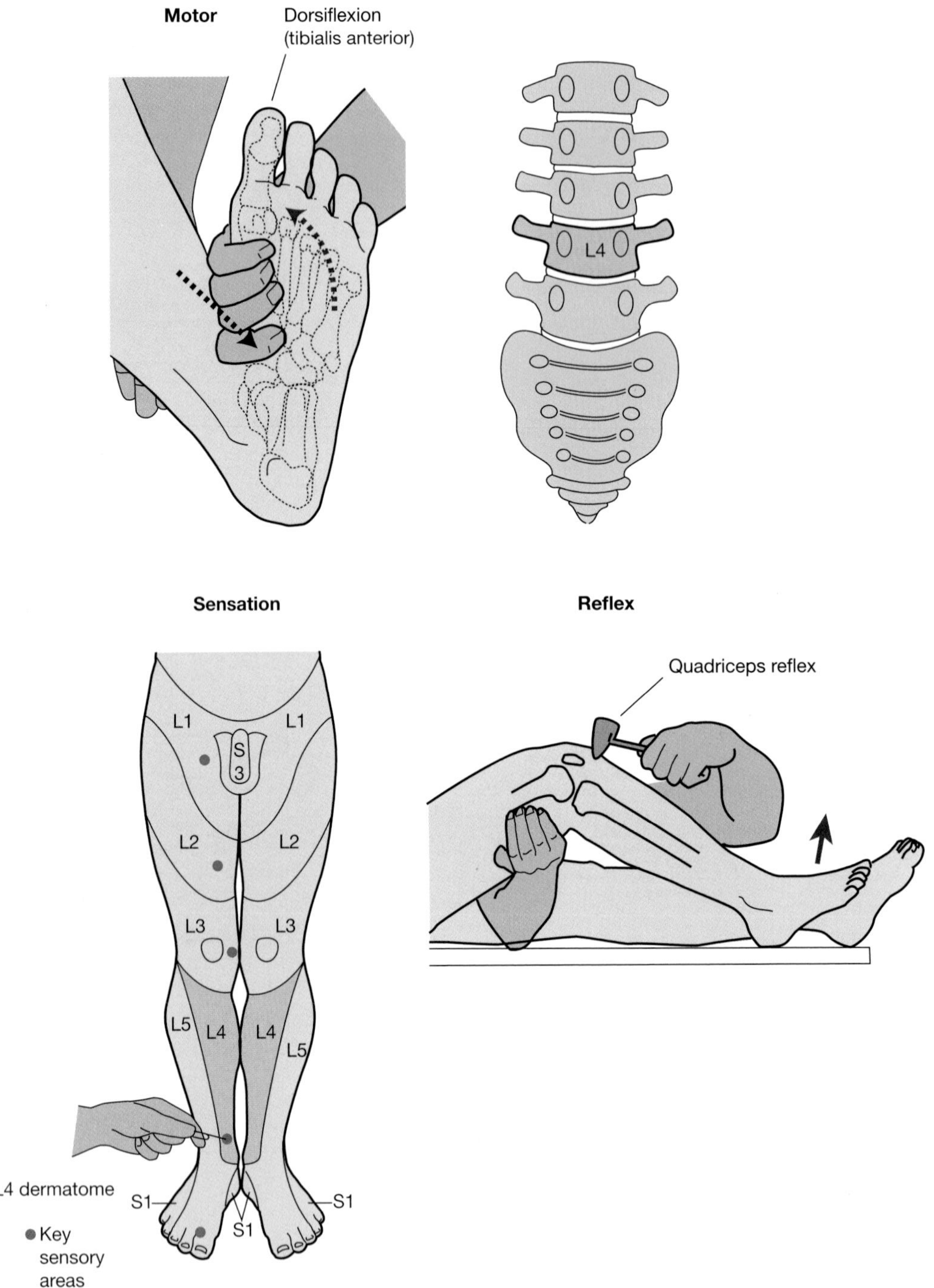

Figure 6.50 The L4 root level.

Reflex Testing

L4 is tested by examining the quadriceps reflex. The patient is sitting with the legs over the edge of the table. Tap the patellar tendon with a reflex hammer and observe for quadriceps contraction and extension of the knee.

The L5 Level

Muscle Testing

The L5 nerve root (Figure 6.51) is best tested by examining the extensor hallucis longus muscle, which extends the great toe's distal phalanx. The patient is

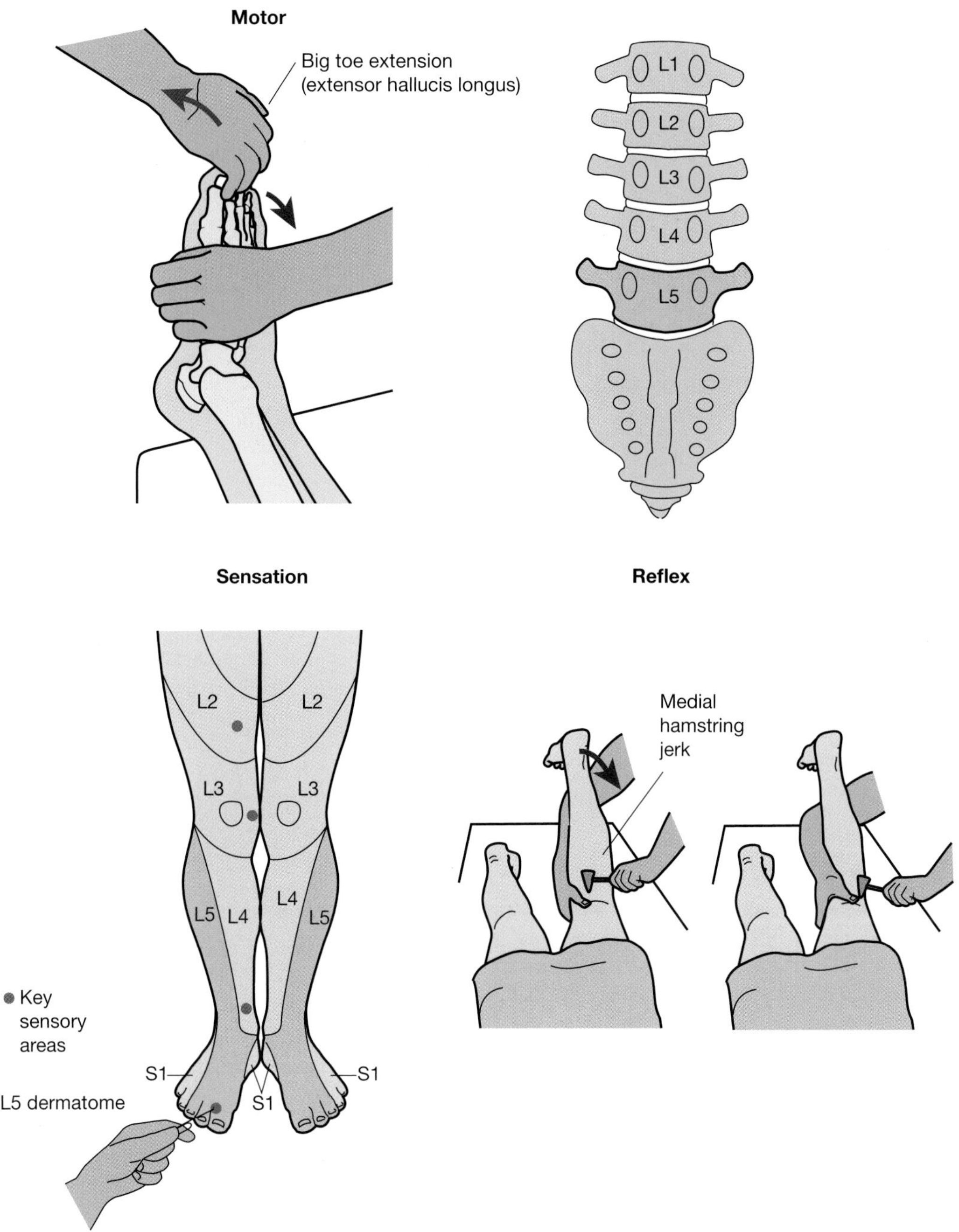

Figure 6.51 The L5 root level.

sitting or supine. Ask the patient to raise the great toe as you apply resistance to the distal phalanx.

Sensation Testing

The L5 dermatome is located on the anterolateral region of the leg and extends onto the dorsal aspect of the foot. The L5 key sensory area is located just proximal to the second web space on the dorsal aspect of the foot.

Reflex Testing

The medial hamstring jerk can be used to test the L5 nerve root. This is performed with the patient supine. Support the lower leg with your forearm and place

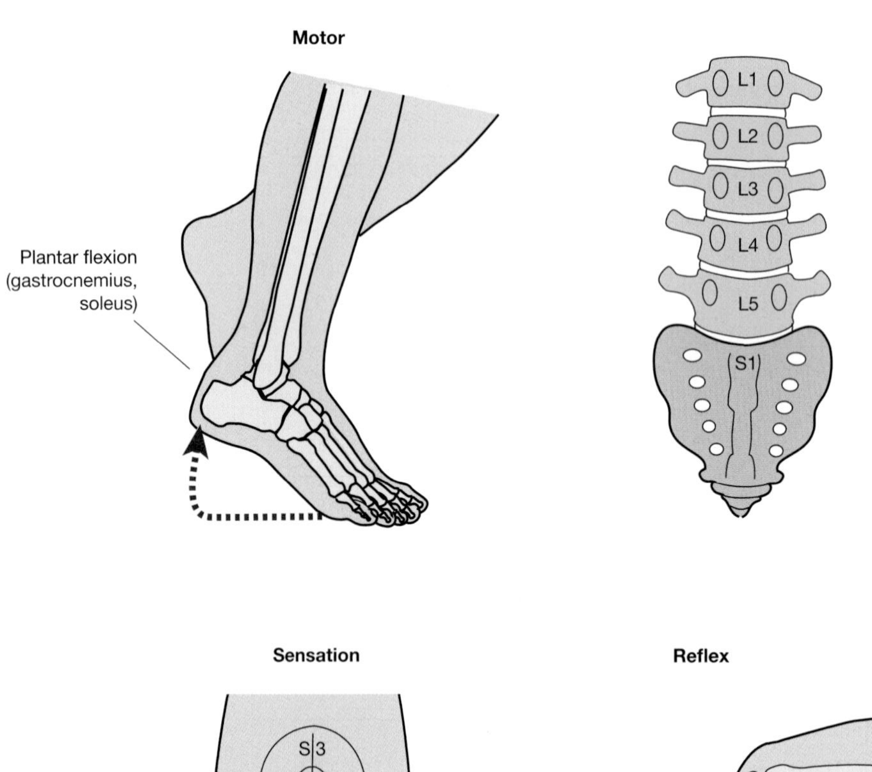

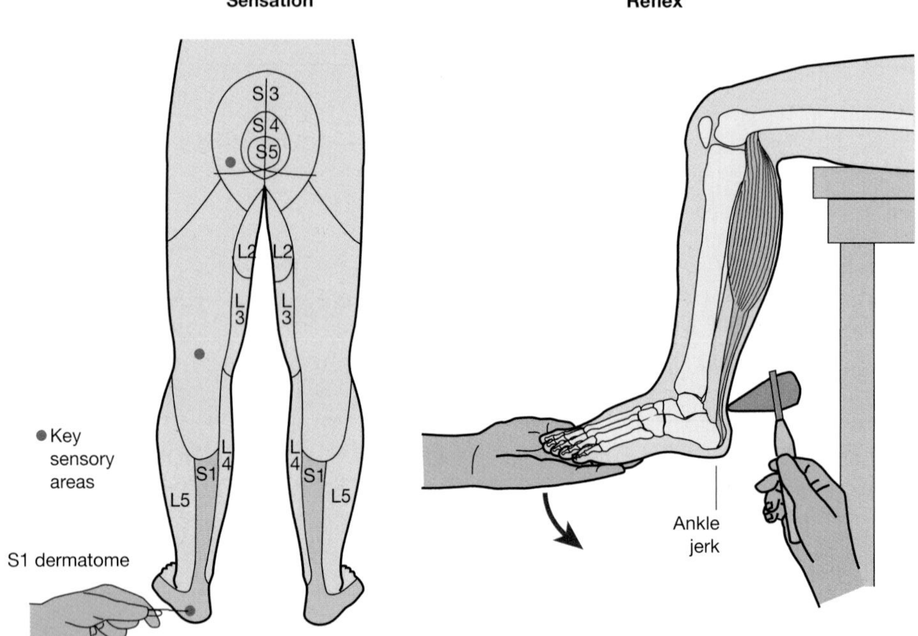

Figure 6.52 The S1 root level.

your thumb over the distal medial hamstring tendon in the popliteal fossa. Tap your thumb with the reflex hammer and observe for knee flexion.

The S1 Level

Muscle Testing

The S1 nerve root (Figure 6.52) is best tested by examining plantar flexion of the foot by the gastrocnemius and soleus muscles. This is performed by asking the patient to stand up on the toes (see p. 410, Figure 13.66 for further information).

Sensation Testing

The S1 dermatome is located on the posterior aspect of the calf and extends distally to the heel and then laterally along the dorsum of the foot. The key sensory area for S1 is located lateral to the insertion of the Achilles tendon on the foot.

Reflex Testing

The S1 nerve root is tested by examining the ankle jerk. The patient is sitting with the legs hanging over the edge of the table. Gently apply light pressure to the plantar aspect of the foot and ask the patient to relax as you tap the Achilles tendon with the reflex hammer. Observe the patient for plantar flexion of the foot and contraction of the calf muscles.

The S2–S5 Levels

Muscle Testing

The S2 through S4 nerve roots supply the urinary bladder and the intrinsic muscles of the foot.

Sensation Testing

The S2 dermatome is located on the posterior aspect of the thigh and extends distally to the mid calf. The key sensory area is located in the center of the popliteal fossa. The S3, S4, and S5 dermatomes are located concentrically around the anus, with the S3 dermatome forming the outermost ring.

The Superficial Reflexes

The upper, middle, and lower abdominal skin reflexes, the cremasteric reflex, and Babinski's reflex are tested to examine the upper motor neurons of the pyramidal tract. These reflexes are exaggerated in upper motor neuron diseases, such as strokes and proximal spinal cord injuries.

Upper Abdominal Skin Reflex (T5–T8)

The patient is in a supine position and relaxed with the arms at the sides and the knees gently flexed (Figure 6.53). The skin over the lower part of the rib cage is stroked with a fingernail or key from laterally to medially. Observe the patient for contraction of the upper abdominal muscles on the same side. You may also note movement of the umbilicus to the same side as the scratch.

Mid-Abdominal Skin Reflex (T9–T11)

Perform the test above, but this time at about the level of the umbilicus (Figure 6.54). The response is similar to that for the upper abdominal skin reflex.

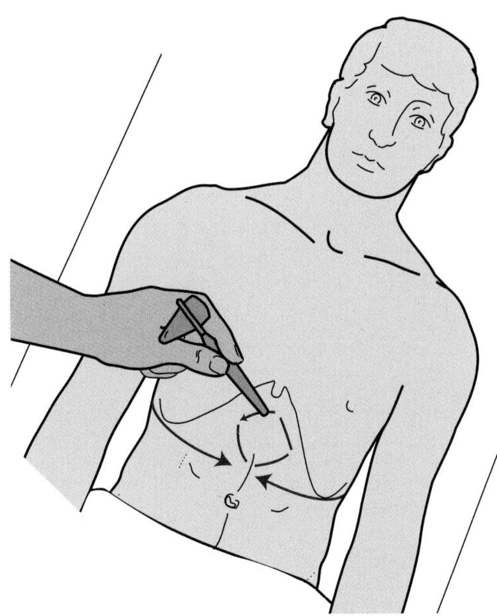

Figure 6.53 The upper abdominal skin reflex (T5–T8).

Lower Abdominal Skin Reflex (T11–T12)

Perform the test as above, but this time over the level of the iliac crest to the hypogastric region (Figure 6.55). Again observe for contraction of the lower abdominal muscles on the same side and movement of the umbilicus in the direction of the scratch.

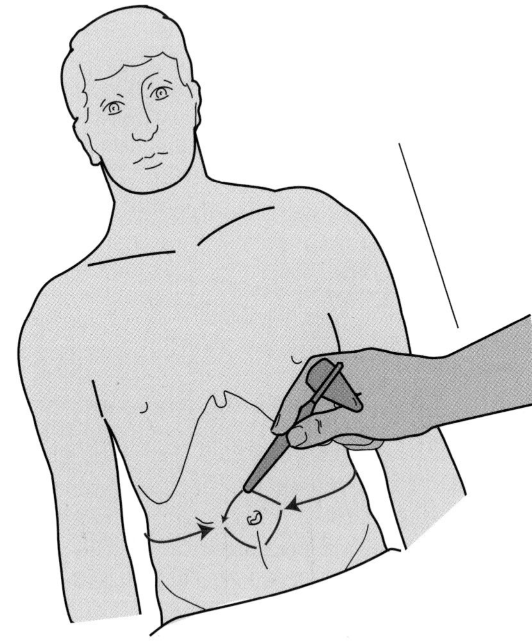

Figure 6.54 The mid-abdominal skin reflex (T9–T11).

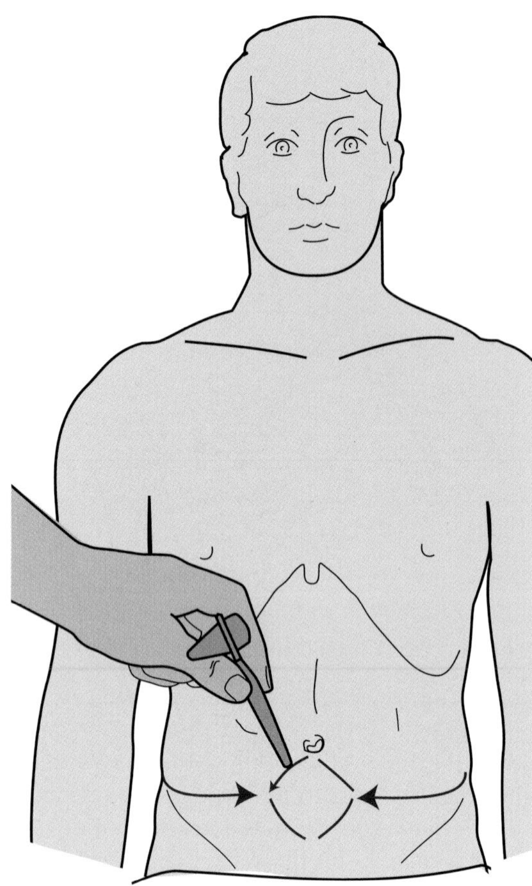

Figure 6.55 The lower abdominal skin reflex (T11, T12).

Cremasteric Reflex (L1–L2)

This test is performed in men only (Figure 6.56). The inner aspect of the thigh is scratched with the handle of the reflex hammer from the pubis downward. You will note an immediate contraction of the scrotum upward on the same side. An irregular or slow rise of the testis on the same side is not a positive response.

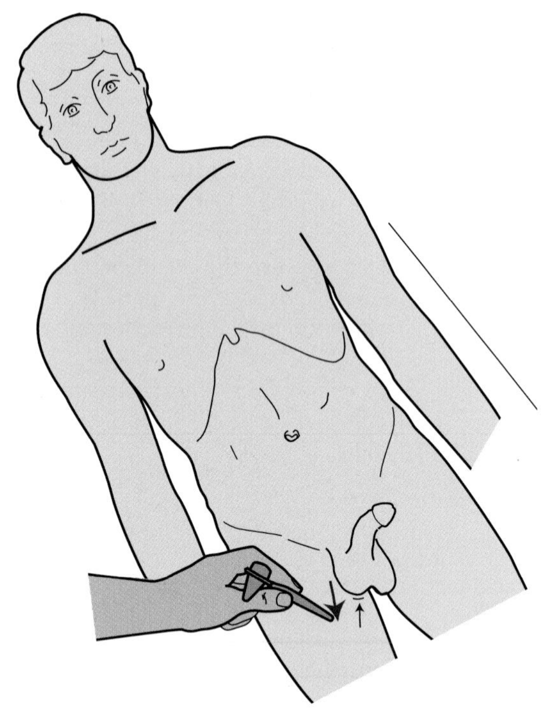

Figure 6.56 The cremasteric reflex. Note that immediate movement of the scrotum upward is a positive test result.

Special Tests

Straight-Leg-Raise (Lasegue) Test

This test is performed to stretch the sciatic nerve and its dural covering proximally. In patients who have a herniated disc at L4–L5 or L5–S1 (Figures 6.57 and 6.58) that is causing pressure on the L5 or S1 nerve roots, stretching the sciatic nerve will frequently cause worsening of the lower-extremity pain or paresthesias or both. The test is performed by asking the patient to lie supine (Figure 6.59). With the patient's knee extended, take the patient's foot by the heel and elevate the entire leg 35–70 degrees from the examining table. As the leg is raised beyond approximately 70 degrees, the sciatic nerve is being completely stretched and causes stress on the lumbar spine. The patient will complain of increased lower-extremity pain or paresthesias on the side that is being examined. This is a positive response on the straight-leg-raising test. If the patient complains of pain down the opposite leg, this is called a positive crossed response on the straight-leg-raising test and is very significant for a herniated disc. The patient may also complain of pain in the posterior part of the thigh, which is due to tightness of the hamstrings.

You can determine whether the pain is caused by tight hamstrings or is of a neurogenic origin by raising the leg up to the point where the patient complains of leg pain, and then lowering the leg slightly (Figure 6.60). This should reduce the pain in the leg. Now passively dorsiflex the patient's foot to increase the stretch on the sciatic nerve. If this maneuver causes pain, the pain is neurogenic in origin. If this movement is painless, the patient's discomfort is caused by hamstring tightness (http://www.youtube.com/watch?v=nWsQWSqfgh4).

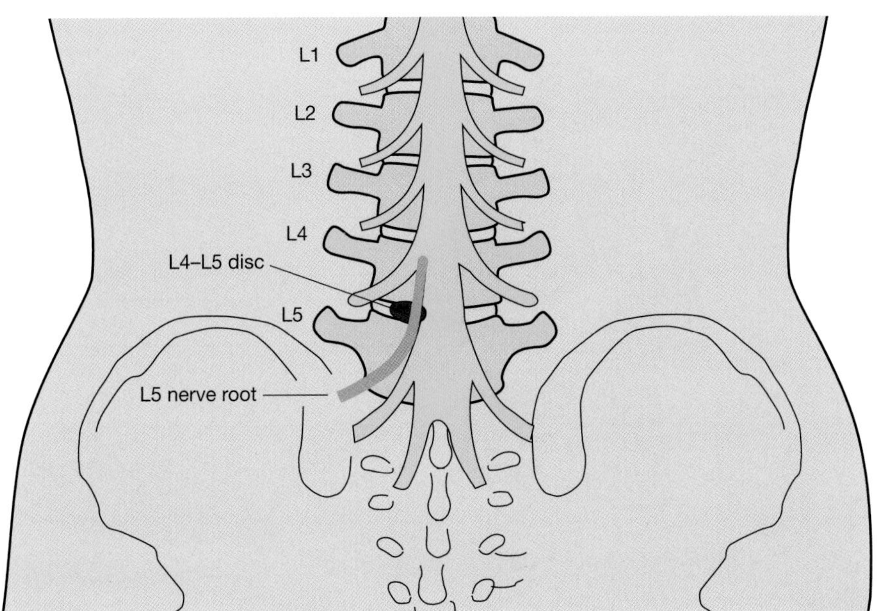

Figure 6.57 A posterolateral herniation of the L4–L5 disc can cause pressure and injury to the L5 nerve root.

Variations on the Straight-Leg-Raise Test

The tibial nerve can be stretched by first dorsiflexing the ankle and everting the foot, and then performing a straight-leg-raise test. The test is abnormal if the patient complains of pain or numbness in the plantar aspect of the foot that is relieved by returning the foot to the neutral position.

The peroneal nerve can be stretched by first plantar flexing the ankle and inverting the foot, and then performing a straight-leg-raise test. The test is abnormal if the patient complains of pain or numbness on the

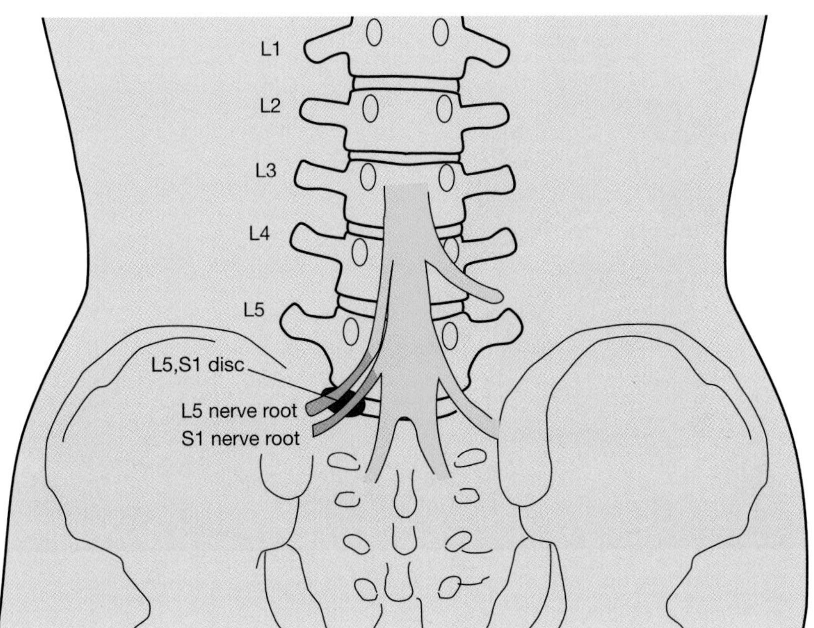

Figure 6.58 A posterolateral herniation of the L5–S1 disc can cause pressure and injury to the L5 and S1 nerve roots.

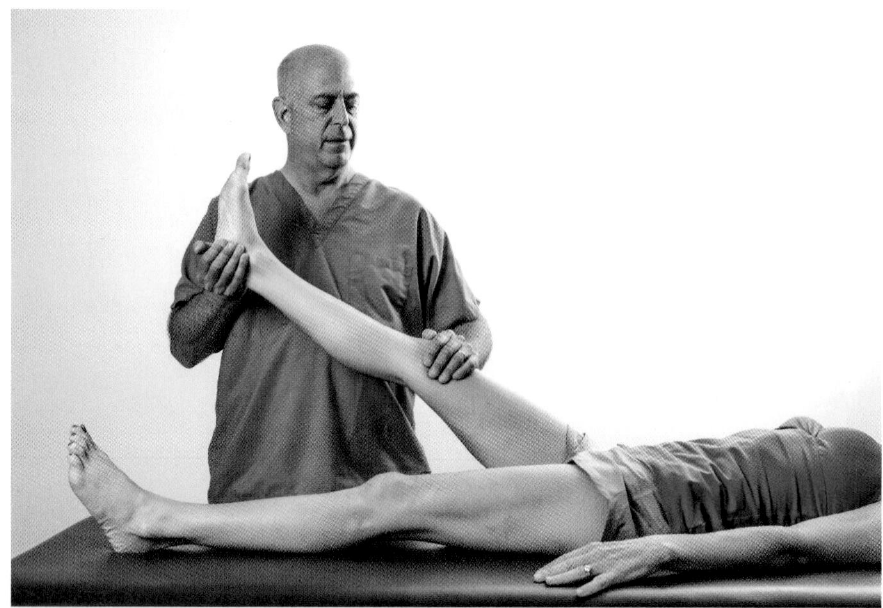

Figure 6.59 Straight-leg-raising test. Between 35 and 70 degrees, the L5 and S1 nerve roots may be stretched against an intervertebral disc. Flexing the hip more than 70 degrees causes stress on the lumbar spine.

dorsum of the foot that is relieved by returning the foot to the neutral position.

The test can be conducted in two ways: either the ankle or the leg can be positioned first. You choose what order to perform the test by first positioning the body part closest to the symptoms. For example, if the pain is in the buttock, use the straight-leg-raise test first and position the ankle afterward. If the pain is in the foot, position the ankle first (Butler, 1991).

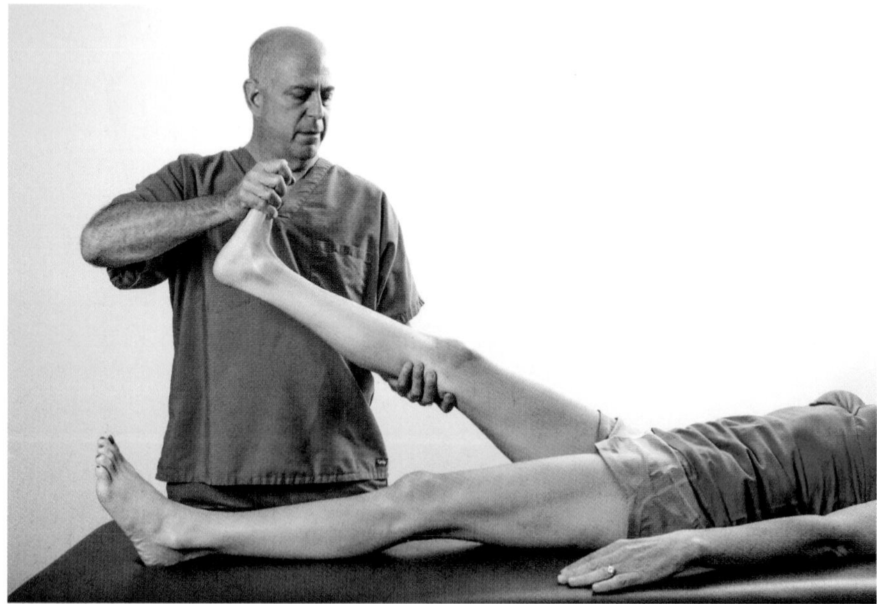

Figure 6.60 By lowering the leg slightly to the point where the patient stops feeling pain or paresthesias in the leg, and then dorsiflexing the ankle, you can determine whether the pain in the leg is due to tight hamstrings or has a neurogenic origin. If the pain is reproduced on dorsiflexion of the ankle after the hamstrings have been relaxed by lowering the leg slightly, the pain has a neurogenic origin.

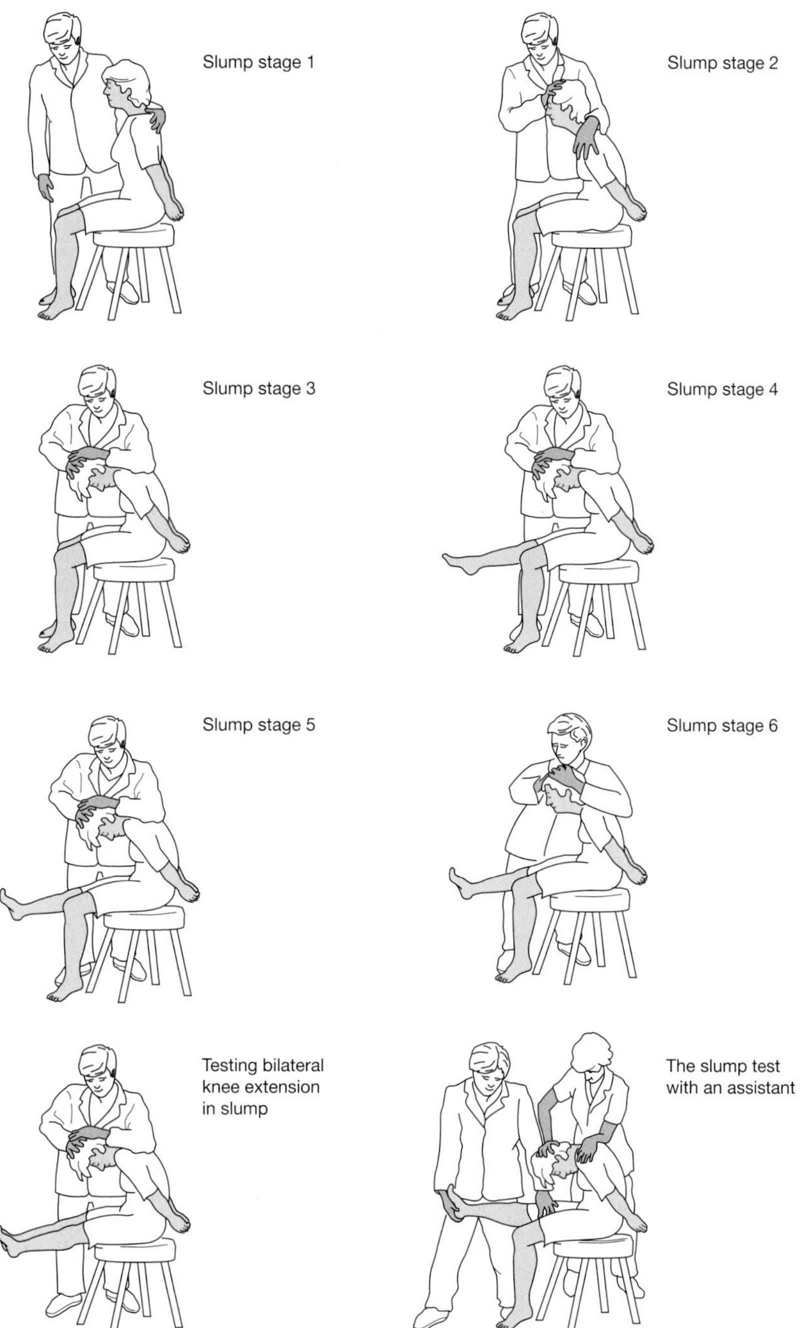

Figure 6.61 The slump test. (Adapted from Butler, 1991.)

The Slump Test

The slump test (Figure 6.61) is a neural tension test which is indicated when the patient complains of spinal symptoms. The test is conducted as follows:

- Patient's position: The patient is sitting with both lower extremities supported with the upper extremities behind the back and the hands clasped.
- Instruct the patient to "sag." Overpressure can be added to increase the degree of flexion. Maintain flexion and then ask the patient to bend the neck toward the chest. Overpressure can be added and the symptoms are reassessed. While maintaining the position, instruct the patient to extend one knee and reassess. Then ask the patient to dorsiflex

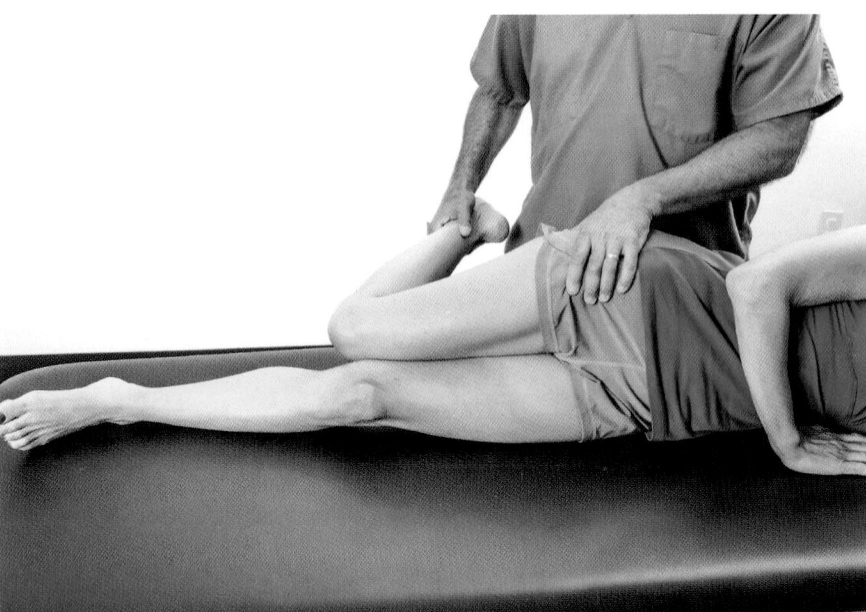

Figure 6.62 The femoral stretch test. The test leg is extended at the hip first, and then the knee is flexed.

the ankle and reassess. Release neck flexion and reassess. Ask the patient to flex the neck again and repeat the process on the other leg. Finally, both legs can be extended simultaneously. The test is terminated when the symptoms are produced.

Normal responses can include pain at T8–T9 in approximately 50% of patients, pain on the posterior aspect of the extended knee, decreased ROM in dorsiflexion, and a release of symptoms and an increase in range when neck flexion is released (Butler, 1991). Worsening of neurological symptoms can be indicative of pathology secondary to tension in the nervous system (http://www.youtube.com/watch?v=nWsQWSqfgh4).

Femoral Nerve Stretch (Prone Knee Bend) Test

This test (Figure 6.62) is useful in determining whether the patient has a herniated disc in the L2–L4 region. The purpose of the test is to stretch the femoral nerve and the L2–L4 nerve roots. The patient is lying on the side, with the test side up. The test can also be performed with the patient lying prone. Support the patient's lower extremity with your arm, cradling the knee and leg. The test leg is extended at the hip and flexed at the knee. If this maneuver causes increased pain or paresthesias in the anterior medial part of the thigh or medial part of the leg, it is likely that the patient has a compressive lesion of the L2, L3, or L4 nerve roots, such as an L2–L3, L3–L4, or L4–L5 herniated disc. You can determine whether the pain is caused by tight rectus femoris or is of neurogenic origin by releasing some of the knee flexion and then extending the hip. If the pain increases with hip extension, it is neurogenic in origin (http://www.youtube.com/watch?v=h5YjDsngTN8).

Hoover Test

This test is useful in identifying a malingering patient who is unable to raise the lower extremity from the examining table while lying supine. The test is performed by taking the patient's heels in your hands while the legs are flat on the table. Ask the patient to raise one of the legs off the table while maintaining the knee in an extended position. Normally, the opposite leg will press downward into your hand. If the patient states that he or she is trying to raise the leg and there is no downward pressure in your opposite hand, it is likely that the patient is malingering. http://www.youtube.com/watch?v=_B3_DcEL84I

Tests to Increase Intrathecal Pressure

These tests are performed in an effort to determine whether the patient's back pain is caused by intrathecal pathology, such as a tumor. By increasing the volume of the epidural veins, the pressure within the intrathecal compartment is elevated.

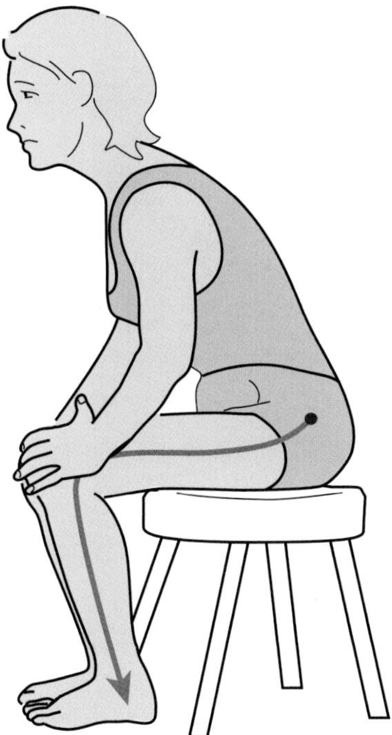

Figure 6.63 Valsalva maneuver.

Valsalva Maneuver

The patient is seated. Ask the patient to take a full breath and then bear down as if he or she were trying to have a bowel movement. This increases intrathecal pressure and may cause the patient to have increased back pain or increased pain down the legs. This is a positive Valsalva maneuver (Figure 6.63).

Sacroiliac Joint Tests

Gaenslen's Sign

This test is used to determine ipsilateral sacroiliac joint disease by stressing the sacroiliac joint. The test is performed with the patient supine on the examining table with both knees flexed and drawn toward the chest. Move the patient toward the edge of the examining table so that one buttock (the test side) is off the table (Figure 6.64). Support the patient carefully and ask him or her to lower the free thigh and leg down to the floor (Figure 6.65). This stresses the sacroiliac joint, and if it is painful, the patient probably has sacroiliac joint dysfunction or pathology (http://www.youtube.com/watch?v=qrt2yPAeT0I).

Patrick's (Fabere) Test

This test (Figure 6.66) is described in more detail in p. 328. It is useful in determining whether there is sacroiliac joint pathology, as well as hip pathology. The patient is supine in a figure-of-four position. Press downward on the patient's bent knee with one hand and with your other hand apply pressure over the iliac bone on the opposite side of the pelvis. This compresses the sacroiliac joint, and if it is painful, the patient has sacroiliac joint pathology. If pressure on the knee alone is painful, this indicates hip pathology on the same side (http://www.youtube.com/watch?v=p1jo3puFDAU).

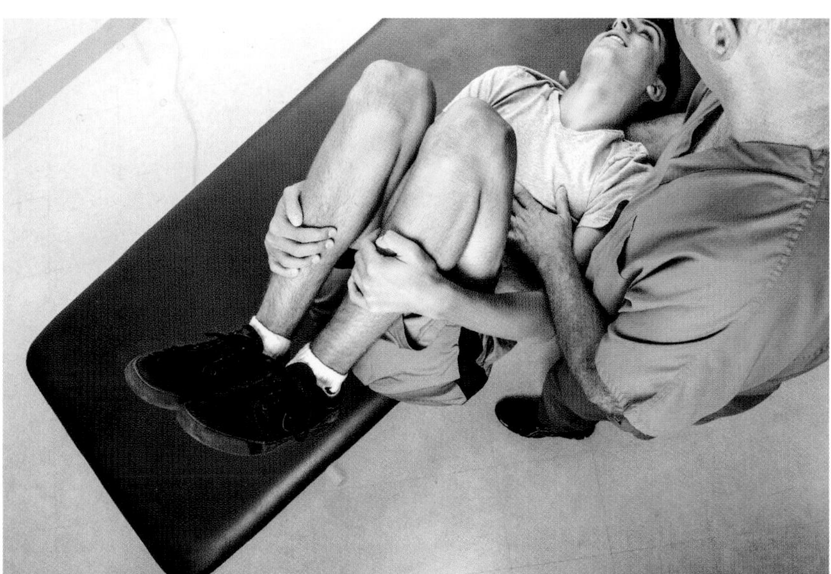

Figure 6.64 Gaenslen's sign. Bring the patient to the edge of the table with the test-side buttock over the edge.

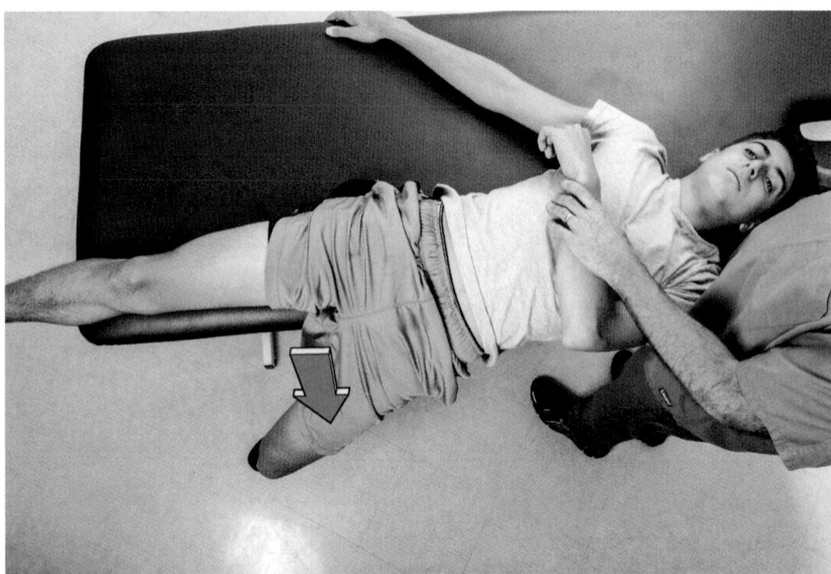

Figure 6.65 Allow the patient's thigh and leg to move downward to stress the sacroiliac joint on that side. Pain on this maneuver reflects sacroiliac joint pathology.

Sacroiliac Distraction–Compression Test

This test is performed to distract the sacroiliac joints. The patient is lying supine and your thumbs are placed over the anterolateral aspect of the iliac crest bilaterally. With both hands, compress the pelvis toward the midline. Place your hands on the medial aspect of the ASIS bilaterally and push laterally. This causes compression of the sacroiliac joints. The test result is positive for sacroiliac joint pathology if the patient complains of pain in the region of the sacroiliac joint (Figure 6.67) (http://www.youtube.com/watch?v=9iHoIjeYqv0).

Spondylolysis Test (Extension in One-Leg Standing)

This test (Figure 6.68) is performed to identify a stress fracture of the pars interarticularis, which may cause spondylolisthesis. Ask the patient to stand on one

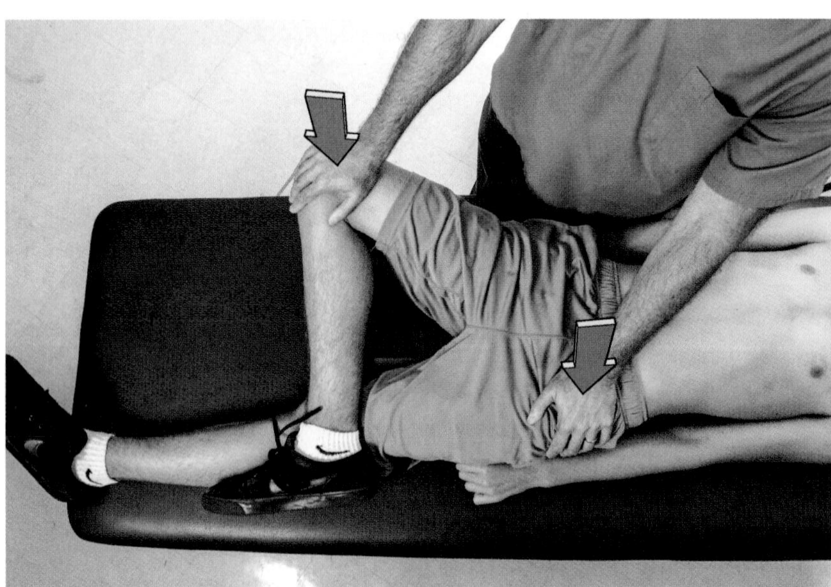

Figure 6.66 Patrick's or Fabere test. The hip is flexed, abducted, externally rotated, and extended.

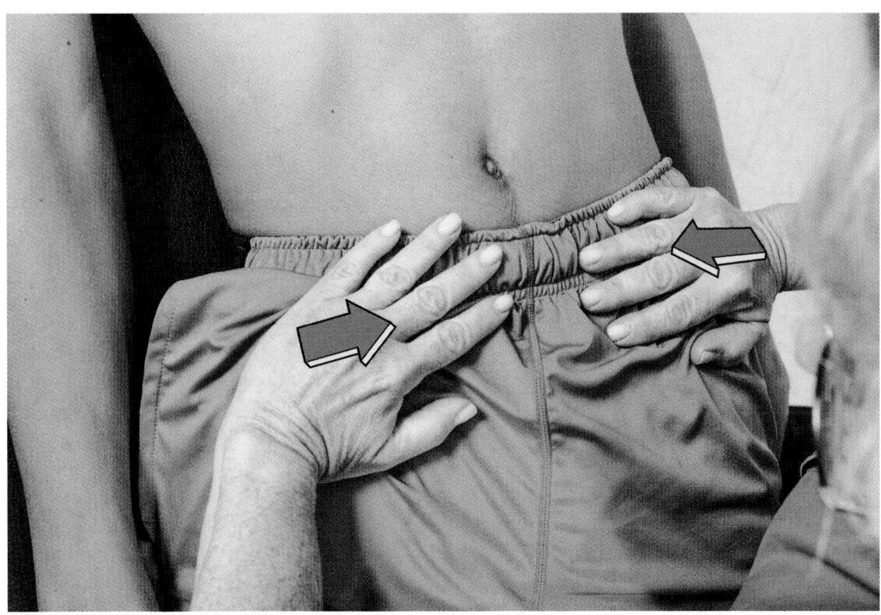

Figure 6.67 The sacroiliac distraction test. By compressing the pelvis medially and distracting the sacroiliac joints, this test determines whether sacroiliac pathology is present.

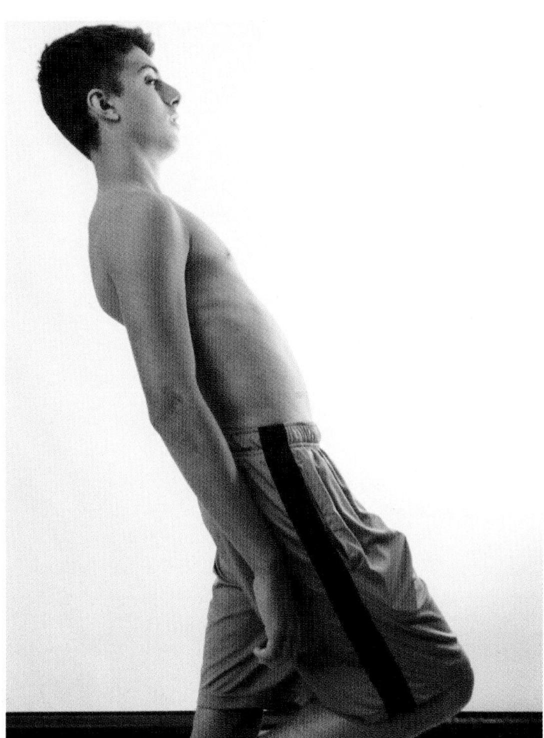

Figure 6.68 Test for spondylolysis (extension in one-leg standing).

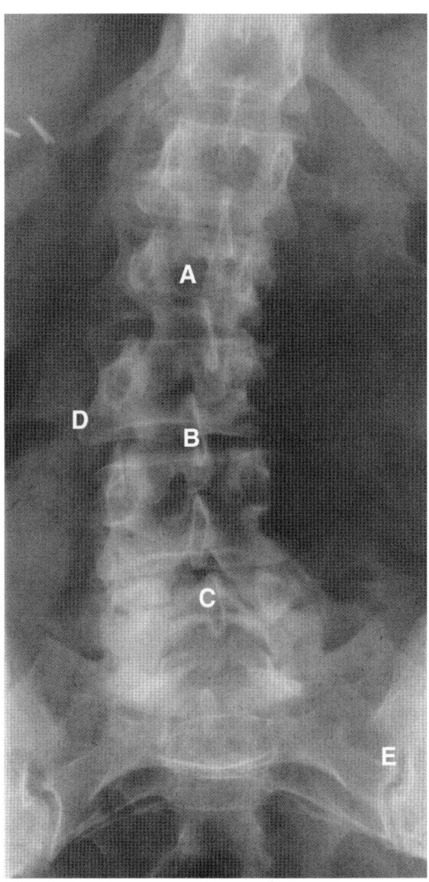

Figure 6.69 Anteroposterior view of the lumbosacral spine.

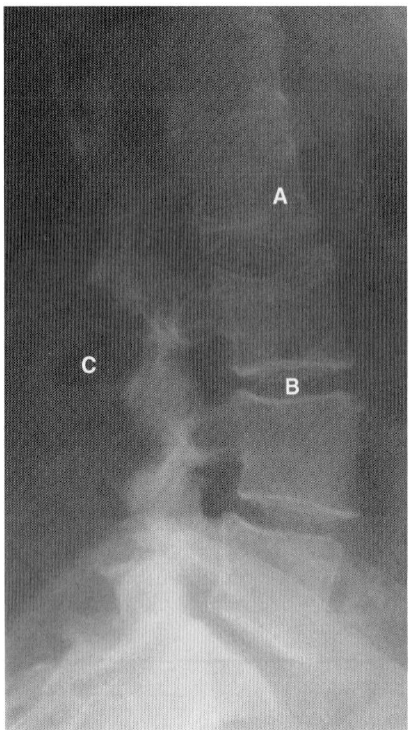

Figure 6.70 Lateral view of the lumbosacral spine.

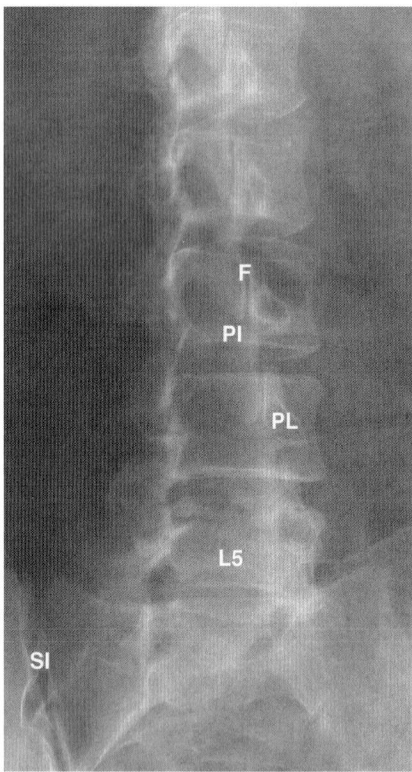

Figure 6.71 Oblique view of the lumbosacral spine.

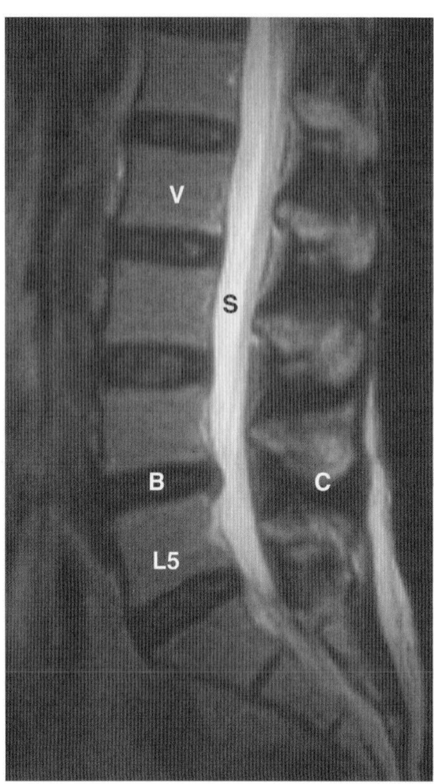

Figure 6.72 Magnetic resonance image of the lumbosacral spine, sagittal view.

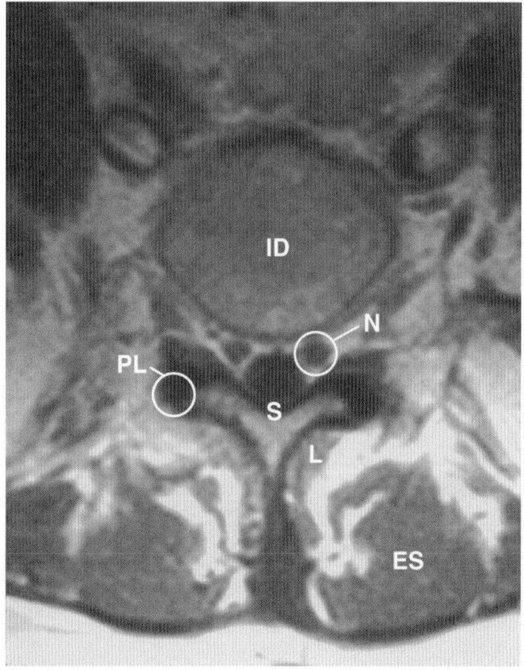

Figure 6.73 Magnetic resonance image of the lumbosacral spine, transverse view.

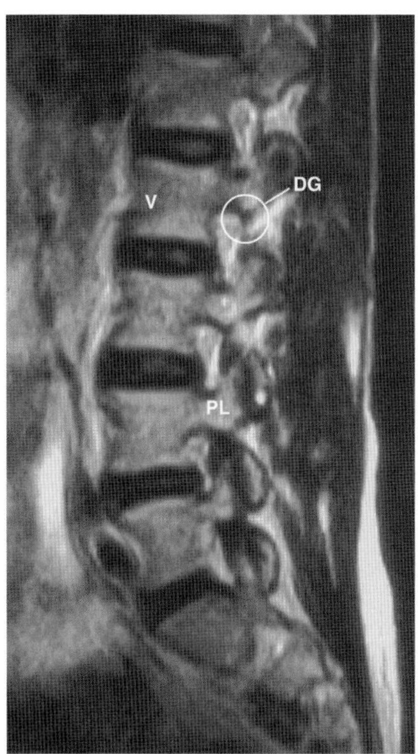

Figure 6.74 Magnetic resonance view of the lumbosacral spine, sagittal view. DG, dorsal root ganglion.

leg and extend the lumbar spine. If the patient complains of pain in the back, the test result is positive and may represent a stress fracture (spondylolysis). This posture stresses the facet joints and will also be painful if there is pathology of the facet joints (http://www.youtube.com/watch?v=ey0y1uWy05s).

Radiological Views

Radiological views are shown in Figures 6.69, 6.70, 6.71, 6.72, 6.73, and 6.74.

A = L2 vertebral body
B = L3/4 disc space
C = Spinous process
D = Transverse process
DG = Dorsal root ganglion of L2 in intervertebral foramen
E = Sacroiliac (S–I) joint
ES = Erector spinae muscle
F = Articular facet
ID = Intervertebral disc
L = Lamina of vertebral arch
L5 = L5 vertebral body
N = Nerve root
PI = Pars interarticularis
PL = Pedicle
S = Spinal canal, cauda equina (C)
A = L2 vertebral body
SI = Sacroiliac joint
V = Vertebral body

PARADIGM FOR A NEOPLASM OF THE LUMBAR SPINE

A 65-year-old bank executive presents with acute pain in the mid low-back region. There has been a slow insidious increasing discomfort for the past 3 months, which has become severe during the past week. There has been no history of trauma. He describes his pain as being worse at night and relieved with standing. His pain is not made worse by coughing, sneezing, or straining during a bowel movement.

On physical examination, the patient appears to be in mild discomfort while seated. He is independent in transfer to and from the examination table and dressing. He has no tension signs with straight leg raise, reflexes are equal bilaterally, as is strength.

There is pain on percussion over the mid lumbar spinous processes. X-rays suggest an absence of the right pedicle of the third lumbar vertebrae.

This paradigm is characteristic of a spinal neoplasm because of:

No history of a trauma
Pain at rest, relieved on standing
No evidence of nerve involvement

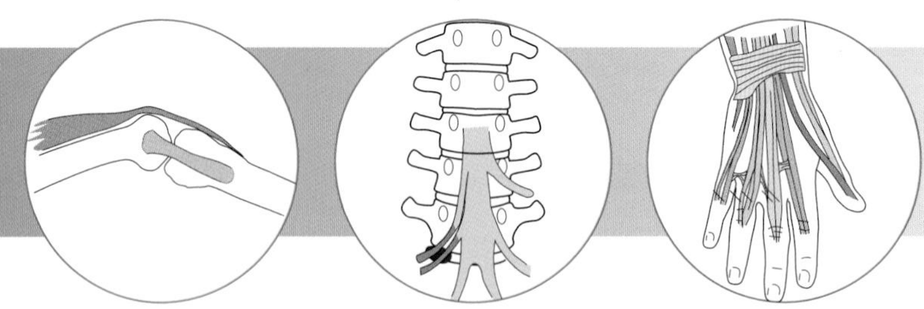

CHAPTER 7

Overview of the Upper Extremity

The usefulness of the human upper extremity is defined by its complex end organ, the hand. The sole purpose of the upper extremity is to position and move the hand in space. The upper extremity is attached to the remainder of the body through only one small articulation, called the sternoclavicular joint. Otherwise, it is suspended from the neck and held fast to the torso by soft tissues (muscles and fasciae). The clavicle, or collarbone, acts as a cantilever, projecting the upper extremity laterally and posteriorly from the midline. The upper extremity gains leverage against the posterior aspect of the thorax by virtue of the broad, flat body of the scapula. The scapula lies flatly on the posterior aspect of the thorax; as such, it is directed approximately 45 degrees forward from the midsagittal plane. At the superolateral corner of the scapula is a shallow socket, the glenoid. The glenoid is aligned perpendicularly to the body of the scapula. The socket faces obliquely forward and laterally. The spherical head of the humerus is normally directed posteromedially (retroverted 40 degrees) so as to be centered within the glenoid socket. The result is that the shoulder is a highly mobile, but extremely unstable configuration that permits a tremendous degree of freedom of movement in space (Figure 7.1).

Midway along the upper extremity, there is a complex modified hinge articulation called the elbow. As will be discussed, the elbow accommodates flexion as well as rotation movements of the forearm. Unlike the shoulder, the elbow has a much more stable configuration. The primary purpose of the elbow is

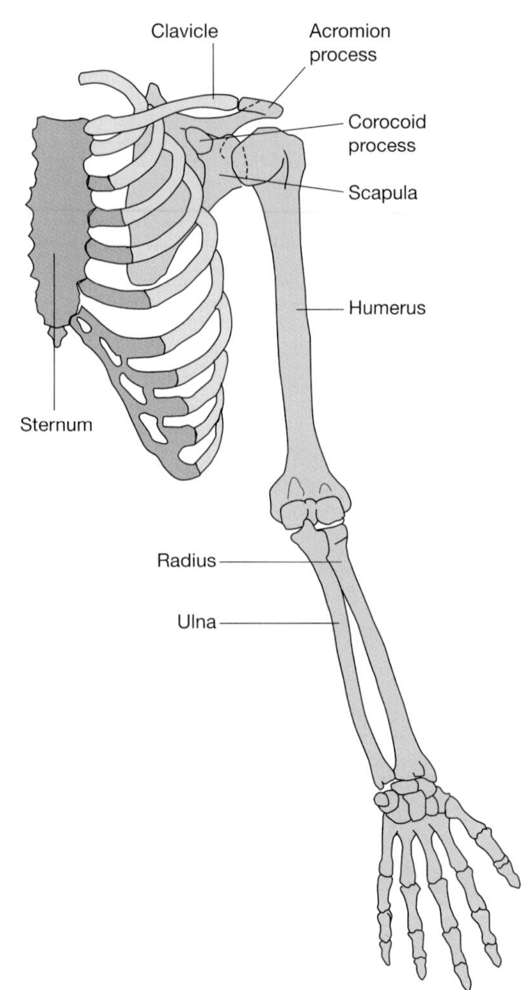

Figure 7.1 Overview of the upper extremity.

Musculoskeletal Examination, Fourth Edition. Jeffrey M. Gross, Joseph Fetto and Elaine Rosen.

Companion website: www.wiley.com/go/musculoskeletalexam

to approximate the hand to other parts of the body, particularly the head.

At the terminus of the upper extremity is the hand. It is connected to the upper extremity by a complex hinge articulation termed the wrist. The wrist serves to modify the grosser movements of the elbow and shoulder. The importance of the wrist and complexity of the hand can best be appreciated when its function has been compromised. There is no single tool or appliance that can duplicate the function of the hand. The disproportionate amount of motor cortex that the brain has allocated to control hand movements emphasizes both the hand's importance and its complexity.

CHAPTER 8

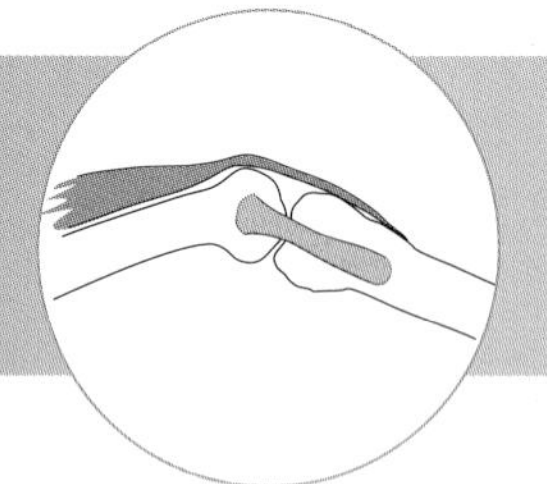

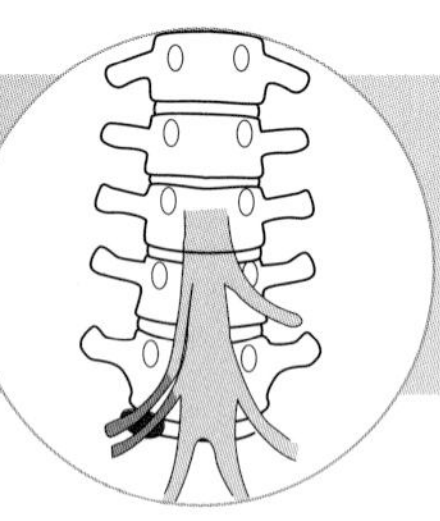

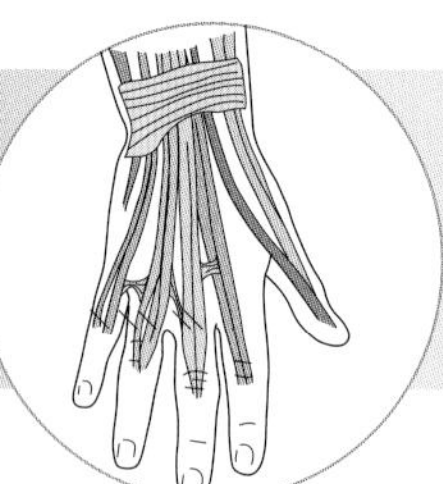

The Shoulder

FURTHER INFORMATION

Please refer to Chapter 2 for an overview of the sequence of a physical examination. For purposes of length and to avoid having to repeat anatomy more than once, the palpation section appears directly after the section on subjective examination and before any section on testing, rather than at the end of each chapter. The order in which the examination is performed should be based on your experience and personal preference as well as the presentation of the patient.

Functional Anatomy

The shoulder contains four articulations: the sternoclavicular, the acromioclavicular, the scapulothoracic, and the glenohumeral.

The shoulder girdle facilitates the placement of the hand in space. It accomplishes this through the complementary movements of the scapula on the thorax and the glenohumeral articulation. This complementary movement is termed the *scapulohumeral rhythm.*

Historically, movements of the shoulder girdle have been subdivided into the specific responsibilities of each of the shoulder's four articulations. However, such an artificial fragmentation of shoulder function is not an accurate portrayal of reality. In fact, under normal circumstances, the articulations work in synchrony, not isolation. The corollary of this fact is that the pathology of any single articulation will have significant adverse consequences on the functioning of the other remaining articulations and the entire upper extremity.

The entire upper extremity is attached to the torso through the small sternoclavicular articulation. It affords limited movement but must withstand significant loads. Therefore, it is not unusual to observe osteoarthritic degeneration of this joint, associated with significant soft-tissue swelling and osteophyte formation.

The acromioclavicular joint, like the sternoclavicular, is a small synovial articulation that has limited range of motion and frequently undergoes osteoarthritic degeneration. More importantly than in the case of the sternoclavicular joint, enlargement of the acromioclavicular articulation has significant adverse consequences on shoulder movement and integrity.

The scapulothoracic articulation is a nonsynovial articulation. It is composed of the broad, flat, triangular scapula overlying the thoracic cage and is separated from the thoracic cage by a large bursa. Its stability is strictly dependent on the soft-tissue attachments of the scapula to the thorax. The plane of the scapula lies 45 degrees forward from the midcoronal plane of the body. Thus, the scapulothoracic articulation serves to supplement the large ball-and-socket articulation of the true shoulder joint.

The glenohumeral joint, or shoulder joint, is a shallow ball-and-socket articulation. As such, it enjoys tremendous freedom of movement. However, this freedom comes at a cost. It is inherently an unstable

Musculoskeletal Examination, Fourth Edition. Jeffrey M. Gross, Joseph Fetto and Elaine Rosen.

Companion website: www.wiley.com/go/musculoskeletalexam

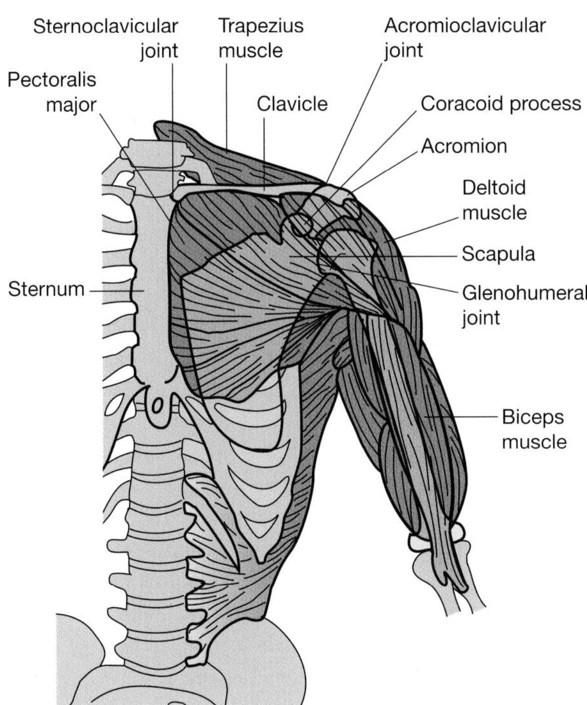

Figure 8.1 Overview of the shoulder showing the importance of the soft tissues in maintaining the round humeral head in the flattened glenoid process of the scapula. The other joints of the shoulder are also shown.

joint. The glenoid is so shallow that the ball (humeral head), if unprotected, can easily slip inferiorly out of the socket, creating a shoulder dislocation.

Normally, this is prevented by soft tissues (Figure 8.1). Anteriorly, there is the subscapularis tendon. Superiorly, there are the tendons of the supraspinatus and long head of the biceps. Posteriorly are the tendons of the infraspinatus and teres minor muscles. These tendons surround the humeral head, forming a "cuff," and the corresponding muscles are responsible for rotating the humeral head within the glenoid socket. Hence, they are referred to as the *rotator cuff*. The purpose of the rotator cuff is to stabilize the humeral head within the glenoid socket, thereby creating a stable pivot point on which the larger shoulder muscles (deltoid and pectoralis major) can efficiently exert force.

The rotator cuff does not extend to the inferior (axillary) aspect of the glenohumeral articulation. Here, the only soft-tissue connection between the ball and socket is the capsular ligaments, the strongest of which is the inferior glenohumeral ligament. This ligament is important because as the arm moves overhead, abduction and external rotation of the humerus

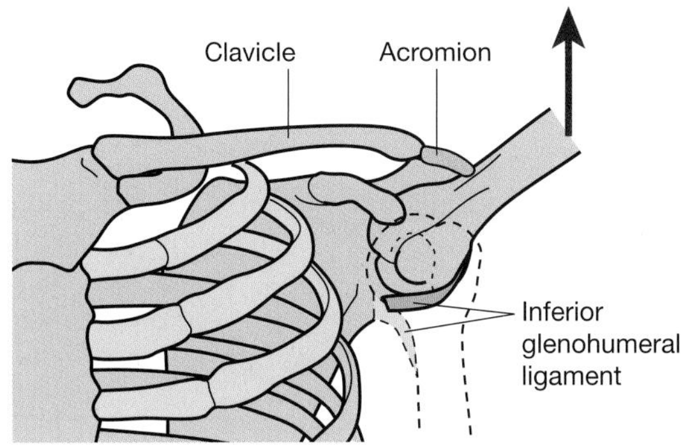

Figure 8.2 The inferior glenohumeral ligament prevents further inferior movement of the humeral head as the arm abducts.

are limited by the acromion process (Figure 8.2). When the shaft of the humerus reaches the acromion, a fulcrum is created. Further attempts to abduct the arm will force the humeral head out of the glenoid socket inferiorly against the glenohumeral ligament. If the tolerance of the inferior capsular ligament to resist this movement is exceeded, either due to the magnitude of the acute force being applied or due to the inherent stretchability of a genetically determined lax ligament, a classic anterior–inferior shoulder dislocation will result (Figure 8.3). The consequent elongation of the inferior glenohumeral ligament is irreversible. Unless corrected, the glenohumeral joint becomes vulnerable to repeat episodes of instability with movement of the arm above the shoulder height (apprehension sign).

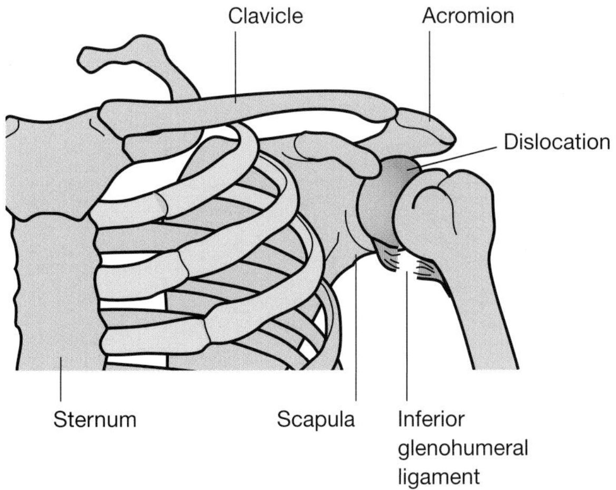

Figure 8.3 Inferior dislocation of the glenohumeral articulation, with attenuation of the inferior glenohumeral ligament.

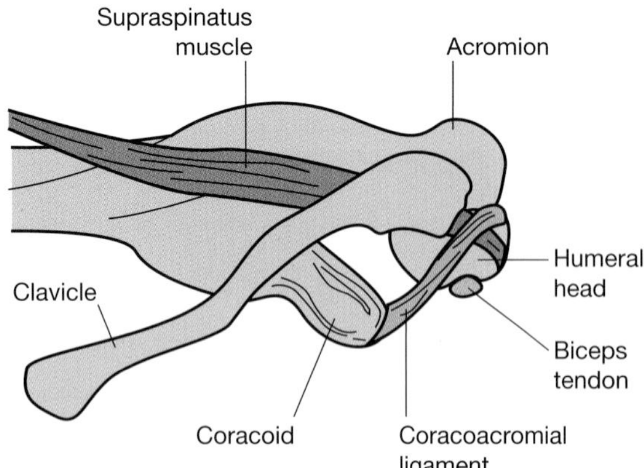

Figure 8.4 Superior view of the shoulder, showing the acromioclavicular joint and the coracoacromial ligament overlying the humeral head.

The superior aspect of the shoulder is protected by the acromioclavicular bony arch and the coracoacromial ligament (Figure 8.4). The latter represents the fibrous vestigial remnant of the coracoacromial bony arch of quadripeds. Beneath this protective roof passes the superior portion of the rotator cuff, the supraspinatus tendon, and the long head of the biceps tendon. The biceps is the only part of the rotator cuff that depresses the humeral head. As the humerus moves, these tendons slide through a space defined by the bony-ligamentous roof above and the humeral head below (Figure 8.5). To reduce friction, there is a bursal sac, the subacromial bursa, positioned between the tendons below and the roof above.

The subacromial space can be absolutely narrowed by osteophytes extending inferiorly from the clavicle, acromion, or acromioclavicular joint. Swelling of the soft tissues within the space (i.e., bursitis and tendinitis) can also relatively narrow the space. These soft-tissue swellings may arise as the result of acute injuries or chronic overuse syndromes. In either case, the result is insufficient space for the free passage of the rotator cuff beneath the coracoacromial arch. This creates a painful pinching of the tissues between the roof above and the humeral head below. This condition has been termed an *impingement syndrome*. The resulting pain from this condition can lead not only to a chronically disabling condition, with erosion of the rotator cuff tissues, but also to an attempt to compensate for the loss of glenohumeral motion with scapulothoracic movement. Excessive stress can be created on the cervical spine due to the muscular effort of the proximal back and shoulder muscles to compensate for the lack of glenohumeral movement.

When the biceps tendon has become chronically inflamed by either frictional wear beneath the acromial arch or chronic tendinitis, it is at risk of rupture. If this occurs, the humeral head depression is compromised. The humerus will then ride superiorly within the glenoid, increasing pressure between the humeral head and the acromial arch. This will also prevent clearance of the greater tuberosity of the humerus beneath the acromion during abduction and will result in limited shoulder motion. The resultant cycle of pain and guarded range of motion produces an increasing pattern of upper-extremity dysfunction.

Shoulder movement therefore represents a complex interplay of multiple articulations and soft tissues, which must be recognized and appreciated for their delicate interrelationship.

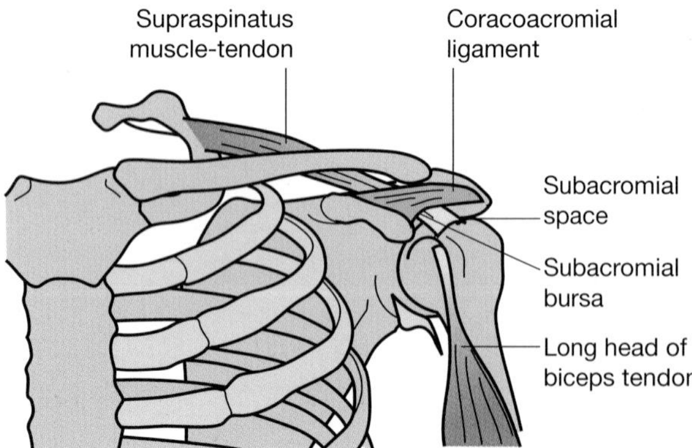

Figure 8.5 The subacromial space is defined superiorly by the acromioclavicular bony arch and the coracoacromial ligament. Inferiorly, it is defined by the humeral head. Within this space lies the subacromial bursa and the tendons of the supraspinatus and long head of the biceps muscles.

Observation

Note the manner in which the patient is sitting in the waiting room. Notice how the patient postures the upper extremity. Is the arm relaxed at the side or is the patient cradling it for protection? How willing is the patient to use the upper extremity? Will the patient extend the arm to you to shake your hand? Pain may be altered by changes in position. Therefore, it is important to watch the patient's facial expression, which may give you insight into the patient's pain level.

Observe the patient as he or she assumes the standing position and note their posture. Pay particular attention to the position of the head and cervical and thoracic spine. Note the height of both shoulders and their relative positions. Once the patient starts to ambulate, observe whether he or she is willing to swing their arms, as pain or loss of motion can limit arm swing. Once the patient is in the examination room, ask him or her to disrobe. Observe the ease with which the patient uses the upper extremities and the rhythm of the movements. Observe for symmetry of bony structures. From the front, observe the clavicles. An uneven contour may be present secondary to a healed fracture. Follow the clavicle and determine whether the acromioclavicular and sternoclavicular joints are at equal heights. From the back, observe the scapulae and determine whether they are equidistant from the spine and lying flat on the rib cage. Is one scapula structurally higher, as in Sprengel's deformity (congenital high scapula)? Is a visible subluxation present at the glenohumeral joint? Notice the size and contour of the deltoid and compare both sides for atrophy or hypertrophy.

Subjective Examination

The glenohumeral joint is a flexible joint held by muscles that allow a wide range of movements. The shoulder is non-weight-bearing; therefore, problems are most commonly related to overuse syndromes, inflammation, and trauma. You should inquire about the nature and location of the patient's complaints as well as their duration and intensity. Note if the pain travels below the elbow. This may be an indication that the pain is originating from the cervical spine. The behavior of the pain during the day and night should also be addressed. Is the patient able to sleep on the involved shoulder or is he or she awakened during the night? Is the patient able to lie down to sleep or is he or she forced to sleep in a reclining chair? This will give you information regarding the patient's reaction to changes in position, activity, and swelling.

You want to determine the patient's functional limitations. Question the patient regarding the use of the upper extremity. Is the patient able to comb his hair, fasten her bra, bring his hand to his mouth to eat, or remove her jacket? Can the patient reach for objects that are above shoulder height? Can the patient lift or carry? Does the patient regularly participate in any vigorous sports activity that would stress the shoulder? What is the patient's occupation? Are there job-related tasks that involve excessive or improper shoulder use?

If the patient reports a history of trauma, it is important to note the mechanism of injury. The direction of the force and the activity being participated in at the time of the injury contribute to your understanding of the resulting problem and help you to better direct your examination. The degree of pain, swelling, and disability noted at the time of the trauma and within the first 24 hours should be noted. Does the patient have a previous history of the same type of injury or other injury to the same location?

The patient's disorder may be related to age, gender, ethnic background, body type, static and dynamic posture, occupation, leisure activities, hobbies, and general activity level. Therefore, it is important to inquire about any change in daily routine and any unusual activities in which the patient has participated.

The location of the symptoms may give you some insight as to the etiology of the complaints. Pain located over the lateral part of the shoulder may be referred from C5. The temporomandibular joint and elbow can also refer pain to the shoulder. In addition, particular attention should be paid to the possibility of referred pain from the viscera, especially the heart, gallbladder, and pancreas. (Please refer to Box 2.1, see page 15 for typical questions for the subjective examination.)

Gentle Palpation

The palpatory examination is started with the patient in the supine position. You should first examine for areas of localized effusion, discoloration, birthmarks, open sinuses or drainage, incisions, bony contours, muscle girth and symmetry, and skinfolds. You should not have to use deep pressure to determine areas of tenderness or malalignment. It is important to use a firm but gentle pressure; this will enhance your palpatory skills. If you have a sound basis of cross-sectional anatomy, you will not need to physically penetrate through several layers of tissue to have a good sense of the underlying structures. Remember that if you increase the patient's pain at this point in the examination, the patient will be very reluctant to allow you to continue, and his or her ability to move may become more limited.

Palpation is best performed with the patient in a relaxed position. Although palpation may be performed with the patient standing, the sitting position is preferred for ease of shoulder examination. While

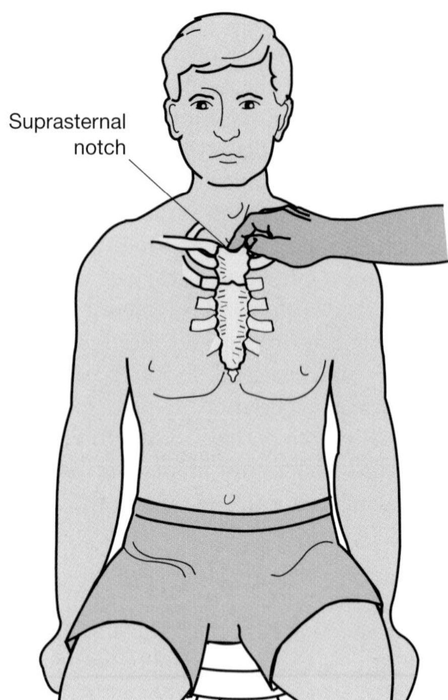

Figure 8.6 Palpation of the suprasternal notch.

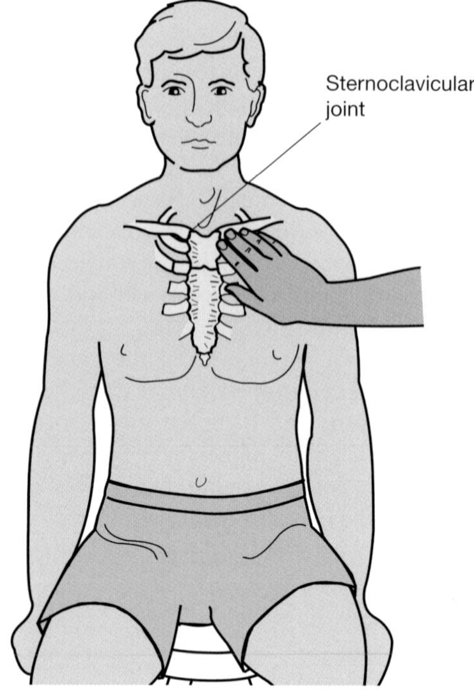

Figure 8.7 Palpation of the sternoclavicular joint.

locating the bony landmarks, you should pay attention to areas of increased or decreased temperature and moisture to identify areas of acute or chronic inflammation.

Anterior View

Bony Structures

Suprasternal Notch

Stand facing the seated patient and use your middle or index finger to locate the triangular notch between the two clavicles. This is the suprasternal notch (Figure 8.6).

Sternoclavicular Joint

Move your fingers slightly superiorly and laterally from the center of the suprasternal notch until you feel the joint line between the sternum and the clavicle (Figure 8.7). The joints should be examined simultaneously to allow for comparison of heights and location. A superior and medial displacement of the clavicle may be indicative of dislocation of the sternoclavicular joint. You can get a better sense of the exact location and stability of the sternoclavicular joint by having the patient shrug the shoulders while you palpate the joint and the upward motion of the clavicles.

Clavicle

Continue to move laterally from the sternoclavicular joint along the superiorly and anteriorly curved bony surface of the clavicle. The bony surface should be smooth and continuous. Any area of increased prominence, sense of motion, crepitus, or pain along the shaft may be indicative of a fracture. In addition, the platysma muscle passes over the clavicle as it courses up the neck and can be palpated by having the patient strongly pull the corners of the mouth in a downward direction (Figure 8.8). The supraclavicular lymph nodes are found on the superior surface of the clavicle, lateral to the sternocleidomastoid. If you notice any enlargement or tenderness, an infection or malignancy should be suspected.

Acromioclavicular Joint

Continue to palpate laterally along the clavicle from the convexity to where it becomes concave to the most lateral aspect of the clavicle, just medial to the acromion. You will be able to palpate the acromioclavicular joint line where the clavicle is slightly

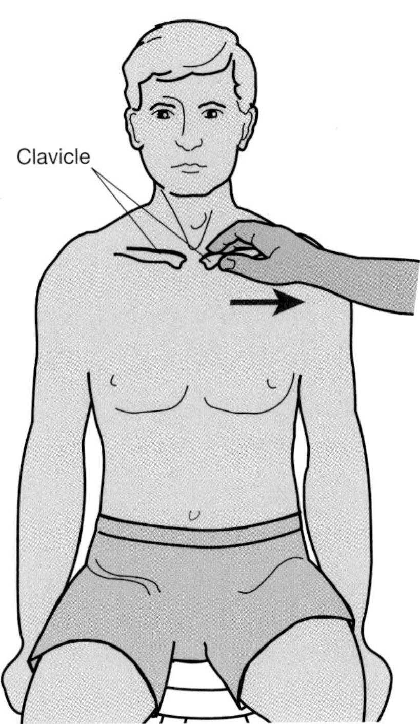

Figure 8.8 Palpation of the clavicle.

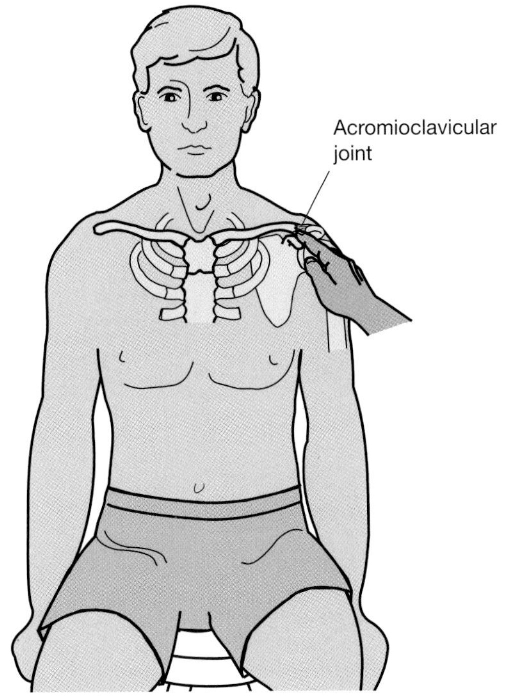

Figure 8.9 Palpation of the acromioclavicular joint.

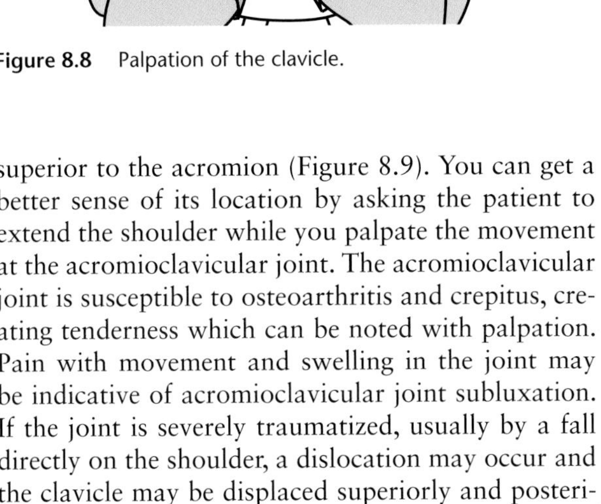
superior to the acromion (Figure 8.9). You can get a better sense of its location by asking the patient to extend the shoulder while you palpate the movement at the acromioclavicular joint. The acromioclavicular joint is susceptible to osteoarthritis and crepitus, creating tenderness which can be noted with palpation. Pain with movement and swelling in the joint may be indicative of acromioclavicular joint subluxation. If the joint is severely traumatized, usually by a fall directly on the shoulder, a dislocation may occur and the clavicle may be displaced superiorly and posteriorly. The acromioclavicular joint is one area in which the pain is felt locally and is not referred.

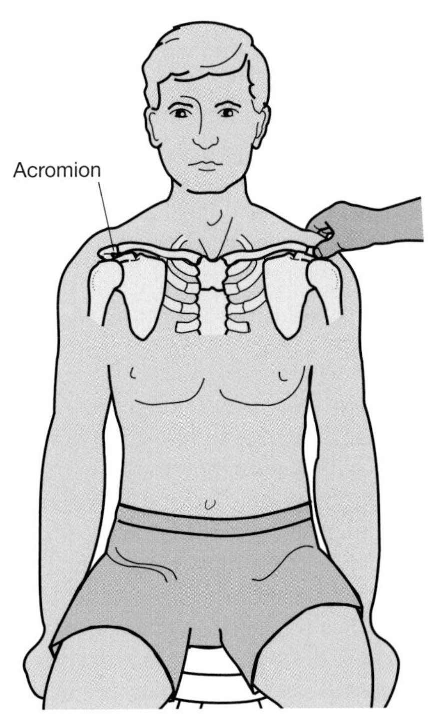

Figure 8.10 Palpation of the acromion process.

Acromion Process

Palpate past the lateral aspect of the acromioclavicular joint and palpate the broad, flattened surface of the acromion between your index finger and thumb (Figure 8.10).

Greater Tuberosity of the Humerus

Allow your fingers to follow to the most lateral aspect of the acromion and they will drop off inferiorly onto the greater tubercle of the humerus (Figure 8.11).

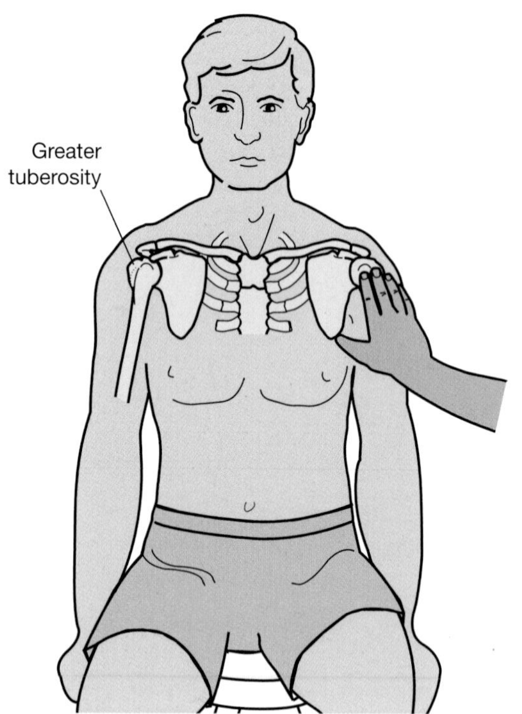

Figure 8.11 Palpation of the greater tubercle of the humerus.

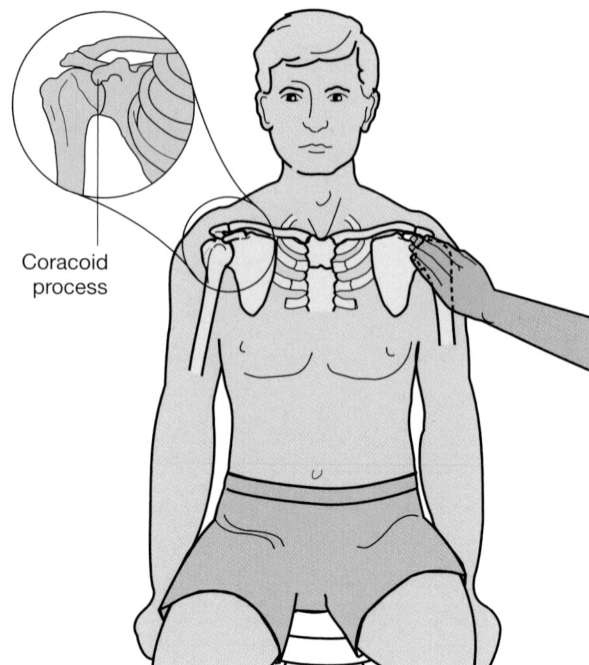

Figure 8.12 Palpation of the coracoid process.

Coracoid Process

Move your fingers on a diagonal inferiorly and medially from the acromioclavicular joint. Gently place your middle finger deep into the deltopectoral triangle until you locate the bony prominence of the coracoid process, which is normally tender to palpation (Figure 8.12). The coracoid process is the attachment of the pectoralis minor, the coracobrachialis, and the short head of the biceps.

Bicipital Groove

Have the patient position the upper extremity at the side so that the arm is in mid-position between internal and external rotation, and the forearm is in mid-position between pronation and supination. Move your fingers laterally from the coracoid process, onto the lesser tubercle of the humerus, and finally into the bicipital groove. The groove can be difficult to palpate if the patient has a hypertrophied deltoid. It may be helpful to locate the medial and lateral epicondyles of the humerus, making sure that they are in the frontal plane. Find the midpoint of the humerus and trace proximally to find the bicipital groove. The groove contains the tendon of the long head of the biceps and its synovial sheath and can therefore be tender to palpation. Ask the patient to internally rotate the arm and you will then feel your finger roll out of the groove and onto the greater tubercle of the humerus (Figure 8.13).

Soft-Tissue Structures

Sternocleidomastoid

To facilitate palpating the sternocleidomastoid muscle, have the patient bend the neck toward the side you are palpating and simultaneously rotate away. This movement allows the muscle to be more prominent and therefore easier to locate. Palpate the distal attachments on the manubrium of the sternum and the medial aspect of the clavicle and follow the muscle superiorly and laterally to its attachment on the mastoid process. The sternocleidomastoid is the anterior border of the posterior triangle of the neck and is a useful landmark for palpating enlarged lymph nodes (Figure 8.14).

Trapezius

Stand behind the seated patient. Differences in contour and expanse can be easily noted as you observe the patient prior to palpation. To enable you to palpate the fibers of the upper trapezius, allow your

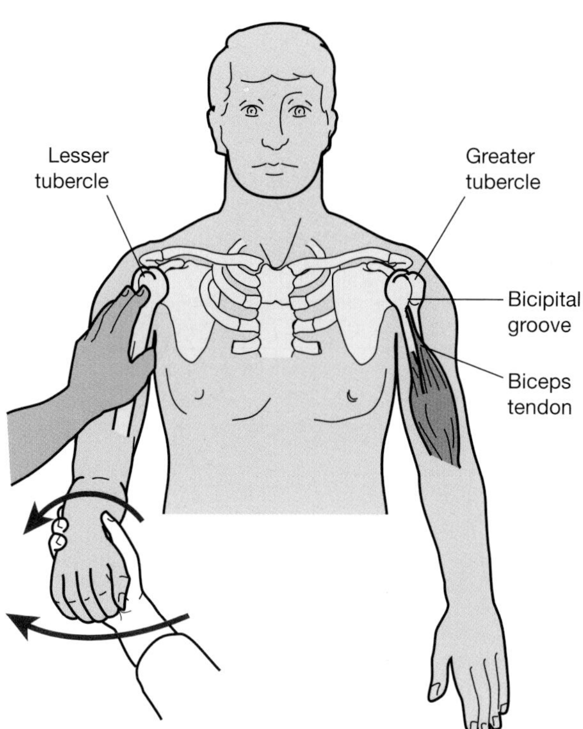

Figure 8.13 Palpation of the bicipital groove.

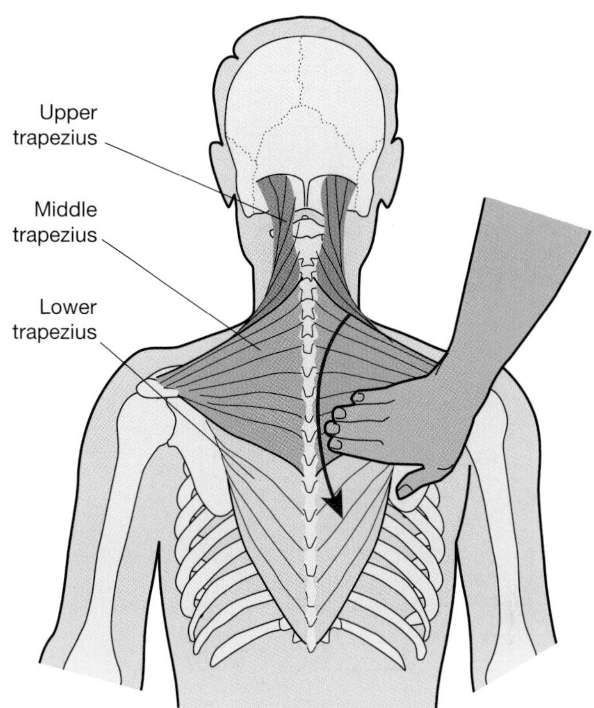

Figure 8.15 Palpation of the trapezius muscle.

fingers to travel laterally and inferiorly from the external occipital protuberance to the lateral third of the clavicle. The muscle is a flat sheet but feels like a cord-like structure because of the rotation of the fibers. It is frequently tender to palpation and often very tight,

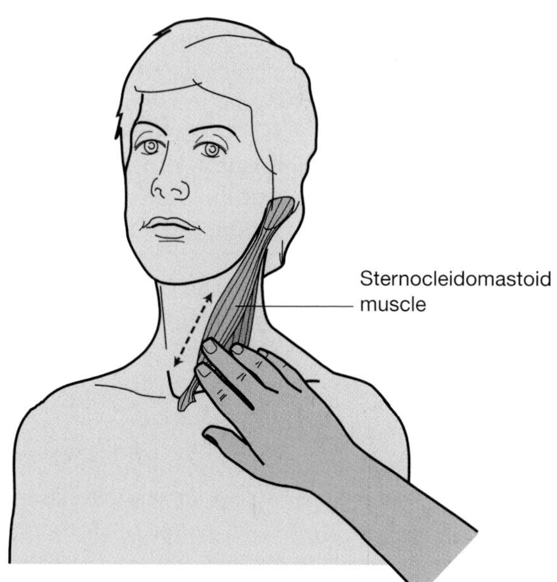

Figure 8.14 Palpation of the sternocleidomastoid muscle.

secondary to tension or trauma. You can palpate the muscle using your thumb on the posterior aspect and your index and middle fingers anteriorly. The fibers of the lower trapezius can be traced as they attach from the medial aspect of the spine of the scapula, running medially and inferiorly to the spinous processes of the lower thoracic vertebrae. The fibers can be made more prominent by asking the patient to depress the scapula. The fibers of the middle trapezius can be palpated from the acromion to the spinous processes of the seventh cervical and upper thoracic vertebrae. The muscle is made more prominent by asking the patient to adduct the scapulae (Figure 8.15).

Pectoralis Major

The pectoralis major is located on the anterior surface of the shoulder girdle. It is palpated from its attachment on the sternal aspect of the clavicle and along the sternum to the sixth or seventh rib, to its lateral attachment to the crest of the greater tubercle of the humerus. It creates the inferior aspect of the deltopectoral groove where it lies next to the deltoid muscle. The muscle forms the anterior wall of the axilla (Figure 8.16).

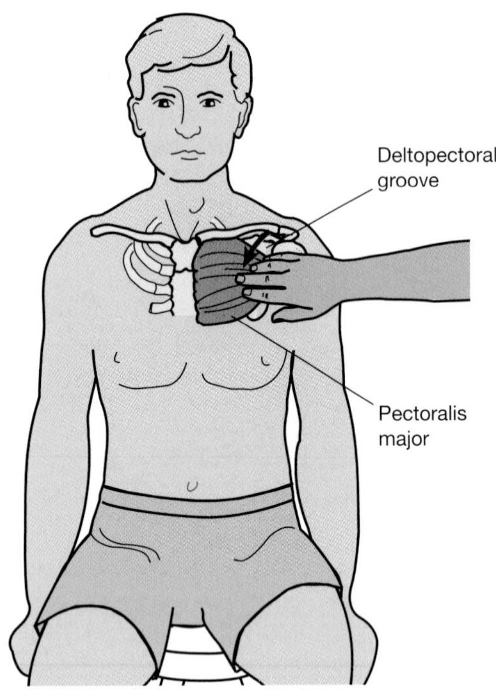

Figure 8.16 Palpation of the pectoralis major muscle.

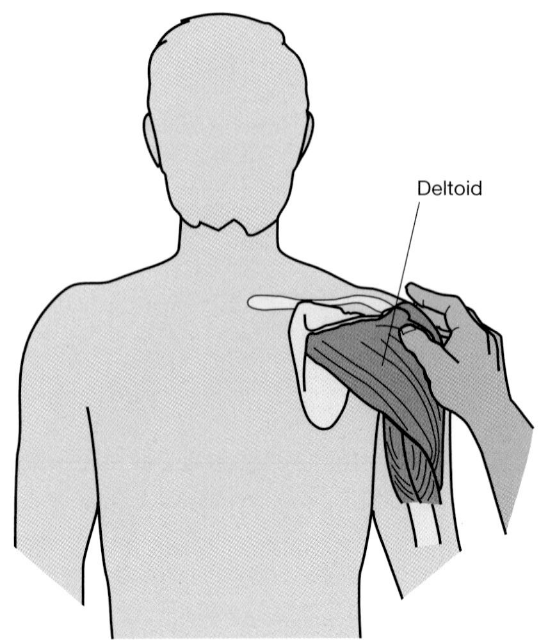

Figure 8.17 Palpation of the deltoid muscle.

Deltoid

The deltoid has proximal attachments to the lateral clavicle, acromion, and spine of the scapula. The fibers then converge and insert onto the deltoid tuberosity of the humerus. The deltoid has a large rounded mass, creating the full contour of the shoulder (Figure 8.17). Atrophy can be caused by injury to the upper trunk of the brachial plexus or to the axillary nerve, following fracture or dislocation of the humerus. Start your examination by standing in front of the patient. Allow your hand to travel from the clavicle inferiorly and laterally as you feel the fullness of the muscle. Take note that the anterior fibers are superficial to the bicipital groove, making it difficult to distinguish whether tenderness in this area is from the muscle itself or the underlying structures. Continue by following the middle fibers from the acromion to the deltoid tuberosity. Note that the middle fibers overlie the subdeltoid bursa. If the patient has bursitis, careful examination of the area will help differentiate the tender structures. A neoplasm affecting the diaphragm or cardiac ischemia can refer pain to the deltoid.

Biceps

Stand in front of the seated patient. Palpate the bicipital groove as described previously. Trace the long head of the biceps tendon inferiorly through the groove as it attaches to the muscle belly. Tenderness of the biceps tendon on palpation may indicate tenosynovitis. This is also a site for subluxation or dislocation of the biceps tendon. The tendon of the short head can be palpated on the coracoid process as previously described. The muscle belly is more prominent when the patient is asked to flex the elbow. The distal aspect of the belly and the biceps tendon can be palpated at its insertion on the bicipital tuberosity of the radius. Palpate for continuity of the belly and tendon (Figure 8.18). If a large muscle bulge is noted on the distal anterior aspect of the humerus with a concavity above it, you should suspect a rupture of the long head of the biceps. A subluxation of the biceps tendon secondary to a rupture of the transverse humeral ligament is known as a snapping shoulder.

Posterior Aspect

Bony Structures

Spine of the Scapula

Palpate the posterior aspect of the acromion medially along the ridge of the spine of the scapula as it tapers at the medial border. The spine of the scapula is located at the level of the spinous process of the third thoracic vertebra (Figure 8.19). The spine of the scapula separates the supraspinous and infraspinous

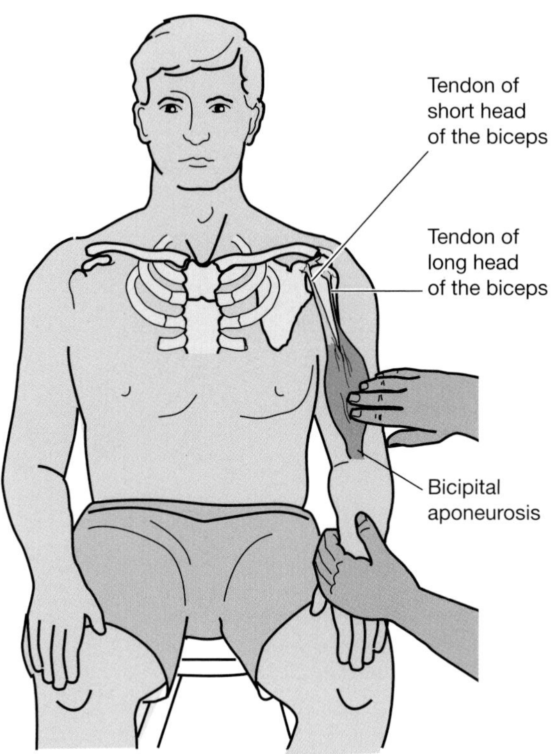

Figure 8.18 Palpation of the biceps muscle.

fossae and serves as the attachment of the supraspinatus and infraspinatus muscles.

Medial (Vertebral) Border of the Scapula

Move superiorly from the medial aspect of the spine of the scapula until you palpate the superior angle, which is located at the level of the second thoracic vertebra. This area serves as the attachment of the levator scapulae and is often tender to palpation. In addition, it is frequently an area of referred pain from the cervical spine. Continue inferiorly along the medial border and note whether it lies flat on the rib cage. If the border wings away from the cage, it may be indicative of a long thoracic nerve injury. Notice the attachment of the rhomboideus major along the length of the medial border from the spine to the inferior angle. The inferior angle of the scapula is located at the level of the seventh thoracic vertebra and serves as the attachment of the latissimus dorsi and serratus anterior (Figure 8.20).

Lateral Border of the Scapula

Continue superiorly and laterally from the inferior angle along the lateral border of the scapula. The lateral border is less defined than the medial border

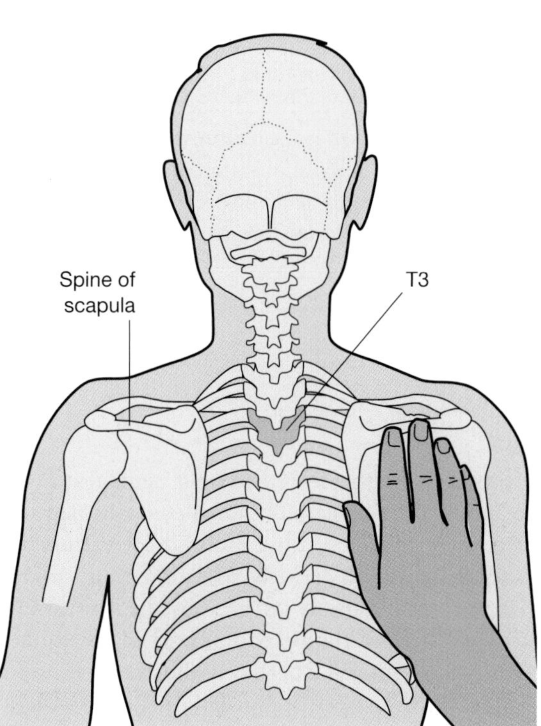

Figure 8.19 Palpation of the spine of the scapula.

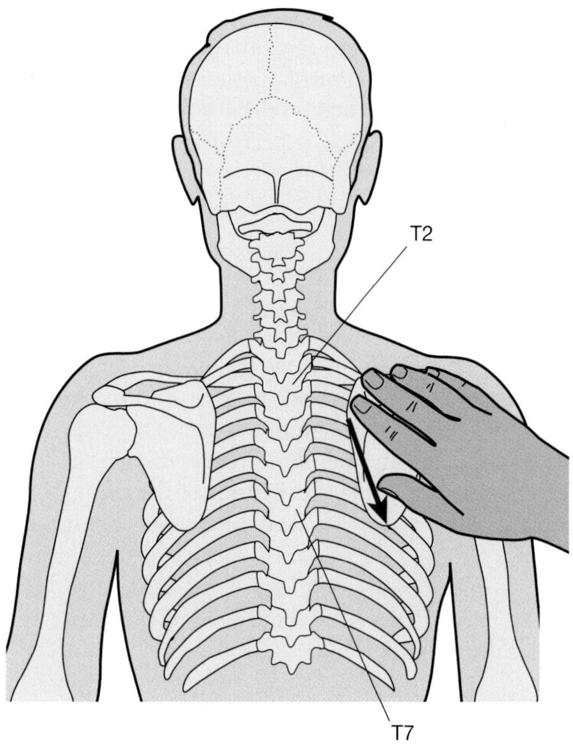

Figure 8.20 Palpation of the medial border of the scapula.

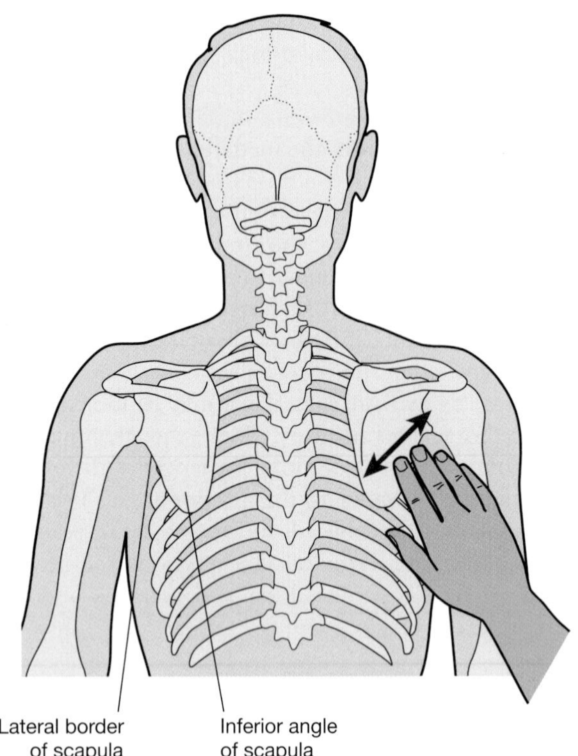

Figure 8.21 Palpation of the lateral border of the scapula.

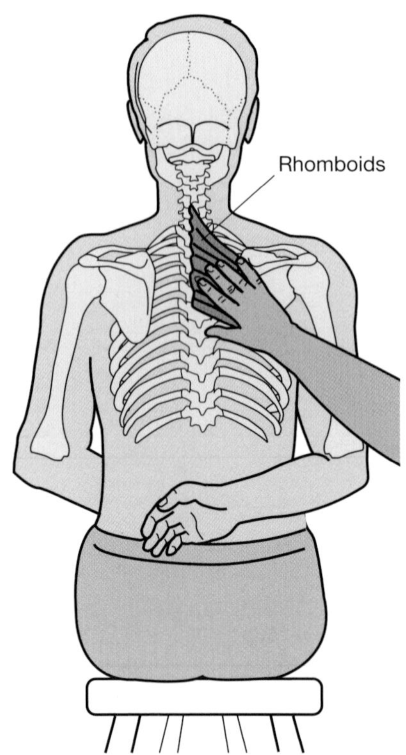

Figure 8.22 Palpation of the rhomboideus major and minor muscles.

because of the muscle attachments of the subscapularis anteriorly and the teres major and minor posteriorly. The attachment of the long head of the triceps can also be palpated on the infraglenoid tubercle, which is at the superior aspect of the lateral border (Figure 8.21).

Soft-Tissue Structures

Rhomboideus Major and Minor

The rhomboideus major originates from the spinous processes of T2–T5 and inserts on the medial border of the scapula between the spine and the inferior angle. The rhomboideus minor attaches from the ligamentum nuchae and the spinous processes of C7 and Tl to the medial border at the root of the spine of the scapula. Stand behind the seated patient. The muscles can be located at the vertebral border of the scapula. You can more easily distinguish the muscle by having the patient place the hand behind the waist and adduct the scapula (Figure 8.22).

Latissimus Dorsi

The latissimus dorsi attaches distally to the spinous processes of T6–T12, inferior three or four ribs, the inferior angle of the scapula, thoracolumbar fascia, iliac crest, and converges proximally to the intertubercular groove of the humerus. Palpation of the superior portion is discussed in the section on the posterior wall of the axilla. Continue to slide your hand along the muscle belly in an inferior and medial direction until you reach the iliac crest. The fibers are much harder to differentiate as you move inferiorly (Figure 8.23).

Medial Aspect

Soft-Tissue Structures

Axilla

The axilla has been described as a pentagon (Moore and Dalley, 1999) created by the pectoralis major and minor anteriorly; the subscapularis, latissimus dorsi, and teres major posteriorly; the first four ribs with their intercostal muscles covered by the serratus anterior medially; and the proximal part of the humerus laterally. The interval between the outer border of the first rib, the superior border of the scapula, and the posterior aspect of the clavicle forms the apex. The axillary fascia and skin make up the base. To examine

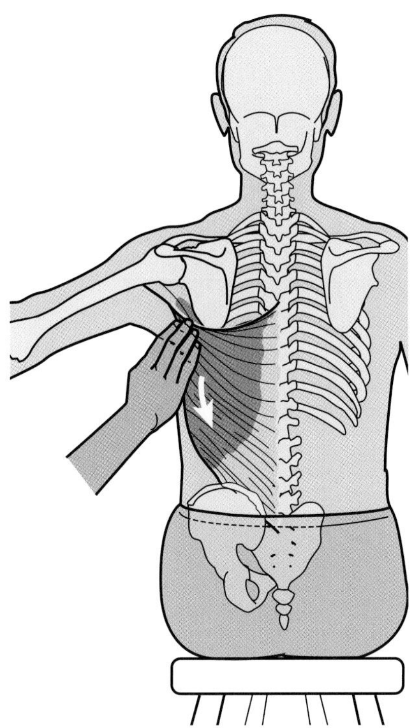

Figure 8.23 Palpation of the latissimus dorsi muscle.

the axilla, face the seated patient. Support the patient's abducted upper extremity by supporting the forearm with the elbow flexed. Allow your opposite hand to gently but firmly palpate. Remember that this area is especially ticklish to palpation. The axilla is clinically significant because it allows for passage of the brachial plexus and the axillary artery and vein to the upper extremity.

Allow your fingers to palpate the anterior wall and grasp the pectoralis major between your thumb, index, and middle fingers. Move to the medial aspect of the axilla and palpate along the ribs and serratus anterior. Move superiorly into the axilla and gently pull the tissue inferiorly, rolling it along the rib cage, to palpate the lymph nodes. Normal lymph nodes should not be palpable in an adult. If palpable nodes are found, they should be noted since they are indicative of either an inflammation, infection, or a malignancy. Continue to palpate laterally and you will note the brachial pulse as you press against the proximal aspect of the humerus, located between the biceps and triceps muscles. Continue to palpate the posterior wall and grasp the latissimus dorsi between your thumb, index, and middle fingers. While palpating the muscles, pay attention to their tone and size. Note whether they are symmetrical bilaterally (Figure 8.24).

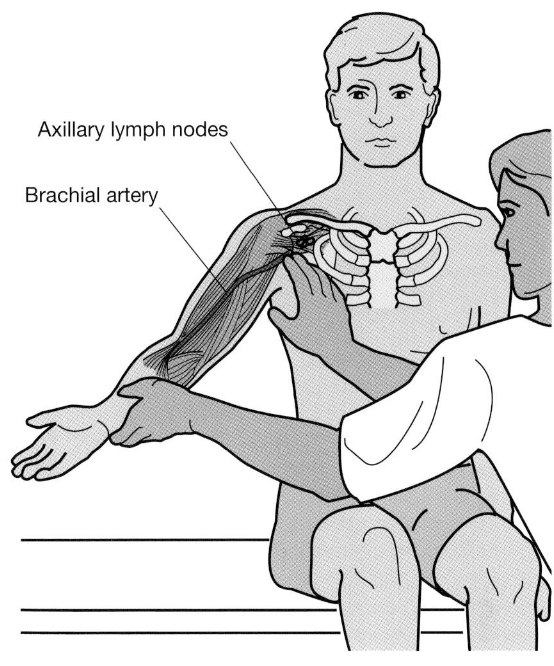

Figure 8.24 Palpation of the axilla.

Serratus Anterior

The description of this palpation is found in the previous section on the axilla. The serratus anterior is important since it secures the medial border of the scapula to the rib cage (Figure 8.25). Weakness or

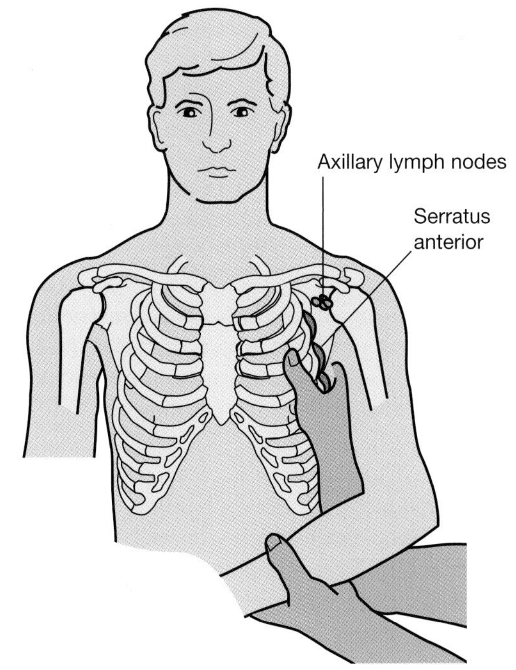

Figure 8.25 Palpation of the serratus anterior muscle.

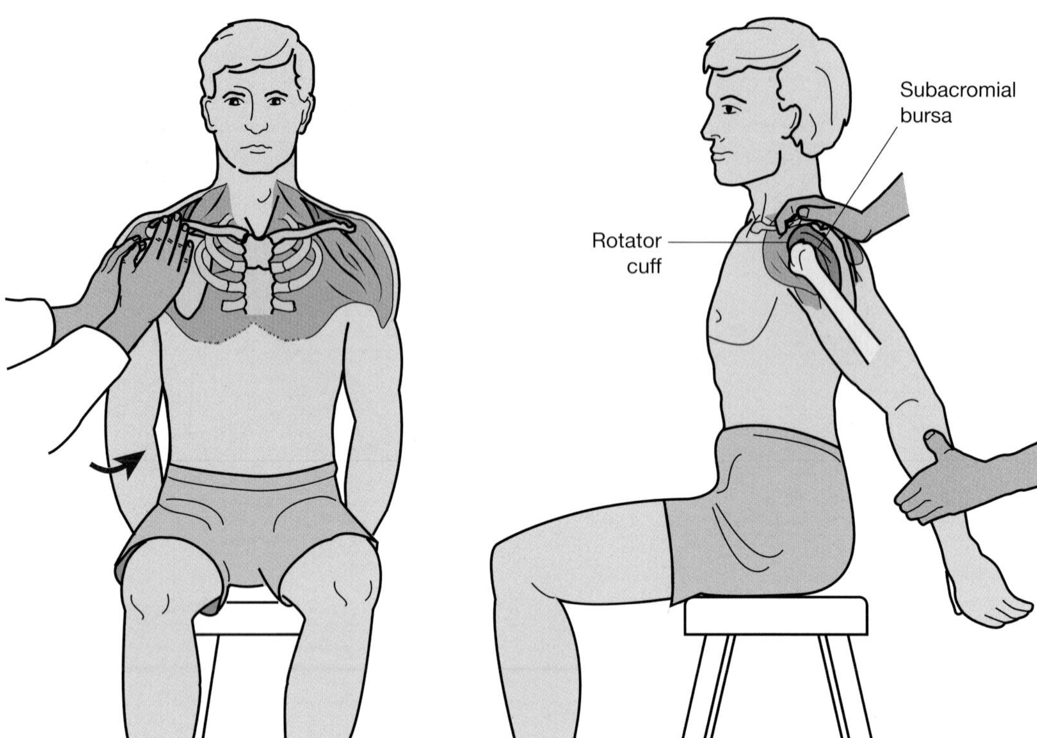

Figure 8.26 Palpation of the rotator cuff muscles.

denervation will be observed as a winged scapula (See section on Possible Deviations from the Norm in the Posterior View in Chapter 2; See Figure 2.8).

Lateral Aspect

Soft-Tissue Structures

Rotator Cuff

When the patient rests the arm at the side, the rotator cuff tendons are located under the acromial arch at the point of their attachment to the greater tubercle of the humerus. These tendons are referred to as the supraspinatus, infraspinatus and teres major (SIT) muscles by virtue of the order of their attachment from anterior to posterior: supraspinatus, infraspinatus, and teres minor. The remaining muscle of the rotator cuff is the subscapularis and is not palpable in this position. To gain easier access to the tendons, ask the patient to bring the arm behind the waist in internal rotation and extension (Figure 8.26). You will be able to distinguish the tendons as a unit over the anterior aspect of the greater tubercle. If an inflammation is present, palpation of the tendons will cause pain.

Cyriax (1984) described a more specific method of palpation of the individual tendons. To locate the supraspinatus tendon, have the patient bend the elbow to 90 degrees and place his or her forearm behind the back. Then ask the patient to lean back onto the elbow in a half-lying position. This fixes the arm in adduction and medial rotation. You can localize the tendon by palpating the coracoid process and moving laterally to the greater tubercle, under the edge of the acromion (Figure 8.27).

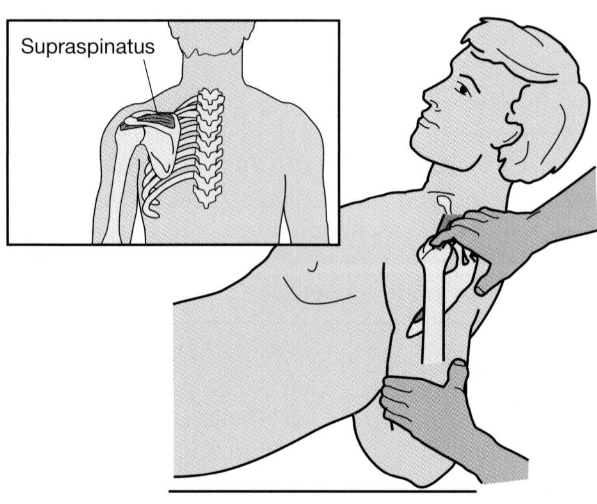

Figure 8.27 Palpation of the supraspinatus tendon.

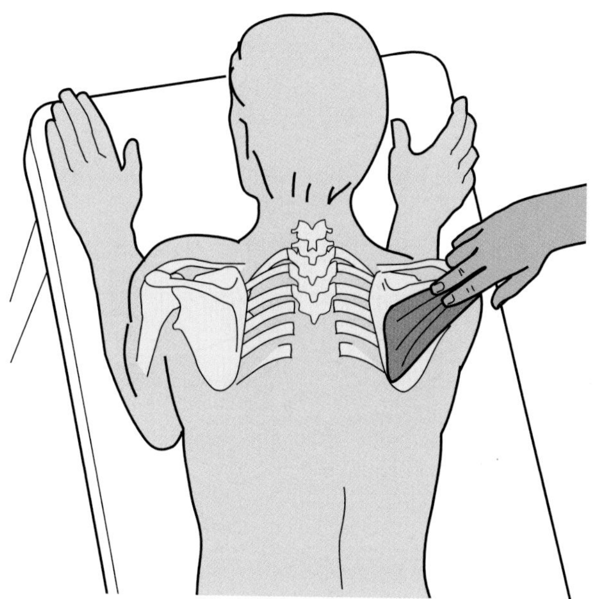

Figure 8.28 Palpation of the infraspinatus tendon.

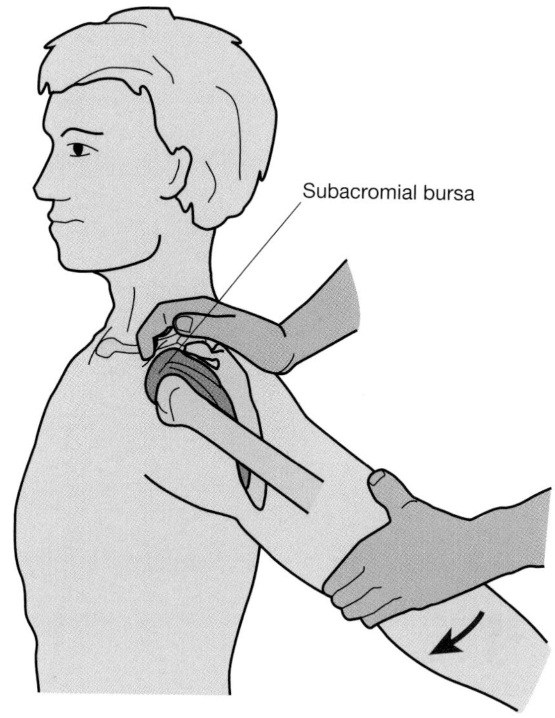

Figure 8.29 Palpation of the subacromial bursa.

To locate the infraspinatus tendon, have the patient prop himself or herself up on the elbows. Ask the patient to hold onto the edge of the treatment table to maintain lateral rotation. Instruct the patient to shift his or her weight over the arm being examined. The weight of the trunk will help to uncover the greater tubercle. The combination of flexion, adduction, and lateral rotation brings the greater tubercle out laterally. Palpate along the spine of the scapula laterally and palpate the infraspinatus tendon on the head of the humerus (Figure 8.28).

Subacromial (Subdeltoid) Bursa

The subacromial bursa is located between the deltoid and the capsule. It is elongated under the acromion and coracoacromial ligament. This bursa does not communicate with the joint. The subacromial bursa can be easily inflamed and become impinged under the acromion by virtue of its position. It will be very tender to palpation if it is inflamed and a thickening may be noted. It can be more easily palpated if it is brought forward from under the acromion by extending and internally rotating the shoulder (Figure 8.29).

Trigger Points of the Shoulder Region

Myofascial pain of the shoulder girdle is extremely common, especially because of the occupational overuse that occurs in many patients. Trigger points around the shoulder can mimic the symptoms of cervical radiculopathy or angina.

The common locations and referred pain zones for trigger points for the levator scapulae, supraspinatus, infraspinatus, deltoid, subscapularis, rhomboideus major and minor, and pectoralis major are illustrated in Figures 8.30 through 8.36.

Active Movement Testing

Active movement testing can be performed either by having the patient perform individual specific movements or by functionally combining the movements. The patient can perform the following movements: flexion and extension on the transverse axis, abduction and adduction on the sagittal axis, and medial and lateral rotation on the longitudinal axis. These should be quick, functional tests designed to clear the joint. If the motion is pain free at the end of the range, you can add an additional overpressure to "clear" the joint. Be aware, however, that overpressure in external rotation can cause anterior dislocation of an unstable shoulder. If the patient experiences pain in any of these movements, you should continue to explore whether

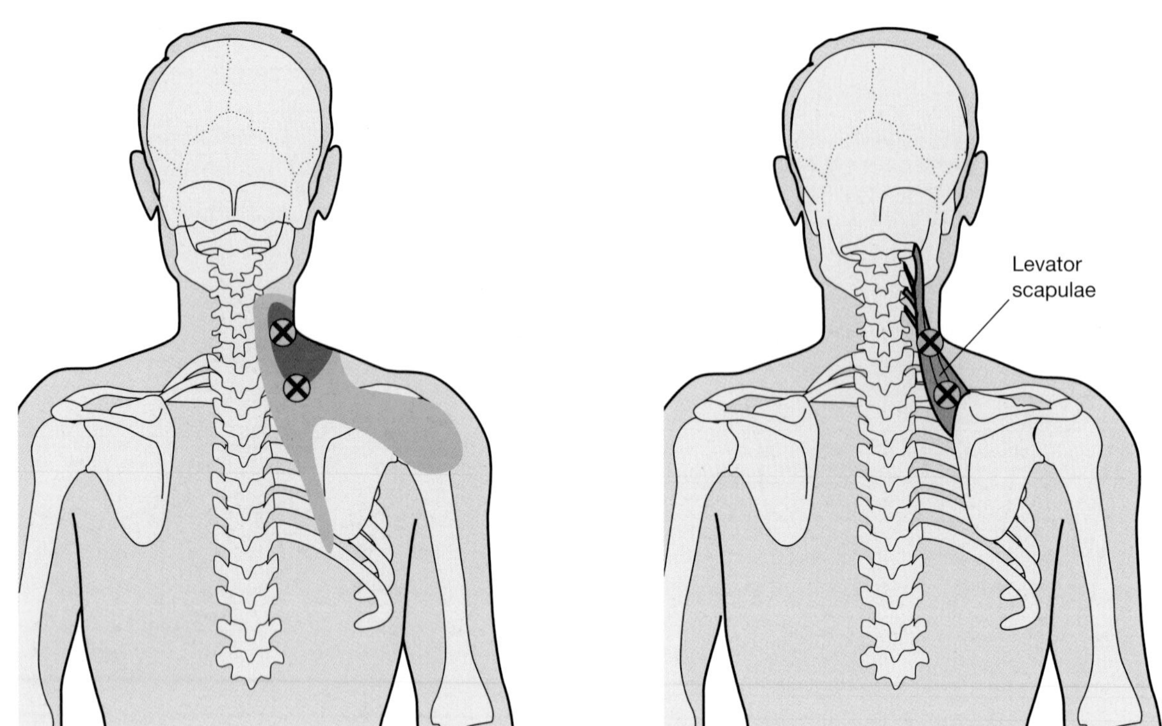

Figure 8.30 Trigger points in the levator scapulae, shown with common areas of referred pain. (Adapted with permission from Travell and Rinzler, 1952.)

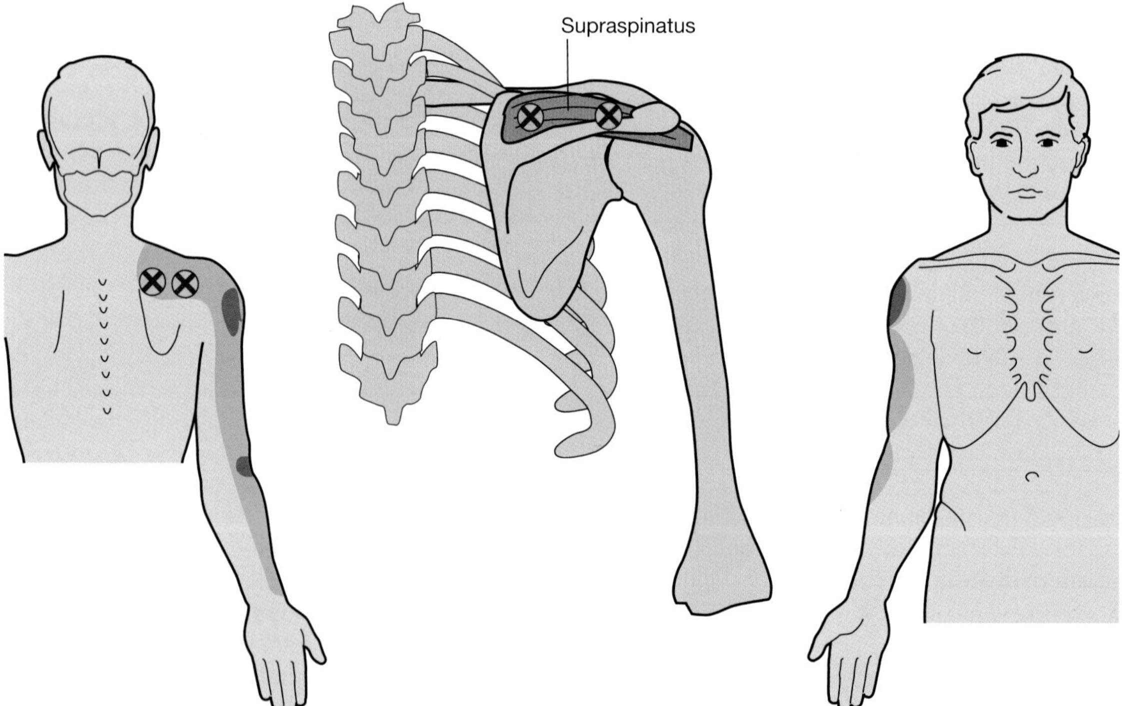

Figure 8.31 Trigger points of the supraspinatus muscle, shown with common areas of referred pain. (Adapted with permission from Travell and Rinzler, 1952.)

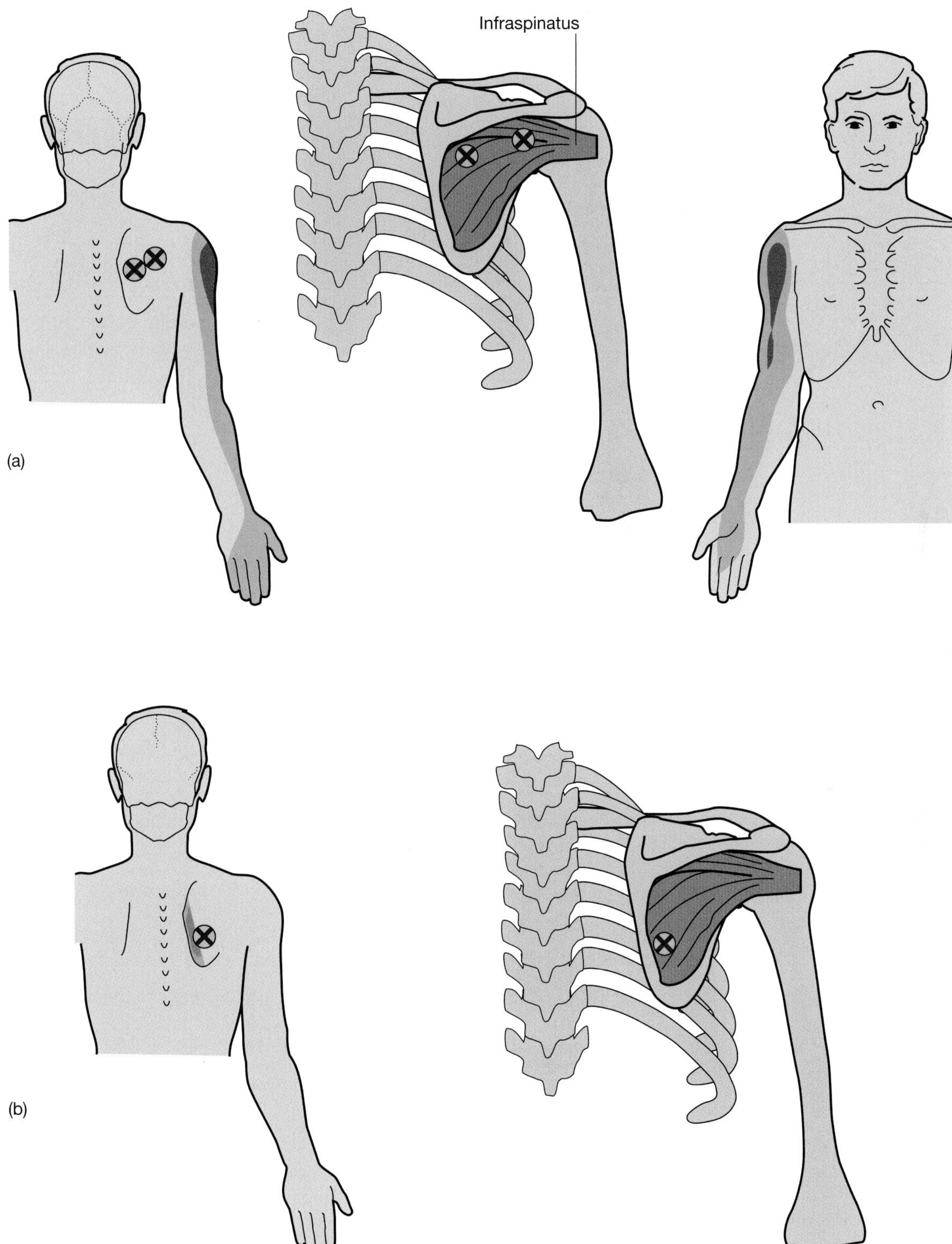

Figure 8.32 Trigger points of the infraspinatus muscle, shown with common areas of referred pain. (Adapted with permission from Travell and Rinzler, 1952.)

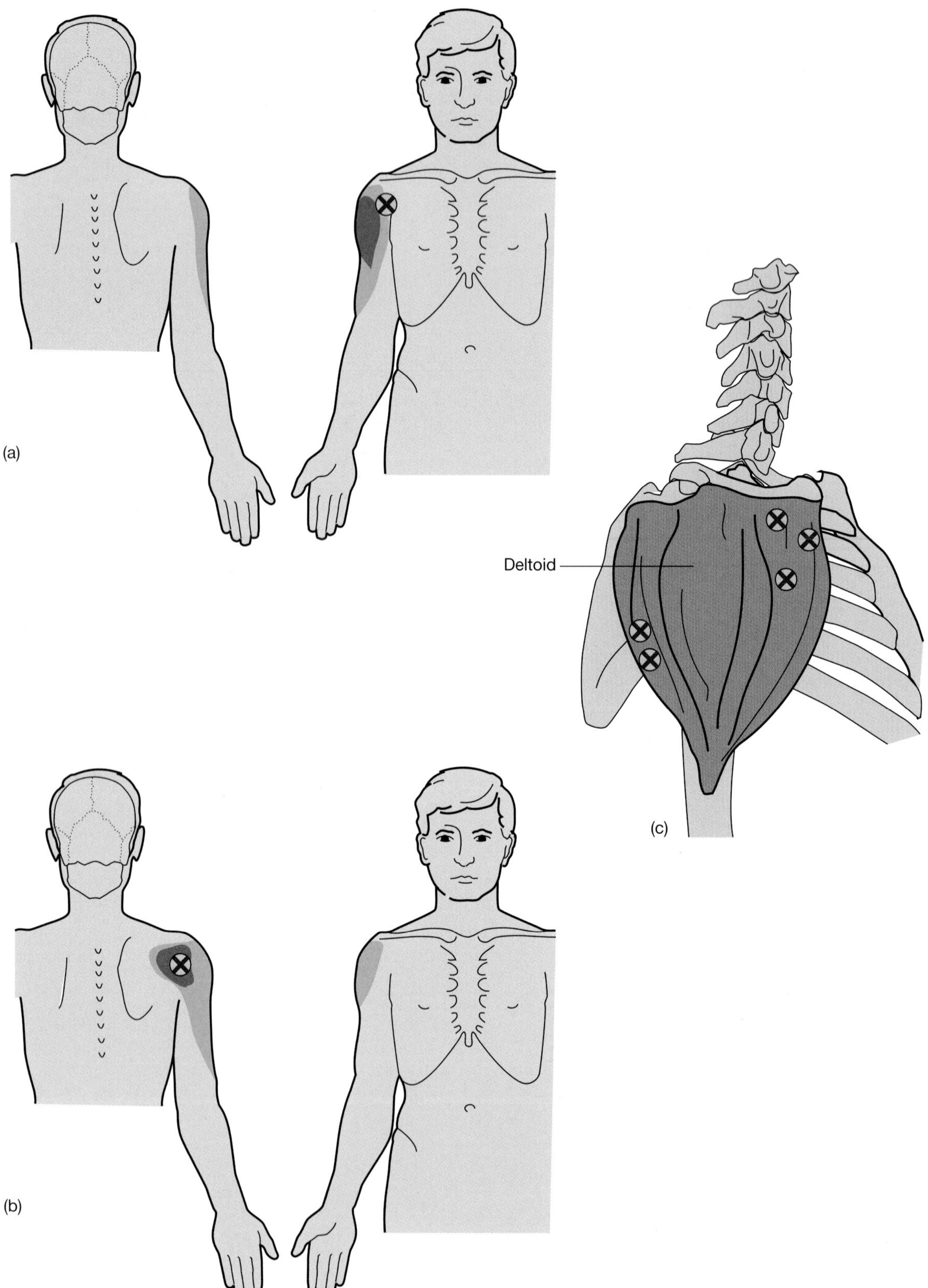

Figure 8.33 Trigger points of the deltoid muscle, shown with common areas of referred pain. (Adapted with permission from Travell and Rinzler, 1952.)

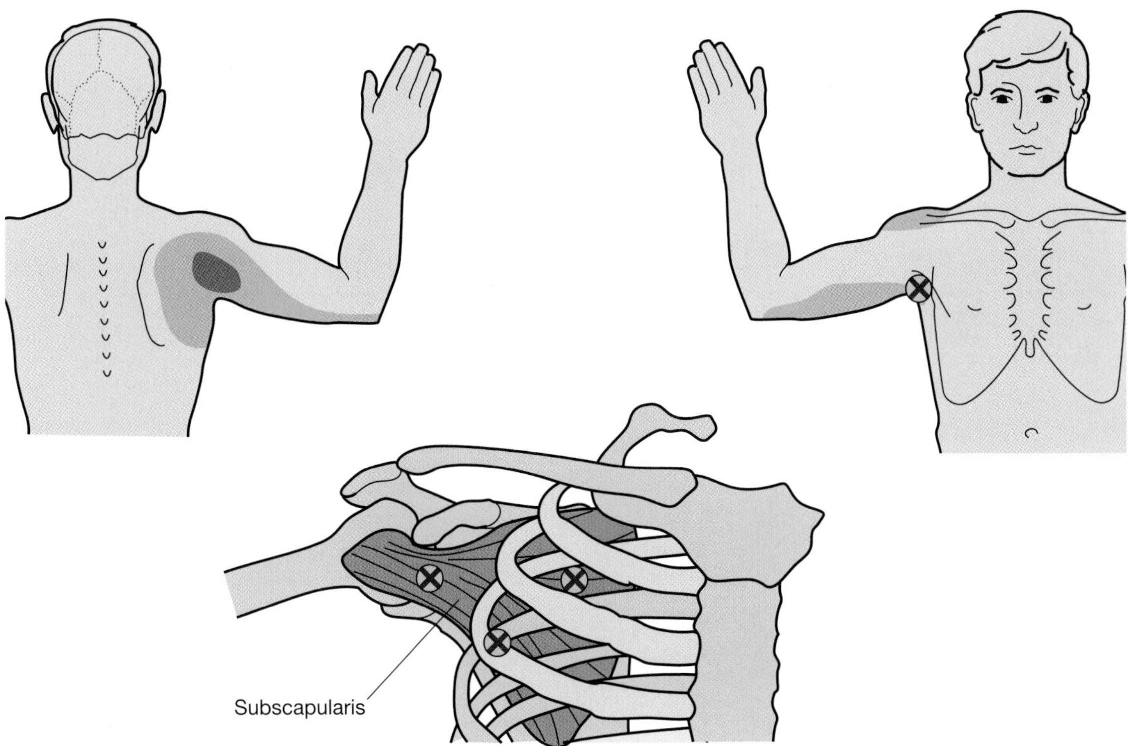

Figure 8.34 Trigger points of the subscapularis muscle, shown with common areas of referred pain. (Adapted with permission from Travell and Rinzler, 1952.)

the etiology of the pain is secondary to contractile or noncontractile structures by using passive and resistive tests.

Place the patient in either the sitting or standing position. Have the patient repeat the movement so that you can observe from both the anterior and posterior aspect. Have the patient place the arms next to the body. Ask the patient to abduct both arms out to 90 degrees with the palms facing the floor. Direct the patient to externally rotate the arms and bring the palms together overhead (Figure 8.37), which achieves the end of range for forward flexion and abduction. Observe the patient for symmetry of movement and the actual available range. Does the patient present with a painful arc (Cyriax, 1984) (pain-free movement is present before and after the pain occurs) secondary to bursitis or tendinitis? Note that the dominant arm may be more limited even in normal activity. Is the patient willing to move or is the patient apprehensive because of instability? From the posterior view, notice how the scapulae move. Is winging present? Mark the inferior angle of the scapula with your thumbs and observe them rotate upward. Note the scapulohumeral rhythm. If a reverse scapulohumeral rhythm is noted, the patient may have a major shoulder dysfunction such as an adhesive capsulitis or rotator cuff tear. From the anterior view, note the symmetry and movement of the sternoclavicular and acromioclavicular joints. From the lateral view, note whether the patient is attempting to substitute by extending the spine, so that it appears that the range is greater than it actually is.

Some clinicians prefer to have patients perform abduction in the neutral plane or plane of the scapula. This is located with the arm in approximately 30–45 degrees of horizontal adduction from the midcoronal plane. This plane is less painful for the patient and represents a more functional movement. There is less stress on the capsule, making the movement easier to perform (Figure 8.38).

Have the patient abduct the shoulder to 90 degrees with the elbow flexed to 90 degrees. Instruct the patient to reach across and touch the opposite acromion. This movement will test for horizontal adduction (cross-flexion). Then instruct the patient to bring the arm into extension while maintaining the 90 degrees of abduction. This will test for horizontal abduction (cross-extension) (Figure 8.39).

Combined functional movements may save you time in the examination process. Be aware, however,

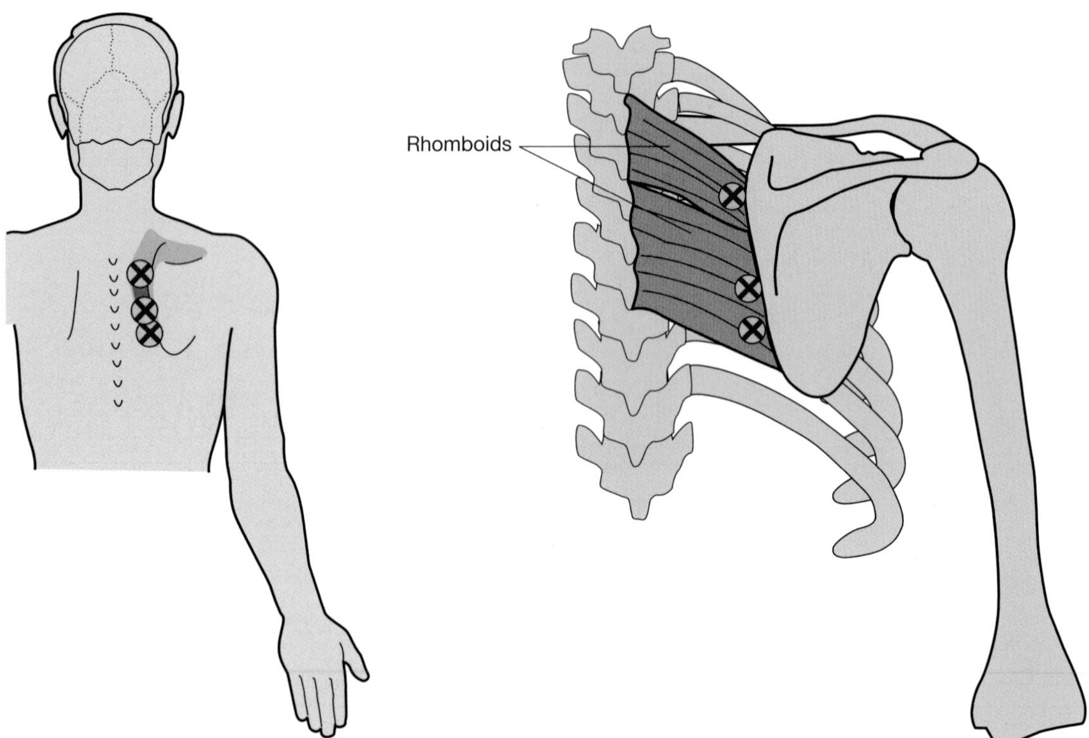

Figure 8.35 Trigger points of the rhomboid muscles, shown with common areas of referred pain. (Adapted with permission from Travell and Rinzler, 1952.)

that since you are testing several movements simultaneously, determining the source of the limitation is more difficult. Using the Apley "scratch" test (Magee, 2008) will give you the most information most efficiently. Ask the patient to bring one hand behind the head and reach for the superior border of the scapula on the opposite side. This movement combines abduction and external rotation. Then ask the patient to bring the opposite hand behind the back and reach up to touch the contralateral inferior angle of the scapula. This movement combines adduction and internal rotation. Then have the patient reverse the movements to observe the combination bilaterally (Figure 8.40).

Passive Movement Testing

Passive movement testing can be divided into two areas: physiological movements (cardinal plane), which are the same as the active movements, and mobility testing of the accessory (joint play, component) movements. You can determine whether the noncontractile (inert) elements are causative of the patient's problem by using these tests. These structures (ligaments, joint capsule, fascia, bursa, dura mater, and nerve root) (Cyriax, 1984) are stretched or stressed when the joint is taken to the end of the available range. At the end of each passive physiological movement, you should sense the end feel and determine whether it is normal or pathological. Assess the limitation of movement and see whether it fits into a capsular pattern. The capsular pattern of the shoulder is lateral (external) rotation, abduction, and medial (internal) rotation (Kaltenborn, 2011).

Physiological Movements

You will be assessing the amount of motion available in all directions. Each motion is measured from the anatomical starting position, which is zero degrees of flexion-extension, with the upper arm lying parallel to the trunk, the elbow in extension, and the thumb pointing anteriorly (Kaltenborn, 2011). The patient should be relaxed to enable you to perform the tests with greater ease. Testing can be performed with the patient in the sitting position, but the supine position and the prone position offer more stability by supporting the patient's trunk.

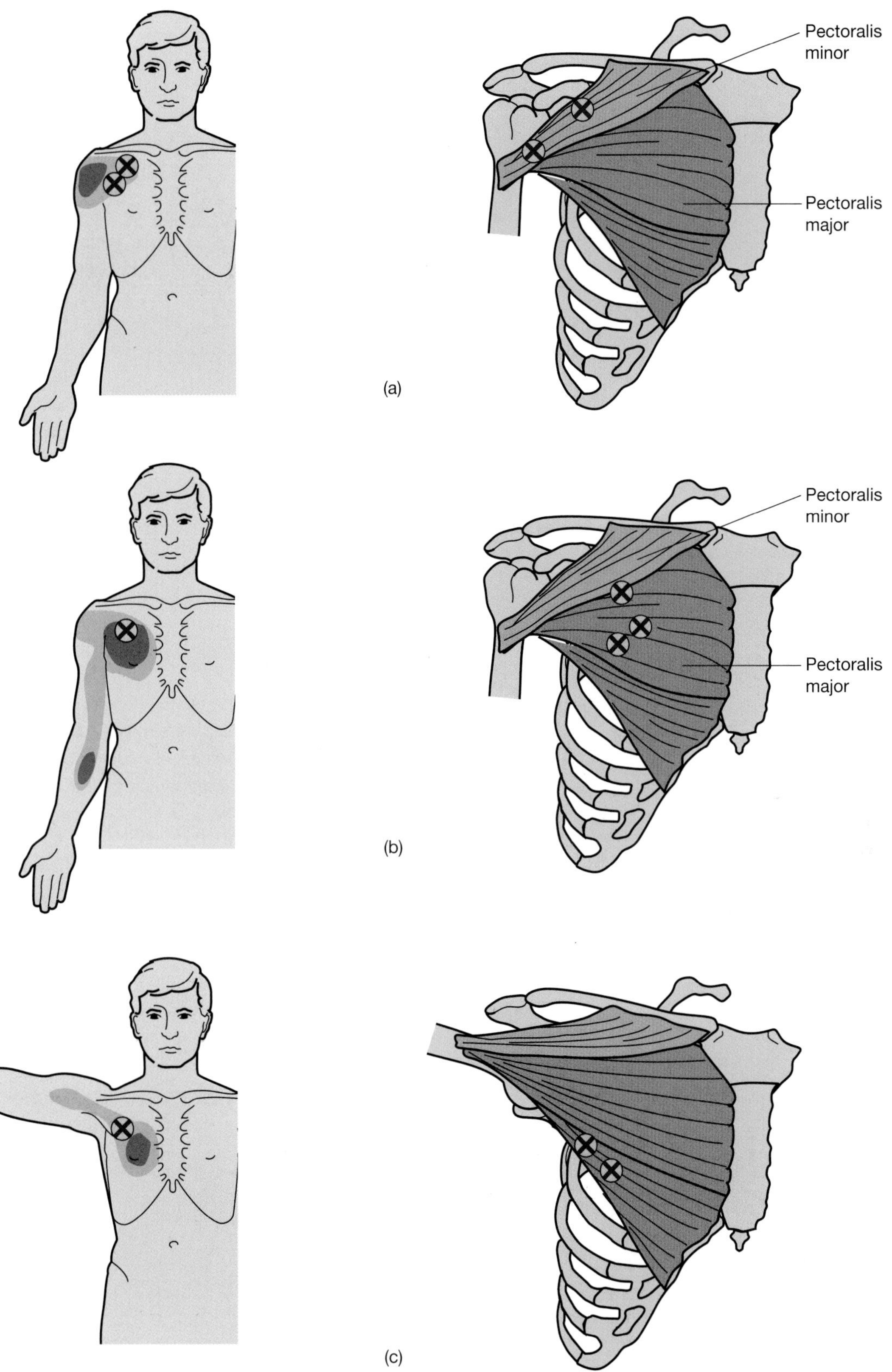

Figure 8.36 Trigger points of the pectoralis major muscle, shown with common areas of referred pain. (Adapted with permission from Travell and Rinzler, 1952.)

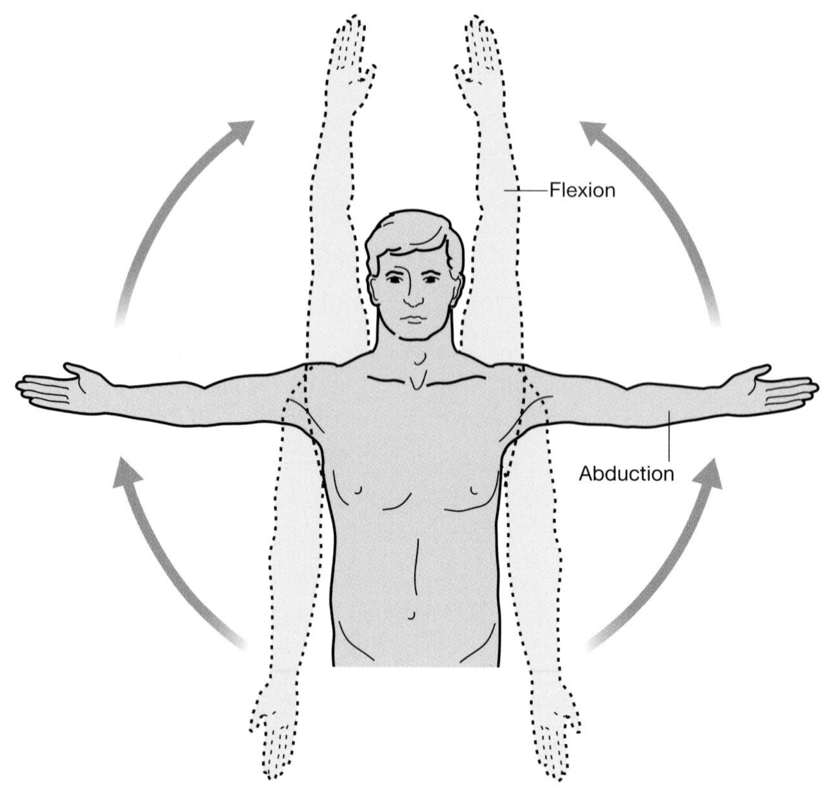

Figure 8.37 Active movement testing of shoulder abduction and flexion.

Flexion

The patient is placed in the supine position with the hip and knees flexed to 90 degrees to flatten the lumbar lordosis. The shoulder is placed in the anatomical starting position. Place your hand over the lateral border of the scapula to stabilize it and thereby accurately assess only glenohumeral movement. Place your hand over the lateral part of the rib cage to stabilize the thorax and prevent spinal extension when you assess shoulder complex movement. Face the patient's side and stabilize either the scapula or the thorax with your left hand. Hold the distal part

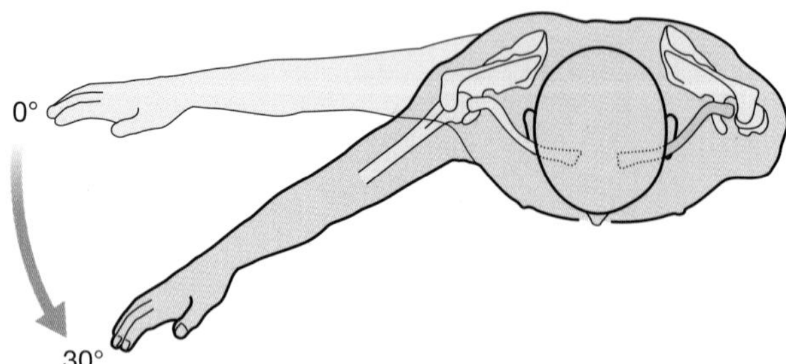

Figure 8.38 Active movement testing of shoulder flexion in the plane of the scapula.

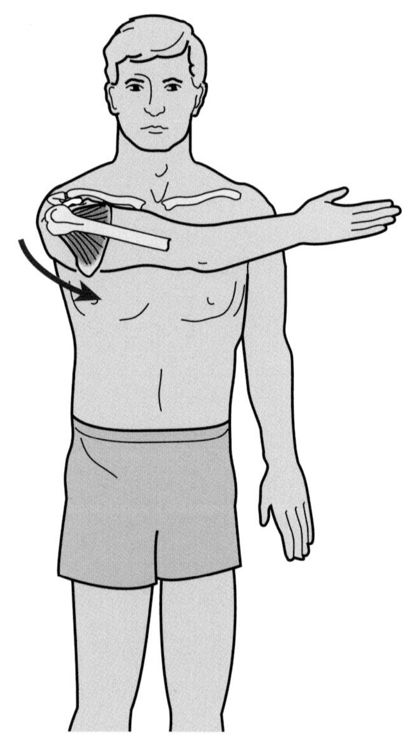

Figure 8.39 Active movement testing of shoulder in horizontal adduction and abduction.

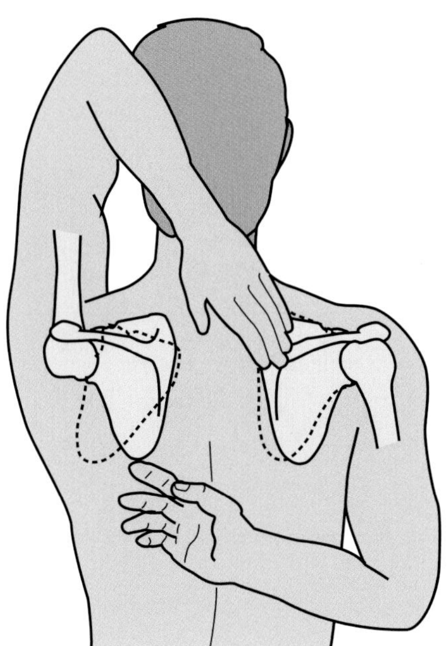

Figure 8.40 Active movement testing using the Apley "scratch" test.

of the patient's forearm, just proximal to the wrist joint, and move the upper extremity in an upward direction. When you sense movement in the scapula, you will know that you have reached the end of the available glenohumeral movement. Continue to move the upper extremity until the end feel is noted for the entire range of motion of the shoulder complex. The normal end feel of glenohumeral flexion is abrupt and firm (ligamentous) (Magee, 2008; Kaltenborn, 2011) because of the tension in the posterior capsule, muscles, and ligaments. The normal end feel of the shoulder complex is also abrupt and firm (ligamentous) due to tension in the latissimus dorsi. The normal range of motion for flexion of the shoulder complex is 0–180 degrees (Figure 8.41) (American Academy of Orthopedic Surgeons, 1965).

Extension

The patient is placed in the prone position with the head and neck in neutral and the shoulder in the anatomical position. Do not place a pillow under the patient's head. The elbow should be slightly flexed so that the long head of the biceps brachii is slack and does not decrease the available range. Place your hand over the superior and posterior aspect of the scapula to stabilize it, and thereby accurately assess glenohumeral movement. Place your hand over the lateral part of the rib cage to stabilize the thorax and prevent spinal flexion while you assess shoulder complex movement. Face the patient's side and stabilize either the scapula or the thorax with your right hand. Place your hand under the distal anterior aspect of the humerus and lift the upper extremity toward the ceiling. The normal end feel is abrupt and firm (ligamentous) due to tension from the anterior capsule and ligaments. The normal end feel of the shoulder complex is also abrupt and firm (ligamentous) due to tension in the pectoralis major and serratus anterior. Normal range of motion is 0–60 degrees (Figure 8.42) (American Academy of Orthopedic Surgeons, 1965).

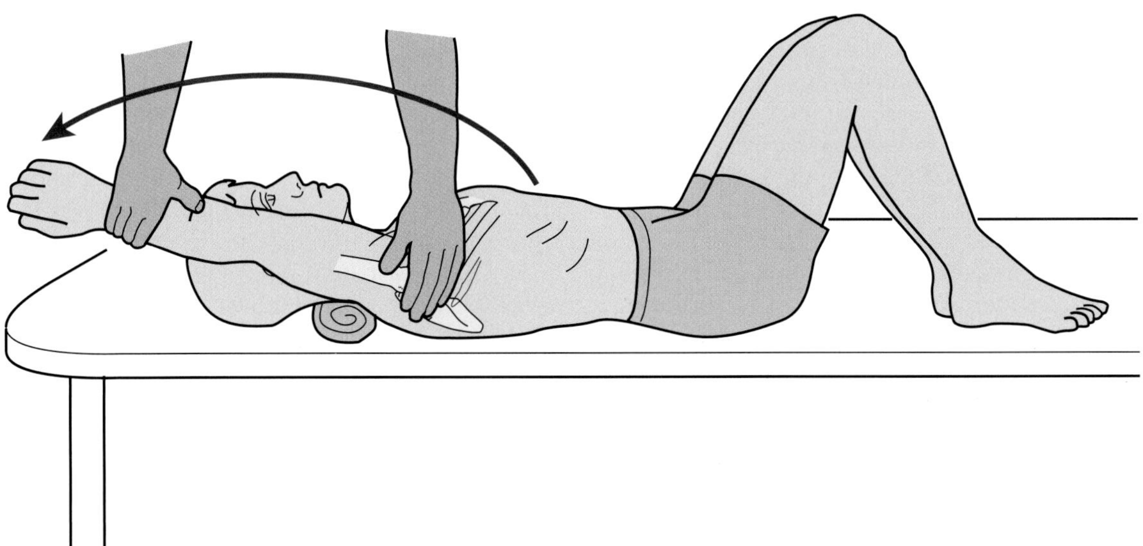

Figure 8.41 Passive movement testing of shoulder flexion.

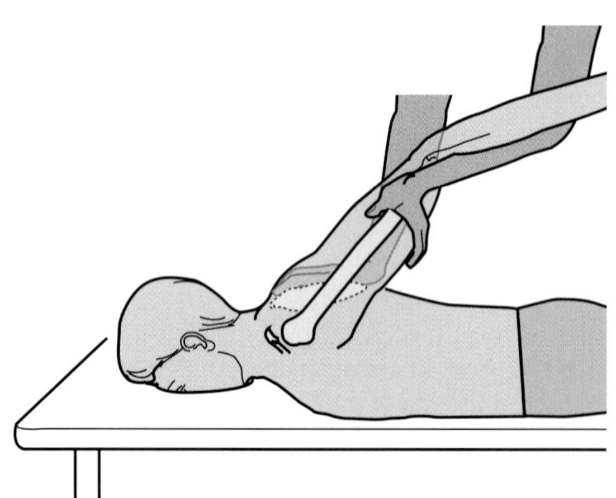

Figure 8.42 Passive movement testing of shoulder extension.

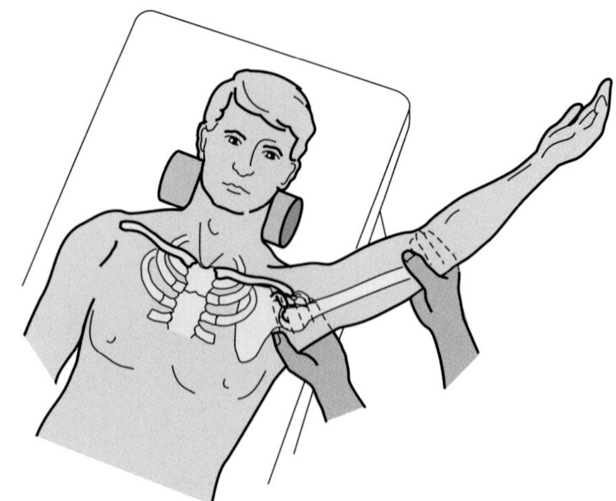

Figure 8.43 Passive movement testing of shoulder abduction.

Abduction

The patient is placed in the supine position with the shoulder in the anatomical starting position. The elbow should be in extension to prevent limitation of motion from tension in the long head of the triceps. Place your hand over the lateral border of the scapula, stabilizing it for accurate assessment of glenohumeral movement. Place your hand over the lateral part of the rib cage to stabilize the thorax and to prevent spinal lateral flexion while you assess shoulder complex movement. Face the patient's side and stabilize either the scapula or the thorax with your left hand. Hold the distal aspect of the patient's arm, just proximal to the elbow joint, and move the upper extremity in an outward direction. You must rotate the humerus laterally before you reach 90 degrees to allow for the greater tubercle of the humerus to pass more easily under the acromion and prevent impingement. When you sense movement in the scapula, you will know that you have reached the end of the available glenohumeral movement. Continue to move the upper extremity until the end feel is noted for the entire range of motion of the shoulder complex. The normal end feel of glenohumeral abduction is abrupt and firm (ligamentous) (Magee, 2008; Kaltenborn, 2011) because of the tension in the inferior capsule and anterior and posterior muscles and ligaments. The normal end feel of the shoulder complex is also abrupt and firm (ligamentous) due to tension in the posterior muscles. The normal range of motion for abduction of the shoulder complex is 0–180 degrees (Figure 8.43) (American Academy of Orthopedic Surgeons, 1965).

Internal (Medial) Rotation

The patient is placed in the supine position with the hip and knees flexed to 90 degrees to flatten the lumbar lordosis. The shoulder is placed at 90 degrees of abduction, with neutral position between supination and pronation of the forearm, with the forearm at a right angle to the treatment table, and the patient's hand facing inferiorly. Support the elbow with a small folded towel so that the shoulder is not extended. Stabilize the elbow to maintain 90 degrees of abduction during the beginning of the movement. Toward the end of the movement, you should stabilize the scapula by placing your hand over the acromion to prevent anterior tilting. Place your hand over the anterior part of the rib cage, just medial to the shoulder, to stabilize the thorax and prevent spinal flexion while you assess shoulder complex movement. Face the patient's side and stabilize either the scapula or the thorax with your right hand. Hold the distal aspect of the patient's forearm, just proximal to the wrist joint, and move the upper extremity so that the palm moves toward the table. When you sense movement in the scapula, you will know that you have reached the end of the available glenohumeral movement. Continue to move the upper extremity until the end feel is noted for the entire range of motion of the shoulder complex. The normal end feel of glenohumeral medial rotation is abrupt and firm (ligamentous) (Magee, 2008; Kaltenborn, 2011) because of the tension in the posterior capsule, muscles, and ligaments. The normal end feel of the shoulder complex is also abrupt and firm (ligamentous) due to tension in the posterior muscles. The normal range of motion for internal rotation of

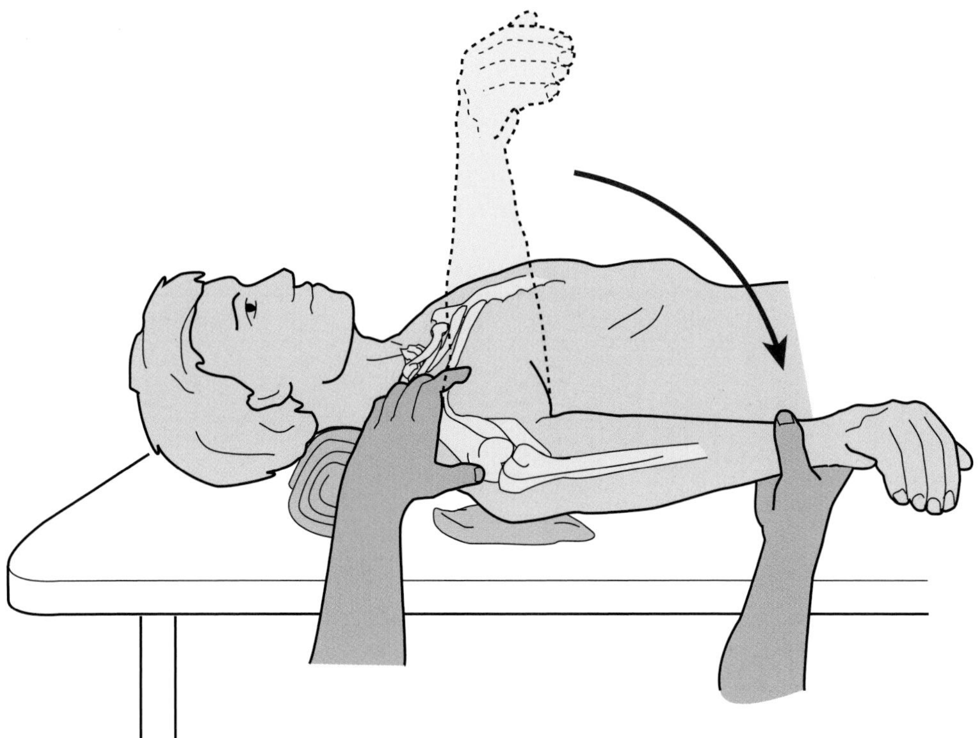

Figure 8.44 Passive movement testing of shoulder internal rotation.

the shoulder complex is 0–70 degrees (Figure 8.44) (American Academy of Orthopedic Surgeons, 1965).

External (Lateral) Rotation

External rotation is performed with the body in the same starting position as for medial rotation. Hold the distal aspect of the patient's forearm, just proximal to the wrist joint, and move the upper extremity so that the dorsum of the hand moves toward the table. When you sense movement in the scapula, you will know that you have reached the end of the available glenohumeral movement. Continue to move the upper extremity until the end feel is noted for the entire range of motion of the shoulder complex. The normal end feel of glenohumeral external rotation is abrupt and firm (ligamentous) (Magee, 2008; Kaltenborn, 2011) because of the tension in the anterior capsule, muscles, and ligaments. The normal end feel of the shoulder complex is also abrupt and firm (ligamentous) due to tension in the anterior muscles. The normal range of motion for external rotation of the shoulder complex is 0–90 degrees (Figure 8.45) (American Academy of Orthopedic Surgeons, 1965).

Mobility Testing of Accessory Movements

Mobility testing of accessory movements will give you information about the degree of laxity in the joint. The patient must be totally relaxed and comfortable to allow you to move the joint and obtain the most accurate information. The joint should be placed in the maximal loose packed (resting) position to allow for the greatest degree of joint movement. The resting position of the shoulder is abduction to approximately 55 degrees and horizontal adduction to 30 degrees (Kaltenborn, 2011).

Traction (Lateral Distraction)

Place the patient in the supine position with the shoulder in the resting position and the elbow in flexion. Stand on the side of the table so that your body is turned toward the patient. Place your hand over the acromion and the superior posterior aspect of the scapula for stabilization. Place your hand on the medial superior aspect of the humerus. Pull the humerus away from the patient (laterally) until all the slack is taken up. This creates a lateral traction force

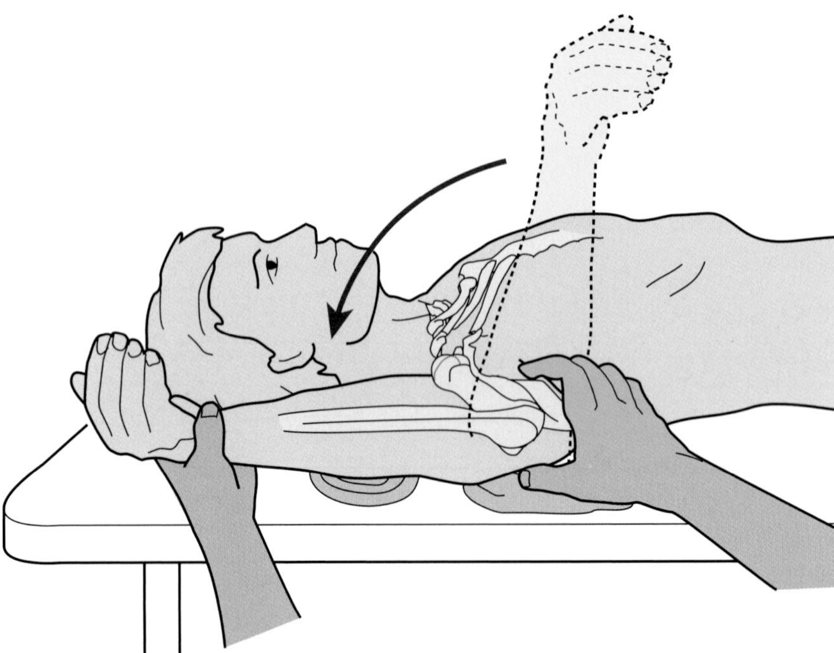

Figure 8.45 Passive movement testing of shoulder external rotation.

and a separation of the humerus from the glenoid fossa (Figure 8.46).

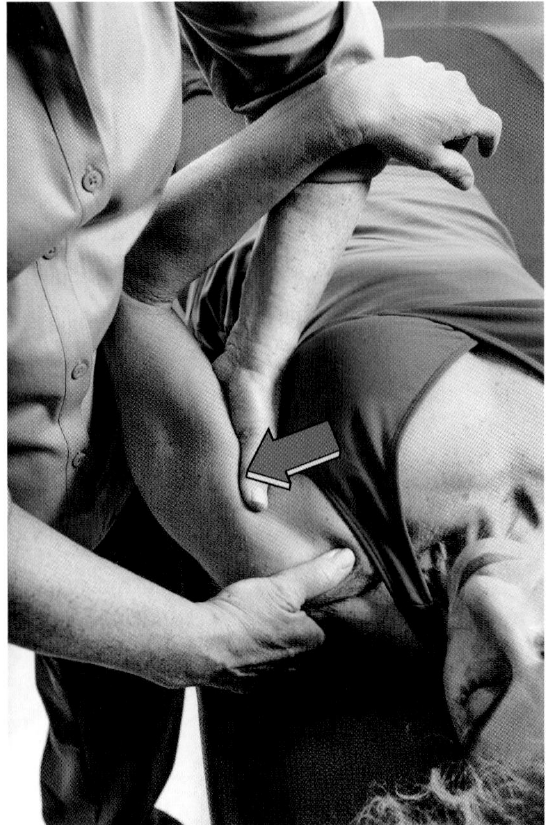

Figure 8.46 Mobility testing of shoulder lateral distraction.

Caudal Glide (Longitudinal Distraction)

Place the patient in the supine position with the shoulder in the resting position. Stand on the side of the table so that your body is turned toward the patient. Cup your hand over the lateral border of the scapula with your thumb located up to the coracoid process for stabilization. Place your other hand around the distal aspect of the humerus, proximal to the elbow joint. Pull the humerus in a caudal direction until all the slack is taken up. This creates a caudal glide or longitudinal traction force and a separation of the humerus from the glenoid fossa (Figure 8.47).

Ventral Glide of the Humeral Head

Place the patient in the prone position so that the humerus is just off the table. Place a small folded towel under the coracoid process to stabilize the scapula. The shoulder is placed in the resting position. Stand at the side of the table so that you are between the patient's arm and trunk and your body is turned toward the patient's shoulder. Hold the patient's humerus with one hand placed over the distal aspect. Place the other hand over the proximal

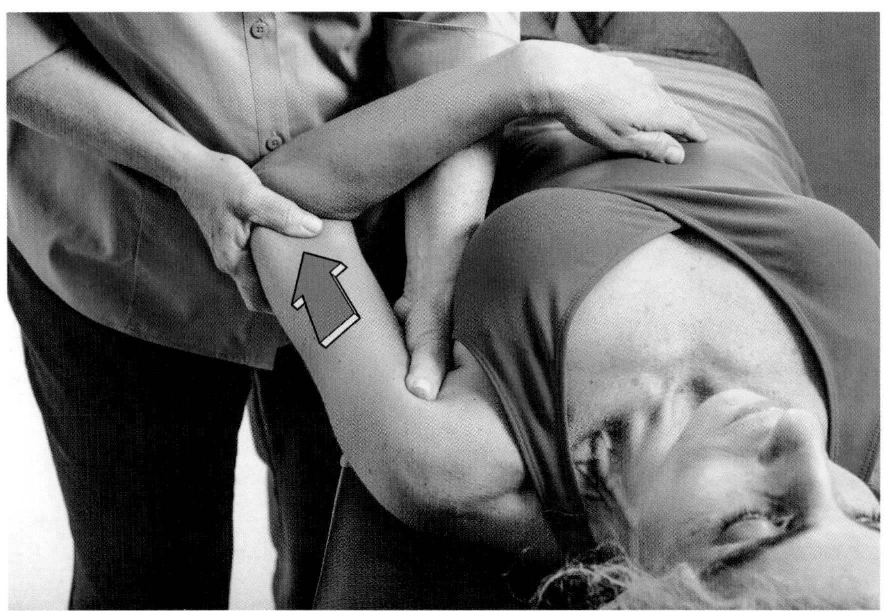

Figure 8.47 Mobility testing of shoulder caudal glide.

aspect of the humerus, just distal to the glenohumeral joint. Move the humerus as a unit in an anterior direction until you take up all the slack. This creates an anterior glide of the humeral head (Figure 8.48).

Dorsal Glide of the Humeral Head

Place the patient in the supine position so that the humerus is just off the table. Place a small folded towel under the scapula to stabilize it. The shoulder is placed in the resting position. Stand at the side of the table so that you are between the patient's arm and trunk and your body is turned toward the patient's shoulder. Hold the patient's humerus with one hand over the distal aspect and support the patient's forearm by holding it between your arm and trunk. Place your other hand at the proximal end of the humerus just distal to the glenohumeral joint. Move

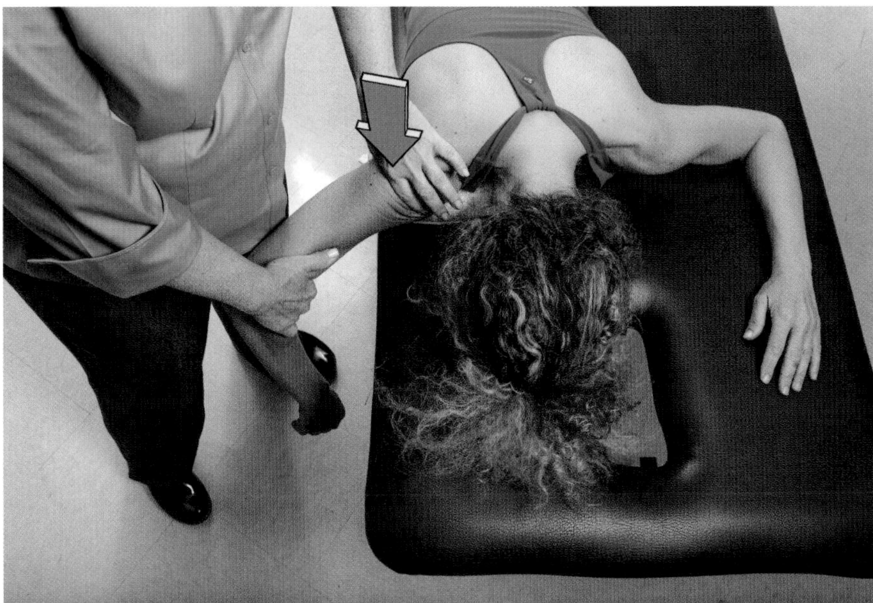

Figure 8.48 Mobility testing of ventral glide of the humeral head.

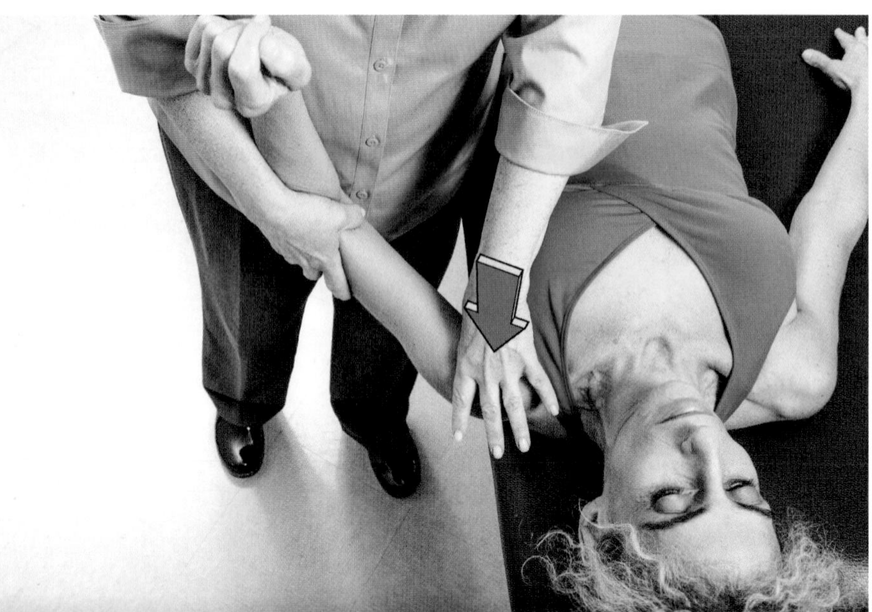

Figure 8.49 Mobility testing of dorsal glide of the humeral head.

the humerus as a unit in a posterior direction until you take up all the slack. This creates a posterior glide of the humeral head (Figure 8.49).

Sternoclavicular Joint Mobility

Place the patient in the supine position. Stand at the side of the table so that you are facing the patient's head. Palpate the joint space of the sternoclavicular joint with the index finger of one hand. Place your index finger and thumb of the other hand around the medial aspect of the clavicle. Move the clavicle in cranial, caudal, anterior, and posterior directions. Take up the slack in each direction. This creates a glide of the clavicle in the direction of your force (Figure 8.50).

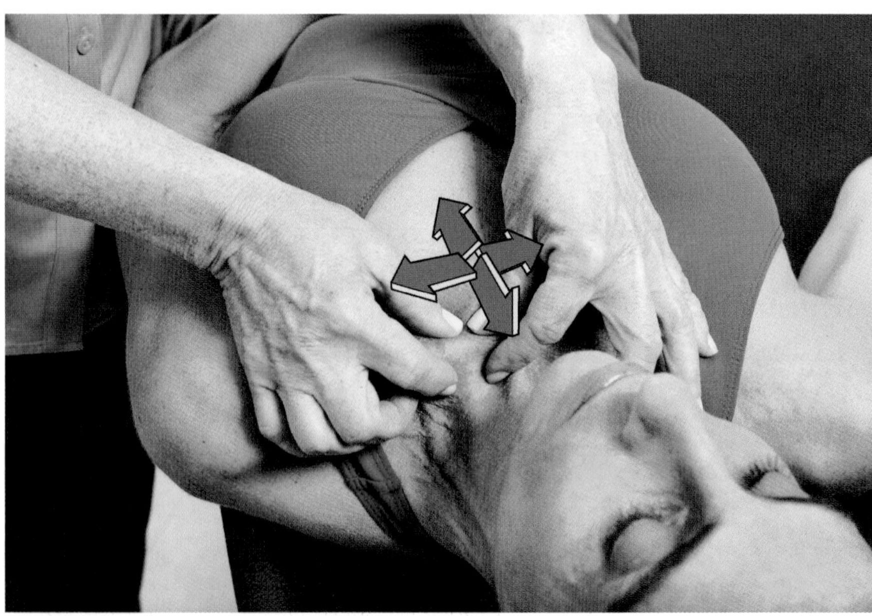

Figure 8.50 Mobility testing of the sternoclavicular joint.

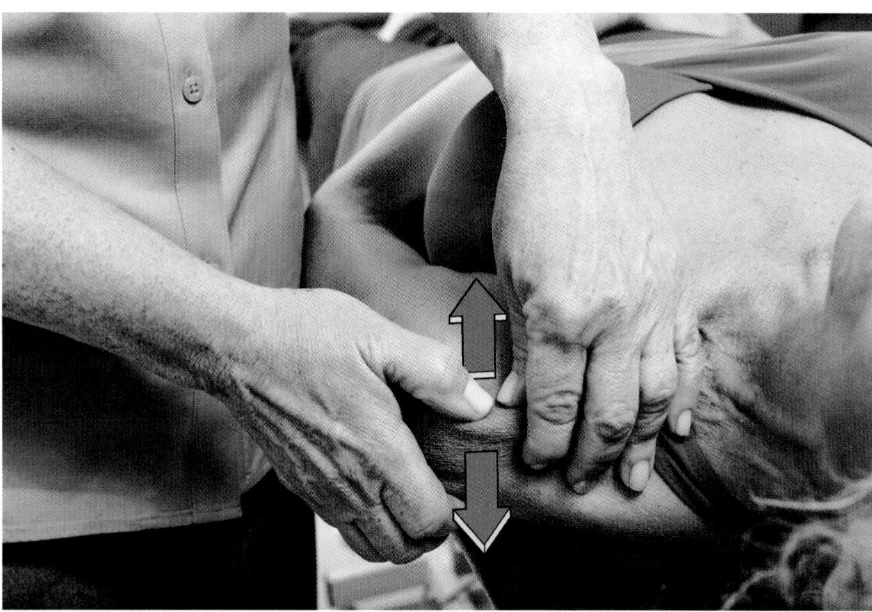

Figure 8.51 Mobility testing of the acromioclavicular joint.

Acromioclavicular Joint Mobility

Place the patient in the supine position. Stand at the side of the table so that you are facing the patient's head. Palpate the joint space of the acromioclavicular joint with the index finger of one hand. Place your index finger and thumb on the anterior and posterior surfaces of the acromion to stabilize it. Place your index finger and thumb around the lateral aspect of the clavicle. Move the clavicle in an anterior and posterior direction. Take up the slack in each direction. This creates a glide of the clavicle in the direction of your force (Figure 8.51).

Scapular Mobilization

Place the patient in the side-lying position. Stand so that you are facing the patient. Place one hand between the patient's upper extremity and trunk. Hold the inferior angle of the scapula by placing your hand so that your fingers grasp the medial border and your thumb rests on the lateral border of the scapula (your webspace should be under the inferior angle). Place your other hand so that your thenar eminence is over the acromion and your fingers surround the superior posterior aspect of the scapula. Move the scapula in cranial, caudal, medial, lateral, upward, and downward directions. Take up the slack in each direction. This creates a glide of the scapula on the thorax in the direction of your force. The scapula can be distracted away from the thorax by retracting the scapula with the medial border coming over the lateral border of your hand (Figure 8.52).

Resistive Testing

The muscles of the shoulder joint, in addition to being responsible for the movement of the arm, are necessary to maintain coaptation of the humeral head to the glenoid fossa of the scapula. For example, during heavy lifting with the extremity, the long muscles that include the triceps, coracobrachialis, and long and short heads of the biceps contract in an effort to raise the humeral head up to the scapula and prevent its inferior dislocation.

As with most joints, weakness of a particular movement may be compensated for by other muscles. This is accomplished by substitution and is generally noticeable on examination as irregular or abnormal movement of the body part. For example, weakness or restricted abduction of the glenohumeral joint may be compensated for by greater lateral rotation, elevation, and abduction of the scapulothoracic joint (i.e., shrugging of the shoulder). To test the strength of the shoulder, you will have to examine flexion, extension, abduction, adduction, internal (medial) rotation, and external (lateral) rotation.

The following movements of the scapula should also be tested: elevation, retraction, protraction, and adduction with depression.

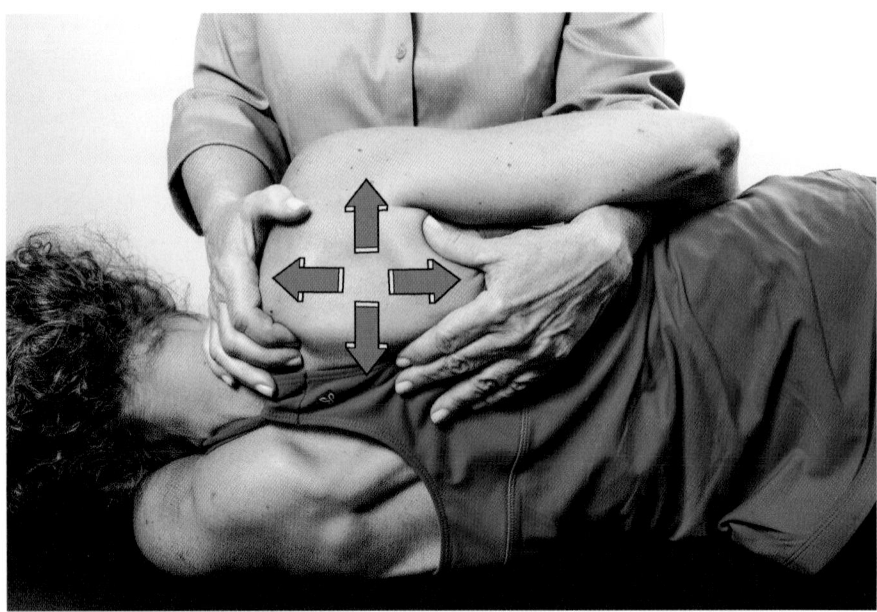

Figure 8.52 Mobility testing of the scapula.

Shoulder Flexion

The primary flexors of the shoulder are the anterior part of the deltoid and the coracobrachialis (Figure 8.53). Secondary flexors include the clavicular head of the pectoralis major, the middle fibers of the deltoid, the biceps brachii, the serratus anterior, and the trapezius.

- Position of patient: Sitting with the arm at the side and the elbow slightly flexed. The patient should then attempt to flex the shoulder to about 90 degrees without rotation or horizontal displacement.
- Resisted test: Stand beside the patient and place one hand on the upper thorax to stabilize the body, and place your other hand just proximal to the elbow joint so that you can apply a downward force on the lower arm. Ask the patient to attempt to elevate the arm directly upward against your resistance (Figure 8.54).

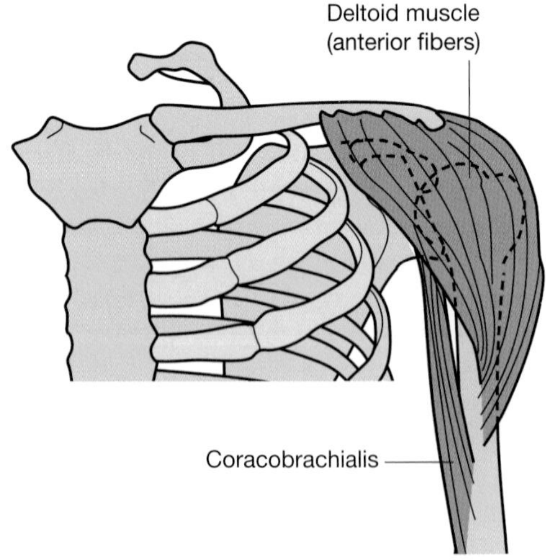

Figure 8.53 The primary flexors of the shoulder are the anterior fibers of the deltoid and the coracobrachialis muscles.

Testing shoulder flexion with gravity eliminated can be performed with the patient lying on the side with the tested arm upward. The arm is placed on a powdered board and the patient is asked to flex through the range of motion in the coronal plane (Figure 8.55).

Painful resisted shoulder flexion may be due to tendinitis of the contracting muscles.

Weakness of shoulder flexion results in an inability to perform many activities of daily living (ADL) and self-care.

Shoulder Extension

The primary extensors of the shoulder are the latissimus dorsi, teres major, and the posterior fibers of the deltoid (Figure 8.56). Secondary extensors include the teres minor and long head of the triceps.

- Position of patient: In the prone position with the shoulder internally rotated and adducted so that the palm is facing upward.

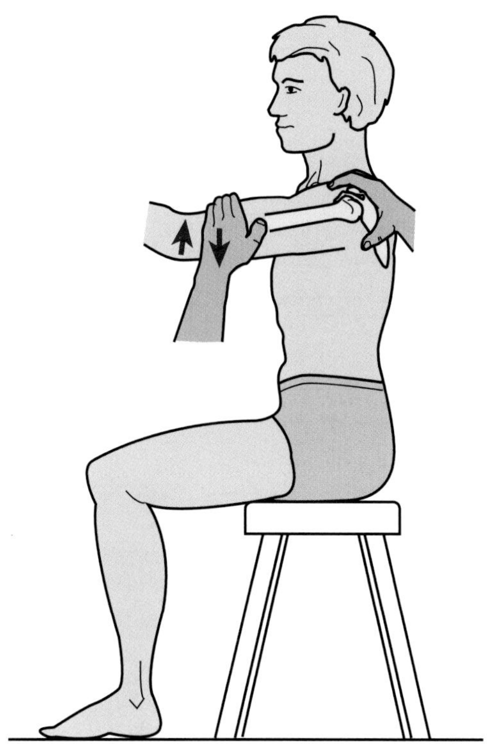

Figure 8.54 Testing shoulder flexion.

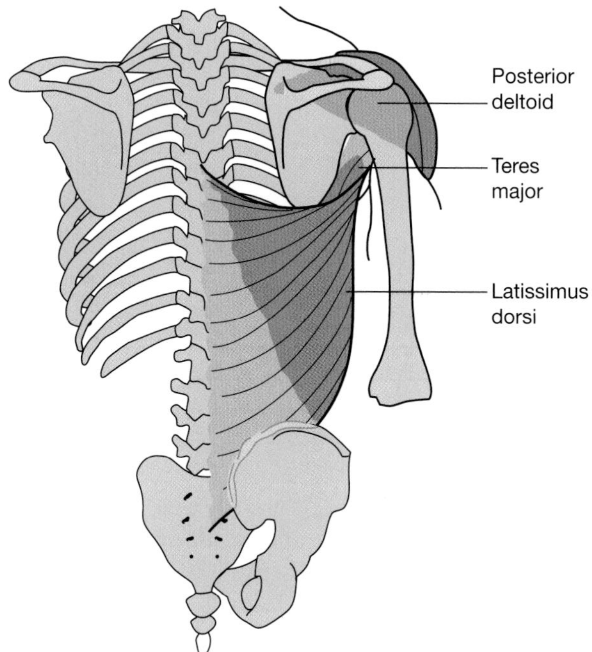

Figure 8.56 The primary extensors of the shoulder are the latissimus dorsi and teres major muscles.

- Resisted test: Stabilize the thorax in its upper portion with one hand and hold the patient's arm proximal to the elbow with your other hand while applying downward resistance as the patient attempts to elevate the arm from the examining table straight upward (Figure 8.57).

Testing shoulder extension with gravity eliminated can be performed with the patient lying on the side with the tested arm upward. The arm is placed

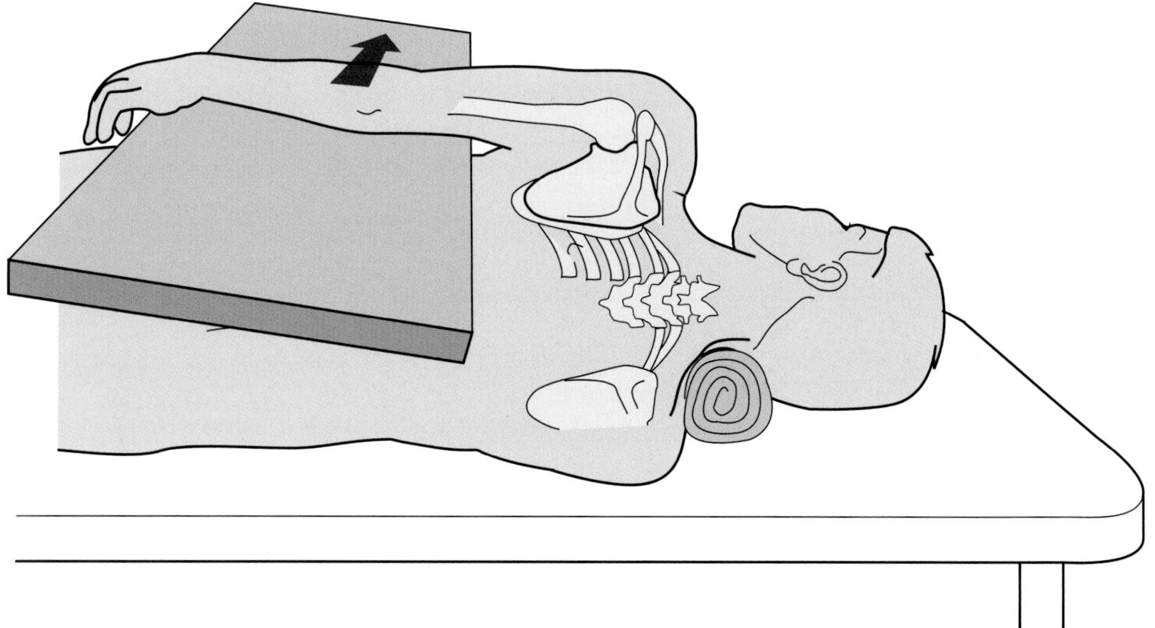

Figure 8.55 Testing shoulder flexion with gravity eliminated.

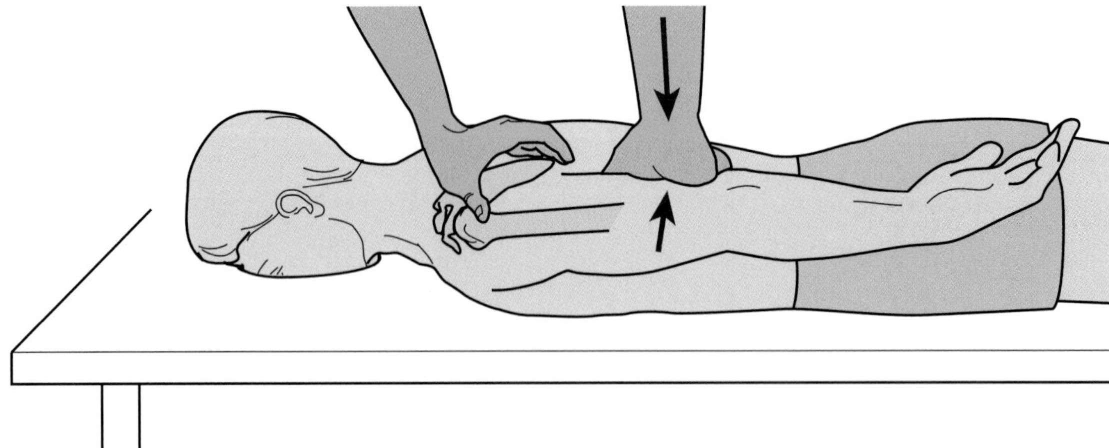

Figure 8.57 Testing shoulder extension.

on a powdered board and the patient attempts to extend the shoulder through the range of motion (Figure 8.58).

Painful shoulder extension may be due to tendinitis of the contracting muscles.

Weakness of shoulder extension will limit the patient's ability to use their arms for climbing, walking with crutches, swimming, or rowing a boat.

Shoulder Abduction

The abductors of the shoulder are primarily the middle portion of the deltoid and supraspinatus muscles (Figure 8.59). Assisting those muscles are the anterior and posterior fibers of the deltoid and the serratus anterior by its direct action on the scapula to rotate it outward and upward.

- Position of patient: Sitting with the arm abducted to 90 degrees and the elbow flexed slightly.
- Resisted test: Stand behind the patient and put one hand over the upper trapezius next to the neck to stabilize the thorax. Take your other hand and place it over the arm just proximal to the elbow joint and apply downward resistance as the patient attempts to abduct the arm upward (Figure 8.60).

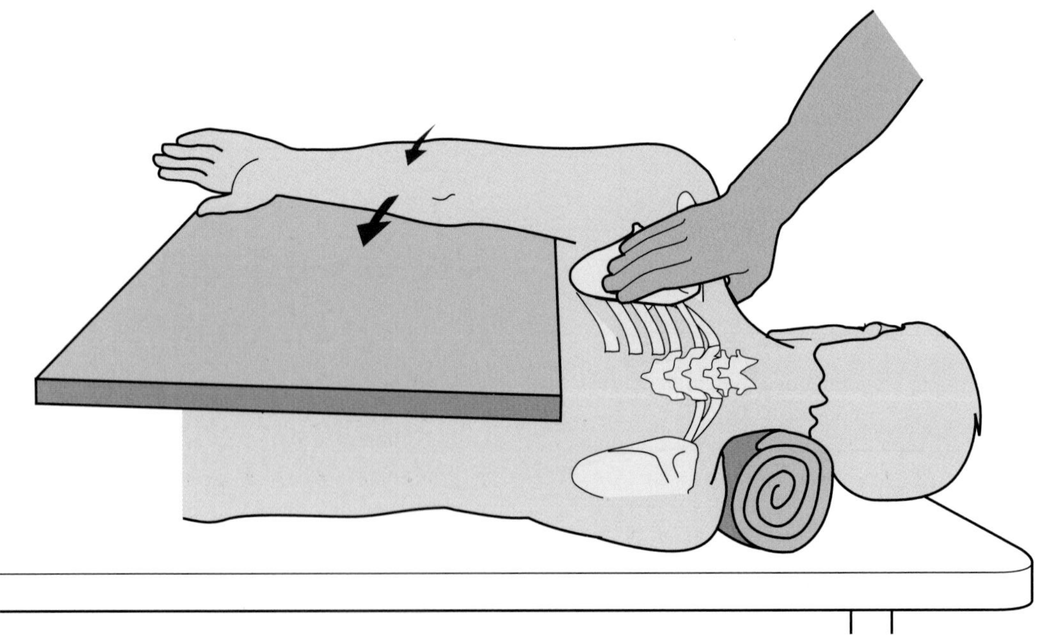

Figure 8.58 Testing shoulder extension with gravity eliminated.

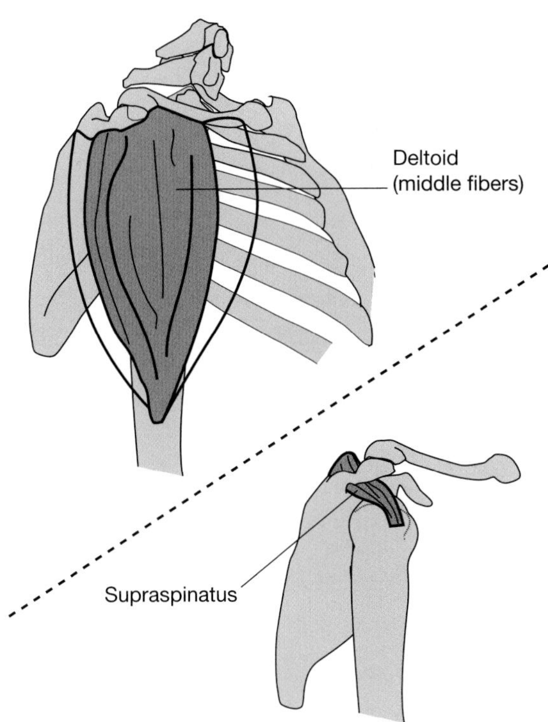

Figure 8.59 The primary abductors of the shoulder are the middle fibers of the deltoid and the supraspinatus muscles.

Testing shoulder abduction with gravity eliminated is performed with the patient in the supine position with the arm at the side and the elbow flexed slightly. The patient attempts to abduct the arm with the weight of the arm supported by the examining table through the range of motion (Figure 8.61).

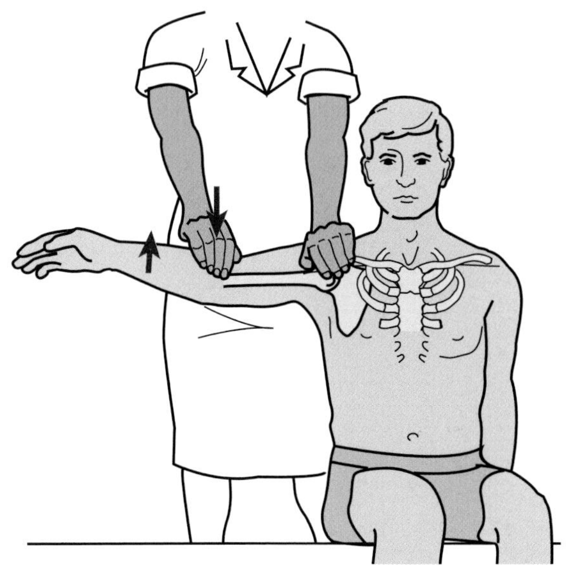

Figure 8.60 Testing shoulder abduction.

Painful resisted shoulder abduction may be due to tendinitis of the contracting muscles.

Weakness of shoulder abduction causes a significant restriction in the patient's ability to perform ADL and self-care.

Shoulder Adduction

The primary adductor of the shoulder is the pectoralis major muscle (Figure 8.62). Accessory muscles include the latissimus dorsi, the anterior portion of the deltoid, and the teres major.

- Position of patient: Supine with the shoulder abducted to about 90 degrees. The patient horizontally adducts the shoulder, bringing the arm across the chest.
- Resisted test: Place one hand behind the patient's shoulder to stabilize the thorax. Take your other hand and hold the patient's arm with your thumb posteriorly so that you can apply a resisting force away from the midline of the patient as the patient attempts to adduct the arm against your resistance (Figure 8.63).

Testing shoulder adduction with gravity eliminated is performed with the patient sitting, with the upper extremity on an examining table and the elbow extended. The patient attempts to bring the arm forward across the body while the weight of the arm is supported by the examining table (Figure 8.64).

Painful resisted shoulder adduction can be caused by tendinitis of the contracting muscles.

Weakness of shoulder adduction can result in restricted bimanual activities. For example, carrying a heavy object at the level of the waist would be difficult.

Shoulder Internal (Medial) Rotation

The primary internal rotators of the shoulder are the latissimus dorsi, teres major, subscapularis, and pectoralis major (Figure 8.65).

- Position of patient: Prone with the arm abducted to 90 degrees and the elbow flexed to 90 degrees.
- Resisted test: Place one hand on the upper arm to stabilize it. Place your other hand above the patient's wrist and push downward as the patient attempts to push your hand upward against your resistance (Figure 8.66).

Testing shoulder internal rotation with gravity eliminated is performed by having the patient lie

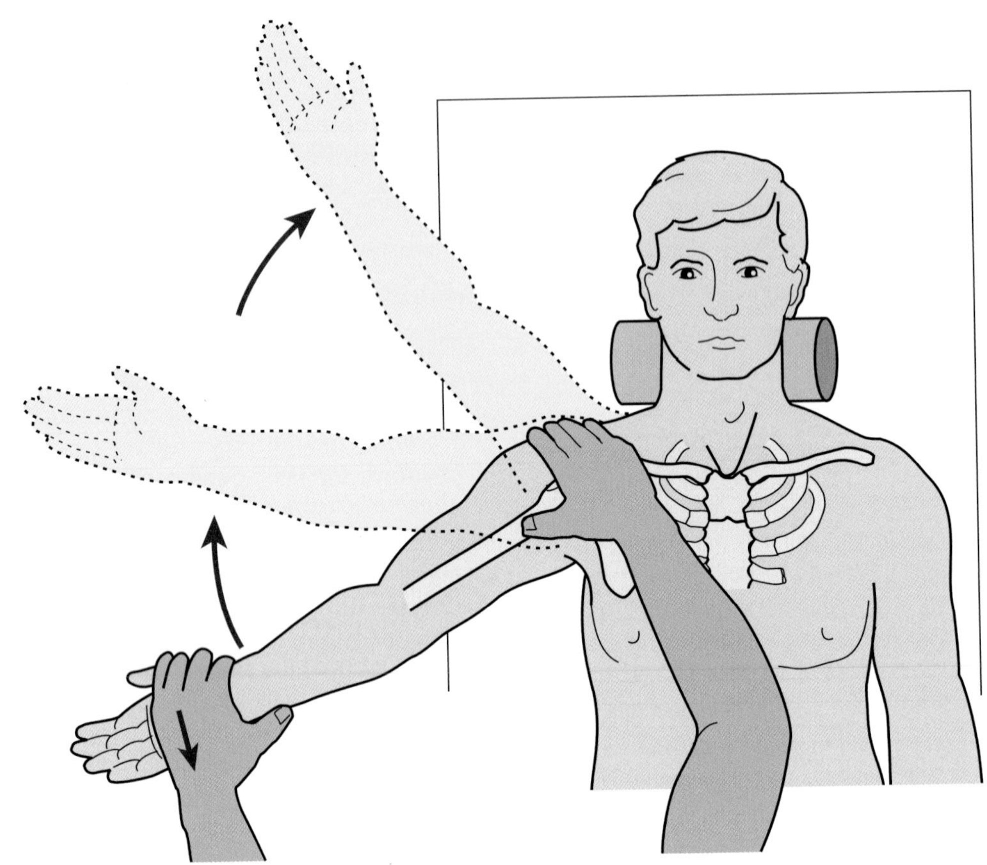

Figure 8.61 Testing shoulder abduction with gravity eliminated.

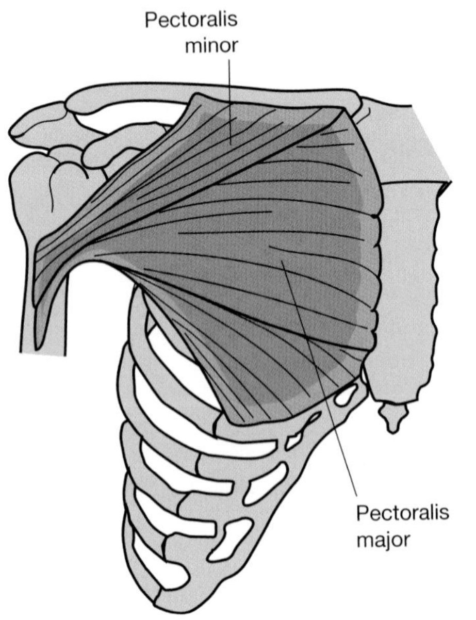

Figure 8.62 The primary adductor of the shoulder is the pectoralis major muscle.

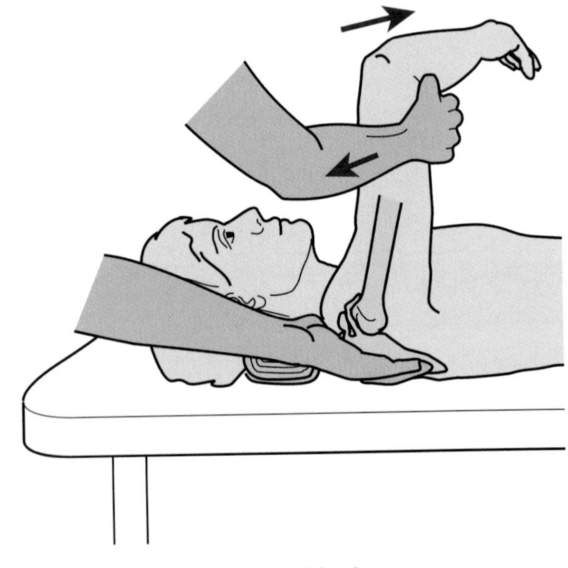

Figure 8.63 Testing shoulder adduction.

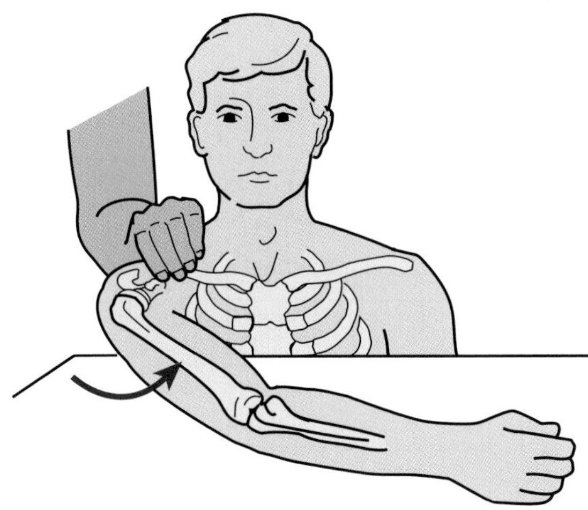

Figure 8.64 Testing shoulder adduction with gravity eliminated.

prone with the tested arm hanging from the table and in external rotation. The patient attempts to internally rotate the arm from the externally rotated position while you support the scapula and thorax with your forearm and hand (Figure 8.67).

Painful internal rotation may be due to tendinitis of the working muscles.

Shoulder External (Lateral) Rotation

The external rotators of the shoulder are the infraspinatus and teres minor muscles (Figure 8.68). The posterior fibers of the deltoid muscle assist in this movement.

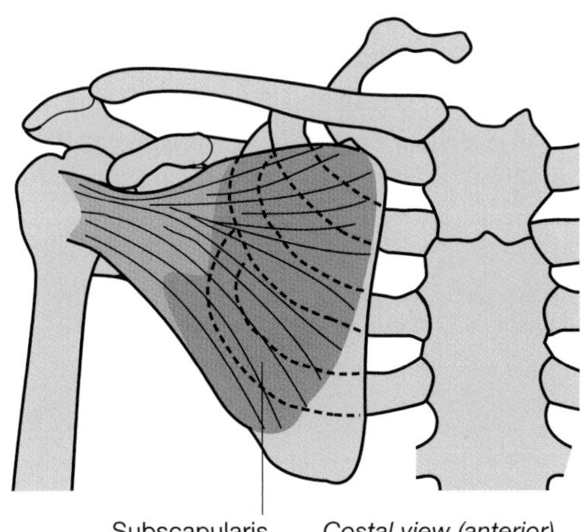

Figure 8.65 The primary shoulder internal rotators are the subscapularis, pectoralis major, and latissimus dorsi.

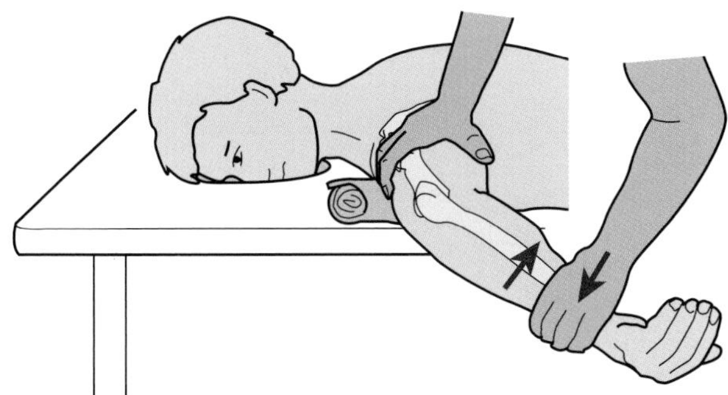

Figure 8.66 Testing shoulder internal rotation.

- Position of patient: Prone with the shoulder abducted to 90 degrees and the elbow bent at 90 degrees. The upper arm is supported by the examining table, with a pillow or folded towel placed underneath the upper arm.
- Resisted test: While stabilizing the scapula with the palm and fingers of one hand, take the patient's arm just above the wrist with your other hand and apply downward resistance as the patient attempts to upwardly rotate the shoulder so that the hand is elevated above the level of the examining table (Figure 8.69).

Testing shoulder external rotation with gravity eliminated is performed with the patient in the prone position, with the test arm dangling over the edge of

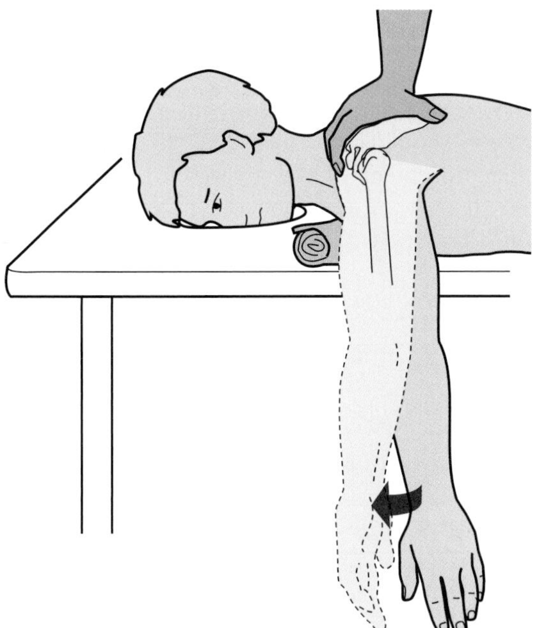

Figure 8.67 Testing shoulder internal rotation with gravity eliminated.

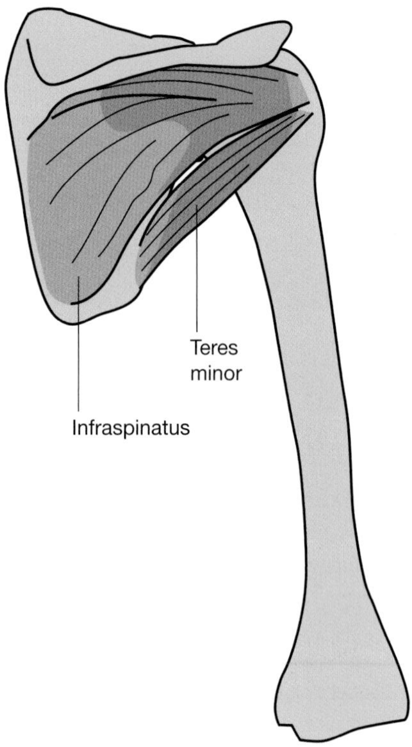

Figure 8.68 The primary external rotators of the shoulder are the infraspinatus and teres minor.

the examining table in internal rotation. The patient attempts to externally rotate the arm while you stabilize the scapula with your hands (Figure 8.70).

Painful resisted external rotation may be due to tendinitis of the working muscles.

Weakness of external rotation will prevent abduction of the shoulder to more than 95 degrees due to the impingement of the greater tubercle of the humerus against the acromion, secondary to inability to depress the humeral head.

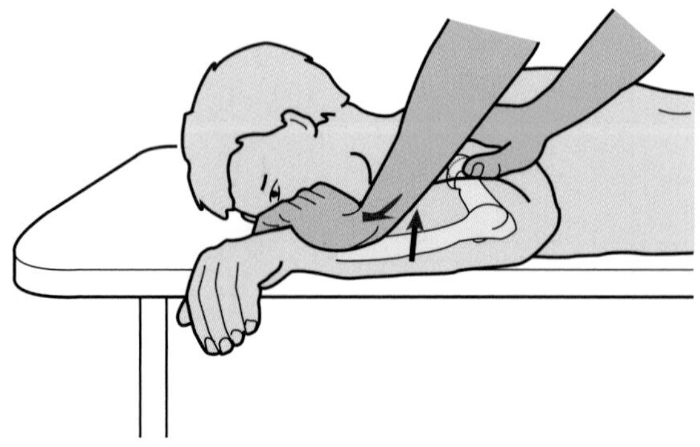

Figure 8.69 Testing external rotation.

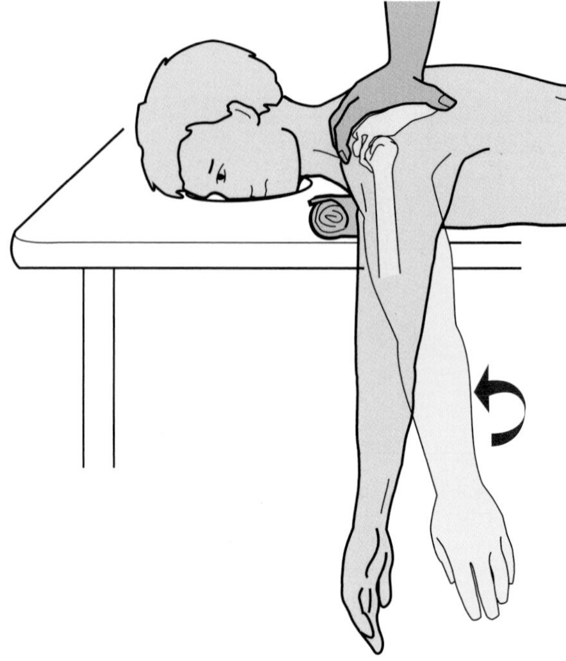

Figure 8.70 Testing external rotation with gravity eliminated.

Scapular Elevation (Shoulder Shrug)

The primary scapular elevators are the upper trapezius and levator scapulae muscles (Figure 8.71). The rhomboid muscles assist in this movement.

- Position of patient: Standing with arms at the sides.
- Resisted test: Stand behind the patient, placing each of your hands over the upper trapezius muscles. Ask the patient to shrug his or her shoulders against your resistance (Figure 8.72).

Testing scapular elevation with gravity eliminated is performed with the patient in the supine position with the arms at the sides. Ask the patient to shrug his or her shoulders in this position (Figure 8.73).

Painful resisted scapular elevation can be due to tendinitis of the working muscles or a sprain of the cervical spine.

Weakness of scapular elevation may be due to cranial nerve damage and other brain stem signs should be searched for. The spinal accessory nerve may be cut during a radical neck dissection.

Scapular Retraction

The scapular retractors are the rhomboideus major and minor muscles, assisted by the middle fibers of the trapezius (Figure 8.74).

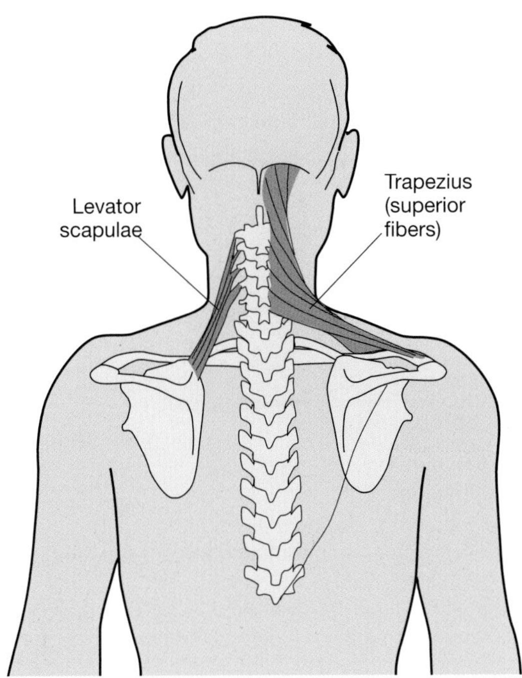

Figure 8.71 The primary scapular elevators are the superior fibers of the trapezius and the levator scapulae muscles.

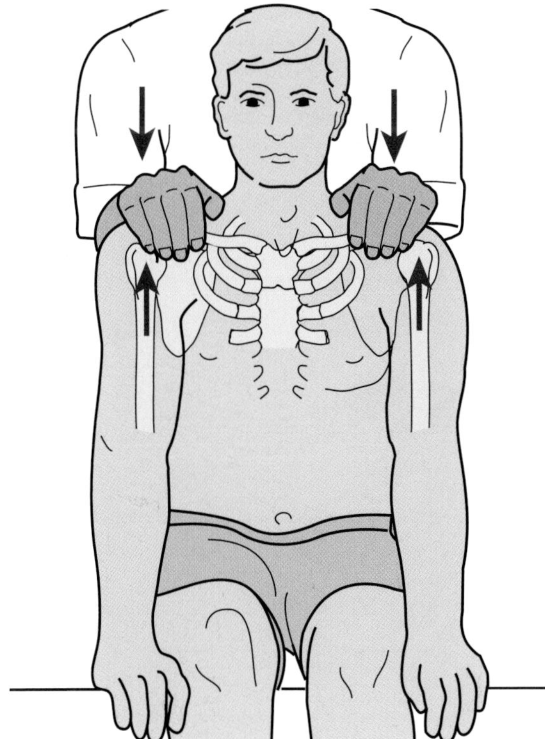

Figure 8.72 Testing scapular elevation.

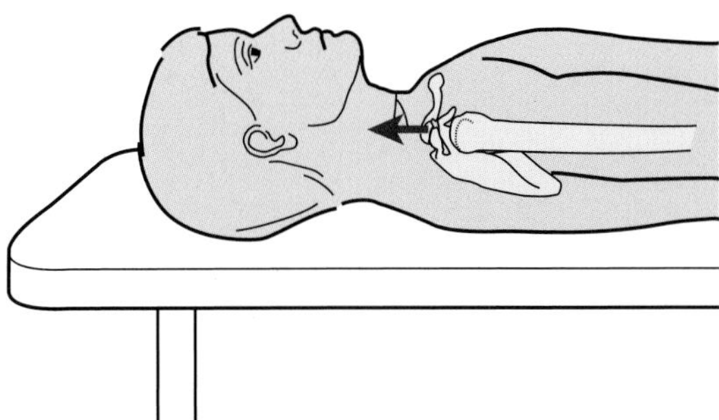

Figure 8.73 Testing scapular elevation with gravity eliminated.

- Position of patient: Standing with the arm adducted and the elbow slightly bent. The humerus is slightly extended.
- Resisted test: Stand beside the patient and place your hand so that you are cupping the elbow. Ask the patient to resist as you attempt to abduct the scapula, using his or her arm as leverage (Figure 8.75).

Testing scapular retraction with gravity eliminated is performed with the patient in the same position.

Painful scapular retraction may be due to tendinitis of the contracting muscles or disorders of the thoracic spine.

Weakness of scapular fixation by the rhomboid muscles leads to weakness of humeral adduction and extension.

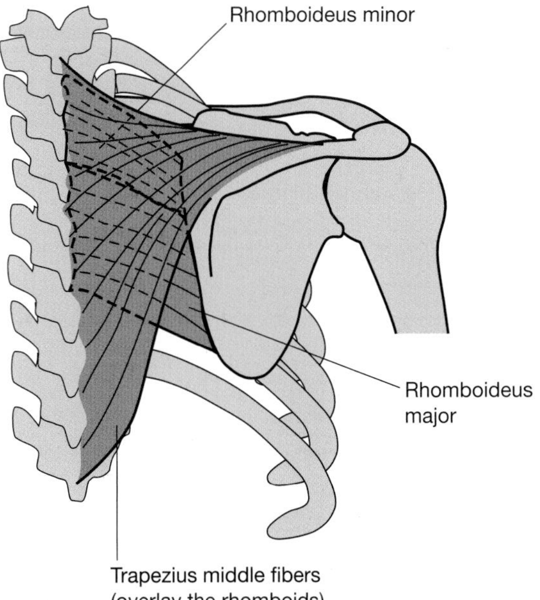

Figure 8.74 The scapular retractors are the rhomboideus major, rhomboideus minor, and the middle fibers of the trapezius muscles.

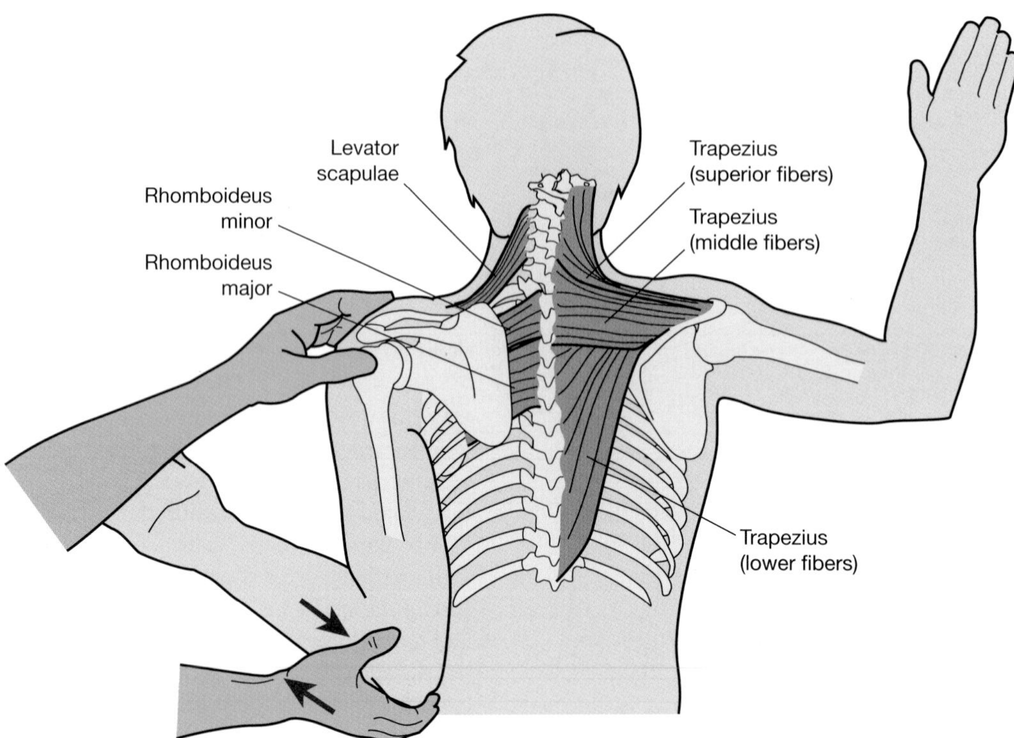

Figure 8.75 Testing scapular retraction.

Scapular Protraction

The serratus anterior muscle is the primary scapular protractor (Figure 8.76). This muscle maintains the inferior angle of the scapula against the thoracic wall and rotates the inferior angle upward.

- Position of patient: Standing with the test arm flexed forward approximately 90 degrees and the elbow bent also about 90 degrees.
- Resisted test: Stand behind the patient and place one hand over the thoracic spine for stabilization. Take your other hand and hold the proximal aspect of the patient's forearm and elbow and attempt to pull the arm backward toward you from this point while the patient attempts to push the arm forward (Figure 8.77).

Testing scapular protraction with gravity eliminated is performed with the patient in the sitting position (Figure 8.78).

Painful scapular protraction may be due to tendinitis of the contracting muscles.

Weakness of the serratus anterior muscle is frequently caused by damage to the long thoracic nerve. This nerve is composed of C5, C6, and C7 nerve roots. The result of weakness of this muscle is a medial winging of the scapula. This can be elicited by asking the

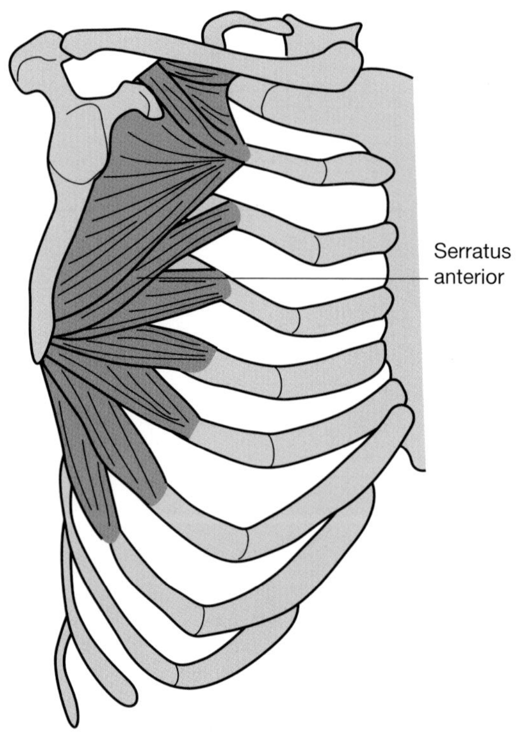

Figure 8.76 The primary scapular protractor is the serratus anterior muscle.

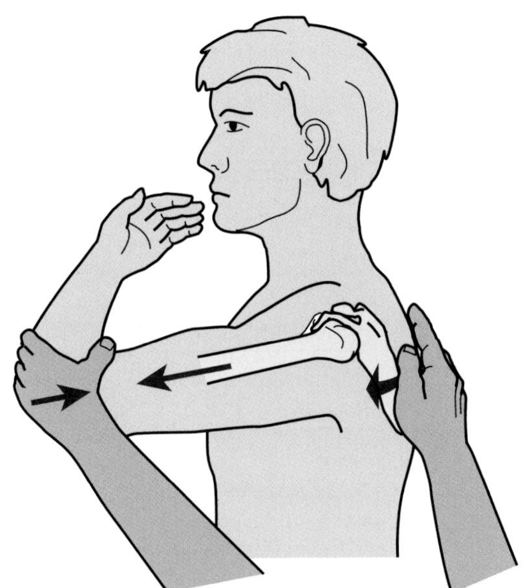

Figure 8.77 Testing scapular protraction.

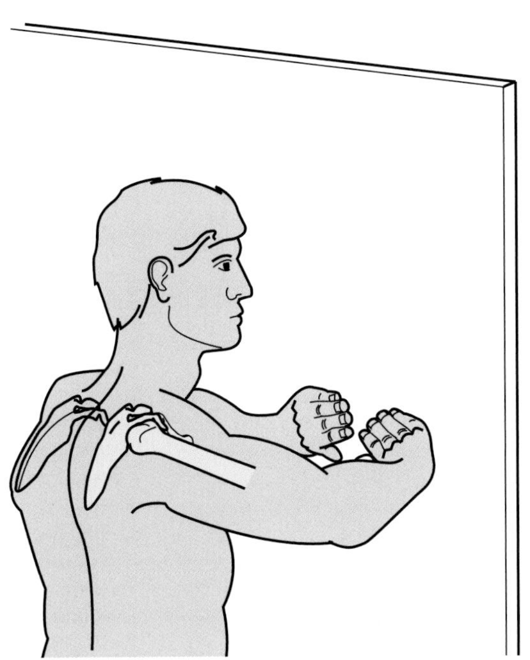

Figure 8.79 Medial winging of the scapula is caused by weakness of the serratus anterior muscle. This is frequently caused by damage to the long thoracic nerve (C5, C6, and C7 nerve roots).

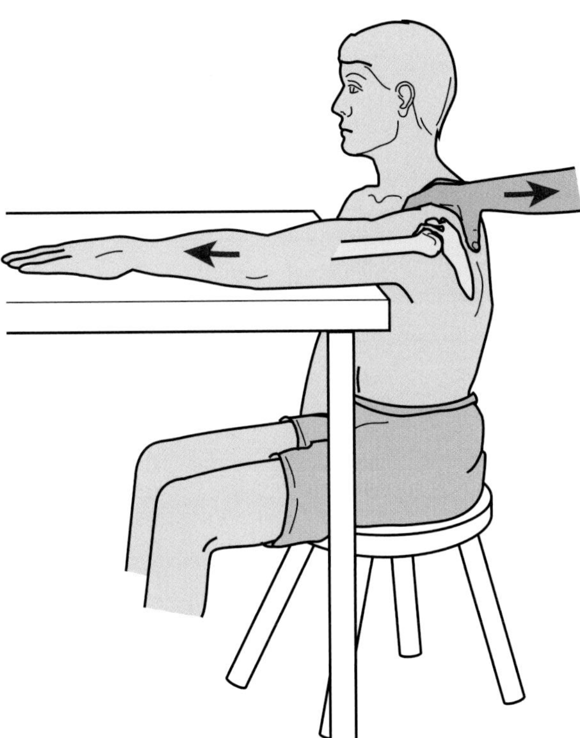

Figure 8.78 Testing scapular protraction with gravity eliminated is performed with the patient in a sitting position with the arm outstretched on a table in front. Ask the patient to bring the entire extremity forward and watch for movement of the scapula away from the midline.

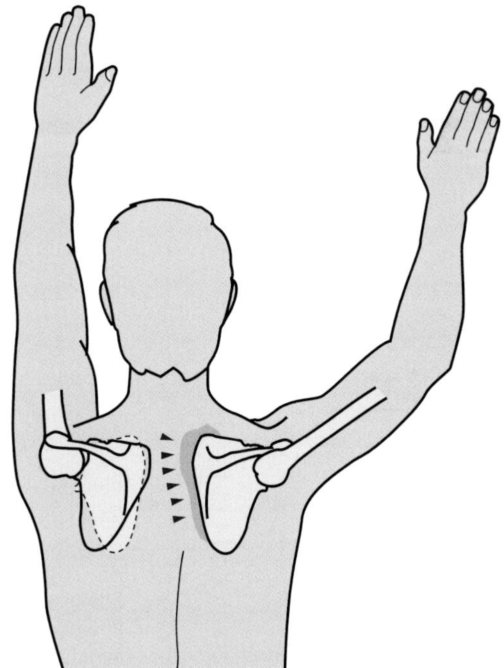

Figure 8.80 Note that with weakness of the right serratus anterior, the patient is unable to fully rotate and abduct the scapula as compared to the left side. The result is an inability to forward flex the arm completely upward.

patient to push against the wall, as shown in Figure 8.79. The scapula wings out medially because the trapezius muscle maintains the medial scapular border close to the vertebral column.

The inability to abduct and rotate the scapula prevents the patient from being able to forward flex the arm to the complete upright position (Figure 8.80).

Neurological Examination

Motor

The innervation and spinal levels of the muscles that function in the shoulder are listed in Table 8.1.

Table 8.1 Movements and Innervation of Shoulder Muscles

Movement	Muscles	Innervation	Root Level
Forward flexion	Deltoid	Axillary	C5, C6
	Pectoralis major (clavicular fibers)	Lateral pectoral	C5, C6, C7
	Coracobrachialis	Musculocutaneous	C6, C7
	Biceps	Musculocutaneous	C5, C6
Extension	Deltoid (posterior fibers)	Axillary	C5, C6
	Teres major	Subscapular	C5, C6
	Teres minor	Axillary	C5
	Latissimus dorsi	Thoracodorsal	C6, C7, C8
	Pectoralis major (sternocostal fibers)	Lateral pectoral	C5, C6, C7
		Medial pectoral	C7, C8, T1
	Triceps (long head)	Radial	C7, C8
Abduction	Deltoid	Axillary	C5, C6
	Supraspinatus	Suprascapular	C5
	Infraspinatus	Suprascapular	C5, C6
	Subscapularis	Subscapular	C5, C6
	Teres major	Axillary	C5
Adduction	Pectoralis major	Lateral pectoral	C5, C6, C7
	Latissimus dorsi	Thoracodorsal	C6, C7, C8
	Teres major	Subscapular	C5, C6
	Subscapularis	Subscapular	C5, C6
Internal (medial) rotation	Pectoralis major	Lateral pectoral	C5, C6, C7
	Deltoid (anterior fibers)	Axillary	C5, C6
	Latissimus dorsi	Thoracodorsal	C6, C7, C8
	Teres major	Subscapular	C5, C6
	Subscapularis	Subscapular	C5, C6
External (lateral) rotation	Infraspinatus	Suprascapular	C5, C6
	Deltoid (posterior fibers)	Axillary	C5, C6
	Teres minor	Axillary	C5
Elevation of scapula	Trapezius (upper fibers)	Accessory	Cranial nerve XI
		C3, C4 nerve roots	C3, C4 roots
	Levator scapulae	C3, C4 nerve roots	C3, C4 roots
		Dorsal scapular	C5
	Rhomboideus major	Dorsal scapular	C5
	Rhomboideus minor	Dorsal scapular	C5
Retraction (backward movement of scapula)	Trapezius	Accessory	Cranial nerve XI
	Rhomboid major	Dorsal scapular	C5
	Rhomboideus minor	Dorsal scapular	C5
Protraction (forward movement of scapula)	Serratus anterior	Long thoracic	C5, C6, C7
	Pectoralis major	Lateral pectoral	C5, C6, C7
	Pectoralis minor	Medial pectoral	C7, C8, T1
	Latissimus dorsi	Thoracodorsal	C5, C6, C7

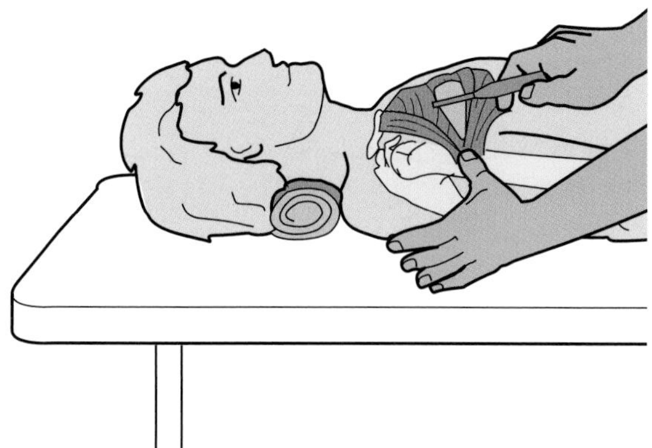

Figure 8.81 Testing the pectoralis reflex (C5 nerve root).

Reflexes

The pectoralis major jerk test is performed to test the C5 nerve root and pectoralis major muscle (Figure 8.81). Perform the reflex test by having the patient lie in the supine position and placing your thumb over the tendon of the pectoralis major muscle just proximal to the shoulder joint. Tap your thumb with the reflex hammer and observe for contraction of the pectoralis major muscle. The shoulder may also adduct somewhat during this reflex. Compare your findings with those from the opposite side. This reflex will be absent if there is severe injury to the pectoralis major muscle, medial and lateral pectoral nerves, upper trunk of the brachial plexus, or C5 nerve root.

Sensation

Light touch and pinprick sensation should be examined after the motor and reflex examination. The dermatomes for the shoulder are C4, C5, C6, and C7. The upper thoracic (T2, T3) dermatomes are responsible for the axilla and medial aspect of the arm (Figure 8.82). Peripheral nerves providing sensation in the shoulder region are shown in Figures 8.83 and 8.84.

Damage to the axillary or the musculocutaneous nerves can result from shoulder dislocation, and the sensory areas of these nerves should be examined carefully when the patient presents with a dislocation (Figure 8.85).

The suprascapular nerve may be damaged due to acromioclavicular joint separation or a ganglion cyst and this will result in pain and atrophy of the supraspinatus and infraspinatus muscles. Forced adduction of the arm across the chest worsens the pain due to stretching of the suprascapular nerve (Figure 8.86).

Damage to the upper trunk of the brachial plexus, which comprises the C5 and C6 nerve roots, leads to an Erb–Duchenne palsy of the upper extremity. This may be caused at birth by trauma due to shoulder dystocia or may be congenital. Characteristic posture and weakness as well as sensory loss result (Figure 8.87).

The spinal accessory nerve may be injured during surgery, and if the branch to the trapezius muscles is destroyed, the patient will present with an inability to shrug the shoulder and a lateral winging of the scapula. The scapula will move posteriorly away from the thorax, as in medial winging. However, the medial border of the scapula is set laterally away from the spinous processes by the strong serratus anterior.

Special Tests

Tests for Structural Stability and Integrity

Many tests have been devised to examine the shoulder for stability in the anterior, posterior, and inferior directions. There are also tests to examine the patient for multidirectional instability. All the tests are performed by applying passive forces to the glenohumeral joint in different directions. A great deal of experience is necessary to evaluate the degree of shoulder instability correctly.

Anterior Instability Tests

Anterior Instability Test (Rockwood Test)

This test is used to evaluate the degree to which the humeral head can be anteriorly subluxed from the glenoid cavity of the scapula (Figures 8.88a–8.88d). The patient is standing or sitting. Stand behind the patient and hold his or her arm just proximal to the wrist with your hand and laterally rotate the shoulder. Then abduct the arm to 45 degrees and again passively rotate the shoulder laterally. This same procedure is repeated at 90 and 120 degrees. At zero degrees, there is rarely any complaint of apprehension or pain. At 45 and 120 degrees, the patient may show some signs of apprehension. The test result is positive when the patient shows marked apprehension and pain posteriorly when the arm is at 90 degrees of abduction. This is due to anterior capsular/labral insufficiency. http://www.youtube.com/watch?v=WC90rwuzOVs

Rowe, Volk, Gerber, and Ganz have described other tests for anterior instability.

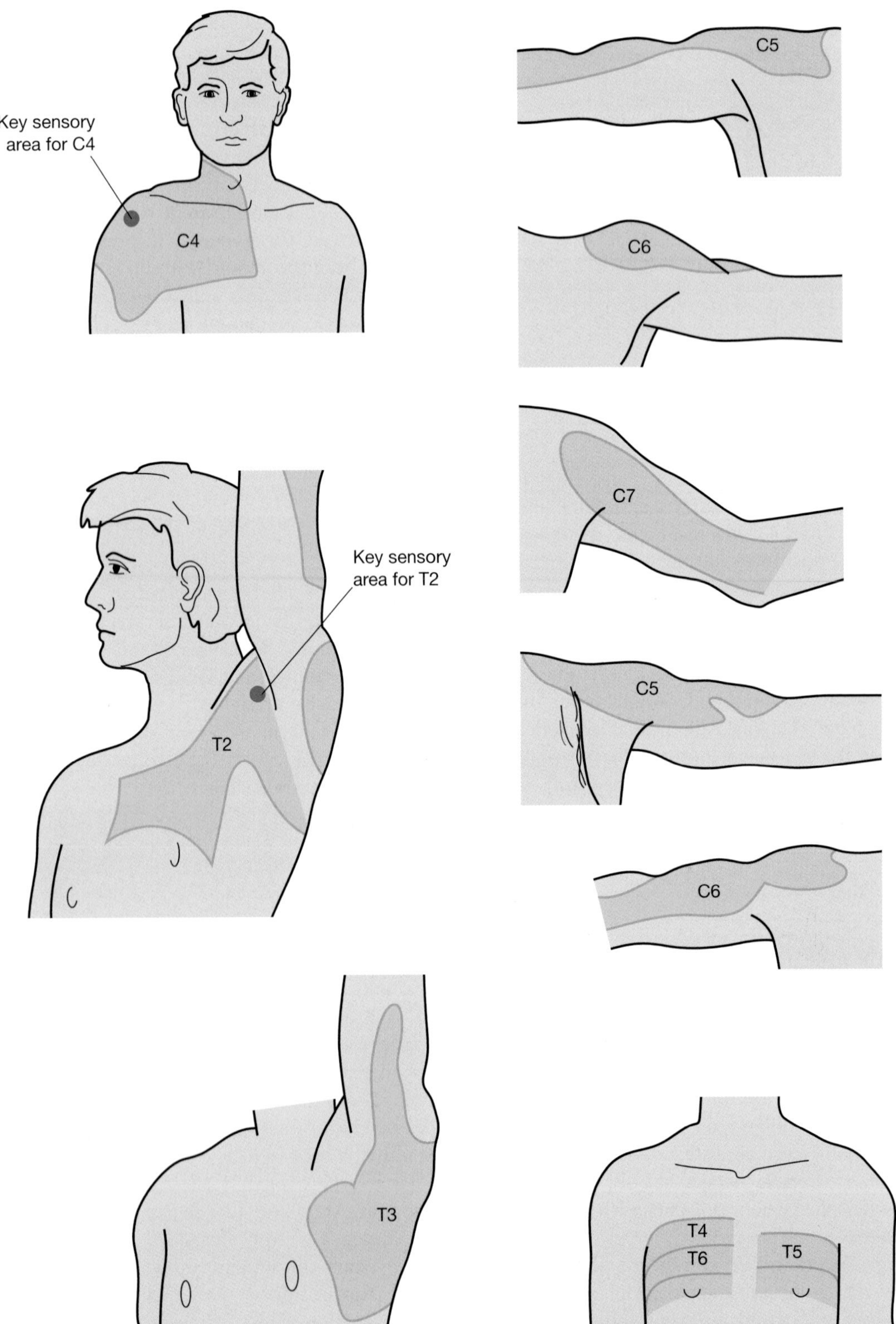

Figure 8.82 The dermatomes of the shoulder and axilla. Note the key sensory areas for the C4 and T2 dermatomes in this region.

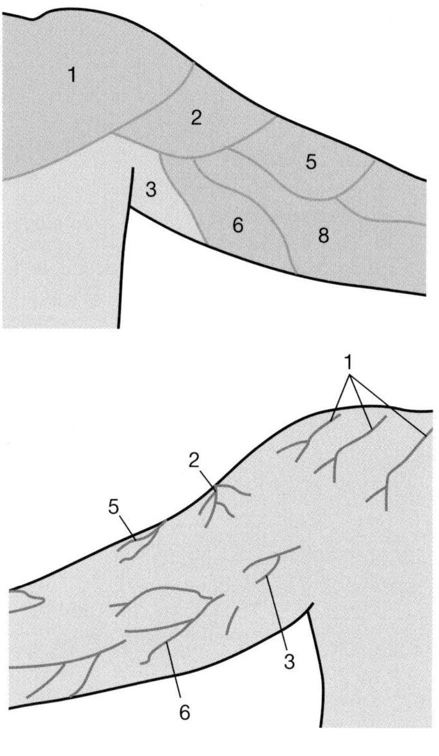

Figure 8.83 The nerve supply and distribution of the shoulder in the anterior view. 1 = supraclavicular nerve (C3, C4); 2 = upper lateral cutaneous (axillary) (C5, C6); 3 = intercostobrachial (T2); 4 = posterior cutaneous nerve of the arm (radial) (C5–C8); 5 = lower lateral cutaneous nerve (radial) (C5, C6); 6 = medial cutaneous nerve of the arm (C8, T1); 7 = posterior cutaneous nerve of the forearm (radial) (C5–C8); 8 = medial cutaneous nerve of the forearm (C8, T1).

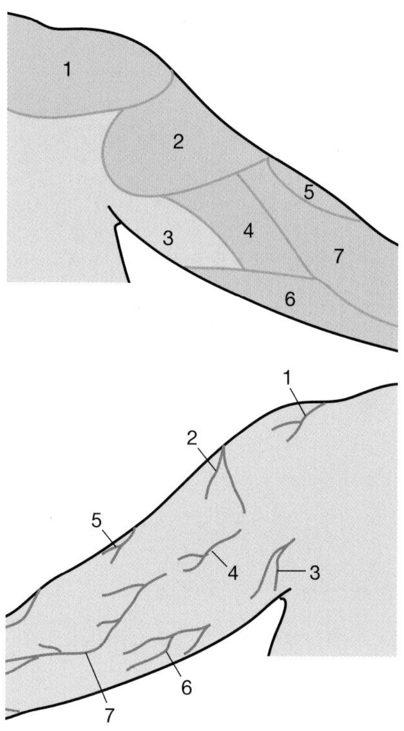

Figure 8.84 The nerve supply and distribution of the shoulder in the posterior view. 1 = supraclavicular nerve (C3, C4); 2 = upper lateral cutaneous (axillary) (C5, C6); 3 = intercostobrachial (T2); 4 = posterior cutaneous nerve of the arm (radial) (C5–C8); 5 = lower lateral cutaneous nerve (radial) (C5, C6); 6 = medial cutaneous nerve of the arm (C8, T1); 7 = posterior cutaneous nerve of the forearm (radial) (C5–C8); 8 = medial cutaneous nerve of the forearm (C8, T1).

Apprehension Test for Anterior Shoulder Dislocation (Crank Test)

The result of this test is frequently positive in patients who have had recent shoulder dislocation or are prone to recurrent shoulder dislocation. Ninety-five percent of shoulder dislocations occur anteriorly. The patient with acute shoulder dislocation shows a characteristic posture of the arm held close to the body, with a prominent acromion and a depression below the deltoid. Any movement of the arm or shoulder is extremely painful.

The apprehension test is performed with the patient in the supine position. Take the patient's forearm with one hand and support the patient's upper arm posteriorly with your other hand. Gently and slowly abduct and externally (laterally) rotate the arm. A positive finding is noted when the patient appears to be afraid

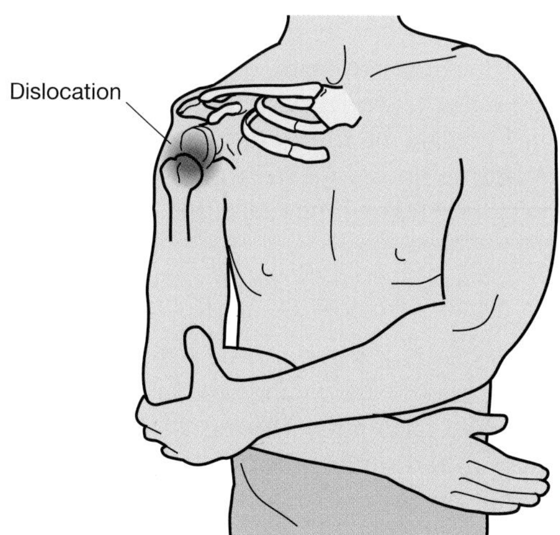

Figure 8.85 Appearance of a dislocated right shoulder. Always assess the patient for neurovascular damage when a dislocation is suspected.

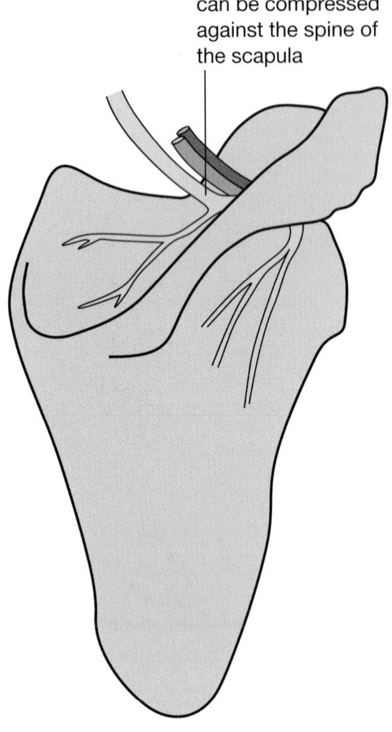

Figure 8.86 The location of the suprascapular nerve close to the skin can cause it to be compressed against the underlying bone.

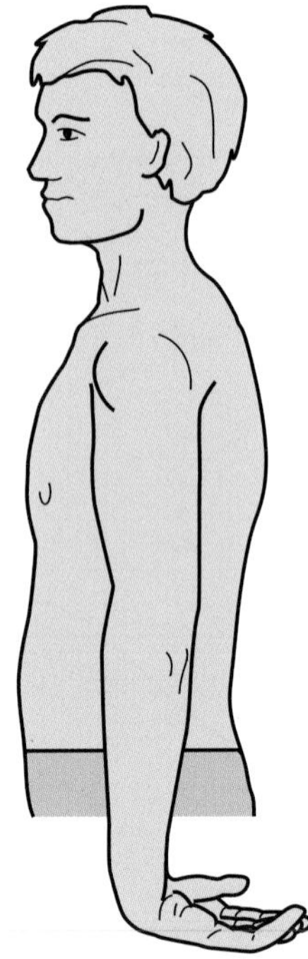

Figure 8.87 Characteristic position of a patient with an Erb–Duchenne palsy of the upper extremity, also referred to as a waiter's tip posture. The shoulder is internally rotated and adducted, and the wrist is flexed.

that the arm may dislocate. The patient may resist further motion and may state that the shoulder feels as though it is going to pop out (see Figure 8.89). http://www.youtube.com/watch?v=WdAqfwzna9 k

As you are performing this test, note the degree of external rotation at which the patient begins to become apprehensive. At this point, put a posterior stress on the humerus with one of your hands by pressing on the proximal part of the humerus anteriorly. You may now be able to further externally rotate the arm with this posterior stress. This is called a *relocation test* (Fowler or Jobe relocation test).

Posterior Instability Tests

Posterior Drawer Test of the Shoulder

This test is used to determine whether there is posterior shoulder instability. The test is performed with the patient in the supine position. Stand next to the patient and grasp the proximal end of the forearm with one hand while allowing the elbow to flex to 120 degrees. Now position the shoulder so that it is in 30 degrees of forward flexion and approximately 100 degrees of abduction. Take your other hand and stabilize the scapula by placing your index and middle fingers on the spine of the scapula and your thumb over the coracoid process. Now flex the shoulder forward to 80 degrees and rotate the forearm medially. While doing this with one hand, move your thumb off the coracoid process and push the head of the humerus posteriorly. You should be able to palpate the head of the humerus with the index finger of your hand. If this test causes apprehension in the patient, or if there is greater posterior mobility of the humeral head than on the opposite side, the test result is positive and indicates posterior instability (Figure 8.90a–8.90d). http://www.youtube.com/watch?v=oH7VdFazEbg

Inferior Instability Tests

Feagin Test

The patient sits on the examination table with their shoulder abducted to 90 degrees, elbow in full extension, and arm resting on your shoulder.

This test is used to assess the presence of humeral head inferior subluxation caused by damage to the inferior glenohumeral ligament. Place both of your hands along the proximal humerus over the deltoid

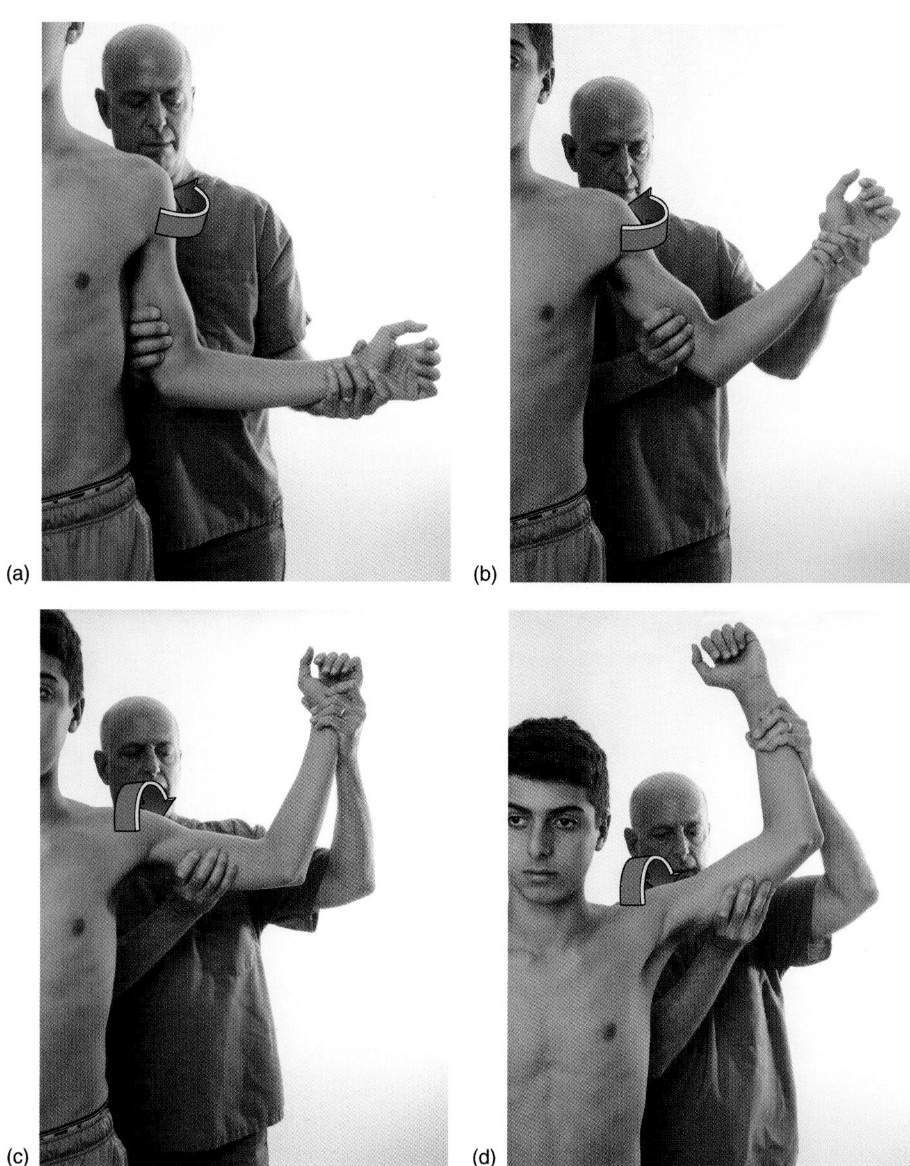

Figure 8.88 Anterior instability test (Rockwood test). This test is used to identify weakness or insufficiency of the anterior capsular and labral structures: (a) with the arms at the sides, (b) with the arm at 45 degrees of abduction, (c) with the arm at 90 degrees of abduction. Look for apprehension and posterior pain in this position, for a positive test result, (d) with the arm at 120 degrees.

while interlocking your fingers. Apply an inferiorly directed force to the humerus and palpate for inferior movement. Also, observe the patient for apprehension or discomfort. Abnormal inferior motion of the humerus and/or patient apprehension is indicative of inferior glenohumeral instability (Figure 8.91). http://www.youtube.com/watch?v=ocCkkuI_6nQ

Sulcus Sign

Instruct the patient to stand with their arm relaxed at their side. Gently distract the arm inferiorly. The presence of a sulcus, space, distal to the acromion may be indicative of inferior glenohumeral instability (Figure 8.92a).

Multidirectional Instability Tests

Rowe Multidirectional Instability Test

While standing, the patient bends forward slightly with the arm relaxed. Palpate using your thumb and index finger around the humeral head. Position the arm in 20–30 degrees of extension and push

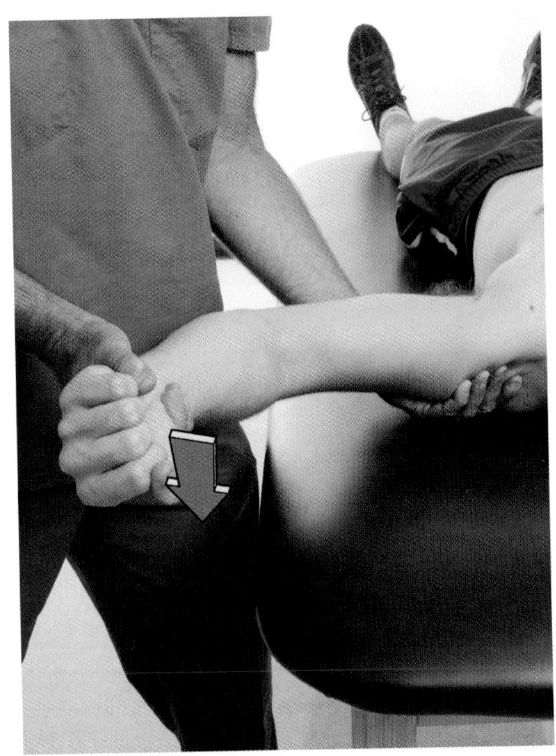

Figure 8.89 The anterior apprehension test.

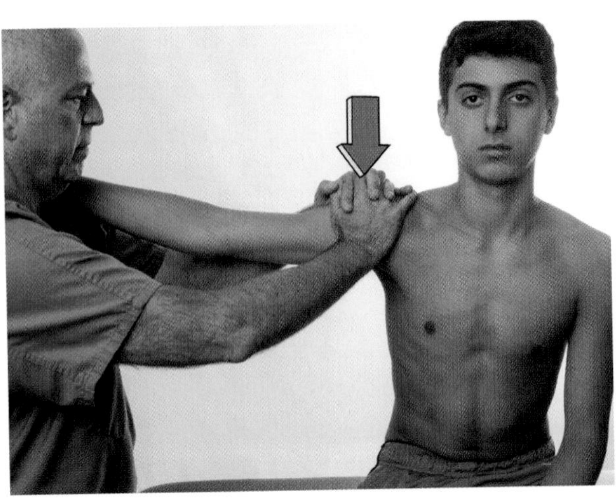

Figure 8.91 Feagin test.

anteriorly on the proximal humerus to determine whether there is anterior instability. Position the arm in 20–30 degrees of flexion and push posteriorly to determine whether there is posterior instability. Distract the arm slightly inferiorly and pull on the forearm to determine if there is inferior instability (Figure 8.93a–8.93c).

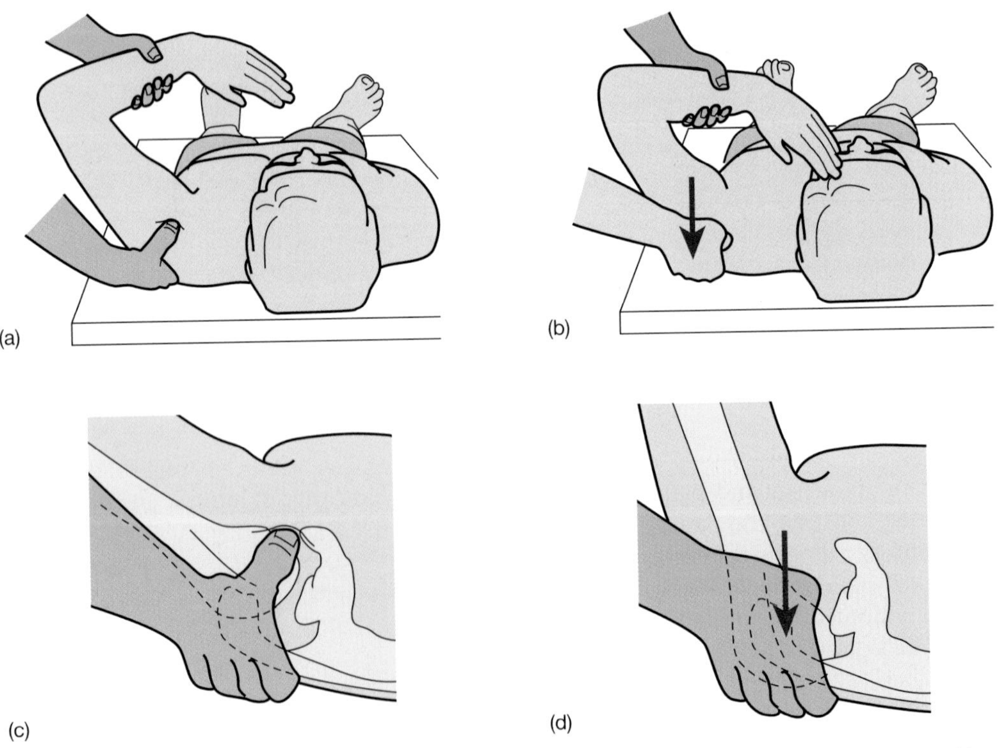

Figure 8.90 Test for posterior drawer of the shoulder: (a and b) how the test is performed and (c and d) the test with a superimposed drawing of the bones on the skin.

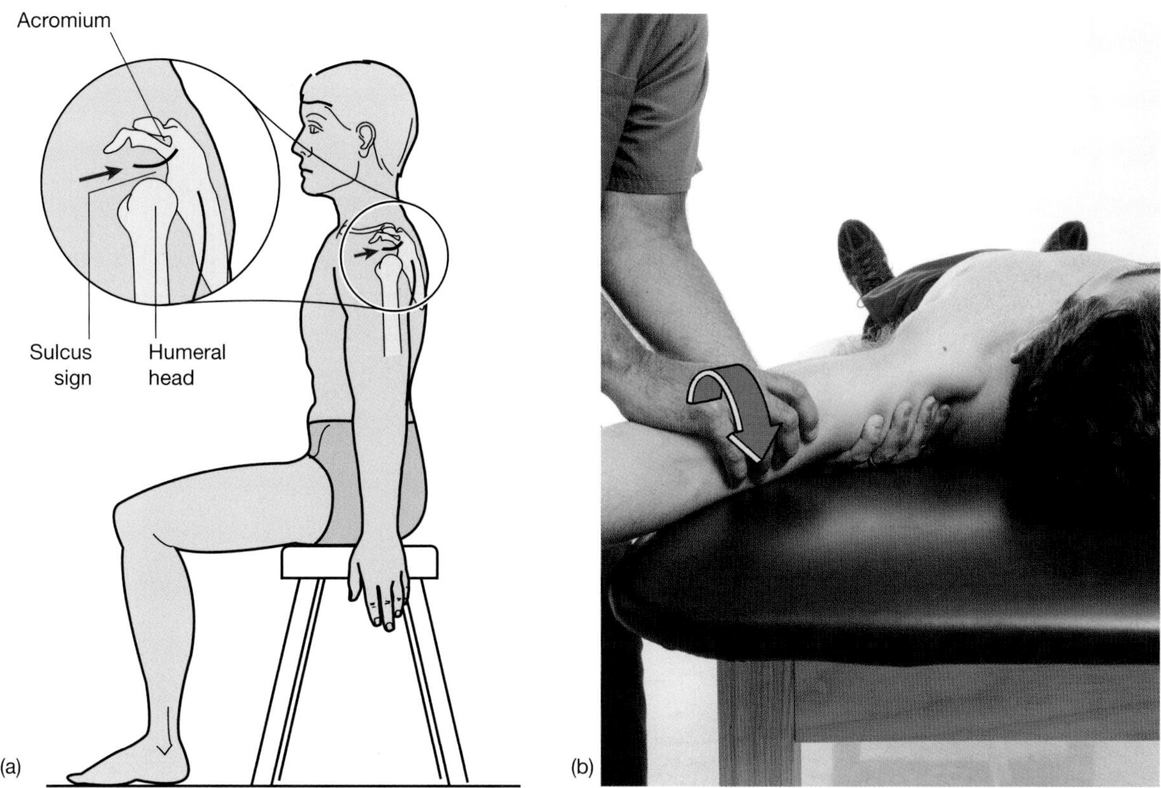

Figure 8.92 (a) The appearance of a gap below the acromion in a patient who has hemiplegia. (b) The clunk test for glenoid labral tears.

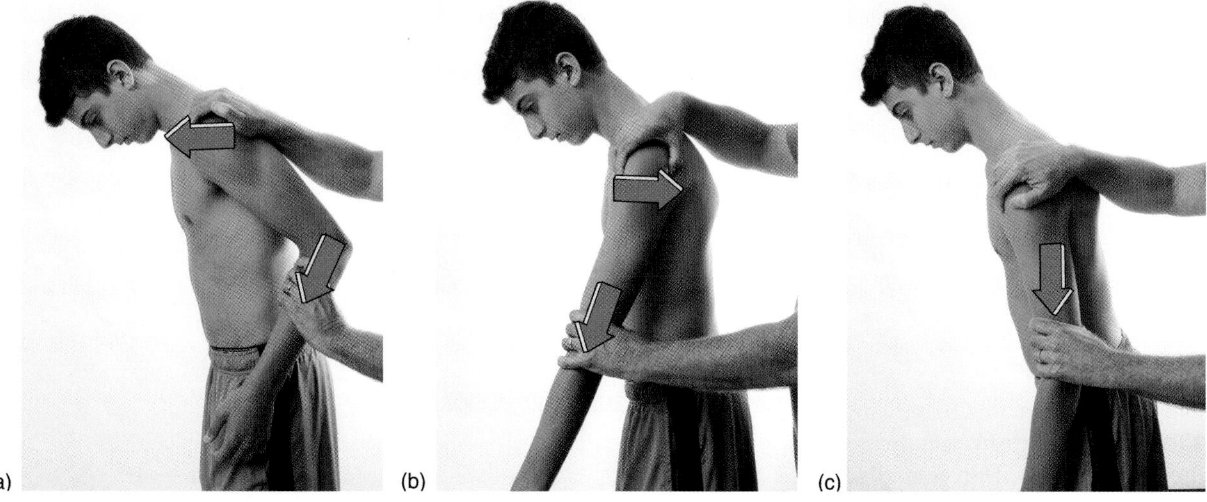

Figure 8.93 Rowe multidirectional instability test. (a) Test for anterior instability. (b) Test for posterior instability. (c) Test for inferior instability.

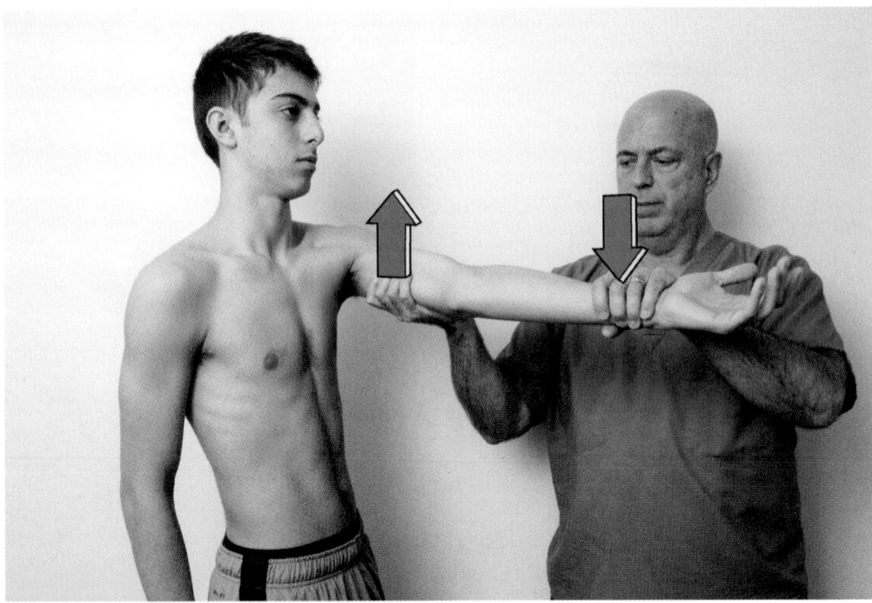

Figure 8.94 Biceps tension test. Apply an eccentric adduction force.

Tests for Labral Tears

Clunk Test

This test is performed to confirm a tear of the glenoid labrum. The patient is in supine. Place one hand on the arm above the elbow and put your other hand over the humeral head. Now, bring the arm into full abduction. Push the humeral head anteriorly while your other hand laterally rotates the humerus. A grinding sound or "clunk" indicates a labral tear (Figure 8.92b).

SLAP Lesions

Biceps Tension Test

Resist forward flexion of the shoulder with the elbow extended and the wrist supinated. If the patient reports pain, the test is considered positive for biceps tendon pathology (Figure 8.94).

Biceps Load Test

Place the patient in supine. Abduct the shoulder to 120 degrees, with maximum external rotation. Flex the elbow to 90 degrees and supinate the forearm. If this test position is painful, ask the patient to flex his elbow against your resistance. Active elbow flexion will increase the pain. The test is negative if the pain is not increased by elbow flexion. A positive test occurs since contraction of the biceps in this shoulder position places increased tension on the torn superior labral tissue by virtue of the biceps attachment, leading to worsening of the pain (Figure 8.95).

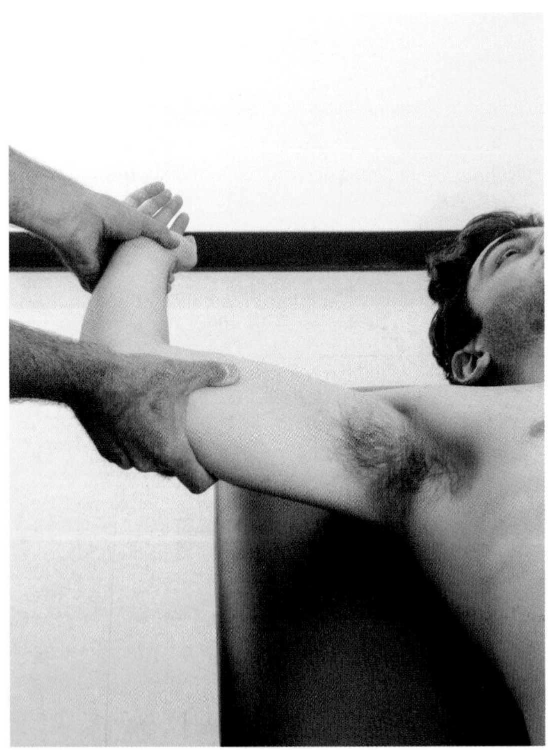

Figure 8.95 Biceps load test. If the starting position is painful, resist active elbow flexion to determine if pain is increased.

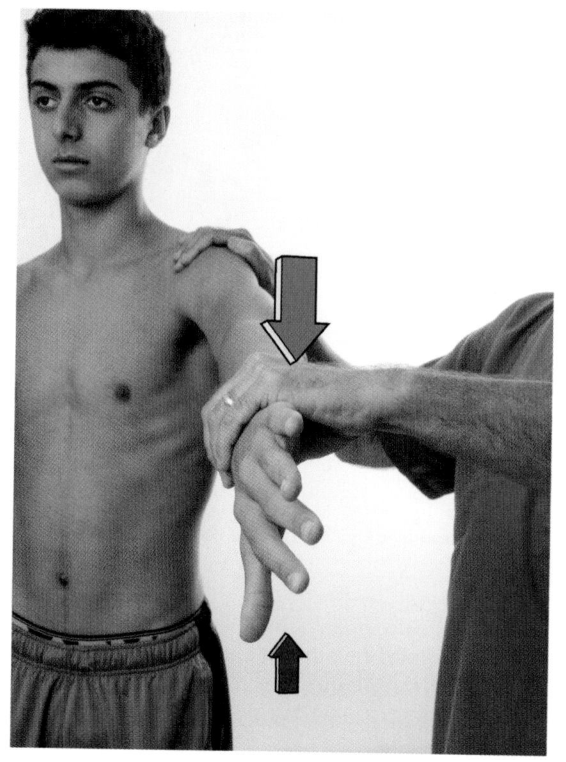
(a)

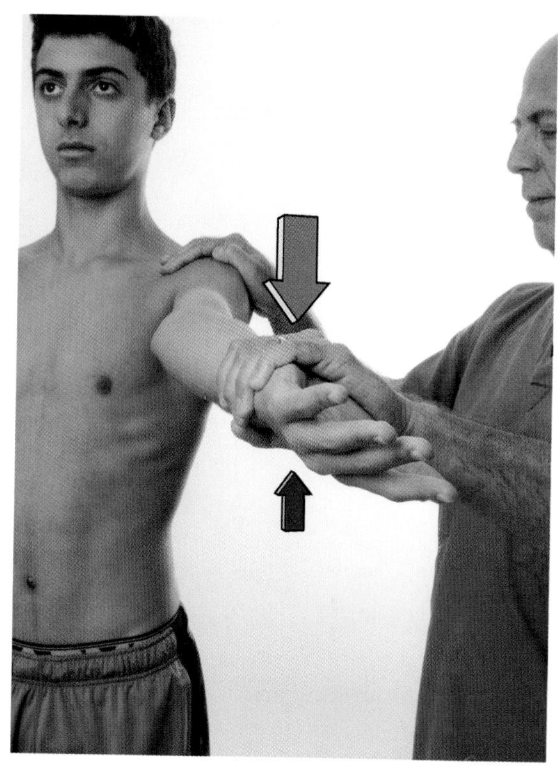
(b)

Figure 8.96 Active compression test of O'Brien. (a) Apply a downward force with shoulder internally rotated. (b) Apply a downward force with shoulder externally rotated.

Active Compression Test of O'Brien

Place the patient in the standing position. Ask the patient to place his arm, with the elbow extended, in 90 degrees of flexion. Adduct the arm 10 degrees from the midline and internally rotate (thumb pointing down). You should stand behind the patient and apply force in a downward direction. Allow the arm to return to the starting position and then repeat the test in full external rotation/supination (palm facing upward). The test is considered to be positive if pain is produced inside the shoulder during the initial part of the test and if the pain is decreased while performing the test in the externally rotated position. If the test is correlated with a positive Speed's test, an anterior type II SLAP (superior labrum anterior–posterior) tear can be diagnosed (Figures 8.96a and 8.96b). http://www.youtube.com/watch?v=0QbNRozDFwY

SLAP Prehension Test

Place the patient in either the sitting or standing position. Ask the patient to place his arm in 90 degrees of abduction with the elbow extended and the forearm pronated (thumb pointing down). This position puts tension on the long head of the biceps and traps the torn labral tissue between the glenoid and humeral head. This may cause pain in the region of the bicipital groove with or without an audible or palpable click. The test should then be repeated with the forearm in supination (thumb pointing up). The test is positive only if the pain is reduced or disappears when the forearm is supinated (Figure 8.97).

Tests for the Acromioclavicular Joint

Cross-Flexion Test

By taking the patient's arm and abducting it to 90 degrees, and flexing the arm across the body, you can exacerbate the pain emanating from the acromioclavicular joint. Palpate the joint with your thumb while forcing cross-flexion of the patient's arm with your other hand (Figure 8.98).

Scapula Stability Tests

Wall Push-Up Test

Ask the patient to stand arm's length from the wall. Instruct them to perform 10–20 repetitions of wall

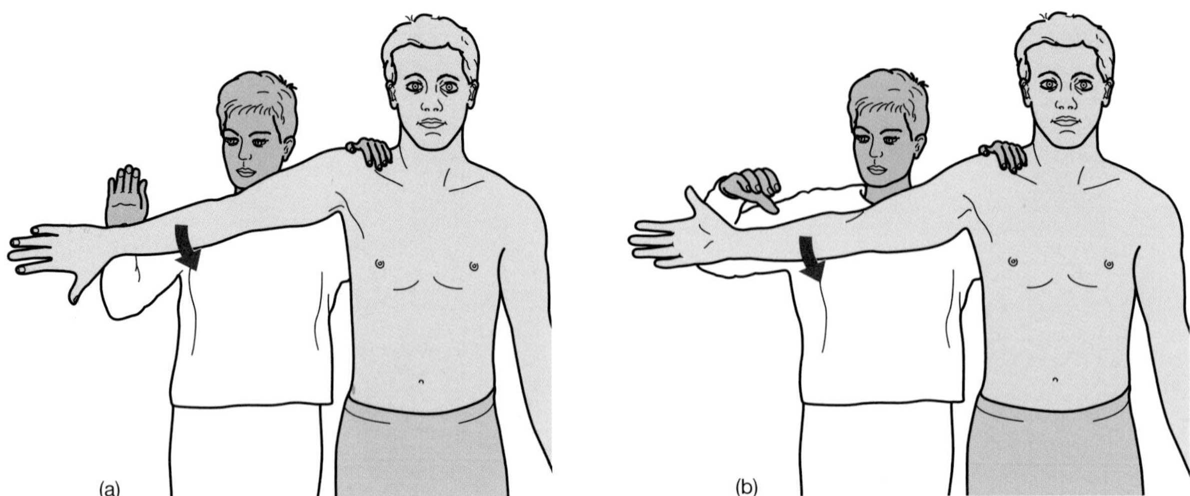

Figure 8.97 SLAP prehension test. (a) If this position is painful, check if pain is reduced by changing to the posture as in (b). The test is positive if pain is reduced.

push-ups. The test is positive if weakness of the scapula muscles or winging of the scapula is noted (Figure 8.99).

Test for Tendinous Pathology

Yergason's Test of the Biceps

This test stresses the long head of the biceps tendon in the bicipital groove to determine if it remains within the groove. The patient is in the standing position with you at the side. Take the patient's elbow with one hand and grasp the forearm with the other. The patient's elbow should be flexed to 90 degrees and the arm should be against the thorax. Ask the patient to resist external rotation of the arm as you pull the forearm toward you. At the same time, push downward as the patient also attempts to flex the elbow. Resistance of attempted supination can also be included. If the biceps tendon is unstable within the bicipital groove, the patient will experience pain and the tendon may pop out of place (Figures 8.100a and 8.100b).

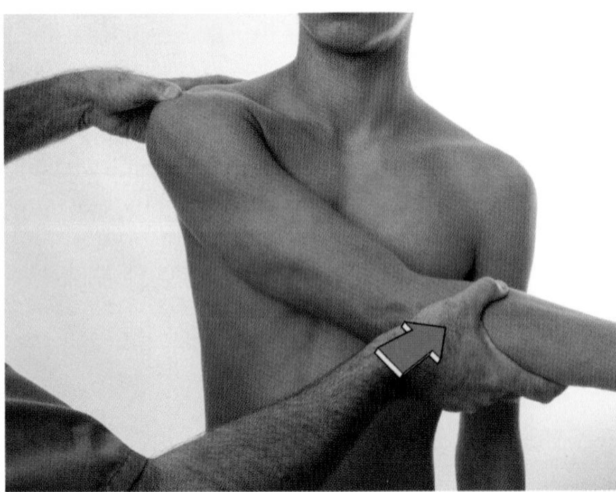

Figure 8.98 The cross-flexion test.

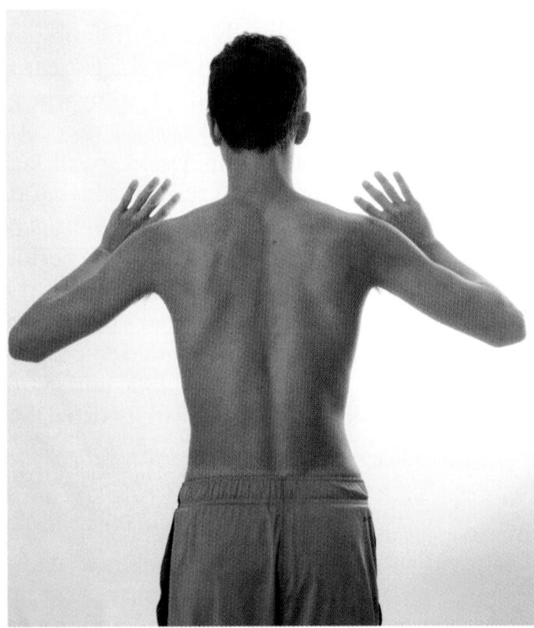

Figure 8.99 Wall push-up test.

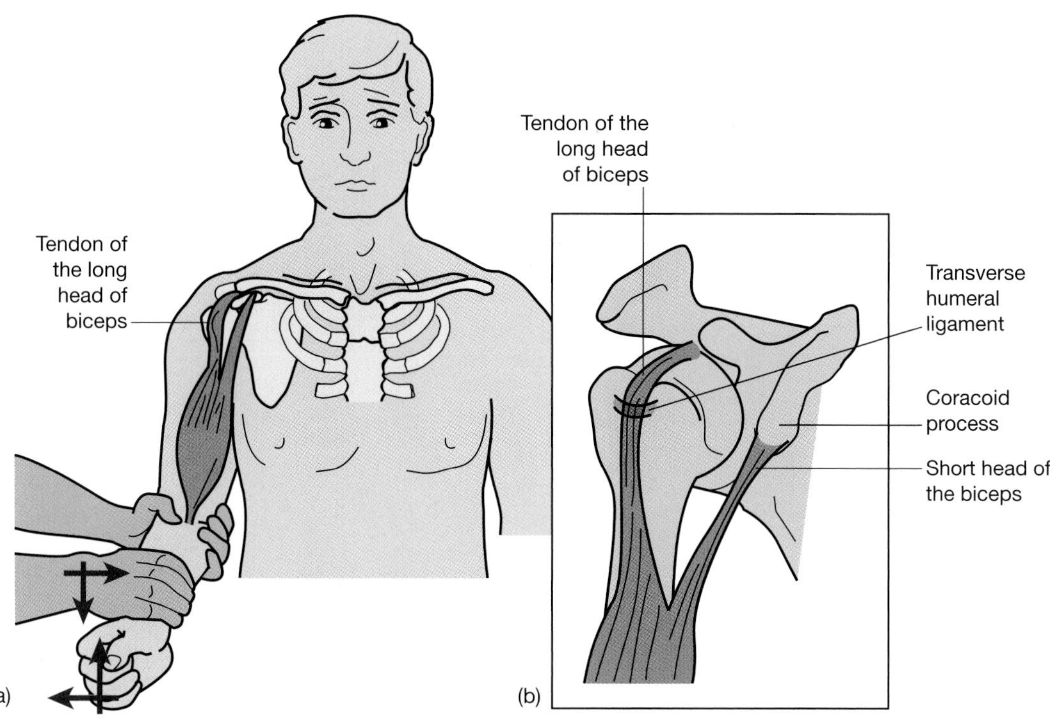

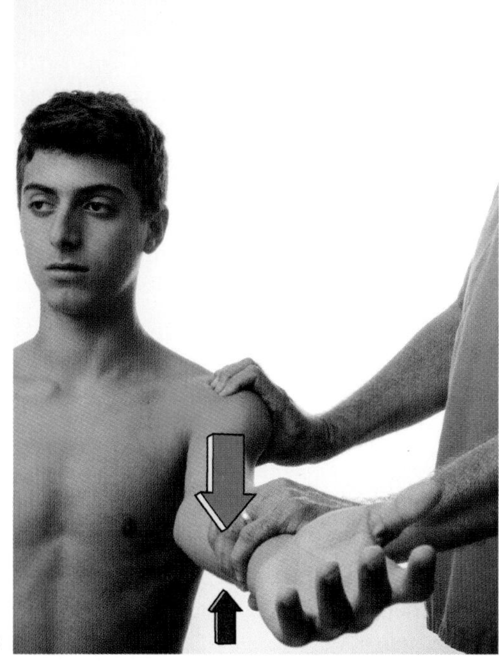

Figure 8.100 (a) The Yergason's test for integrity of the long head of the biceps tendon in the bicipital groove. (b) If the ligament that restrains the long head of the biceps tendon within its groove is damaged, the biceps tendon will sublux, as shown. (c) Speed's test for biceps tendinitis.

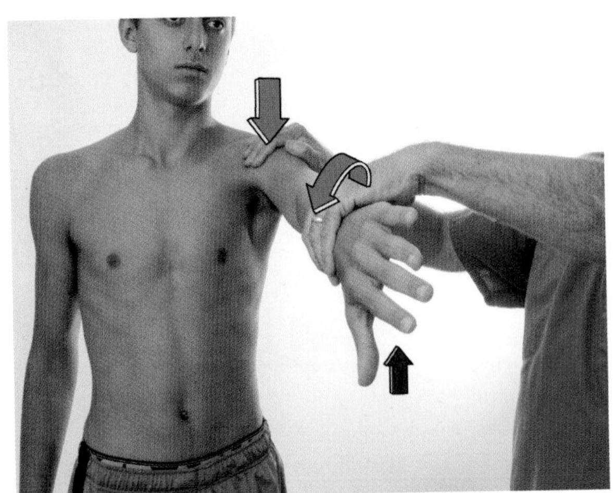

Figure 8.101 The supraspinatus impingement test (Hawkins-Kennedy).

Speed's Test of the Biceps

This test is used to confirm biceps tendinitis or partial rupture of the tendon. The patient is sitting with the elbow fully extended and the shoulder forward flexed to 90 degrees. Resist forward flexion with the forearm in supination. The test is positive when the patient feels pain in the bicipital groove (Figure 8.100c).

Tests for Impingement of the Supraspinatus Tendon

Hawkins–Kennedy Supraspinatus Impingement Test

This test brings the supraspinatus tendon against the anterior portion of the coracoacromial ligament. With the patient standing, take the arm and forward flex the shoulder to 90 degrees. Forcibly internally rotate the shoulder, as the patient tries to elevate the arm. This will cause pain if the patient has supraspinatus tendinitis (Figure 8.101).

Yocum Test

This is a variation of the Hawkins–Kennedy test. Ask the patient to abduct the affected arm to 90 degrees and place their hand on the opposite shoulder. Instruct the patient to elevate the elbow without allowing them to shrug their shoulder. The test is positive if the patient reports pain (Figure 8.102).

Neer Impingement Test

Test the patient in either sitting or standing position. Place one hand on the posterior aspect of the scapula to stabilize the shoulder girdle. With your other hand, internally rotate the patient's arm by grasping it near the elbow and raise it into full forward flexion. The test is positive if the patient reports pain from 70–120 degrees of forward flexion, as the rotator cuff comes into contact with the coracoacromial arch (Figure 8.103).

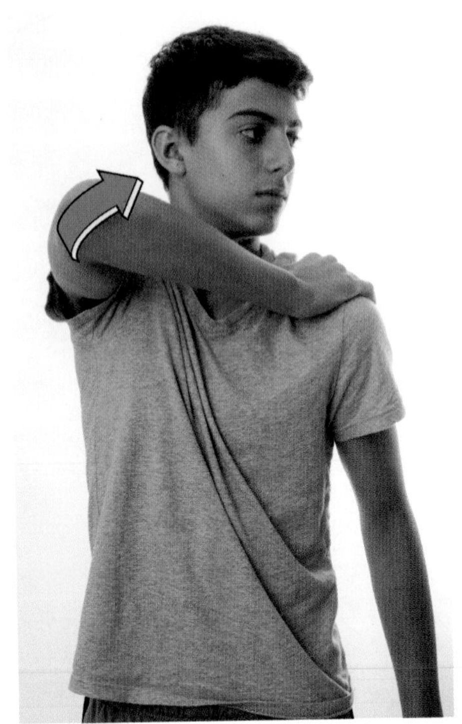

Figure 8.102 Yocum test.

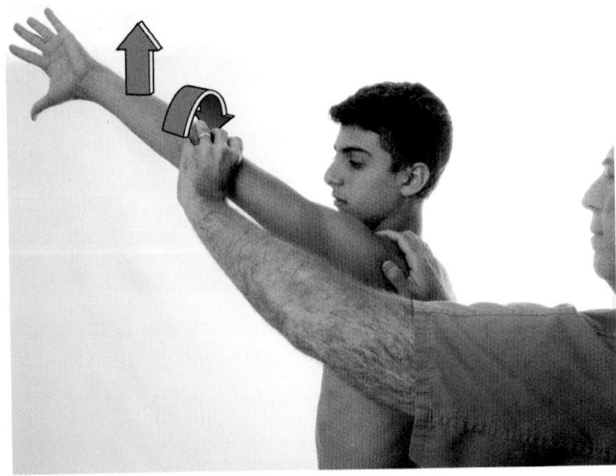

Figure 8.103 Neer impingement test. Flex and internally rotate the patient's shoulder.

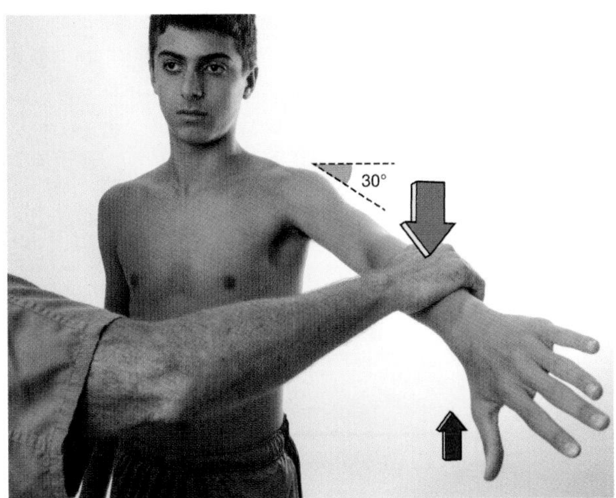

Figure 8.104 The supraspinatus test.

Supraspinatus Test (Empty Can Test)

This test is also performed to examine the supraspinatus tendon for pathology. The patient can be sitting or in the supine position. Stand in front of the patient and have him or her abduct the shoulder to 90 degrees and then forward flex the arm approximately 30 degrees (to the plane of the scapula) with the arm internally rotated so that the thumb points down to the ground. Place your hand over the patient's elbow and apply downward pressure as the patient attempts to raise the arm upward against your resistance. If this is painful, the patient likely has pathology of the supraspinatus muscle or tendon or involvement of the suprascapular nerve (Figure 8.104). A variation of this test is referred to as the full can test. The patient repeats the test as described above with their arm in external rotation. This is thought to allow for a better contraction of the supraspinatus muscle.

Tests for Muscle Pathology

Drop Arm Test

This test is performed to determine whether there is a tear of the rotator cuff tendons. The patient can be standing or sitting. Stand behind the patient and abduct the arm to 90 degrees passively with the elbow extended. Ask the patient to slowly lower the arm back to the side. The test result is positive if the patient is unable to lower the arm slowly (i.e., it drops), or if the patient has severe pain while attempting this maneuver (Figures 8.105a and 8.105b).

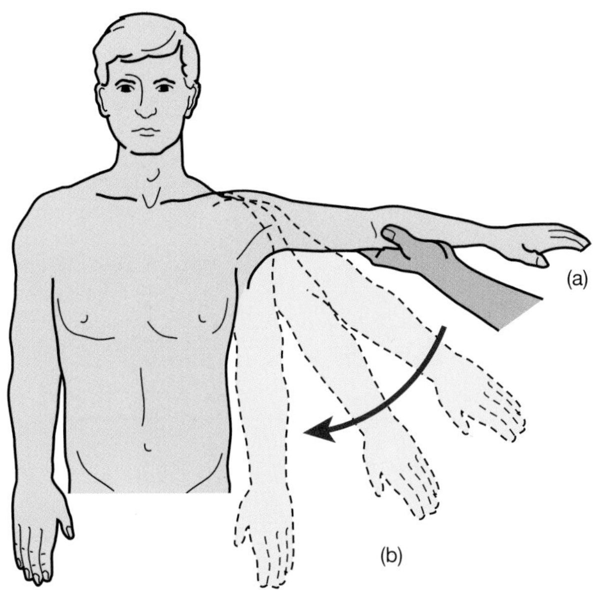

Figure 8.105 (a) The patient's arm is passively elevated by the examiner. (b) The patient's arm drops suddenly due to an inability to hold the arm up as a result of tears in the rotator cuff.

Lift-Off Test (Gerber's Test)

This is a test for the subscapularis muscle. The subscapularis muscle internally rotates and extends the shoulder. This test can only be performed if the patient has full active internal rotation of the shoulder so that he may achieve the starting position. Examine the patient in standing. Ask the patient to place his hand behind his back with the dorsum of the hand resting on the mid-lumbar spine. Then, ask the patient to raise the dorsum of his hand away from his back. The test is normal if the patient can actively lift the dorsum of the hand off the back. If he cannot lift off his hand, there is damage to the subscapularis muscle or tendon (Figures 8.106a and 8.106b).

Lateral Rotation Lag Sign (Infraspinatus Spring Back Test)

This is a test for the posterosuperior rotator cuff. Ask the patient to sit on the examination table with his back to you. Hold the patient's wrist. Passively abduct the shoulder to 90 degrees in the plane of the scapula, flex the elbow to 90 degrees, and move the shoulder to near maximal external rotation. Ask the patient to actively maintain the position. If he or she is unable to, it suggests a larger disruption of the muscles or tendons (Figure 8.107). Continue to

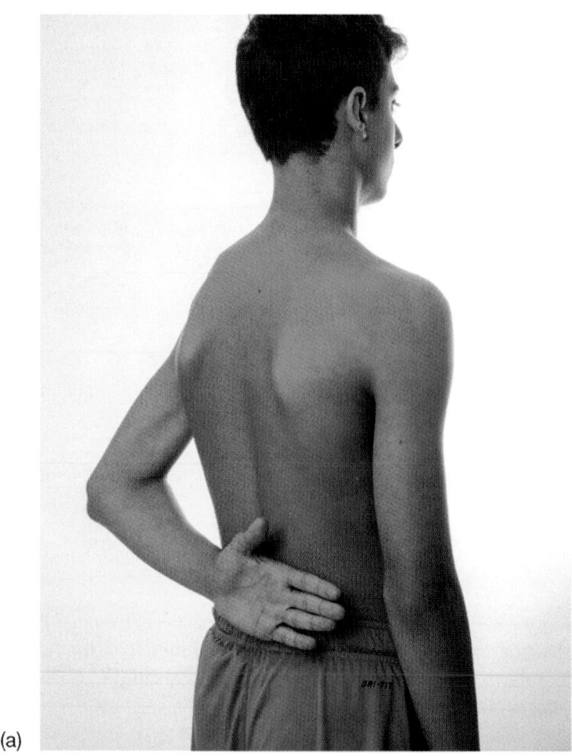
(a)

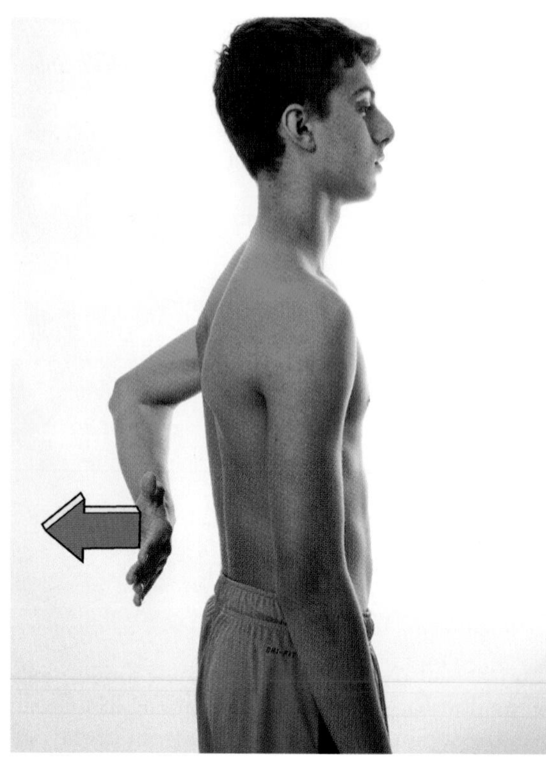
(b)

Figure 8.106 Lift-off test (Cerber's test). (a) Starting position. (b) Patient attempts to lift "off" his hand and wrist away from his back.

support the elbow, but release your hold at the wrist. The degree of movement is estimated and is referred to as the lag. This lag equals the difference between passive and active ROM (range of motion). For small ruptures of the infraspinatus or teres minor, the lag may be as little as 5 degrees.

Figure 8.107 Lateral rotation lag sign (infraspinatus spring back test). This is the starting position. When you release the hand, it will "spring forward."

Hornblower's Sign

This test is used to determine if there is teres minor pathology. The patient can be sitting or standing. Abduct the shoulder to 90 degrees and support the arm in the scapular plane. Ask the patient to flex the elbow to 90 degrees. The patient then tries to externally rotate the arm against resistance. The sign is positive if the patient is unable to maintain the externally rotated position and the arm drops back to the neutral position. An alternate method is to ask the patient to bring both hands to their mouth, as though they were trying to blow a horn. The test is positive if the patient is unable to reach their mouth without abducting their arm (Figure 8.108).

Tests for Thoracic Outlet Syndrome

The tests used for diagnosis of thoracic outlet syndrome attempt to narrow the thoracic outlet and reproduce symptoms or signs of neurovascular

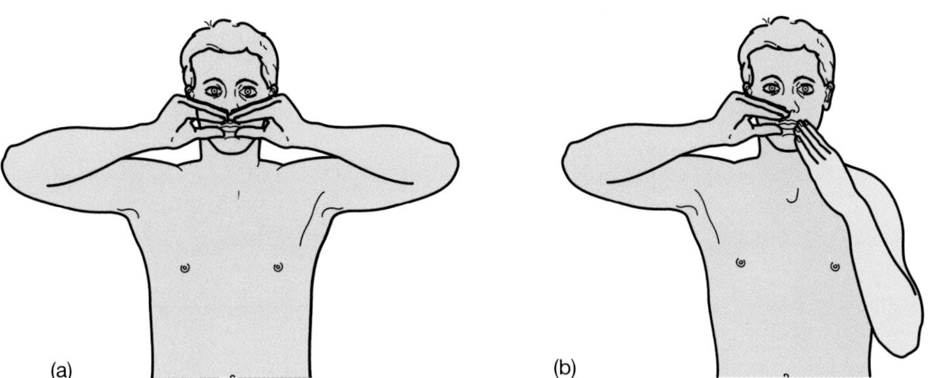

Figure 8.108 Hornblower's sign. (a) Normal result. (b) Patient is unable to abduct the left upper extremity to reach the same level as the mouth.

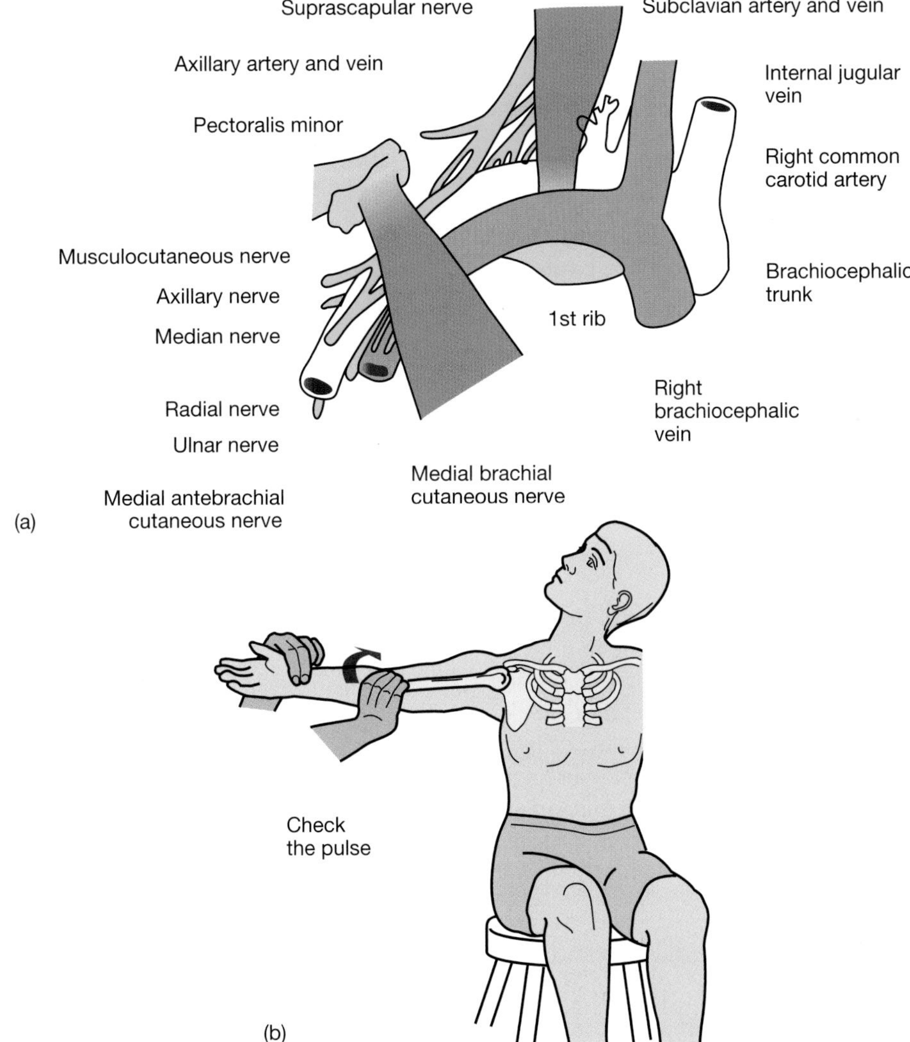

Figure 8.109 (a) The structures of the thoracic outlet. Note the position of the nerves, arteries, and veins as they pass over the first rib and beneath the pectoralis minor muscle. (b) Adson's maneuver for testing for thoracic outlet syndrome.

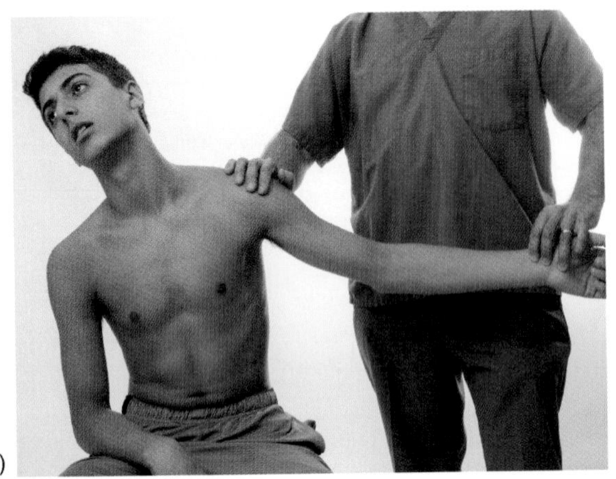

(a)

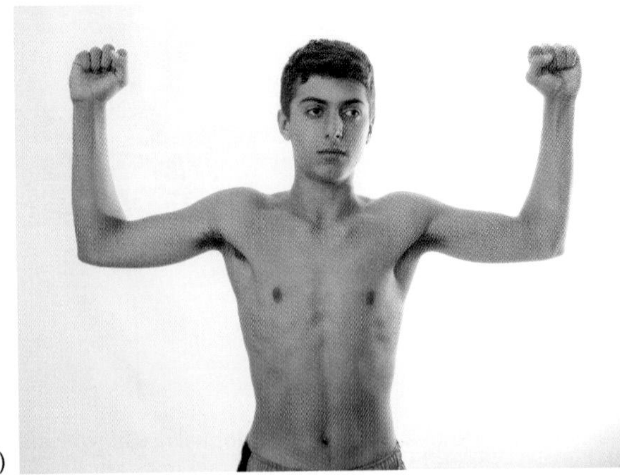

(b)

Figure 8.110 (a) Wright's maneuver for testing for thoracic outlet syndrome. (b) Roos test for thoracic outlet syndrome.

compression (numbness, tingling, pain, loss of palpable pulses) (Figure 8.109a).

Adson's Maneuver

The patient is sitting and the arm is outstretched. Find the patient's radial pulse with one hand. While palpating the pulse, ask the patient to turn his or her head so as to face the test shoulder. Then ask the patient to extend the head while you laterally rotate and extend the patient's shoulder and arm. Now ask the patient to take a deep breath and hold it (Valsalva maneuver). A disappearance of the pulse indicates a positive test result (Figure 8.109b). This occurs because the anterior scalene muscle is being stretched and it pulls the first rib upward, narrowing the thoracic outlet.

Wright's Maneuver

The patient is seated, with you on the side to be tested. Palpate the patient's radial pulse with one hand. Ask the patient to rotate the head away from you and the test shoulder. Ask the patient, at the same time, to elevate the chin in a torsional manner, again away from the side that is being tested. Now ask the patient to take a deep breath and hold it in (Valsalva maneuver). The test result is positive if symptoms are aggravated or precipitated, or if the pulse is no longer palpable (Figure 8.110a).

Roos Test

The patient stands and abducts and externally rotates their arms. The elbows are flexed to 90 degrees. The patient then opens and closes their fists for 3 minutes. If they experience ischemic pain in the arm, numbness or tingling in the hand, or extreme weakness, the test is positive for thoracic outlet syndrome on the affected side (Figure 8.110b).

Referred Pain Patterns

A painful shoulder may be due to irritation of the diaphragm that can occur with hepatobiliary or pancreatic disease. An apical lung tumor (Pancoast's tumor) may cause pain in the shoulder as well. A C5 or C6 radiculopathy frequently causes shoulder pain. Pain may radiate from the elbow to the shoulder. Cardiac pain is also sometimes felt in the shoulder. Embryologically, there is a common origin of innervation of the diaphragm and adjacent internal organs (liver, gallbladder, and heart). This innervation originates near the midcervical spine (Figure 8.111). For this reason, inflammation of these organs may be perceived as discomfort (referred pain) in the C5 or C6 dermatome.

Radiological Views

Radiological views of the shoulder are presented in Figures 8.112–8.114.

A = Acromion
C = Clavicle
Co = Coracoid process
D = Acromioclavicular joint
G = Glenoid
Gr = Greater tubercle of the humerus
H = Humerus
S = Scapula

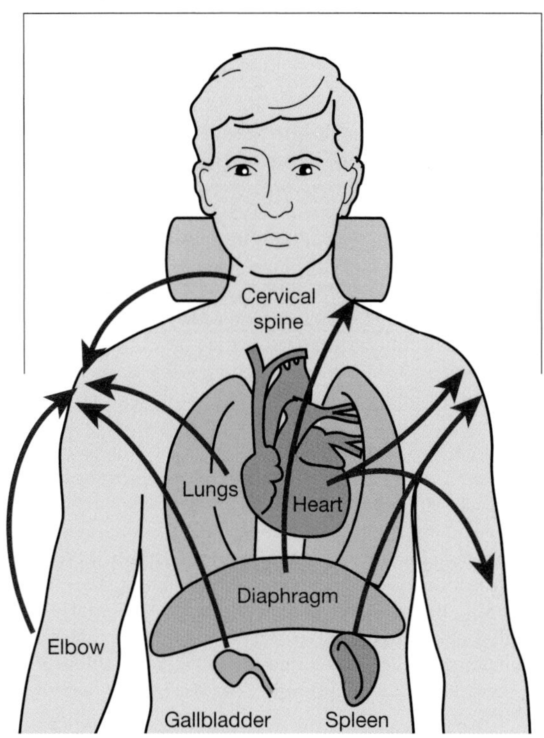

Figure 8.111 Structures referring pain to the shoulder. These organs have a common embryological origin with the midcervical spine and therefore may radiate pain to the shoulder.

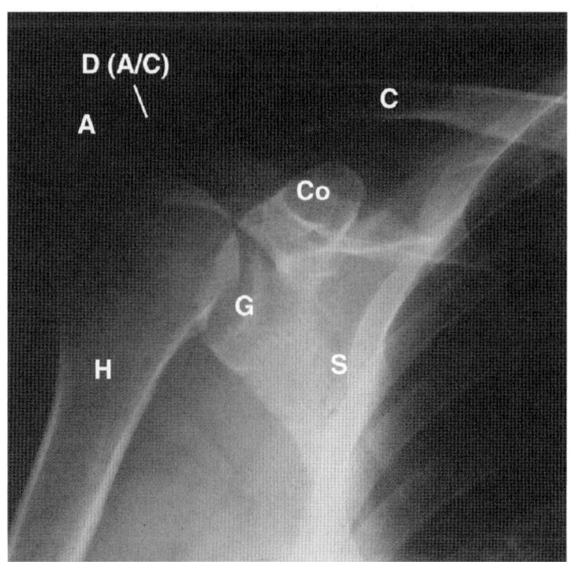

Figure 8.112 Internal rotation view of the shoulder.

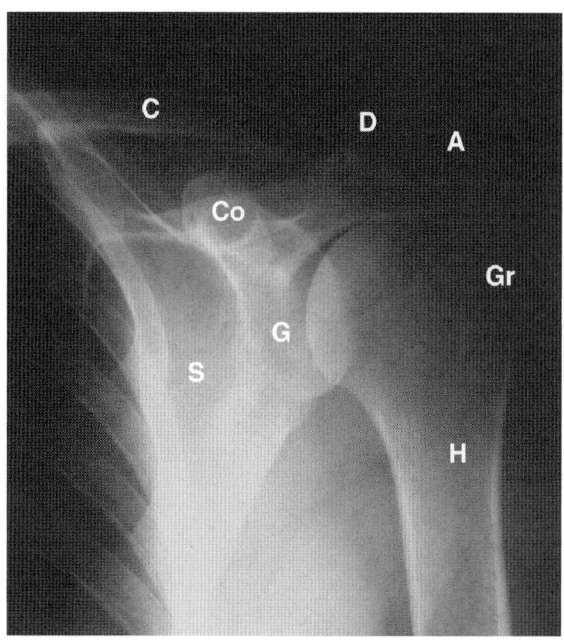

Figure 8.113 External rotation view of the shoulder.

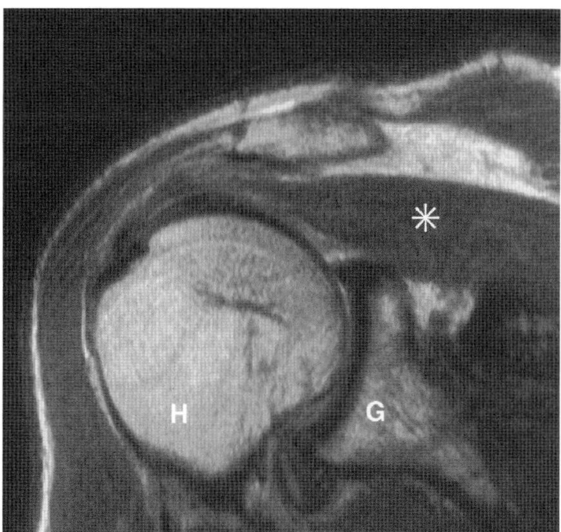

Figure 8.114 Magnetic resonance image of the shoulder (* represents rotator cuff).

SAMPLE EXAMINATION

History: A 50-year-old right-hand-dominant recreational tennis player presents with a chief complaint of 1 week of neck pain. He recently won his dub tournament. There was no trauma. The pain began several days after the event. There had been no neurovascular symptoms.

Physical Examination: Well-developed, well-nourished male with full ROM of the cervical spine. There was tenderness on palpation of the paramedial right scapula. Deep tendon reflexes (DTRs), sensation, and muscle testing of both upper extremities were normal. He had a negative vascular examination of the upper extremities. He had negative compression and distraction of the cervical spine. The patient lacked terminal 20 degrees of forward flexion and external rotation of the right shoulder. The remaining motions were normal. Scapular dyskinesia was noted with shoulder flexion and abduction. Special provocation tests for instability, apprehension, SLAP lesions, and impingement were negative. Mobility testing of the right scapulothoracic joint and glenohumeral joint was mildly restricted. Popping was perceived with passive ROM of the right shoulder above shoulder height.

Presumptive Diagnosis: Overuse syndrome with resultant strain of the trapezius and rhomboid muscles of the right shoulder.

Physical Examination Clues: (1) He had well-localized tenderness and trigger points, identifying injury to a specific anatomical structure. (2) He had negative neurological and vascular signs in the upper extremities, indicating that there was no radicular or vascular component to his injury. (3) He had negative findings with vertical compression and distraction of the cervical spine, full ROM of the cervical spine, and a negative neurovascular examination, indicating no irritation of intervertebral joints or cervical roots exiting from the spinal foramina. (4) Negative special provocation testing of the shoulder ruled out impingement, instability, and labral tears. (5) A popping noise with passive ROM of the right shoulder above shoulder height, decreased scapulothoracic mobility, and scapular dyskinesia indicate scapulothoracic dysfunction. Proper shoulder and neck function requires normal glenohumeral and scapulothoracic movement. Limitation of either, as noted in the restricted mobility examination of the scapulothoracic and glenohumeral joints, will expose the remaining articulation to overuse due to compensation. The lack of full shoulder ROM in the context of a sport such as tennis, which requires repetitive and full ROM of the shoulder, exposes the patient to a compensatory overuse of the otherwise unaffected region.

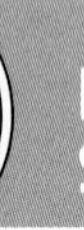

PARADIGM FOR A CHRONIC IMPINGEMENT SYNDROME OF THE SHOULDER

A 45-year-old man presents with a complaint of right shoulder pain. The pain has been episodic for at least 10 years, but has become more severe, constant, and limiting in ADL over the past 3 months. There has been no recent trauma to the upper extremity, but the patient had fallen onto the right shoulder skiing 25 years ago. At that time, he had limited use of his right dominant arm for 4 weeks. Eventually, he recovered "full" use of that limb and has participated in regular athletic activities. Three months ago, the patient had been traveling extensively on business. He developed pain in the superior shoulder and lateral aspect of the arm. It is not aggravated by movement of the head and neck, and is not associated with "pins and needles" or "electric shock" sensations in any part of the upper extremity. He has noticed that there is often a sensation or sound of "rubbing" and "popping" in the area of the shoulder when reaching overhead.

On physical examination, the patient lacks the terminal 20 degrees of shoulder external rotation due to pain. He shows full strength and no evidence of shoulder instability. His right acromioclavicular joint is larger and more tender as compared with that on the opposite side. There are no neurological deficits found and he has a negative cervical spine examination. X-rays show normal glenohumeral alignment; there is hypertrophy of the acromioclavicular joint with elevation of the clavicle. There is slight sclerosis on the superior margin of the greater tubercle and minimal narrowing of the subacromial space. This paradigm is most consistent with chronic subacromial impingement because of

A history of prior injury with apparent full recovery
Delayed onset of symptoms
A history of recent aggravating event(s)
Crepitus on ROM without instability

CHAPTER 9

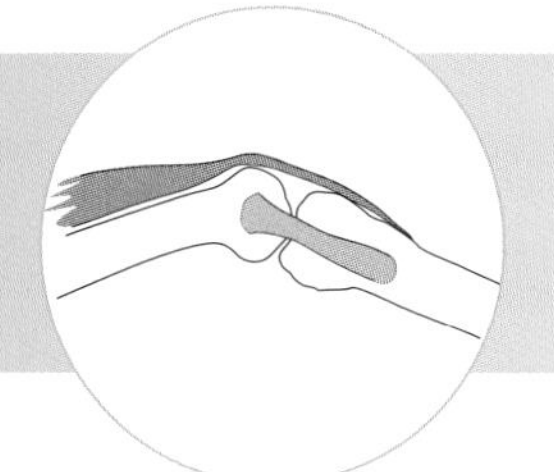

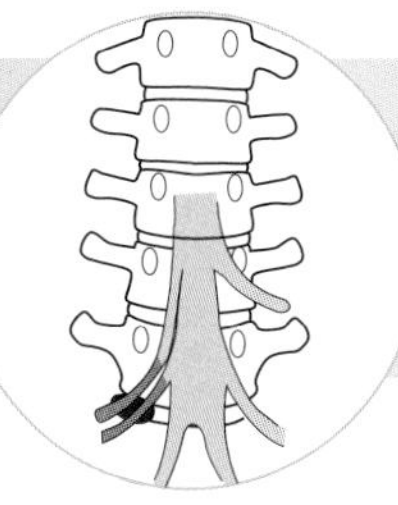

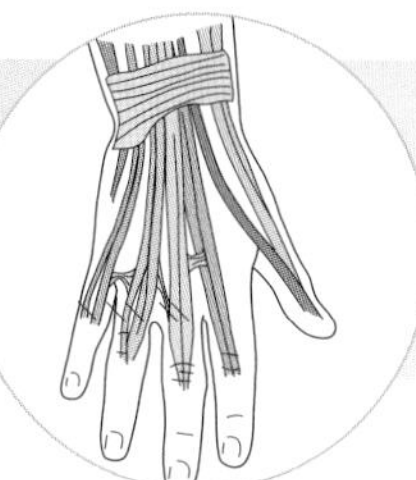

The Elbow

FURTHER INFORMATION

Please refer to Chapter 2 for an overview of the sequence of a physical examination. For purposes of length and to avoid having to repeat anatomy more than once, the palpation section appears directly after the section on subjective examination and before any section on testing, rather than at the end of each chapter. The order in which the examination is performed should be based on your experience and personal preference as well as the presentation of the patient.

Functional Anatomy

The elbow is a complex hinged joint whose function is to facilitate the placement of the hand in space. It allows flexion–extension and pronation–supination of the forearm. It is composed of three bones: the humerus, radius, and ulna, and three articulations: humeroulnar, humeroradial, and the less important proximal radioulnar.

The humeroulnar joint is the largest and most stable of the elbow articulations. It is a simple hinge. Its stability is dependent on the medial collateral ligament. Dislocation at the elbow is pathognomonic of medial collateral ligament compromise. Therefore, after reduction of dislocation, the reduced elbow must be recognized as being potentially unstable until medial collateral ligament integrity has been restored by healing or surgical repair or both.

The humeroradial joint lies lateral to the humeroulnar articulation. It is composed of a shallow disc (radial head) articulating on the spherical humeral capitellum. As such, proximal migration of the radius is prevented throughout the entire arc of elbow flexion and extension (Figure 9.1). Pronation and supination are accomplished by rotation of the radius along its long axis about the ulna (Figure 9.2a). Rotation toward the palm down is *pronation*, whereas rotation toward the palm up is *supination*. At full supination, the radius and ulna lie parallel within the forearm. At full pronation, the radius crosses the ulna at its mid shaft. Although it rotates during pronation and supination, the radial head remains otherwise in a fixed position relative to the ulna. The relative position and movement of the radius about the elbow is crucial to the diagnosis and treatment of injuries to the elbow-arm-wrist complex. A common mechanism of injury of the upper extremity is falling onto the outstretched hand (Figure 9.2b). In this position, the elbow is extended and the forearm is usually pronated by the rotation of the body on the fixed hand. During pronation with the radial head fixed proximally to the ulna by the annular ligament, the shaft of the radius rotates about the long axis of the ulna. Terminal pronation is limited by the contact of the shaft of the radius on the ulna. At maximum pronation, the contact point of the crossed radius (increased

Musculoskeletal Examination, Fourth Edition. Jeffrey M. Gross, Joseph Fetto and Elaine Rosen.

Companion website: www.wiley.com/go/musculoskeletalexam

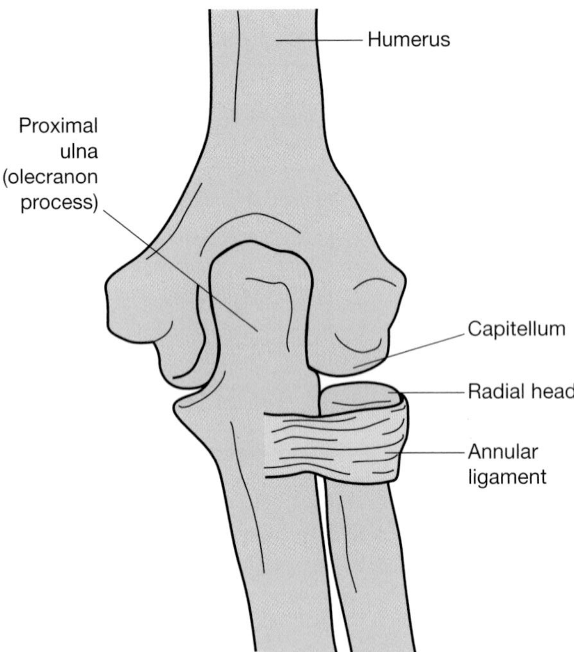

Figure 9.1 The medial humeroulnar joint is a hinge joint. The lateral humeroradial joint is a shallow ball and socket. The proximal radioulnar joint allows for pronation and supination. The radial head is distal to the ulna and is supported against the ulna by the annular ligament.

pronation) places enormous stress on the bones and articulations of the elbow and forearm. The consequences of forcibly pronating the forearm beyond this point will result in the following spectrum of possible injuries:

1. tear of the annular ligament with dislocation of the radial head;
2. fracture of the radial shaft;
3. fracture of the ulnar shaft;
4. fracture of both bones of the mid forearm; or
5. combination or permutation of the above (i.e., Monteggia fracture, a fracture of the ulna with dislocation of the radial head).

Understanding this analysis of the mechanism of injury provides insight into the treatment of such injuries. It is crucial to their resolution. For example, treatment of fractures and dislocations usually requires a maneuver that reverses the mechanism of injury. Therefore, for injuries resulting from hyperpronation of the forearm, an integral part of the manipulative movements performed for treatment involves supination of the forearm.

In addition to bony and articular injuries, the soft tissue about the elbow can also be injured, for example, from excessive movements. As a consequence of the enormous range of motion the elbow must perform during the course of daily activities, the large excursions of bony prominences beneath the overlying soft tissues can create irritations. To permit the elbow its large range of excursion (0–150 degrees of flexion), the skin overlying the posterior aspect of the elbow is very redundant and loosely attached to the underlying hard and soft tissues. Interposed between the skin and underlying tissues is the olecranon bursa. This bursa ensures that the skin will not become adherent to the underlying tissues restricting terminal flexion of the elbow. This function is similar to that which exists on the anterior aspect of the knee and the dorsum of the metacarpophalangeal and interphalangeal joints of the digits of the hand. Like these areas, as a consequence of its location, the posterior elbow bursa (olecranon bursa) is very vulnerable to blunt trauma, the result of which may be hemorrhage, swelling, pain, and inflammation characteristic of traumatic injuries. The lining of a bursal sac is similar to the synovial lining that exists in synovial articulations. As a result, when traumatized and inflamed, it becomes thickened, produces excessive fluid exudates, and is characterized by localized swelling and warmth (bursitis) (Figure 9.2c).

Observation

The examination should begin in the waiting room before the patient is aware of the examiner's observation. Information regarding the degree of the patient's disability, level of functioning, posture, and gait can be observed. The clinician should pay careful attention to the patient's facial expressions with regard to the degree of discomfort the patient is experiencing. The information gathered in this short period can be very useful in creating a total picture of the patient's condition

Note the manner in which the patient is sitting in the waiting room. Notice how the patient is posturing the upper extremity. Is the arm relaxed at the side or is the patient cradling it for protection? If the elbow is swollen, the patient may posture it at 70 degrees of flexion (the resting position), which allows for the most space for the fluid. Swelling may be easily noticed at the triangular space bordered by the lateral epicondyle, radial head, and the olecranon. How willing is the patient to use the upper extremity? Will he or she extend their arm to you to shake your hand? Pain may be altered by changes in position, so watch

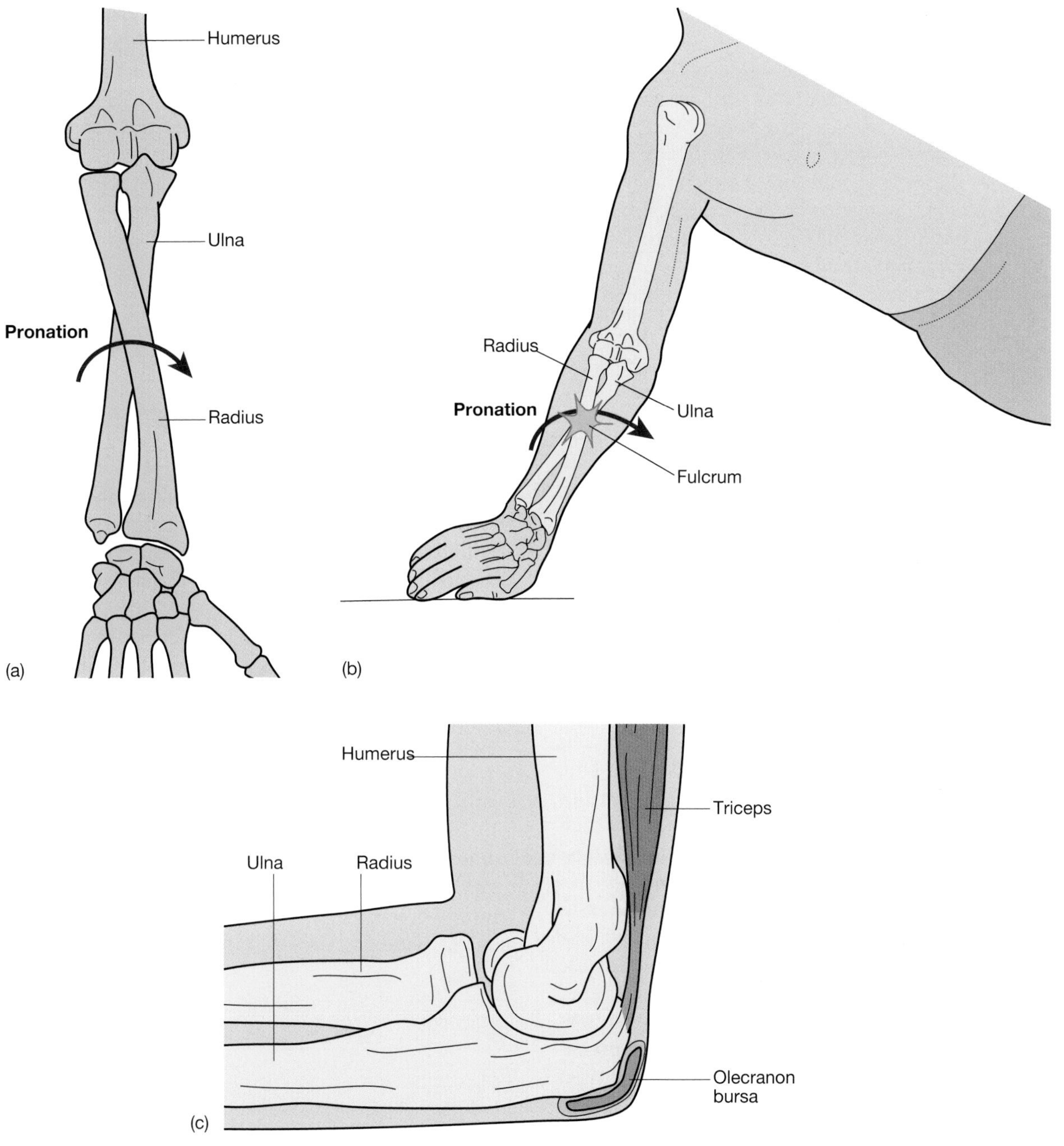

Figure 9.2 (a) Pronation is the medial rotation of the radius anterior to the ulna; this results in a palm-down position of the hand. Supination is the reverse movement, palm-up rotation of the hand. (b) Falling onto an outstretched hand with the forearm pronated results in a fracture of the ulnar shaft due to a fulcrum effect. (c) The olecranon bursa in a flattened sac with synovial lining. It lies between the skin at the posterior aspect of the elbow and the underlying bony and muscular soft tissues.

the patient's facial expression to give you insight into their pain level.

Observe the patient as he or she assumes the standing position. Observe the patient's posture. Pay particular attention to the position of the head, cervical spine, and the thoracic kyphosis. Note the height of the shoulders and their relative positions. Once the patient starts to ambulate, observe whether he or she is willing to swing the arms, which can be limited by either loss of motion or pain.

Once the patient is in the examination room, ask the patient to disrobe. Observe the ease with which the patient uses the upper extremities and the rhythm of the movements. Observe for symmetry of bony structures. Note the carrying angle with the upper extremity postured in the anatomical position. Does the patient present with cubitus valgus or varus (gunstock deformity). Note whether there is any atrophy present in the biceps. This may be secondary to C5 or C6 myotomal involvement. Note the symmetry of the forearms. Atrophy may be secondary to C6, C7, or C8 myotomal involvement.

Subjective Examination

The elbow is a stable joint. Since it is nonweightbearing, problems are most commonly related to overuse syndromes, inflammatory processes, and trauma. You should inquire about the nature and location of the patient's complaints as well as their duration and intensity. Note whether the pain travels either above or below the elbow. Inquire about the behavior of the pain during the day and night to give you better insight into the pain pattern secondary to changes in position, activity level, and swelling.

You want to determine the patient's functional limitations. Question the patient regarding use of their upper extremity. Is the patient able to comb his hair, fasten her bra, bring his arm to his mouth to eat, or remove her jacket? Does the patient regularly participate in any vigorous sports activity that would stress the elbow? What is the patient's occupation?

If the patient reports a history of trauma, it is important to note the mechanism of injury. The direction of the force and the activity in which the patient was participating at the time of the injury contribute to your understanding of the resulting problem and help you to better direct the examination. The degree of pain, swelling, and disability at the time of the trauma and within the initial 24 hours should be noted. Does the patient have a previous history of the same injury? Does the patient report any clicking or locking? This may be due to a loose body in the joint. Is any grating present? This may be due to osteoarthritis.

The patient's disorder may be related to age, gender, ethnic background, body type, static and dynamic posture, occupation, leisure activities, hobbies, and general activity level. Therefore, it is important to inquire about any change in daily routine and any unusual activities in which the patient has participated.

The location of the symptoms may give you some insight into the etiology of the complaints. The cervical spine and the shoulder can refer pain to the elbow. The most common nerve roots that refer pain are C6 and C7. (Please refer to Box 2.1, see p. 15 for typical questions for the subjective examination.)

Gentle Palpation

The palpatory examination is started with the patient in either the supine or sitting positions. You should first search for areas of localized effusion, discoloration, birthmarks, open sinuses or drainage, incisional areas, bony contours, muscle girth and symmetry, and skinfolds. You should not have to use deep pressure to determine areas of tenderness or malalignment. It is important to use a firm but gentle pressure, which will enhance your palpatory skills. By having a sound basis of cross-sectional anatomy, you will not need to physically penetrate through several layers of tissue to have a good sense of the underlying structures. Remember that if you increase the patient's pain at this point in the examination, the patient will be very reluctant to allow you to continue and may become more limited in his or her ability to move.

Palpation is most easily performed with the patient in a relaxed position. Although palpation may be performed with the patient standing, the sitting position is preferred for ease of examination of the elbow. While locating the bony landmarks, it is also useful to pay attention to areas of increased or decreased temperature and moisture. This will help you identify areas of acute and chronic inflammation.

Anterior Aspect

Soft-Tissue Structures

Cubital (Antecubital) Fossa

The anterior surface of the crook of the elbow is referred to as the cubital fossa. This has been described as a triangular structure. The base of the triangle is formed by a line between the medial and lateral epicondyles of the humerus. The medial side is formed by the pronator teres and the lateral side by the brachioradialis. The floor is composed of the brachialis and the supinator. The fossa contains the following structures: biceps tendon, distal part of the brachial artery and veins, the origins of the radial and ulnar arteries, and parts of the median and radial nerves (Figure 9.3).

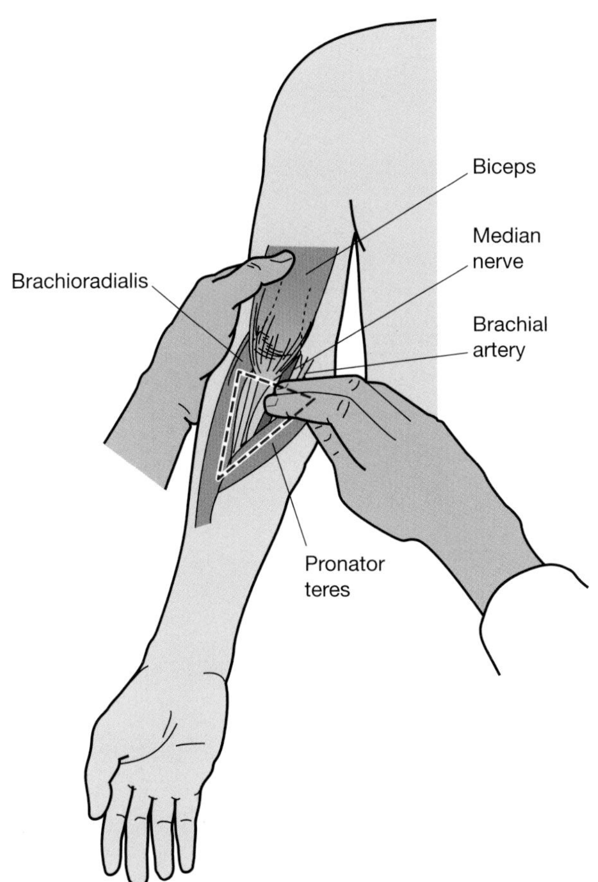

Figure 9.3 Palpation of the cubital fossa and contents.

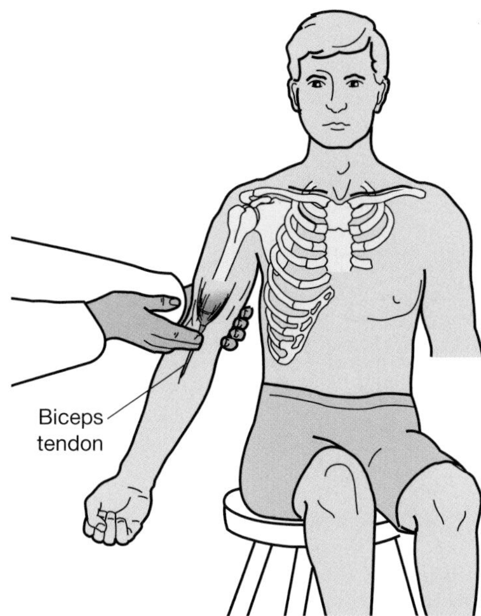

Figure 9.4 Palpation of the biceps muscle and tendon.

Trauma in the cubital fossa can lead to compression of the brachial artery, leading to Volkmann's ischemic contracture.

Biceps Muscle and Tendon

The anterior surface of the middle two-thirds of the humerus is composed of the biceps muscle belly. Follow the fibers distally and you will feel the tapered ropelike structure, which is the biceps tendon just proximal to its distal attachment on the radial tuberosity (Figure 9.4). The tendon becomes more prominent if you resist elbow flexion with the forearm in the supinated position.

The distal tendon or muscle belly can be ruptured following forceful flexion of the elbow. The patient will demonstrate weakness in elbow flexion and supination, pain on passive pronation, and tenderness in the cubital fossa. Rupture of the long head is often asymptomatic and may not be evident clinically, except for a concavity in the upper arm or a bulbous swelling in the anterior lower half of the arm, which is the retracted muscle belly.

Brachial Artery

The brachial artery is located in the cubital fossa medial to the biceps tendon (see Figure 9.3). The brachial pulse can be readily assessed at this point.

Median Nerve

The median nerve crosses in front of the brachial artery and travels medial to it in the cubital fossa. Locate the brachial artery and allow your finger to move slightly medially and you will feel a ropelike structure, which is the median nerve (see Figure 9.3). It travels between the bicipital aponeurosis and the brachialis before it enters the forearm between the heads of the pronator teres.

Medial Aspect

Bony Palpation

Medial Epicondyle and Supracondylar Ridge

Stand next to the patient and make sure the upper extremity is in the anatomical position. Place your fingers along the medial aspect of the humerus and allow them to move distally along the medial supracondylar ridge of the humerus until you reach a very prominent pointed structure. This is the medial epicondyle of the humerus (Figure 9.5). Tenderness in this area can be due to inflammation of the common aponeurosis of

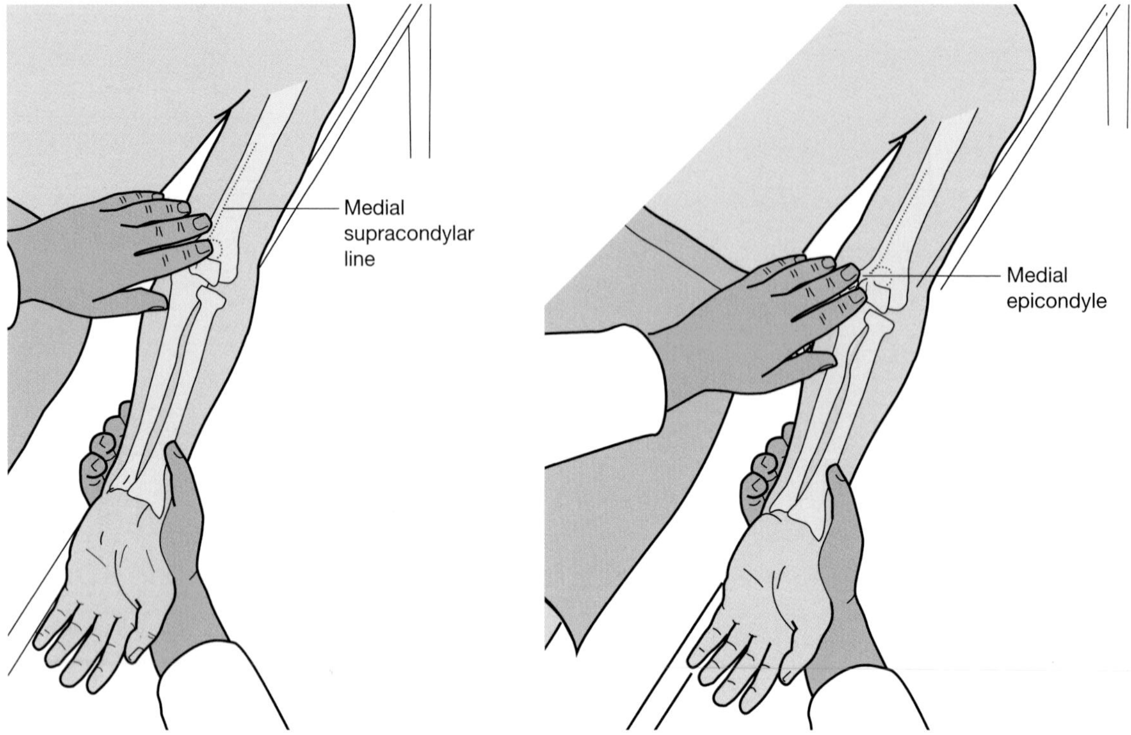

Figure 9.5 Palpation of the medial epicondyle and supracondylar ridge.

the flexor and pronator tendons of the forearm and wrist and is commonly referred to as golfer's elbow (medial epicondylitis).

Soft-Tissue Structures

Medial (Ulnar) Collateral Ligament

The medial collateral ligament consists of anterior and posterior sections that are connected by an intermediate section. The anterior portion attaches from the medial epicondyle of the humerus to the coronoid process. The posterior section attaches from the medial epicondyle to the olecranon. It has been described as a fan-shaped structure (Figure 9.6). The ligament is responsible for the medial stability of the elbow and its integrity can be tested with a valgus stress test (described in pp. 214–216). The ligament is not distinctly palpable, but the medial joint line should be examined for areas of tenderness secondary to sprains.

Ulnar Nerve

Ask the patient to flex the elbow to 90 degrees. Palpate the medial epicondyle and continue to move posteriorly and laterally until you feel a groove between

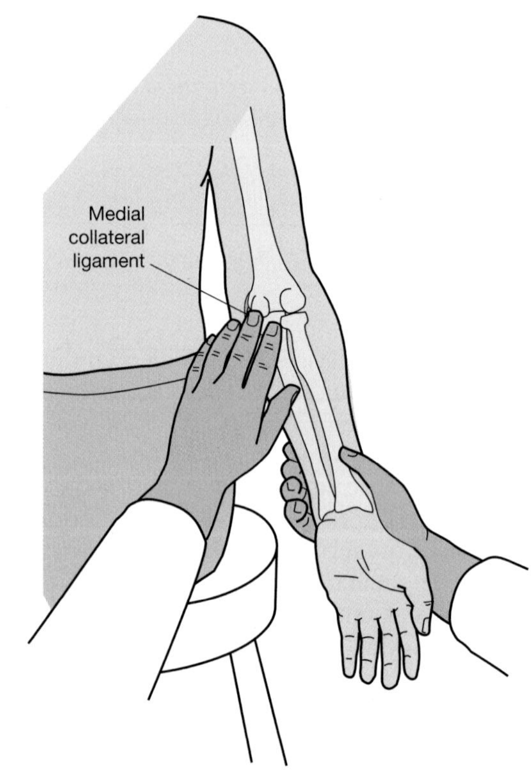

Figure 9.6 Palpation of the medial collateral ligament.

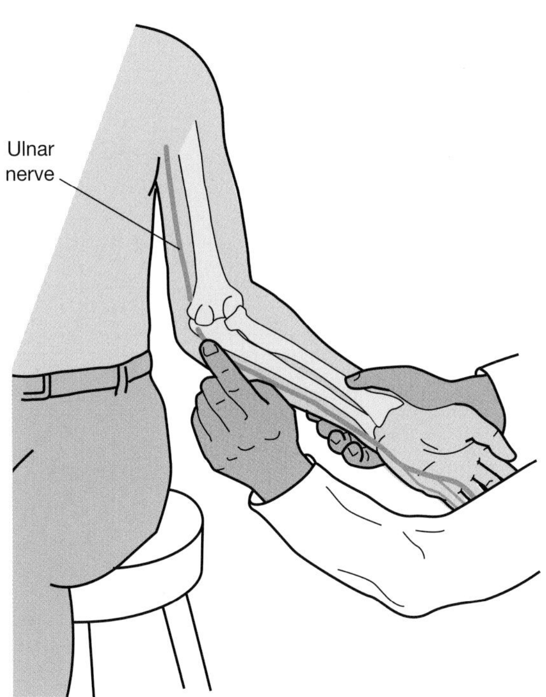

Figure 9.7 Palpation of the ulnar nerve.

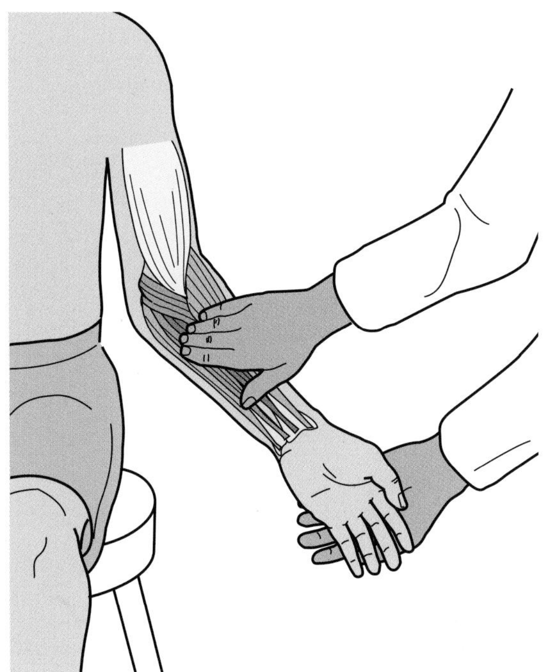

Figure 9.8 Palpation of the wrist flexor–pronator muscles.

the medial epicondyle and the olecranon. Gently palpate in the groove and you will feel a round cordlike structure under your fingers. This is the ulnar nerve (Figure 9.7). Because the nerve is so superficial, be careful not to press too hard; you may cause paresthesias radiating down the forearm and into the hand. It is often referred to as the funny bone since when it is accidentally hit, the person experiences tingling. Because of its close proximity to the bony prominences, the nerve can be injured secondary to fractures of the medial epicondyle and the supracondylar ridge. The ulnar nerve can be entrapped in the cubital tunnel formed by the medial collateral ligament and flexor carpi ulnaris. This can cause a tardy ulnar palsy (see section on "Neurological Examination").

Wrist Flexor–Pronator

The common origin of the flexor–pronator muscle group is found at the medial epicondyle of the humerus. From lateral to medial, this group is composed of the pronator teres, flexor carpi radialis, palmaris longus, and flexor carpi ulnaris (Figure 9.8). The individual muscles are difficult to differentiate by palpation. You can get a sense of their location by resisting the individual muscle's function. Resist pronation of the forearm and you will feel the pronator teres contract under your fingers. Provide resistance while the patient flexes the wrist in radial deviation and you get a sense of the location of the flexor carpi radialis. Provide resistance while the patient flexes the wrist in ulnar deviation and you get a sense of the location of the flexor carpi ulnaris. The tendons are easily distinguishable at the wrist (described in pp. 220–221 in Chapter 9).

The muscle mass should be examined for tenderness and swelling, which can occur after overuse or strain. Inflammation of this area is commonly involved in golfer's elbow. The specific test is described later on in p. 231.

Lateral Aspect

Bony Structures

Lateral Epicondyle and Supracondylar Ridge

Stand next to the patient and make sure the upper extremity is in the anatomical position. Place your fingers along the lateral aspect of the humerus and allow them to move distally along the lateral supracondylar ridge of the humerus until you reach a small rounded structure. This is the lateral epicondyle of the humerus (Figure 9.9). Tenderness in this area can be due to inflammation of the common aponeurosis of

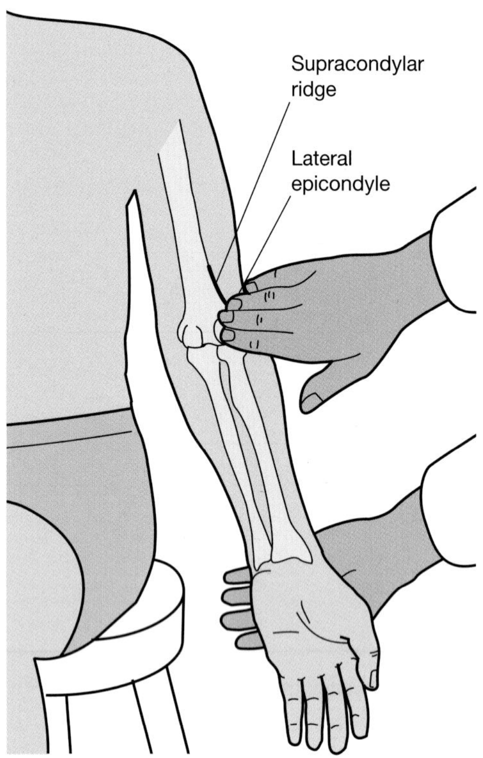

Figure 9.9 Palpation of the lateral epicondyle and supracondylar ridge.

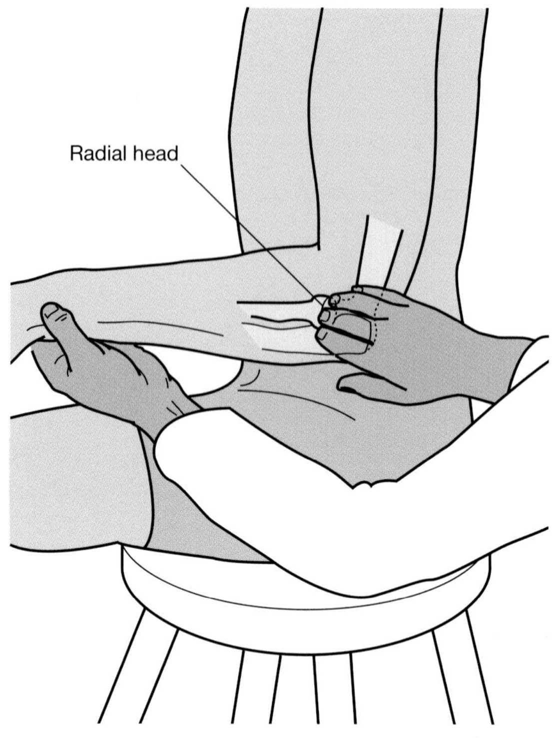

Figure 9.10 Palpation of the radial head.

the extensor tendons of the wrist and is commonly referred to as tennis elbow (lateral epicondylitis).

Radial Head

Ask the patient to flex the elbow to 90 degrees. Place your fingers on the lateral epicondyle and move them distally. You will first palpate a small indentation and then come to the rounded surface of the radial head (Figure 9.10). If you place your fingers more laterally, the radial head is more difficult to locate because it is covered by the thick bulk of the extensor mass.

To confirm your hand placement, ask the patient to supinate and pronate the forearm and you will feel the radial head turning under your fingers.

Soft-Tissue Structures

Lateral (Radial) Collateral Ligament

The lateral collateral ligament attaches from the lateral epicondyle to the annular ligament. It is a cordlike structure (Figure 9.11). The ligament is responsible for the lateral stability of the elbow and its integrity can be tested with a varus stress test (described in pp. 214–216, Figure 9.28). The ligament is not distinctly palpable, but the lateral joint line should be examined for areas of tenderness secondary to sprains.

Annular Ligament

The annular ligament surrounds the radial head and serves to keep it in contact with the ulna. The lateral collateral ligament blends with the superficial fibers. The ligament is not palpable (Figure 9.12).

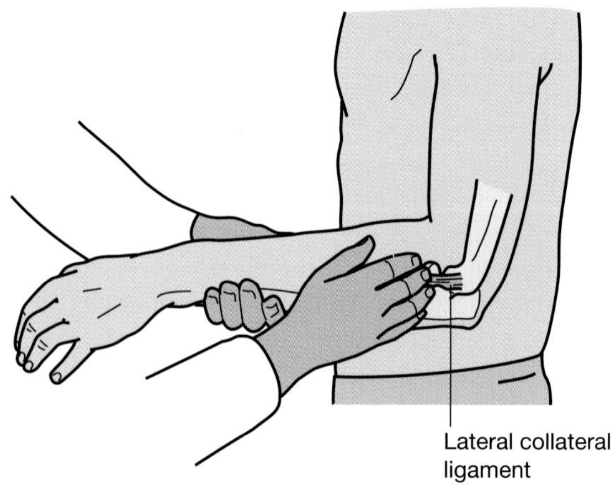

Figure 9.11 Palpation of the lateral collateral ligament.

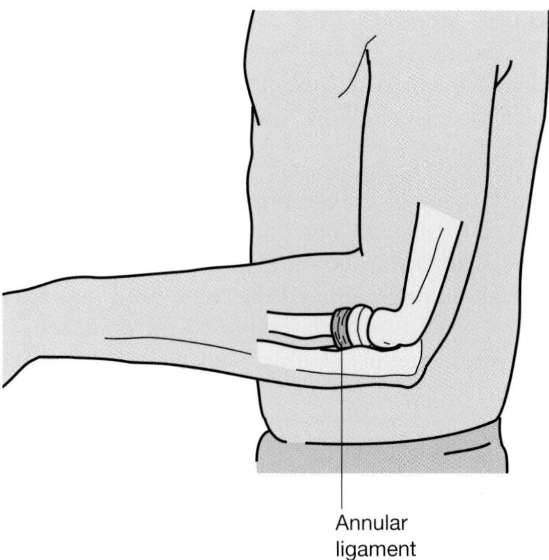

Figure 9.12 The annular ligament.

Humeroradial Bursa

The humeroradial bursa is located over the radial head and under the common aponeurosis of the extensor tendons. It is not normally palpable. It can be inflamed secondary to direct trauma or overuse and should not be confused with lateral epicondylitis. Calcification can be visualized in a radiograph.

Wrist Extensor–Supinator

The common origin of the extensor–supinator muscle group is found at the lateral epicondyle and the supracondylar ridge of the humerus. This group is composed of the brachioradialis, extensor carpi radialis longus, extensor carpi radialis brevis, and extensor digitorum (Figure 9.13). The individual muscles are difficult to differentiate by palpation at the muscle belly. You can get a sense of their location by resisting the muscle function. Provide resistance while the patient flexes the elbow with the forearm in the neutral position and you will see the contour of the brachioradialis on the anterolateral surface of the forearm lateral to the biceps tendon. It forms the lateral border of the cubital fossa. Provide resistance while the patient extends the wrist in radial deviation and you get a sense of the location of the extensor carpi radialis longus and brevis. Resist finger extension and you will feel the extensor digitorum contract under your fingers. The tendons are easily distinguishable at the wrist (described in Chapter 10).

The muscle mass should be examined for tenderness and swelling, which can occur after overuse or strain. Inflammation of this area is commonly involved in tennis elbow. The specific test is described later in this chapter (p. 231).

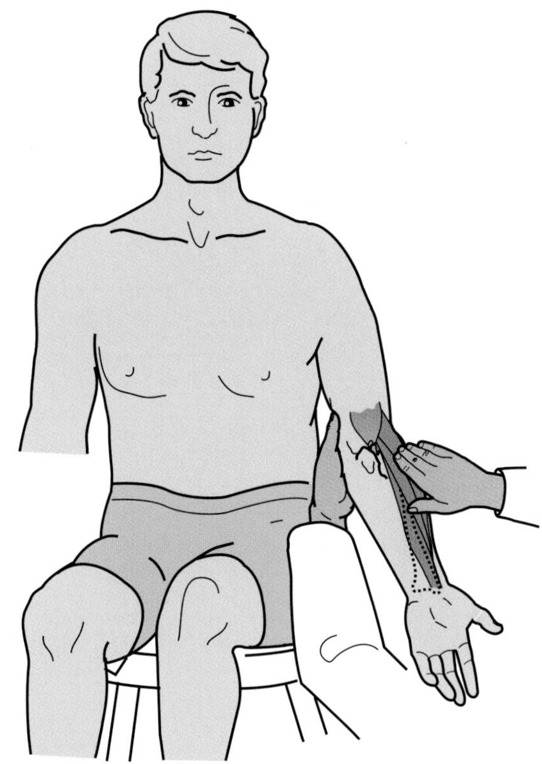

Figure 9.13 Palpation of the wrist extensor–supinator muscles.

Posterior Aspect

Bony Structures

Olecranon

Move your fingers to the posterior surface of the elbow and you will palpate a very prominent process that tapers to a rounded cone. This is the olecranon process (Figure 9.14). The olecranon is more distinct when the patient flexes the arm, bringing the olecranon out of the olecranon fossa. The relationship between the medial and lateral epicondyles and the olecranon can be examined in both the flexed and extended positions. In flexion, as the olecranon moves out of the fossa, it becomes the apex of an isosceles triangle formed by the three structures. As the arm moves back into extension and the olecranon moves back into the fossa, the three structures form a straight line (Figure 9.15). Disruption of these geometric figures can be caused by a fracture of any of the structures, or dislocation of the olecranon.

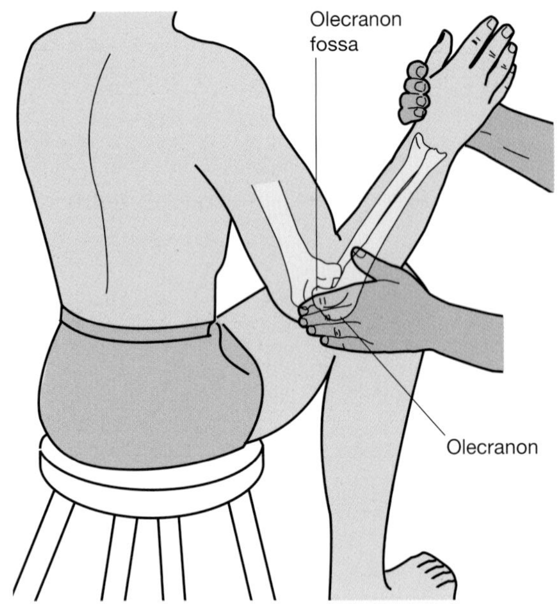

Figure 9.14 Palpation of the olecranon and olecranon fossa.

Olecranon Fossa

Once you have found the olecranon, move your fingers proximally and allow them to drop into a small depression, which is the olecranon fossa (see Figure 9.14). This fossa cannot be palpated when the patient's elbow is in extension, as it is filled by the olecranon process. When the elbow is completely flexed, the fossa is blocked by the tension in the triceps tendon. Therefore, the optimal position for palpation is at 45 degrees of elbow flexion.

Ulna Border

Go back to the olecranon process and allow your fingers to move distally along the superficial ridge of the ulna. The ulna border is easily followed and can be traced along the length of the bone until you reach the ulna styloid process (Figure 9.16). Point tenderness and an irregular surface can be indicative of a fracture.

Soft-Tissue Structures

Olecranon Bursa

The olecranon bursa lies over the posterior aspect of the olecranon process. It is not normally palpable. If the bursa becomes inflamed, you will feel a thickening in the area under your fingers. The inflammation can be so significant that it may appear as a large swelling resembling a golf ball over the posterior olecranon and is sometimes referred to as student's elbow (Figure 9.17).

Triceps

The triceps muscle is composed of three portions. The long head originates from the infraglenoid tubercle of

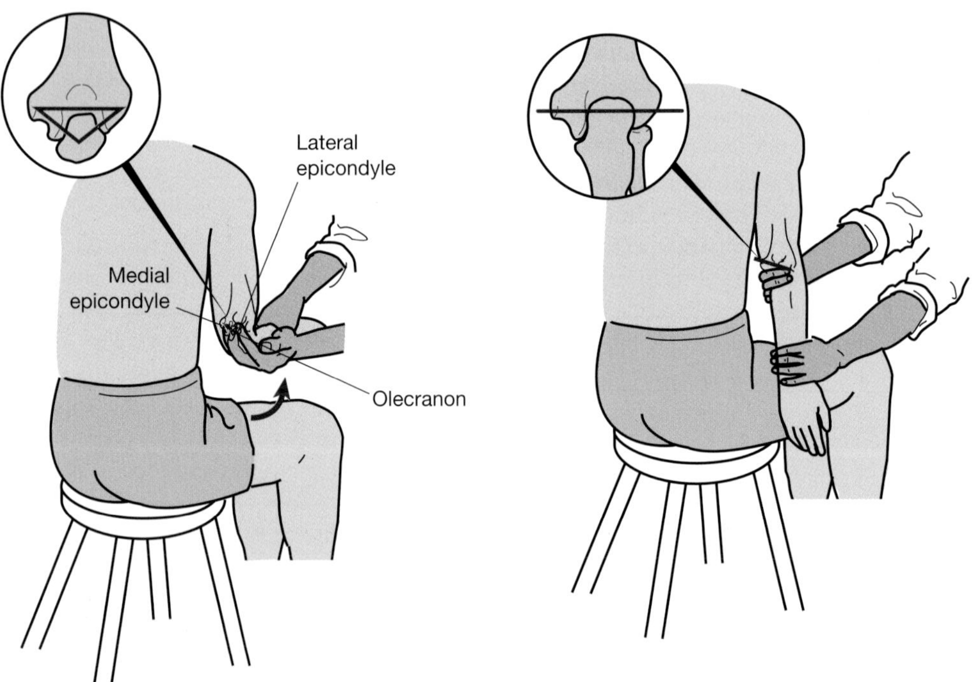

Figure 9.15 Alignment of the medial and lateral epicondyles and olecranon in flexion and extension.

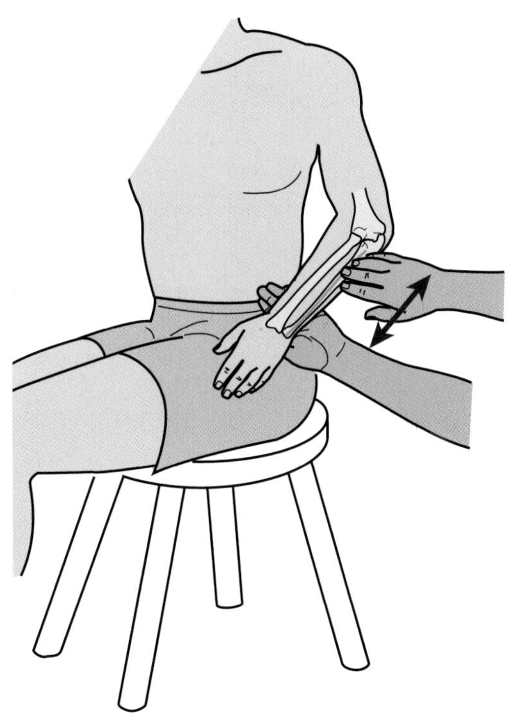

Figure 9.16 Palpation of the ulna border.

the scapula, the lateral head originates from the posterior surface of the humerus, and the medial head originates from the posterior aspect of the humerus below the radial groove. All three heads insert distally by a common tendon to the olecranon.

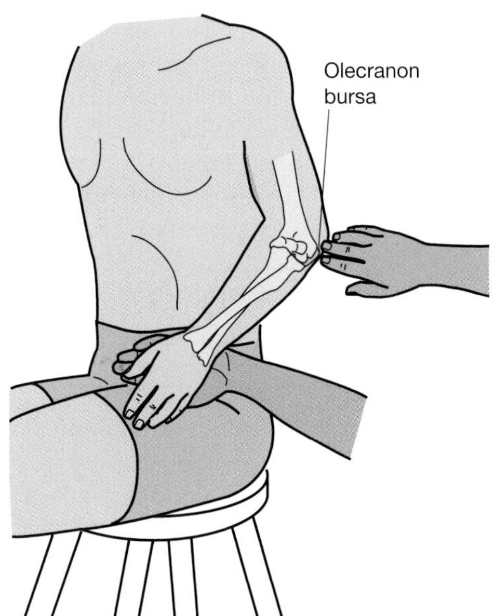

Figure 9.17 Palpation of the olecranon bursa.

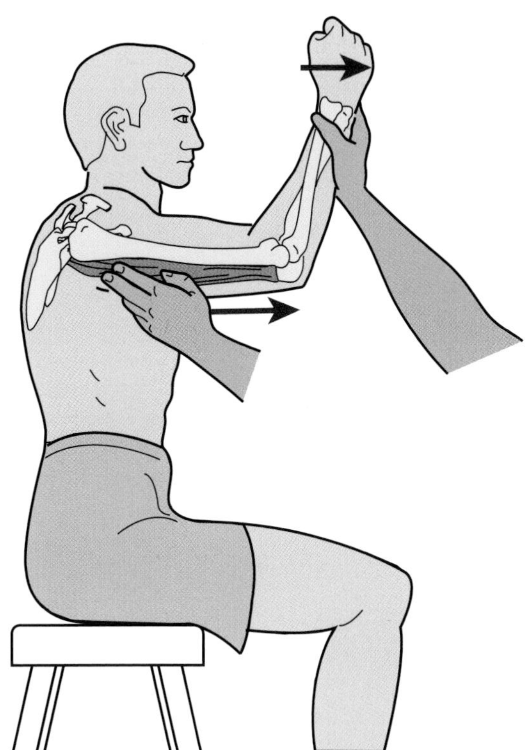

Figure 9.18 Palpation of the triceps muscle.

The superior portion of the long head can be palpated on the proximal posterior aspect of the humerus as it emerges from under the deltoid. The lateral head can be palpated on the middle posterior aspect of the humerus. The medial head can be located on both sides of the triceps tendon just superior to the olecranon. The contour of the muscle can be made much more distinct by resisting elbow extension (Figure 9.18).

Trigger Points

Myofascial pain of the elbow region is relatively uncommon. Referred pain patterns from trigger points in the biceps and triceps muscles are illustrated in Figures 9.19 and 9.20.

Active Movement Testing

The major movements of the elbow (humeroulnar and humeroradial) joint are flexion and extension on the transverse axis. To accomplish the full range of flexion and extension, the radius and ulna must be able to abduct and adduct. The major movements of the superior radioulnar joint are supination and pronation around a longitudinal axis. These should

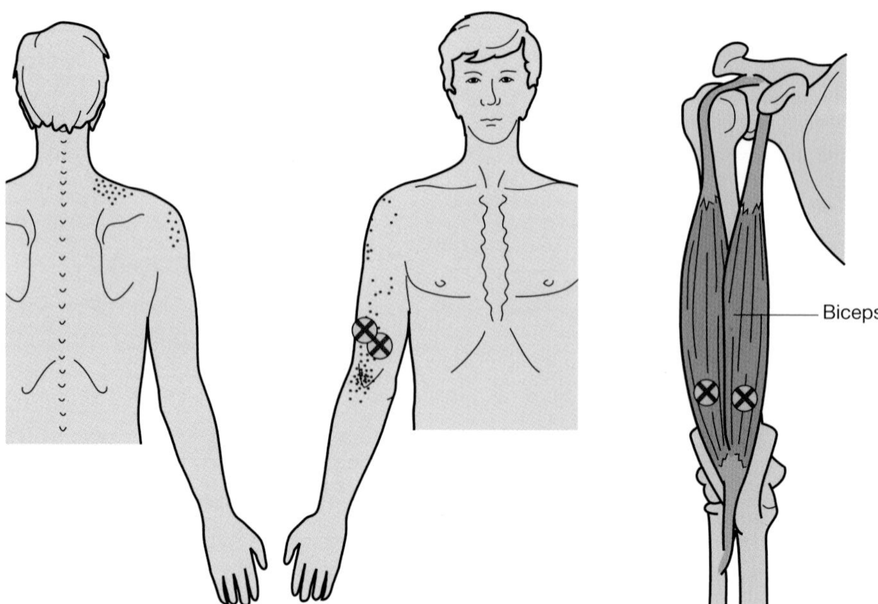

Figure 9.19 Common trigger points and their referred pain patterns within the biceps muscle. (Adapted with permission from Travell and Rinzler, 1952.)

be quick, functional tests designed to clear the joint. If the motion is pain free at the end of the range, you can add an additional overpressure to "clear" the joint. If the patient experiences pain during any of these movements, you should continue to explore whether the etiology of the pain is secondary to contractile or noncontractile structures by using passive and resistive testing.

A quick screening examination of the movements can be accomplished by asking the patient to reach for the back of the neck on the ipsilateral side of the elbow being tested. Then ask the patient to return the arm to the side in the anatomical position. Symmetrical hyperextension of 10 degrees can be considered normal. Pronation and supination can be checked functionally by asking the patient to place the elbow into the angle of the waist and turn the forearm as though he or she is turning a doorknob to the right or left. Observe the patient's wrist as he or she may try to substitute for the movement by abducting or adducting the arm. These tests can be performed with the patient in either the sitting or standing position.

Passive Movement Testing

Passive movement testing can be divided into two areas: physiological movements (cardinal plane), which are the same as the active movements, and mobility testing of the accessory (joint play, component) movements. You can determine whether the noncontractile (inert) elements are causative of the patient's problem by using these tests. These structures (ligaments, joint capsule, fascia, bursa, dura mater, and nerve root) (Cyriax, 1982) are stretched or stressed when the joint is taken to the end of the available range. At the end of each passive physiological movement, you should sense the end feel and determine whether it is normal or pathological. Assess the limitation of movement and see whether it fits into a capsular pattern. The capsular pattern of the elbow is greater restriction of flexion than extension so that with 90 degrees of limited flexion there is only 10 degrees of limited extension (Cyriax, 1982; Kaltenborn, 2011). The capsular pattern of the forearm is equal restriction of pronation and supination, which usually only occurs with significant limitation in the elbow joint (Kaltenborn, 2011).

Physiological Movements

You will be assessing the amount of motion available in all directions. Each motion is measured from the zero starting position. For the elbow, both the arm and the forearm are in the frontal plane, with the elbow extended and the forearm supinated. For the forearm, the elbow should be flexed to 90 degrees with the forearm midway between supination and pronation (Kaltenborn, 2011).

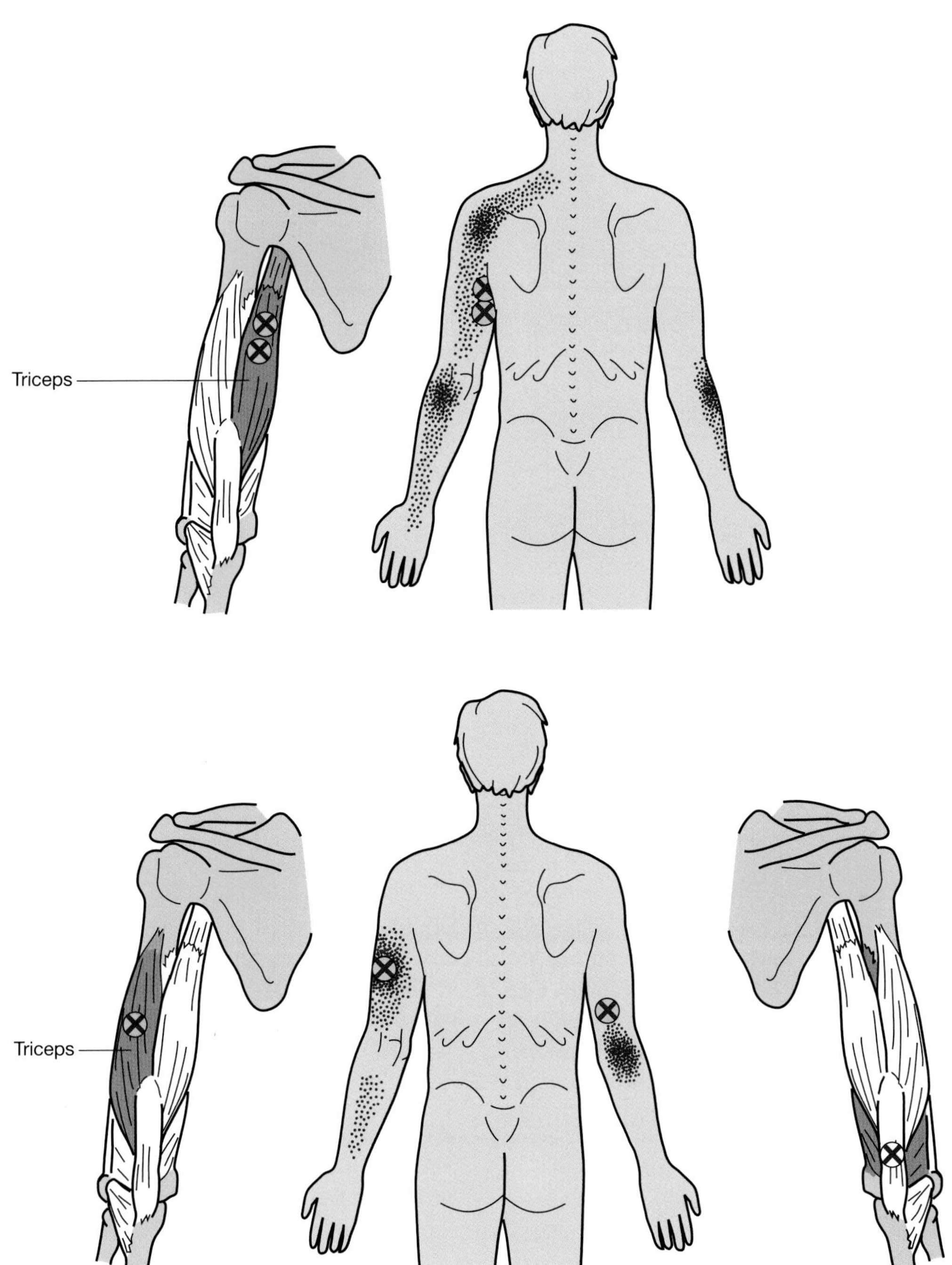

Figure 9.20 Common trigger points and their referred pain patterns within the triceps muscle. (Adapted with permission from Travell and Rinzler, 1952.)

Flexion

The best position for measuring flexion is supine with the patient's elbow in the zero starting position with the shoulder at zero degrees of flexion and abduction. A small towel placed under the distal posterior aspect of the humerus will allow for full extension. Place one hand over the distal end of the humerus to stabilize it, but be careful not to obstruct the patient's range into flexion. Hold the distal aspect of the patient's forearm and bring the hand toward

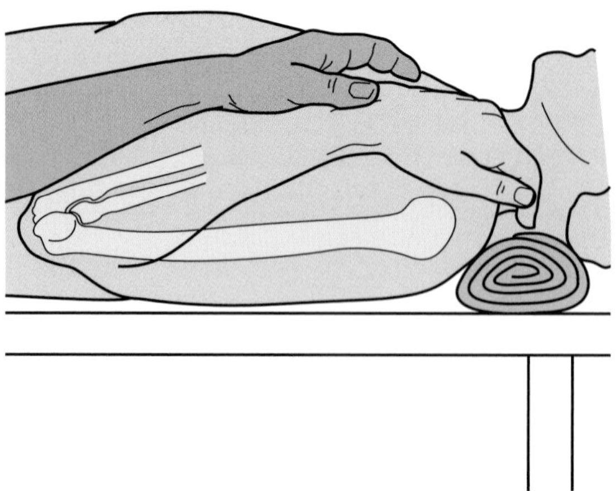

Figure 9.21 Passive movement testing of flexion of the elbow.

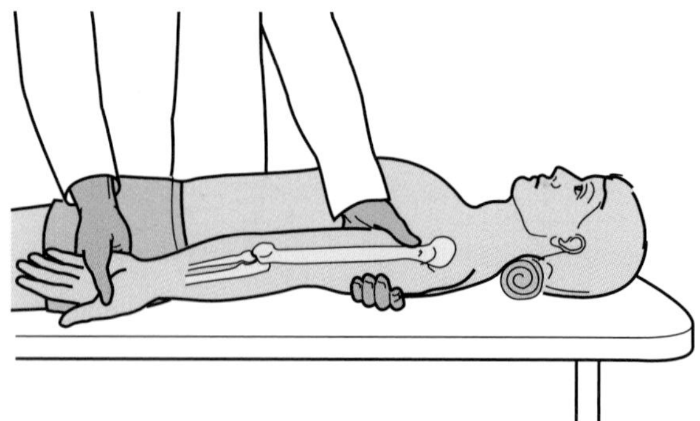

Figure 9.22 Passive movement testing of extension of the elbow.

the shoulder. The normal end feel is soft tissue caused by the muscle bulk of the biceps. If the patient's muscles are very atrophied, a hard end feel can be noted as the coronoid process meets or compresses into the coronoid fossa. This motion can also be restricted by tightness in the triceps muscle and the posterior capsule, producing an abrupt and firm (ligamentous) end feel (Magee, 2008; Kaltenborn, 2011). Normal range of motion is 0–150 degrees (American Academy of Orthopedic Surgeons, 1965) (Figure 9.21).

Extension

Full extension is achieved when the patient is placed in the supine position. The hand placement is the same as for flexion of the elbow. The motion is accomplished by allowing the patient's elbow to return to the zero starting position from flexion. The normal end feel is hard due to the contact between the olecranon and the olecranon fossa. The motion can also be restricted by tightness in the biceps and brachialis muscles and anterior capsule that produces an abrupt and firm (ligamentous) end feel (Magee, 2008; Kaltenborn, 2011). The normal range of motion is zero degree (American Academy of Orthopedic Surgeons, 1965) (Figure 9.22).

Pronation

The best position for measuring pronation is having the patient sitting with their forearm in the zero starting position and the shoulder at zero degrees of flexion and abduction. Stand so that you face the patient. Stabilize the posterior distal aspect of the humerus by cupping your hand around the olecranon to prevent substitution by shoulder medial rotation and abduction. Support the distal end of the forearm with your other hand. Rotate the forearm so that the patient's palm faces the floor. The normal end feel is hard due to the contact of the radius rotating over the ulna. The motion can be restricted by tightness in the supinator muscles, the interosseous membrane, and the inferior radioulnar joint that produces an abrupt and firm (ligamentous) end feel (Magee, 2008; Kaltenborn, 2011). Normal range of motion is 0–80–90 degrees (American Academy of Orthopedic Surgeons, 1965) (Figure 9.23).

Supination

Supination is tested with the patient in the same position as pronation. Substitution can be accomplished by shoulder lateral rotation and adduction. Rotate the patient's forearm so that the palm faces the ceiling. The normal end feel is abrupt and firm (ligamentous) due to tension in the pronator muscles, interosseous membrane, and the inferior radioulnar joint (Magee, 2008; Kaltenborn, 2011). Normal range of motion is 0–80–90 degrees (American Academy of Orthopedic Surgeons, 1965) (Figure 9.24).

Mobility Testing of the Accessory Movements

Mobility testing of accessory movements will give you information about the degree of laxity present in the joint. The patient must be totally relaxed and comfortable to allow you to move the joint and obtain the most accurate information. The joint should be placed in the maximal loose packed (resting) position to allow for the greatest degree of joint movement. The resting position of the elbow is 70 degrees

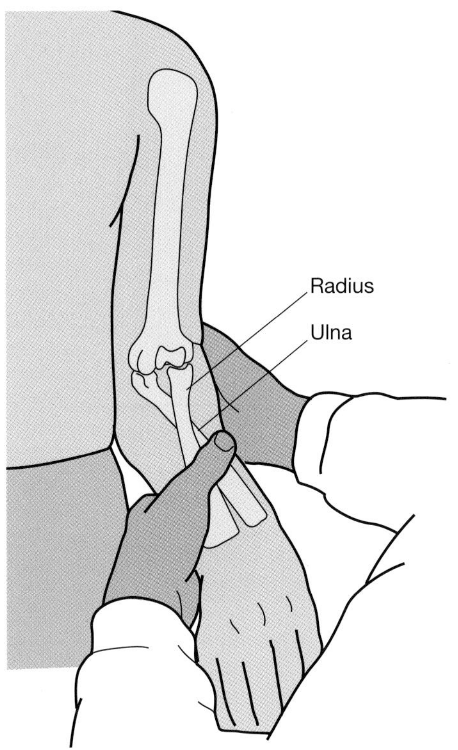

Figure 9.23 Passive movement testing of pronation of the forearm.

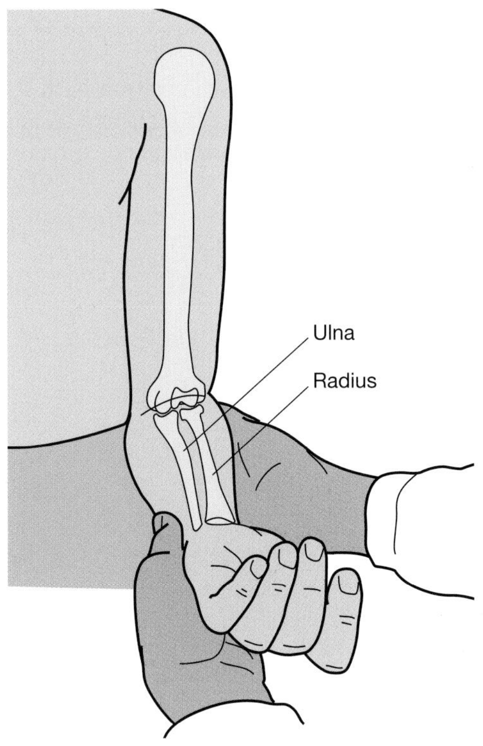

Figure 9.24 Passive movement testing of supination of the forearm.

of flexion and 10 degrees of supination. The resting position of the forearm (superior radioulnar joint) is 70 degrees of flexion and 35 degrees of supination (Kaltenborn, 2011) and the resting position of the humeroradial joint is the forearm fully supinated and the elbow fully extended.

Traction of the Elbow (Humeroulnar) Joint

Place the patient in the supine position with the elbow flexed approximately 70 degrees and the forearm supinated approximately 10 degrees. Stand to the side of the patient facing the posterior aspect of the forearm to be tested. Stabilize by grasping the posterior distal aspect of the humerus. Allow the distal part of the forearm to rest against your trunk. Place your other hand around the anterior proximal portion of the ulna as close as possible to the joint line. Pull the ulna in a longitudinal direction until you have taken up the slack, producing traction in the humeroulnar joint (Figure 9.25).

Lateral Glide of the Ulna

Place the patient in the supine position with the elbow flexed approximately 70 degrees. Stand on the side of the patient with your body facing the patient. Allow the patient's forearm to rest against your chest. Place one hand around the lateral distal aspect of the humerus to stabilize it. Place your other hand around the proximal medial aspect of the ulna. Move the ulna in a lateral direction until all the slack has been taken up. This tests the ability of the ulna to glide laterally on the humerus (Figure 9.26).

Medial Glide of the Ulna

This test is performed with the patient in the same position as the lateral glide of the ulna except that your hand placement is reversed. Stabilize the humerus by placing your hand around the proximal medial aspect. Move the ulna medially, until all the slack has been taken up, by placing your hand around the proximal lateral aspect of the forearm over the radius and ulna (Figure 9.27).

Medial and Lateral Gapping (Varus–Valgus Stress)

Place the patient in the supine position with the patient's elbow in slight flexion and supination. Stand on the side of the table and face the patient. Place your hand around the distal lateral aspect of the

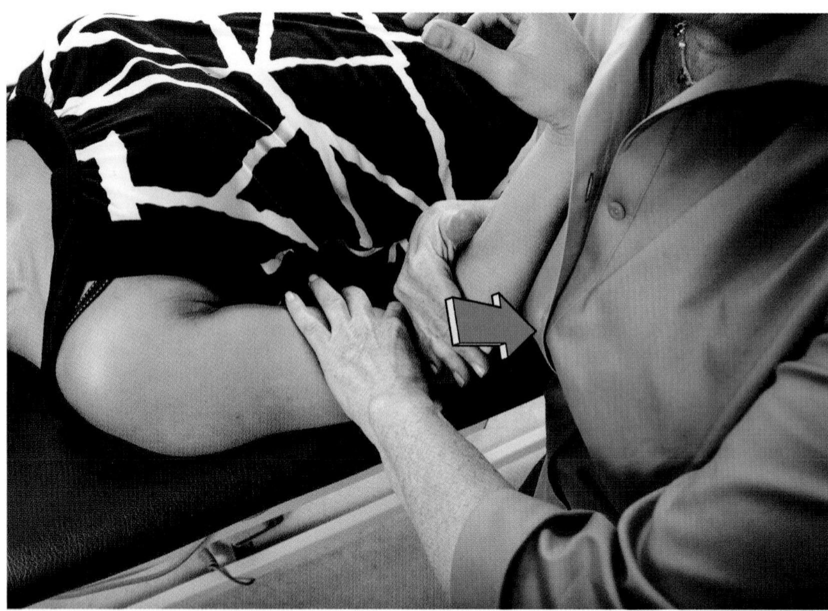

Figure 9.25 Mobility testing of traction of the elbow.

humerus to stabilize it. Place your other hand at the distal medial aspect of the forearm proximal to the wrist. Move the ulna laterally, producing a gapping on the medial aspect of the elbow. This is also referred to as a *medial (valgus) stress.* This tests for the integrity of the medial collateral ligament (Figure 9.28a).

To test the integrity of the lateral collateral ligament, the same test should be repeated by reversing your hand placements. This will allow you to create a varus (lateral) force creating gapping on the lateral aspect of the elbow joint (see Figure 9.28b).

Traction of the Humeroradial Joint

Place the patient in the supine position with the arm resting on the table and the elbow flexed to approximately 70 degrees. Stand on the side of the table and

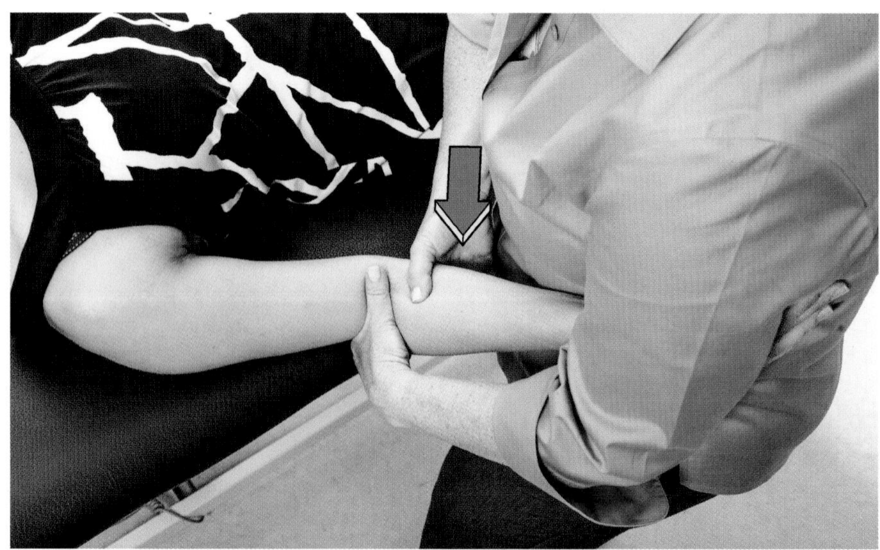

Figure 9.26 Mobility testing of lateral glide of the ulna.

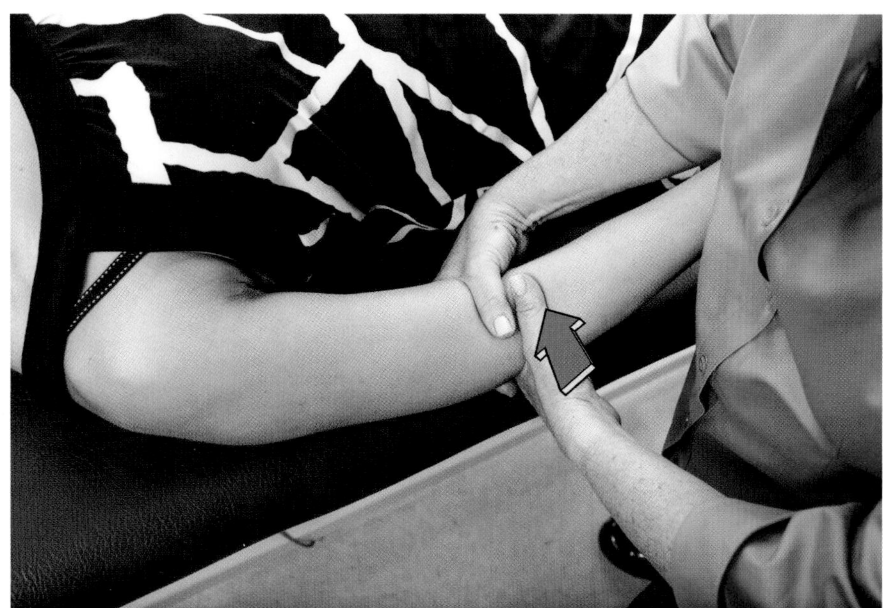

Figure 9.27 Mobility testing of medial glide of the ulna.

face the patient. Place your hand around the distal anterior aspect of the humerus to stabilize it. Place your thumb at the joint space to palpate the movement. Place your other hand at the distal end of the forearm just proximal to the wrist joint. Make sure that you are holding only the radius. Pull the radius in a longitudinal direction until you take up all the slack. This movement produces traction in the humeroradial joint (Figure 9.29).

Ventral and Dorsal Glide of the Radial Head

Place the patient in the seated position so that the arm is supported on the treatment table. Position the patient's arm in the resting position. Stand so that you are facing the patient. Place one hand under the proximal dorsal aspect of the ulna to stabilize it. Place the index finger and thumb of your other hand around the radial head. Move the radial head in a ventral and then a dorsal direction until all the slack is taken up in both directions. This tests for the mobility of the proximal radioulnar joint (Figure 9.30).

Ventral and Dorsal Glide of the Radius

Place the patient in the seated position so that the arm is supported on the treatment table. Position the patient's arm in the resting position. Stand so that you

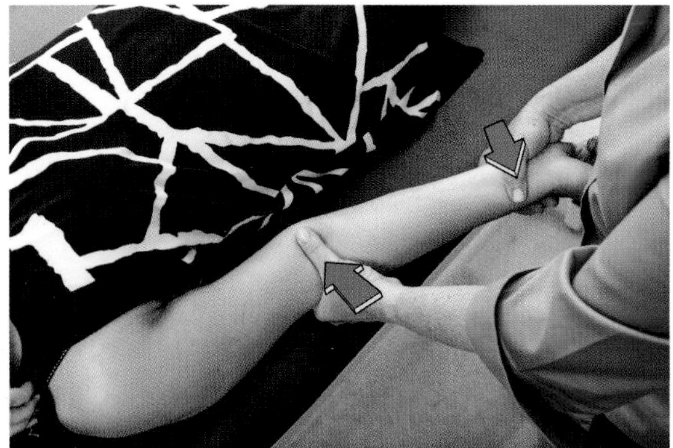

(a)

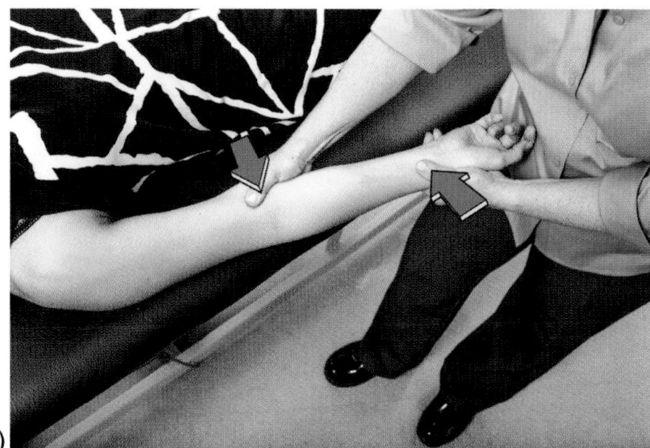

(b)

Figure 9.28 Mobility testing of medial (a) and lateral (b) gapping of the elbow.

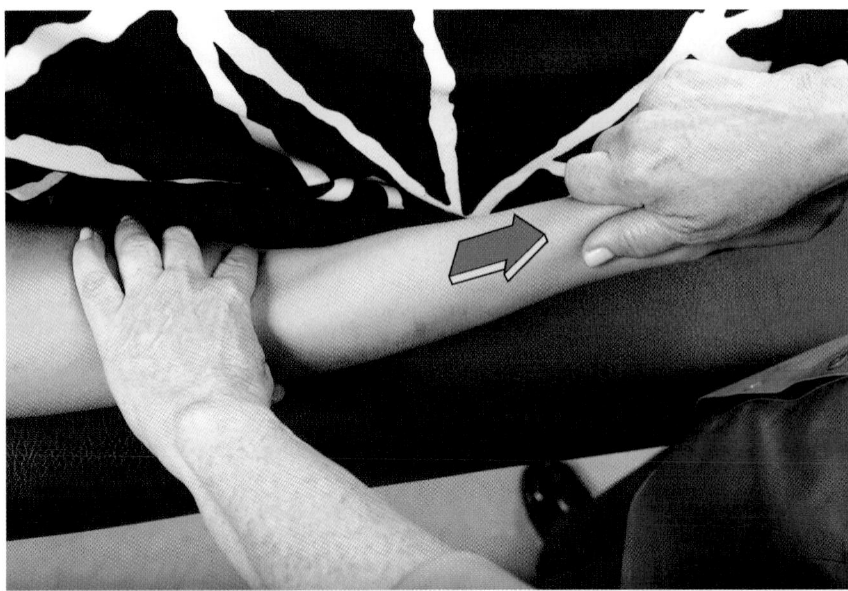

Figure 9.29 Mobility testing of traction of the humeroradial joint.

are facing the patient. Place one hand under the distal dorsal aspect of the ulna to stabilize it. Place the index finger and thumb of your other hand around the distal end of the radius just proximal to the wrist joint. Move the radius in both a ventral and a dorsal direction until all the slack is taken up in both directions. This tests for the mobility of the distal radioulnar joint (Figure 9.31).

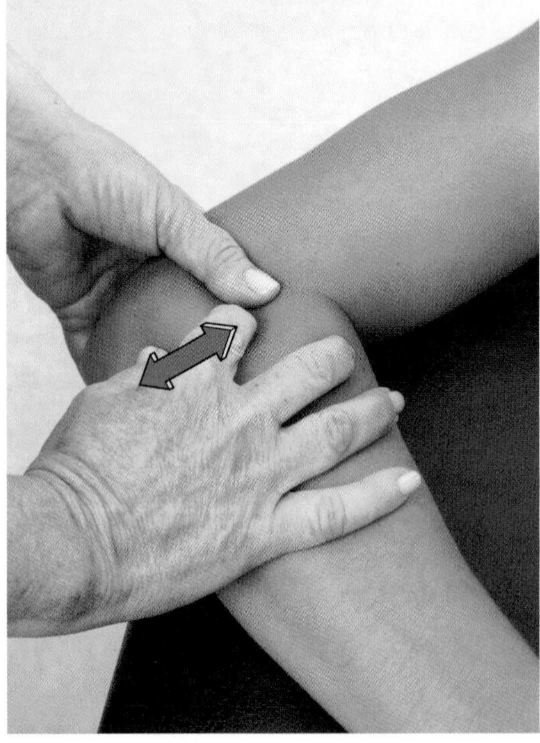

Figure 9.30 Mobility testing of ventral and dorsal glide of the radial head.

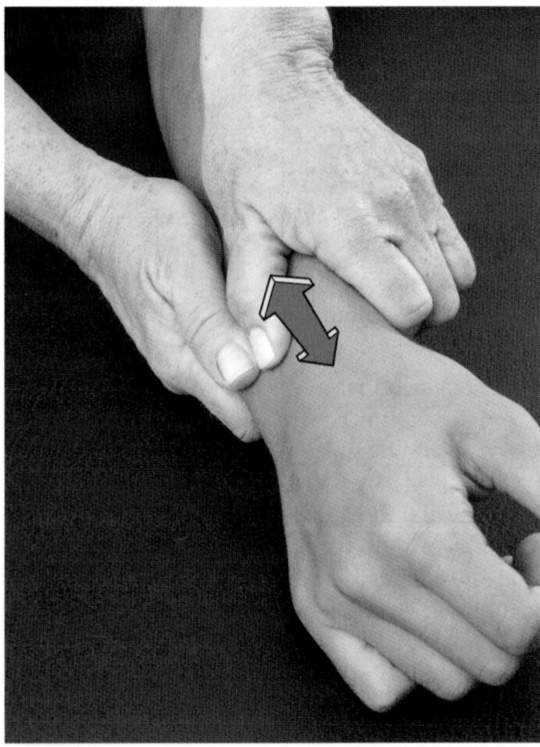

Figure 9.31 Mobility testing of ventral and dorsal glide of the radius.

Resistive Testing

The muscles of the elbow function to position the hand in space. The motions to be tested are flexion, extension, pronation, and supination. The prime movers of the elbow joint are located in the arm.

Although the elbow is analogous to the knee in many respects, unlike the knee, the elbow usually functions as part of an open chain with the hand and wrist. This may be why most of the flexors and extensors of the wrist and fingers also cross the elbow joint, affording more precise control of the fingers and hand in space. Note that none of the muscles of the toes cross the knee joint. The gastrocnemius is the only muscle that crosses the knee and ankle joints.

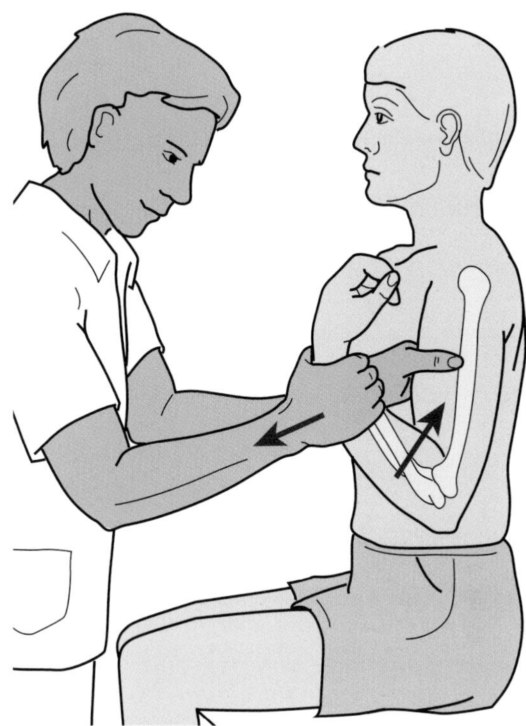

Figure 9.33 Testing elbow flexion.

Elbow Flexion

The flexors of the elbow are the biceps brachii, the brachialis, and brachioradialis (Figure 9.32).

- Position of patient: Sitting with the arm at the side. The forearm is supinated (Figure 9.33).
- Resisted test: Take the patient's wrist with your hand and stabilize his or her upper arm with your other hand. Ask the patient to flex the elbow as you resist this motion by holding the forearm and pulling downward.

Testing elbow flexion with gravity eliminated is performed with the patient in a supine position and the shoulder abducted to 90 degrees and externally rotated (Figure 9.34). Stabilize the upper arm as the patient attempts to slide the forearm along the table into elbow flexion through the complete range of motion.

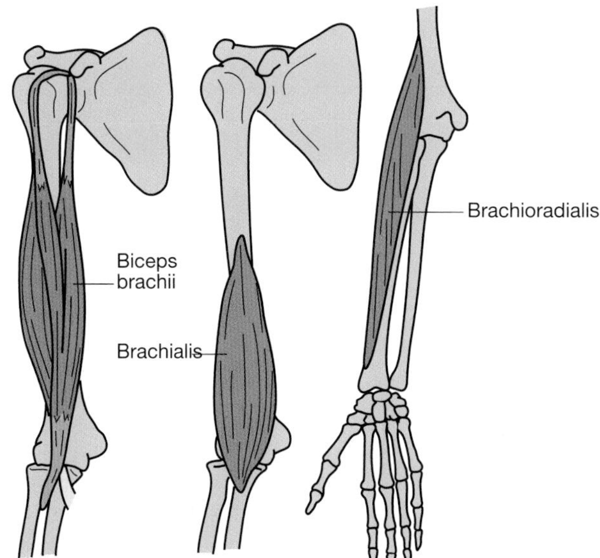

Figure 9.32 The flexors of the elbow.

Painful resisted elbow flexion accompanied by a large bulge in the mid arm may be due to rupture of the biceps tendon.

Weakness of elbow flexion caused by damage to the musculocutaneous nerve, which innervates the biceps and brachialis muscles, will cause the patient to pronate the forearm and substitute for loss of elbow flexion by using the brachioradialis, extensor carpi radialis longus, wrist flexors, and pronator teres. Weakness of elbow flexion causes a substantial restriction in activities of daily living such as feeding and grooming.

Elbow Extension

The elbow extensors are the triceps brachii and anconeus muscles (Figure 9.35).

- Position of patient: Supine with the shoulder flexed to 90 degrees and the elbow flexed (Figure 9.36).
- Resisted test: Stabilize the arm with one hand just proximal to the elbow and apply a downward

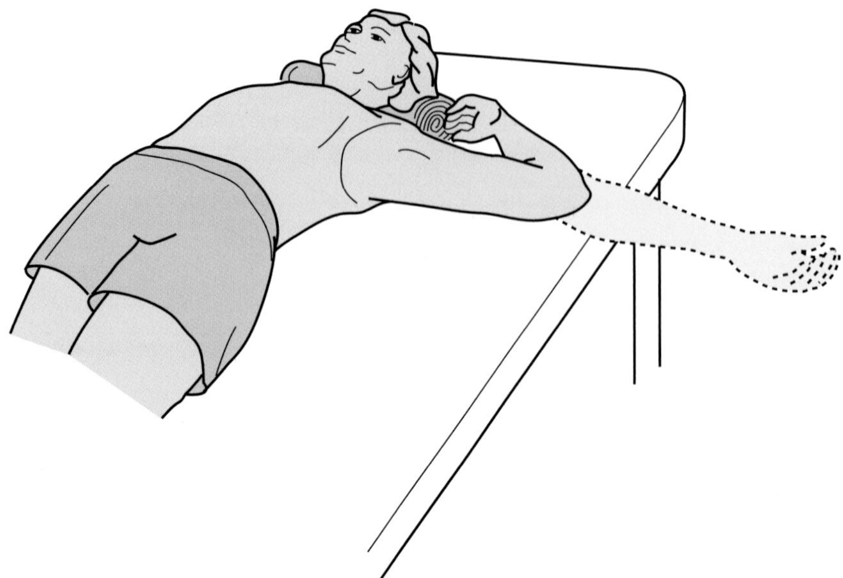

Figure 9.34 Testing elbow flexion with gravity eliminated.

flexing resistive force with your other hand to the forearm just proximal to the wrist. Ask the patient to extend the elbow upward against your resistance.

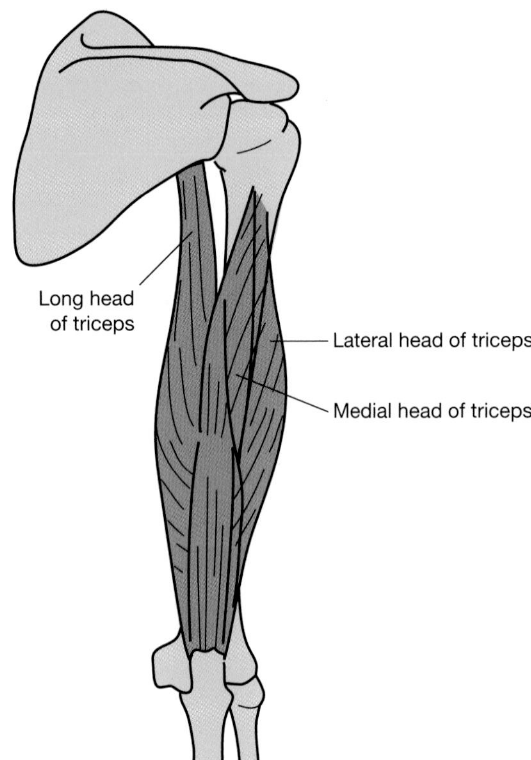

Figure 9.35 The elbow extensors.

Testing elbow extension with gravity eliminated is performed with the patient in the supine position and the shoulder abducted to 90 degrees and internally rotated (Figure 9.37).

Painful resisted elbow extension associated with a swelling over the olecranon process is likely due to olecranon bursitis.

Weakness of elbow extension causes difficulty in using a cane or crutches owing to an inability to

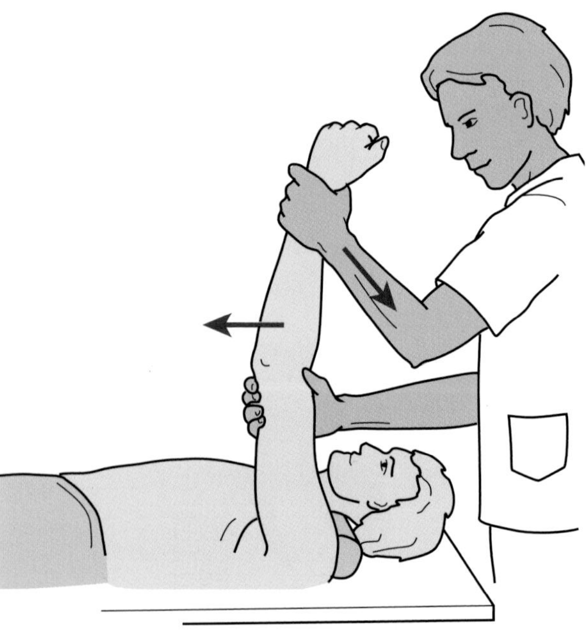

Figure 9.36 Testing elbow extension.

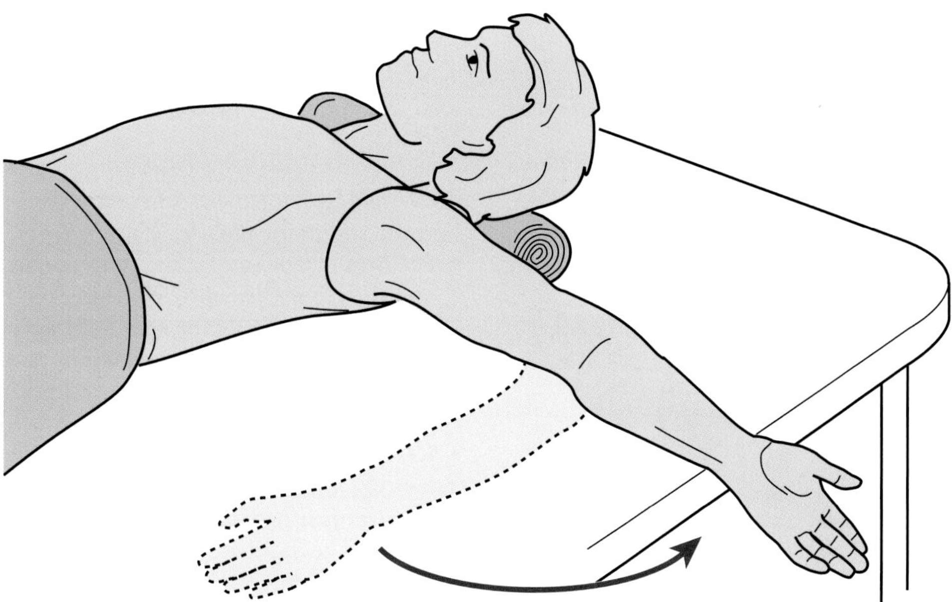

Figure 9.37 Testing elbow extension with gravity eliminated.

bear weight on the extended elbow. Activities such as throwing, reaching upward toward a high object, and doing push-ups are also restricted.

Forearm Pronation

The pronators of the forearm are the pronator teres and pronator quadratus muscles (Figure 9.38).

- Position of patient: Sitting with the arm at the side and the elbow flexed to 90 degrees to prevent rotation at the shoulder. The forearm is initially supinated (Figure 9.39).
- Resisted test: Stabilize the upper arm with one hand placed just proximal to the elbow joint. With your other hand, take the patient's forearm just proximal to the wrist and apply a rotational stress into supination as the patient attempts to pronate the forearm. Do not allow the patient to internally rotate the shoulder in an effort to increase the movement of the forearm.

Testing forearm pronation with gravity eliminated is performed with the patient in the same position. The test is performed without resistance (Figure 9.40).

The pronator quadratus muscle can be isolated by performing the resisted test with the elbow in

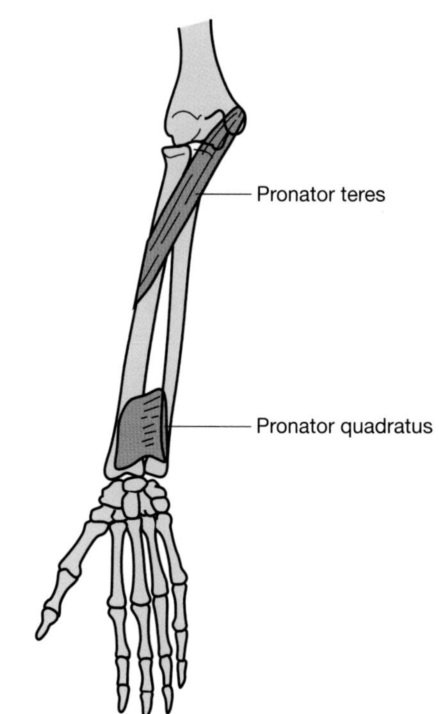

Figure 9.38 The forearm pronators.

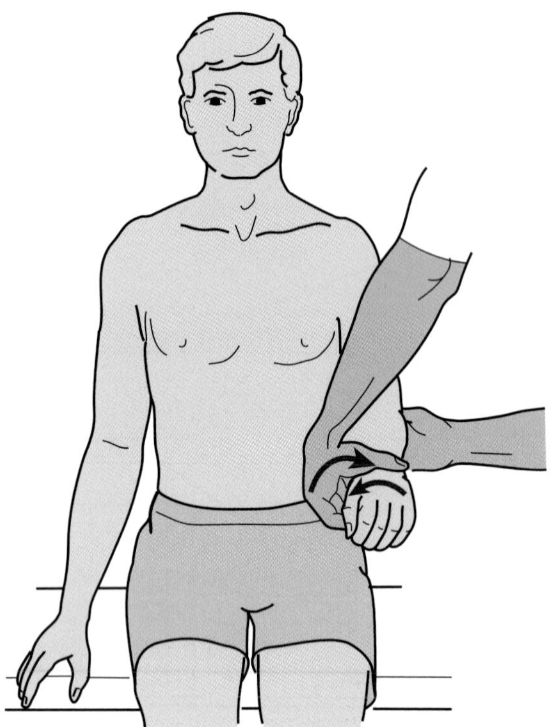

Figure 9.39 Testing forearm pronation.

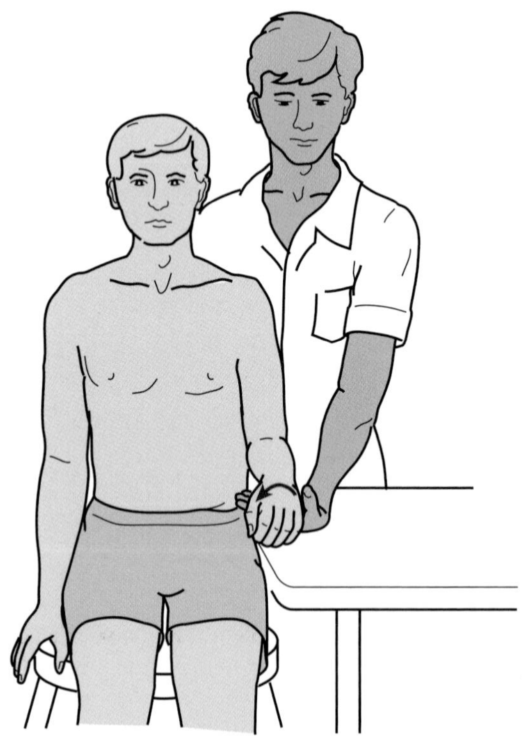

Figure 9.40 Testing forearm pronation with gravity eliminated.

extreme flexion. This puts the pronator teres muscle at a mechanical disadvantage. This is useful in testing for anterior interosseous nerve syndrome (see p. 227, Figure 9.55).

Forearm Supination

The supinators of the forearm are the biceps brachii and the supinator muscles (Figure 9.41).

- Position of patient: Seated with the arm at the side and the elbow flexed to 90 degrees to prevent external rotation of the shoulder, which is used to compensate for lack of supination range of motion. The forearm is in neutral position (Figure 9.42).
- Resisted test: Stabilize the upper arm with one hand placed above the elbow and take the patient's forearm just proximal to the wrist. The patient attempts to supinate the forearm as you apply a rotational force into pronation to resist him or her.

Testing forearm supination with gravity eliminated is performed with the patient in the same position, but without resistance (Figure 9.43).

Painful resisted supination may be due to biceps tendinitis.

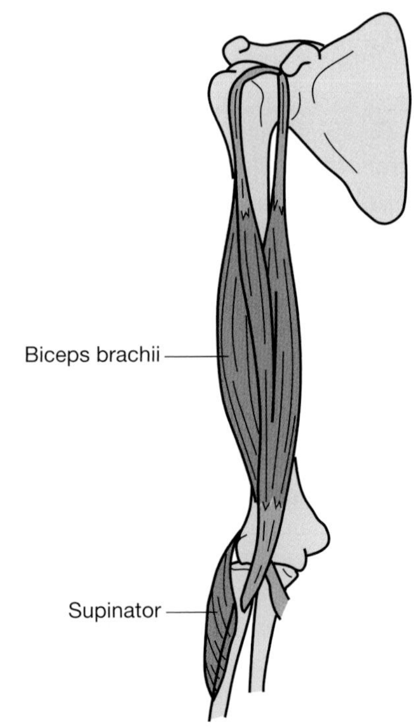

Figure 9.41 The forearm supinators.

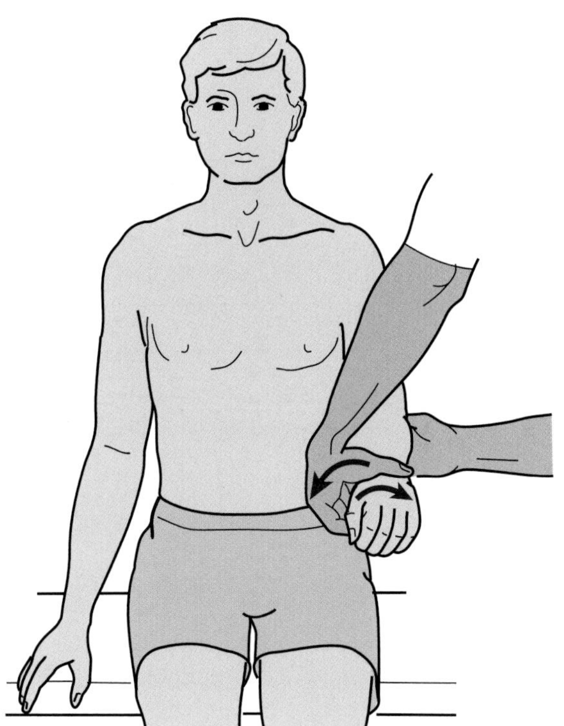

Figure 9.42 Testing forearm supination.

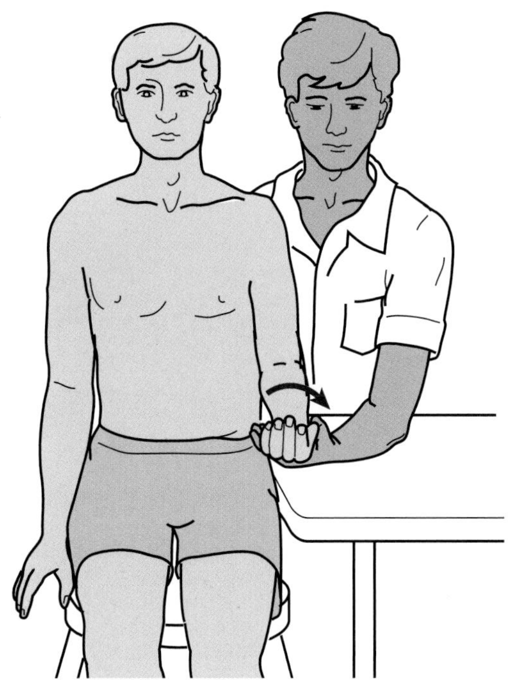

Figure 9.43 Testing forearm supination with gravity eliminated.

Weakness of forearm supination affects many activities of daily living, including feeding oneself and personal hygiene.

Neurological Examination

Motor

The innervation and spinal levels of the muscles that function across the elbow are listed in Table 9.1.

Reflexes

Biceps Reflex

The biceps reflex (Figure 9.44) is used to test the C5, and to a lesser extent, the C6 neurological levels. The test is performed by having the patient rest their forearm on your forearm as you take the patient's elbow in your hand with your thumb pressing downward on the biceps tendon. The tendon becomes more prominent as the patient flexes the elbow slightly. Ask the patient to relax and take the reflex hammer with your other hand and tap onto your thumbnail. The biceps

Table 9.1 Muscles, Innervation, and Root Levels of the Elbow

Movement	Muscles	Innervation	Root Levels
Flexion of elbow	Biceps brachii	Musculocutaneous	C5, C6
	Brachialis	Musculocutaneous	C5, C6
	Brachioradialis	Radial	C5, C6
	Pronator teres	Median	C6, C7
	Flexor carpi ulnaris	Ulnar	C7, C8, T1
Extension of elbow	Triceps	Radial	C7, C8
	Anconeus	Radial	C7, C8
Pronation of forearm	Pronator teres	Median	C6, C7
	Pronator quadratus	Anterior interosseous (median)	C8, T1

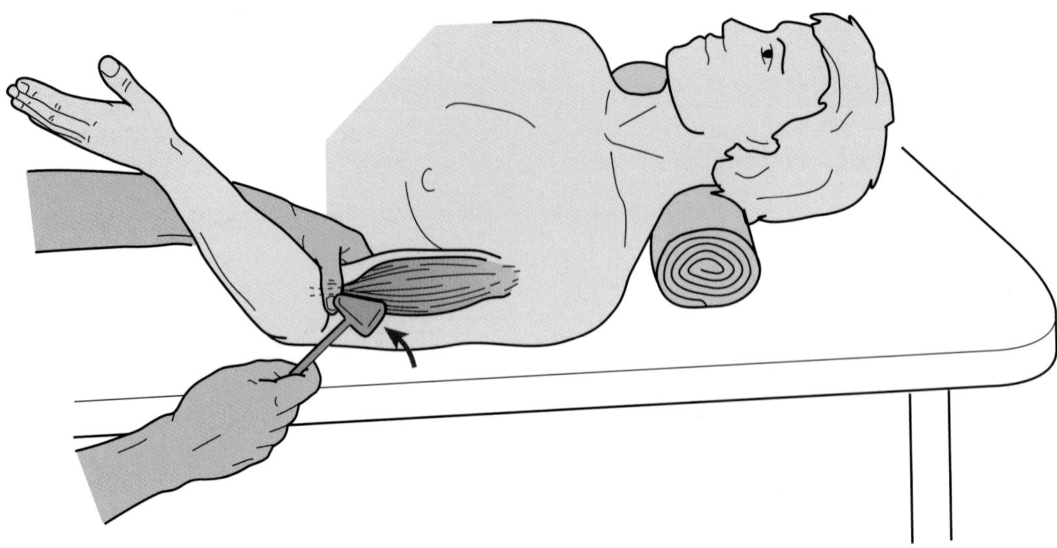

Figure 9.44 Testing the biceps reflex.

will contract and the arm may jump slightly. Absence of this reflex indicates damage to the C5 nerve root level, the upper trunk or lateral cord of the brachial plexus, musculocutaneous nerve, or biceps musculotendinous unit. Always compare the findings to the opposite side.

Brachioradialis Reflex

The brachioradialis reflex (Figure 9.45) is used to test the C6 nerve root level. Have the patient rest their forearm over yours with the elbow in slight flexion. Use the flat end of the reflex hammer to tap the distal end of the radius. The test result is positive when the brachioradialis muscle contracts and the forearm jumps up slightly. Absence of this reflex signifies damage in the C6 nerve root level, the upper trunk or posterior cord of the brachial plexus, the radial nerve, or the brachioradialis musculotendinous unit. Always compare the findings to the opposite side.

Triceps Reflex

The triceps reflex (Figure 9.46) tests the C7 nerve root level. The test is performed by having the patient's forearm resting over yours. Hold the patient's arm

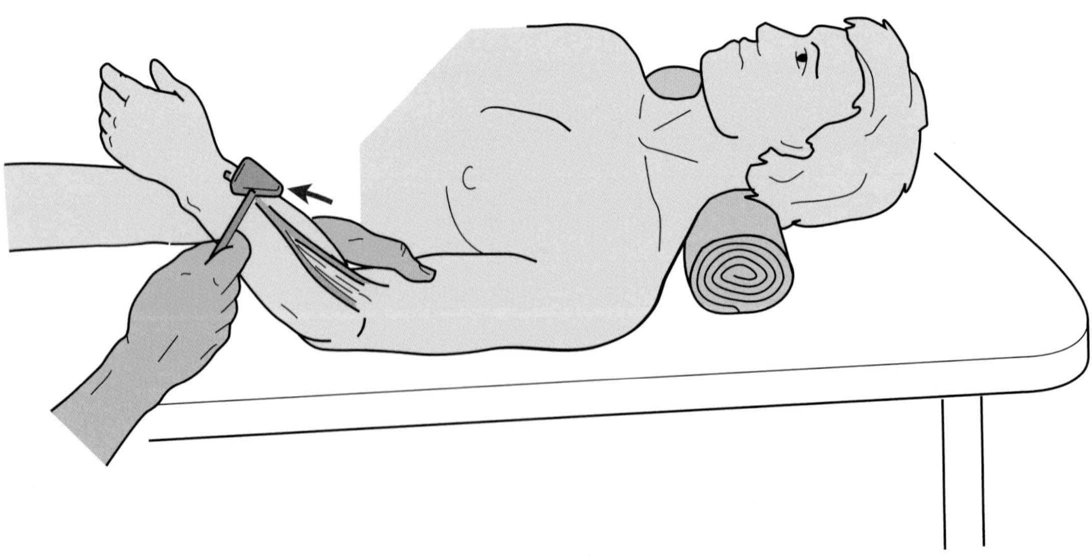

Figure 9.45 Testing the brachioradialis reflex.

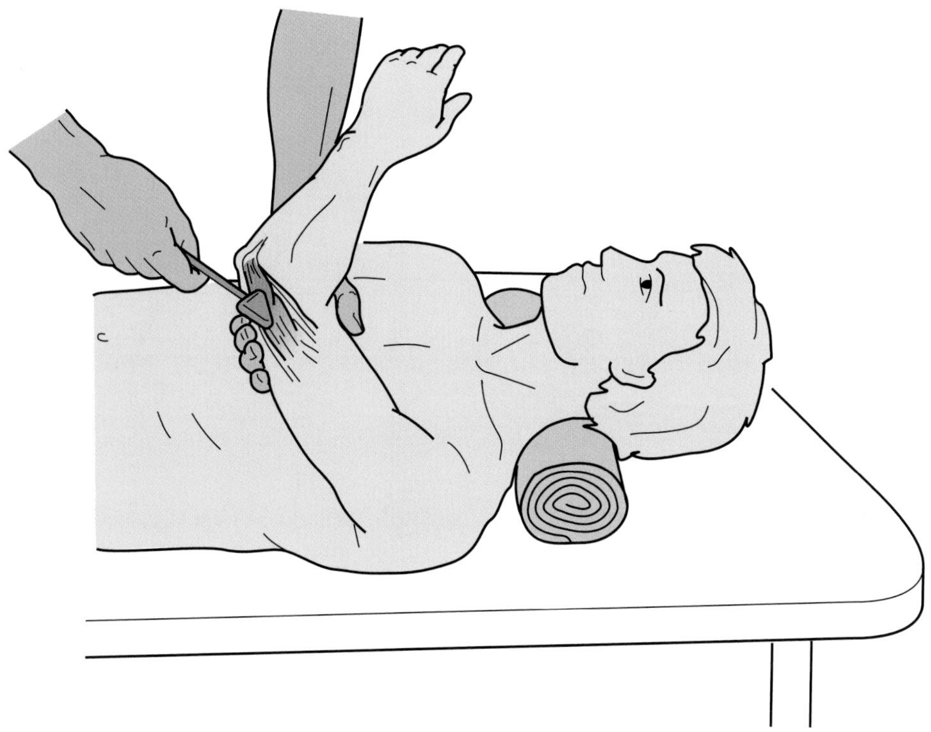

Figure 9.46 Testing the triceps reflex.

proximal to the elbow joint to stabilize the upper arm. Ask the patient to relax, and tap the triceps tendon with the reflex hammer, just proximal to the olecranon process. The test result is positive when contraction of the triceps muscle is visualized. Absence of this reflex signifies damage to the C7 nerve root, middle trunk or posterior cord of the brachial plexus, radial nerve, or triceps musculotendinous unit. Always compare the findings to the opposite side.

Sensation

Light touch and pinprick sensation should be examined after the motor and reflex examination. The dermatomes for the elbow are C5, C6, C7, C8, and T1. Peripheral nerves and their distribution in the elbow region are shown in Figures 9.47, 9.48, and 9.49.

Entrapment Neuropathies

Median Nerve

Median nerve entrapment at the elbow is much less common than at the wrist, as in carpal tunnel syndrome. The median nerve may be compressed above the elbow by an anomalous structure known as the *ligament of Struthers*. At and below the elbow, the median nerve may be compressed by the bicipital aponeurosis (lacertus fibrosus). It may also be compressed at the level of the pronator teres and the flexor digitorum superficialis muscles (Figure 9.50).

The anterior interosseous nerve, which is a branch of the median nerve, may be compressed in the proximal part of the forearm.

Ligament of Struthers

The ligament of Struthers is a relatively rare compression site of the median nerve. The patient usually complains of pain and paresthesias in the index or long finger. You may exacerbate the pain in this condition by having the patient extend the elbow and supinate the forearm. In addition, you may be able to palpate a bony spur proximal to the medial epicondyle of the humerus, which is the attachment site of this anomalous ligament.

Pronator Teres Syndrome

Here, the median nerve is being compressed between the two heads of the pronator teres muscle (Figure 9.51). The other entrapment sites at the bicipital aponeurosis and flexor digitorum superficialis are usually grouped with pronator teres syndrome.

A patient with entrapment of the median nerve at the pronator teres will frequently have tenderness

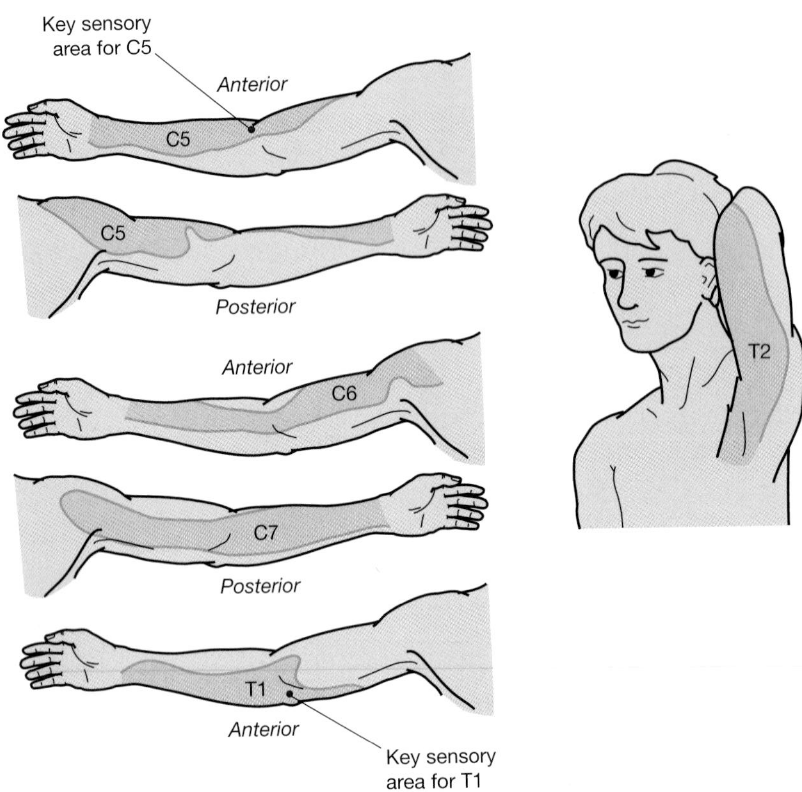

Figure 9.47 The dermatomes of the upper arm and forearm. Note the key sensory areas for C5 and T1, located laterally and medially in the antecubital fossa.

over the proximal portion of the pronator teres muscle. Compression of the pronator teres for 30 seconds, resulting in paresthesias in the thumb and index fingers, is positive for pronator teres syndrome. Reproduction of symptoms of pain or paresthesias during resisted wrist flexion and pronation is also positive for pronator teres syndrome (Figure 9.52).

Reproduction of symptoms of pain or paresthesias in the proximal part of the forearm caused by resisted supination and elbow flexion (biceps muscle) is a positive sign for median nerve compression at the lacertus fibrosus (Figure 9.53).

Reproduction of the symptoms of pain or paresthesias in the forearm or hand following resisted flexion of the long finger is positive for median nerve compression at the flexor digitorum superficialis arch (Figure 9.54).

Anterior Interosseous Nerve

This nerve is a motor nerve to the long flexors of the thumb and index and middle fingers, and the pronator quadratus muscle. There are no cutaneous sensory fibers. However, this nerve does provide some sensation to the joints of the wrist. Examination of a patient with anterior interosseous nerve syndrome characteristically reveals weakness of the long flexor muscles. This can be tested for by asking the patient to make the "OK" sign. An inability to do tip-to-tip pinch of the thumb and index finger results from damage to the anterior interosseous nerve (Figure 9.55).

Ulnar Nerve

The ulnar nerve is susceptible to compression at three sites in the region of the elbow. These include the arcade of Struthers, which is proximal to the elbow; the retrocondylar groove of the humerus at the elbow; and the cubital tunnel just distal to the elbow joint (Figure 9.56). The localization of ulnar neuropathy in the elbow region is best elucidated with electrodiagnostic studies.

Ulnar neuropathy at the elbow results in weakness of the intrinsic muscles of the hand. This can be tested for by having the patient attempt to adduct the little finger to the ring finger. An inability to do this is called a *Wartenberg's sign*. Atrophy may also be noted in the intrinsic muscles of the hand.

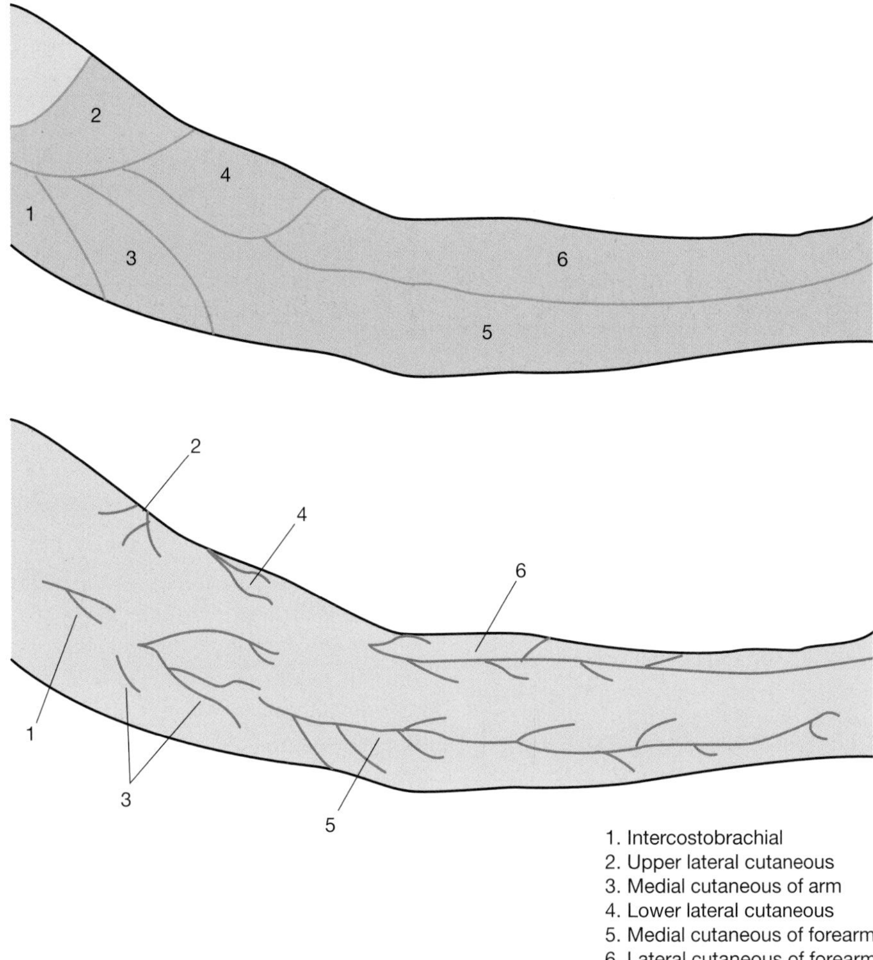

Figure 9.48 Anterior view of the sensory nerves and their distributions in the upper arm and forearm.

Tinel's sign may be elicited at the elbow between the olecranon process and medial epicondyle (Figure 9.57). This is obtained by tapping the ulnar nerve in its groove with your finger. The test result is positive when a tingling sensation is noted in the forearm and medial aspect of the hand. As the nerve regenerates, Tinel's sign is felt more distally by the patient. Beware that false-positive Tinel's signs are common at the elbow.

The patient may have increased symptoms of paresthesias and tingling in the ulnar nerve distribution when asked to flex the elbow for 5 minutes. This is called the *elbow flexion test.*

Radial Nerve

The radial nerve may be compressed within the spiral groove in the proximal part of the humerus, as in Saturday night palsy (Figure 9.58).

The radial nerve (posterior interosseous branch) may also be compressed at the arcade of Frohse (Figure 9.59), which is the proximal tendinous arch of the supinator muscle.

Saturday Night Palsy

The patient will be unable to extend the wrist or fingers. Sensory loss in the distribution of the radial nerve will also be noted. The triceps muscle will be normal because the branch to it arises proximal to the damage to the radial nerve. Therefore, elbow extension will be strong.

Posterior Interosseous Nerve or Supinator Syndrome

The patient will have weakness of wrist and finger extension (see Figure 9.59). Sensation to the posterior lateral hand and brachioradialis and supinator muscle function will all be normal. On wrist extension,

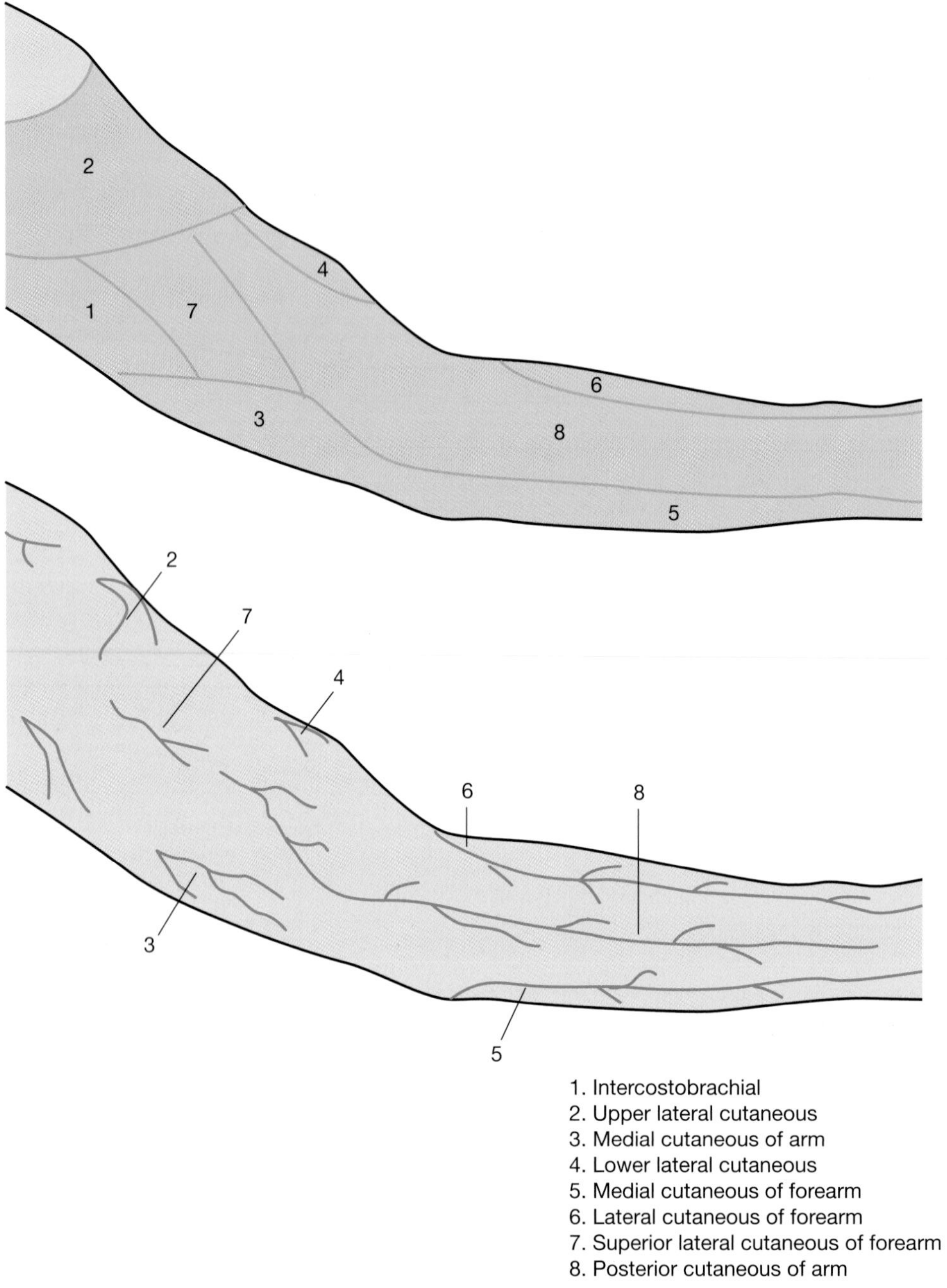

Figure 9.49 Posterior view of the sensory nerves to the arm and forearm, along with their distributions.

the patient may deviate radially due to some sparing of the extensor carpi radialis longus and brevis muscle function, with complete loss of the extensor carpi ulnaris muscle. Note that some interphalangeal joint extension will be present due to preservation of the median and ulnar intrinsic muscles of the hand. A radial nerve lesion should always be ruled out in the presence of lateral elbow pain (tennis elbow).

Special Tests

Tennis Elbow (Lateral Epicondylitis) Test

The various maneuvers used to test for lateral epicondylitis attempt to stress the tendinous attachment of the extensor carpi radialis brevis and longus muscles at the lateral epicondyle of the humerus (Figure 9.60). These muscles can be stretched by

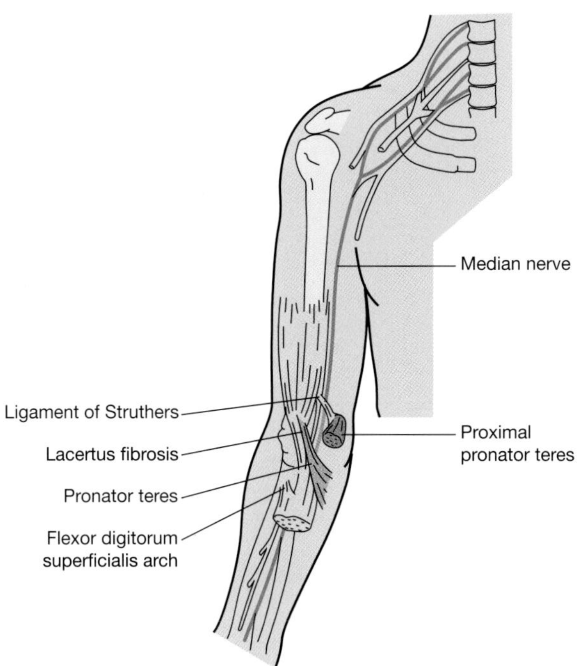

Figure 9.50 Common sites of entrapment of the median nerve near the elbow include the ligament of Struthers, the lacertus fibrosus, pronator teres muscle, and flexor digitorum superficialis arch.

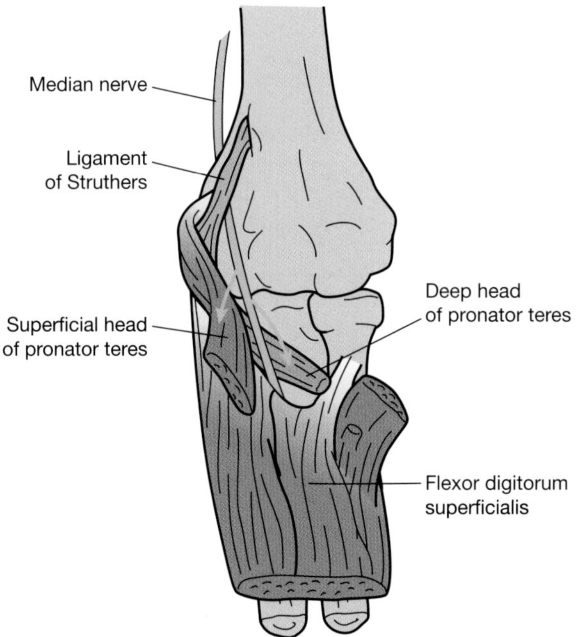

Figure 9.51 In pronator teres syndrome, the median nerve is compressed after its branches are given off to the pronator teres muscles. This muscle is intact. If the nerve is compressed by the ligament of Struthers more proximally, the pronator teres will not be functional. The median nerve is shown coursing between the two heads of the pronator teres muscle.

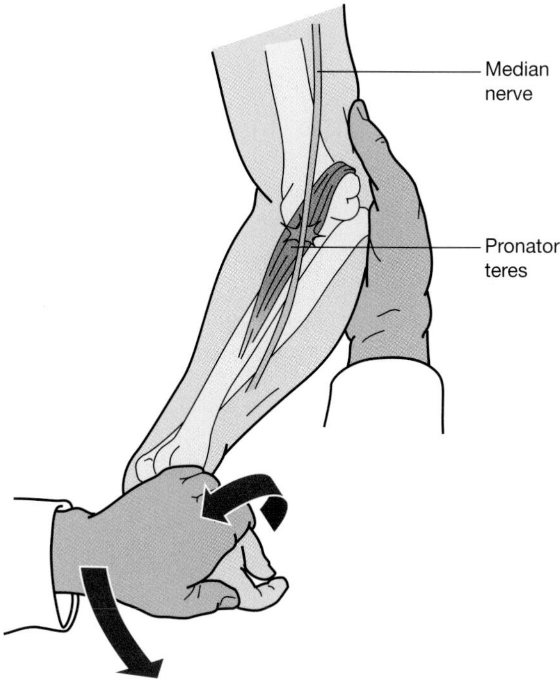

Figure 9.52 Pain that results from resistance of pronation of the forearm and flexion of the wrist may be due to median nerve compression at the level of the pronator teres muscle. This maneuver squeezes the median nerve within the pronator teres muscle.

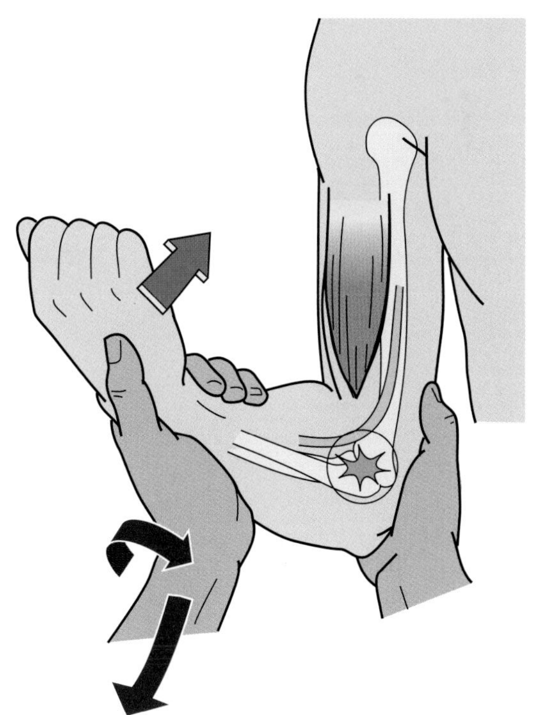

Figure 9.53 The presence of pain in the forearm increased by resistance of forearm supination and elbow flexion is positive for compression of the median nerve at the lacertus fibrosus.

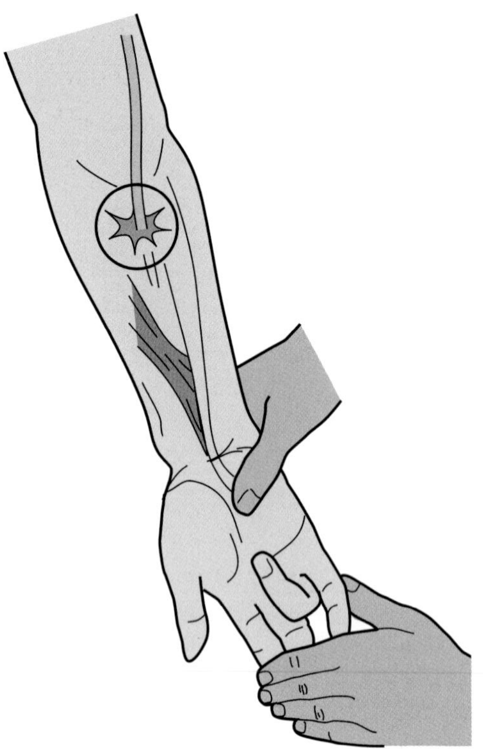

Figure 9.54 Pain in the proximal part of the forearm that is made worse by resisted flexion of the long finger may be due to compression of the median nerve at the level of the flexor digitorum superficialis arch.

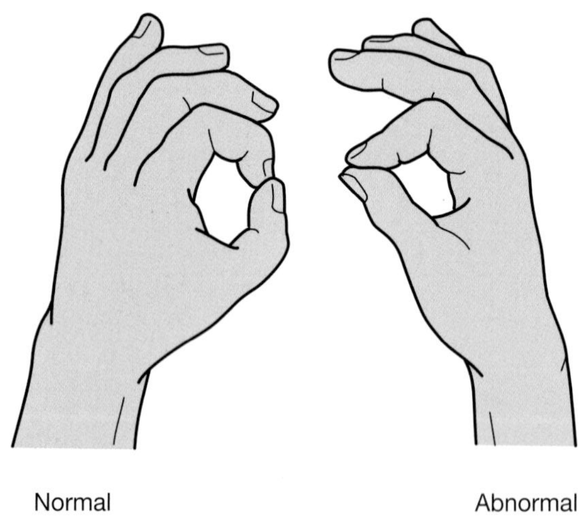

Figure 9.55 The patient with anterior interosseous nerve compression is unable to form the "OK" sign. This is due to weakness of the flexor digitorum profundus to the index finger and the flexor pollicis longus.

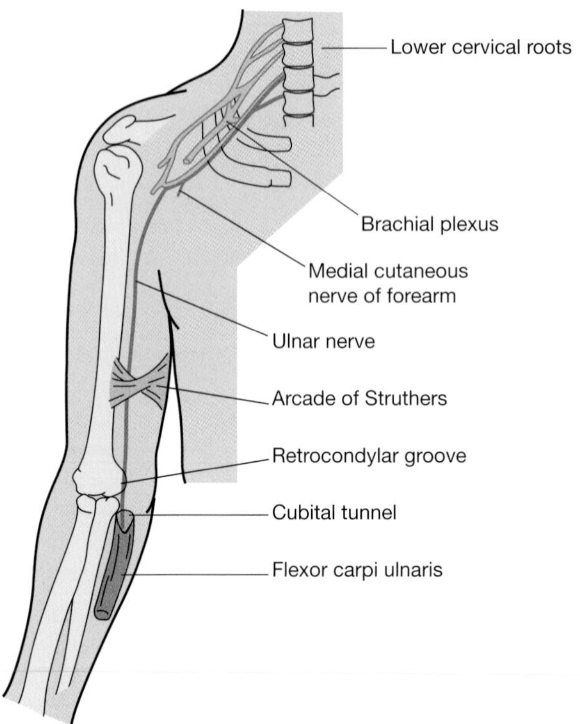

Figure 9.56 Common sites of entrapment of the ulnar nerve include the arcade of Struthers, the retrocondylar groove of the humerus, and the cubital tunnel.

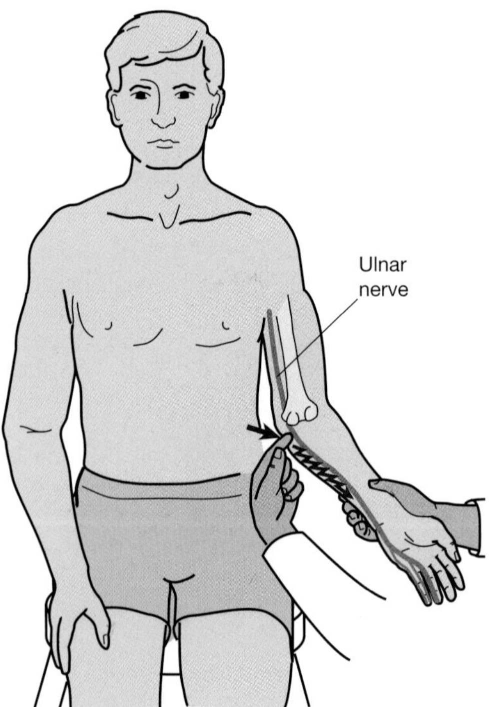

Figure 9.57 Tinel's sign is produced in the ulnar nerve by tapping in the groove between the medial epicondyle of the humerus and the ulna. Similarly, pain may be felt in the medial aspects of the hand and forearm.

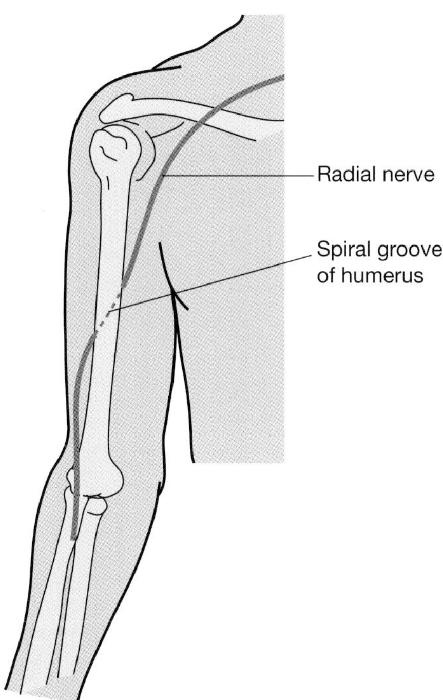

Figure 9.58 The radial nerve may be compressed at the spiral groove of the humerus due to pressure, as in Saturday night palsy.

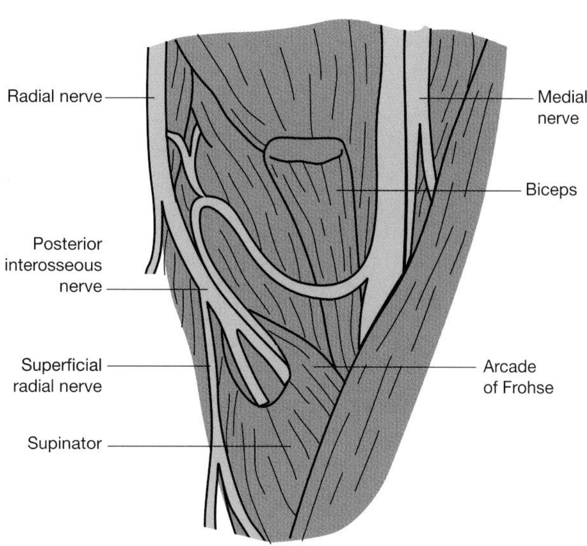

Figure 9.59 The posterior interosseous branch of the radial nerve may be compressed at the level of the arcade of Frohse, which is part of the supinator muscle. Note that the superficial radial nerve, which is a sensory nerve to the hand, is not affected by this compression.

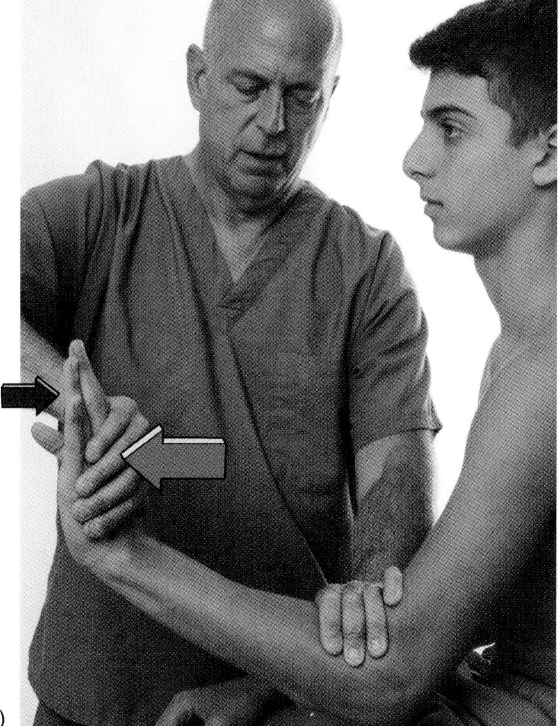

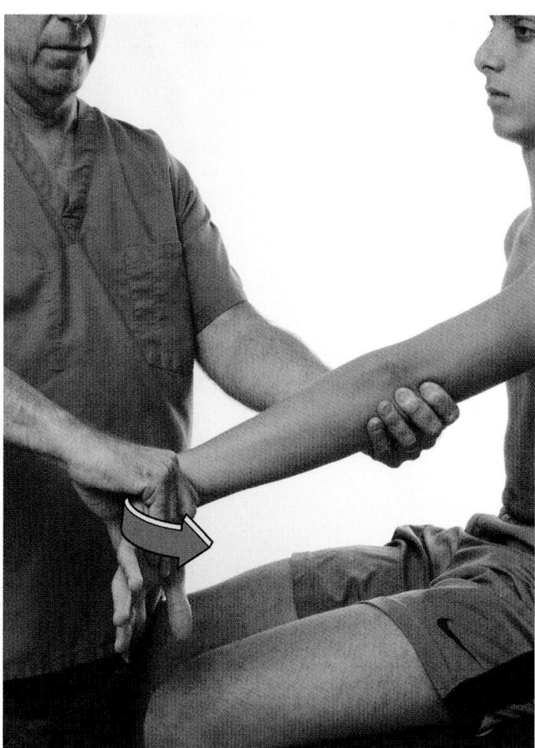

Figure 9.60 Tennis elbow (lateral epicondylitis) can be tested for by resisting wrist extension, as in (a), or by passively extending the elbow and flexing the wrist to stretch the tendons of the wrist extensors, as in (b).

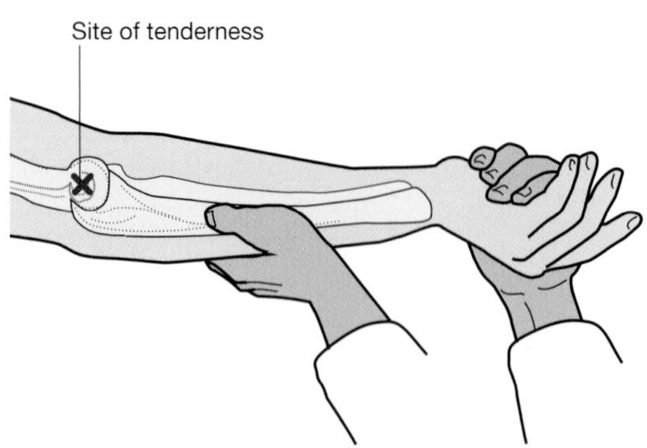

Figure 9.61 Golfer's elbow (medial epicondylitis) will be noted by palpating at the site of tenderness in the medial epicondylar region. The pain is intensified by resisting wrist flexion and forearm pronation with the elbow extended.

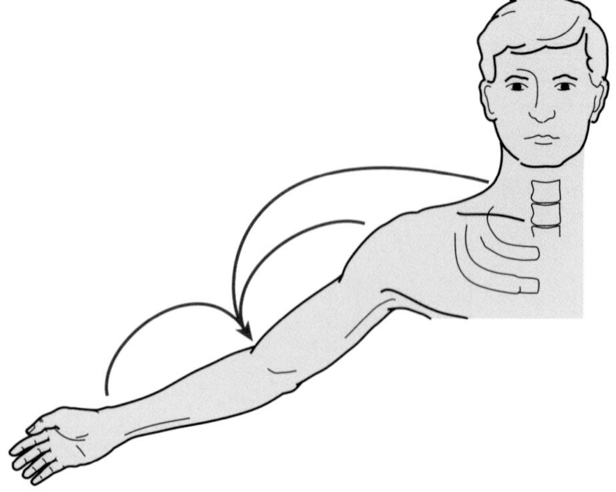

Figure 9.62 Pain may be referred to the elbow from the neck, shoulder, or wrist.

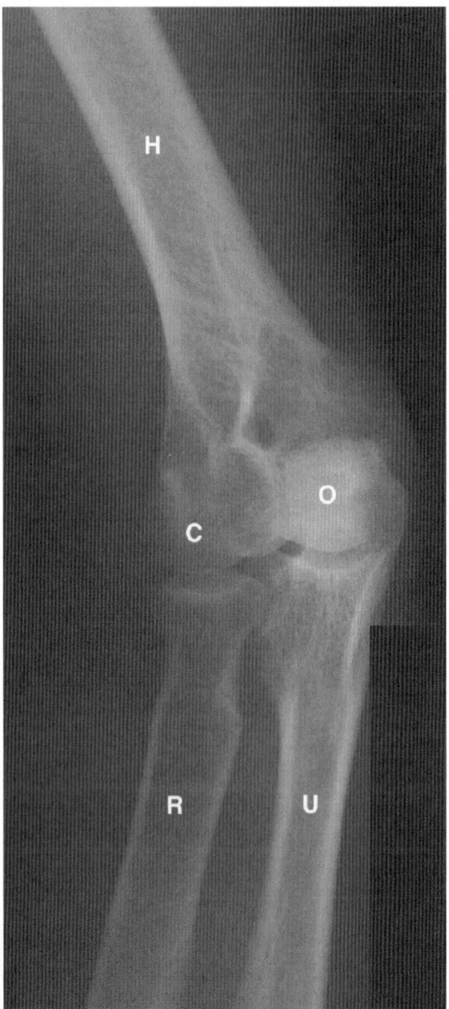

Figure 9.63 Anteroposterior view of the elbow with the forearm supinated.

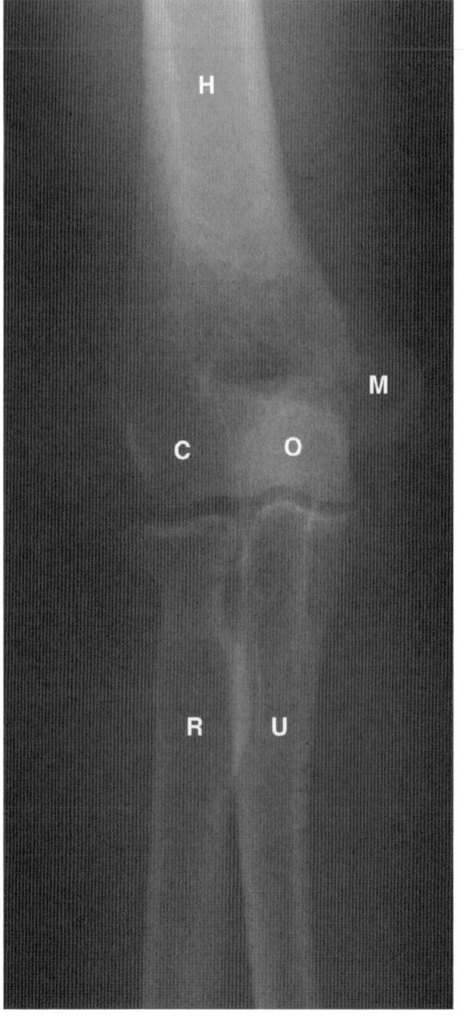

Figure 9.64 View of the elbow with the forearm pronated.

having the patient make a fist, flex the wrist, pronate the forearm, and extend the elbow. Resisted extension of the third metacarpophalangeal joint or of the wrist may also be performed to stress this common attachment site of the extensor muscles (http://www.youtube.com/watch?v=futWq8mXzUo).

Golfer's Elbow (Medial Epicondylitis) Test

The patient's forearm is supinated and the elbow and wrist are extended by the examiner (Figure 9.61). Pain is felt by the patient in the region of the medial epicondyle due to overuse of the wrist flexors. Putting the patient in this position stretches these overused muscles at their tendinous attachment to the medial epicondyle of the humerus. This test will also cause pain in the proximal medial area of the forearm in patients with overuse syndromes due to typing and playing instruments (i.e., strings, piano, and woodwinds) (http://www.youtube.com/watch?v=NW_jH6zx1ac).

Referred Pain Patterns

Pain in the region of the elbow may be referred from the lower cervical spinal segments, the shoulder, and the wrist (Figure 9.62).

Radiological Views

Radiological views are presented in Figures 9.63, 9.64, and 9.65.

H = Humerus
O = Olecranon process of ulna
R = Radius
U = Ulna
T = Trochlea of humerus
M = Medial epicondyle of humerus
C = Capitellum of humerus

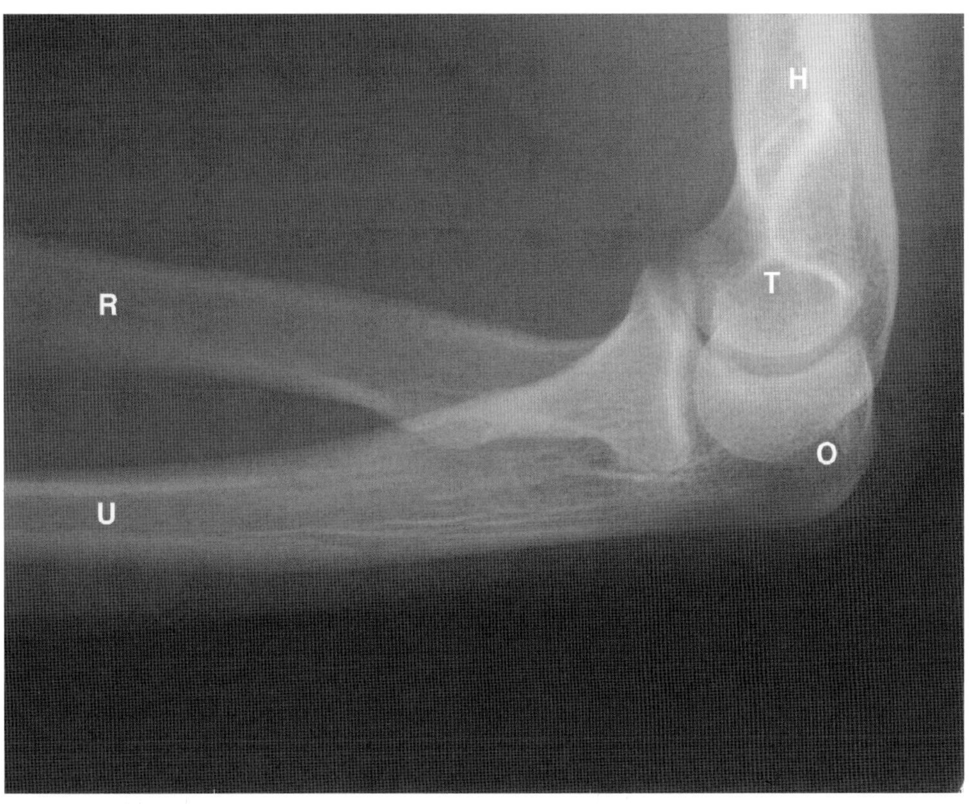

Figure 9.65 Lateral view of the elbow.

PARADIGM FOR INFLAMMATORY DISEASE INVOLVING THE ELBOW

A 25-year-old woman presents with complaints of swelling, pain, and limited motion in her right elbow. She reports no history of recent or prior trauma. She is employed as a secretary and has recently joined a health club. A year ago, her symptoms were initially episodic, but now have become a daily problem.

Upon arising each morning, she notices stiffness in the elbows, wrists, and finger joints of both upper extremities. She has had no recent infections but reports having a low-grade temperature and her face to be "flushed." Her weight has decreased by 10 pounds, and she has noticed an increase in the frequency of her urination. She has no significant prior medical history, but does remember an aunt who became an early invalid because of "arthritis."

Her physical examination demonstrates the patient to be a slender young woman in no acute distress. Her right elbow is slightly swollen, minimally tender, and lacking the terminal 30 degrees of flexion and extension. Her left elbow seems unremarkable, but the metacarpophalangeal and proximal interphalangeal joints of many digits on each hand are moderately enlarged and lack full extension. Her cheeks have a slightly erythematous rash. Laboratory tests report a mild anemia, an increase in the white cell count, increased protein in the urine, and an elevated sedimentation rate. X-rays of the elbows and hands show only soft-tissue enlargement with no bony lesions. Aspiration of the elbow produces a cloudy yellowish viscous fluid, which on analysis shows a large number of inflammatory cells but no organisms.

This is a paradigm of inflammatory disease (rheumatoid arthritis or systemic lupus erythematosus) rather than soft-tissue injury of the elbow because of:

No history of trauma
Age and sex of the patient
Pattern of symptom onset and progression
Symmetrical distribution of signs and symptoms to both upper extremities

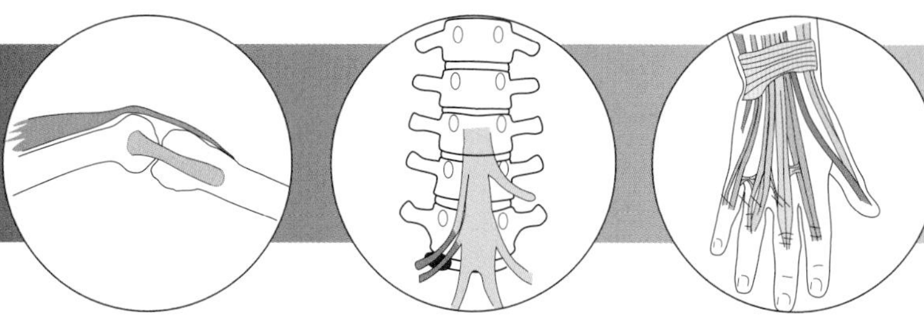

CHAPTER 10

The Wrist and Hand

FURTHER INFORMATION

Please refer to Chapter 2 for an overview of the sequence of a physical examination. For purposes of length and to avoid having to repeat anatomy more than once, the palpation section appears directly after the section on subjective examination and before any section on testing, rather than at the end of each chapter. The order in which the examination is performed should be based on your experience and personal preference as well as the presentation of the patient.

Functional Anatomy

The hand can be divided into two major parts: the wrist and five digits. The carpus, or wrist, is composed of eight small bones. As a unit, the carpus can be thought of as an egg lying on its side, resting in a shallow cup. In this way, it can accommodate movement in three planes, although in unequal amounts. The greatest degree of freedom is in the flexion–extension plane. Next is ulnar–radial deviation. The least movement occurs in rotation about the long axis of the forearm.

The shallow cup is formed by both bony and soft tissues. There are laterally, the distal end of the radius and its styloid, and medially, the distal ulnar styloid and the triangular fibrocartilaginous meniscus. The meniscal soft tissue is interposed between the distal end of the ulna and the wrist bones. The "egg" of the wrist is composed of two rows of small, irregularly shaped bones called the *carpals* (Figure 10.1). These two rows are linked together by many interosseous ligamentous structures and are also connected through the scaphoid navicular bone, which acts as a linkage between the proximal and distal carpal rows. The carpal bones, because of their shape, permit varying amounts of movement. Together, they facilitate and modify placement of the digits in space. Because of its position as linkage between carpal rows, the scaphoid (navicular) (meaning "boat shaped") can be stressed across its midsection or waist, creating a fracture of that bone. Because of its vascular supply following the unusual distal-to-proximal direction, fracture of the scaphoid can lead to avascular necrosis and collapse of the proximal half of that bone. This damage leads to impairment of wrist function and progressive osteoarthritis of the wrist joint.

The five digits can be divided into three groups. The index and long fingers represent a stable central column about which the medial ring and small fingers, and lateral thumb wrap.

The basal joint of the thumb is the most mobile of the hand articulations. Shaped like a saddle, the basal joint permits flexion and extension in two planes. The saddle shape, however, is quite unstable, and possibly the reason for the greater propensity for this joint to undergo osteoarthritic degeneration compared to the other joints of the hand.

Each of the digits of the hand has joints that permit flexion and extension. They can each be thought of as

Musculoskeletal Examination, Fourth Edition. Jeffrey M. Gross, Joseph Fetto and Elaine Rosen.

Companion website: www.wiley.com/go/musculoskeletalexam

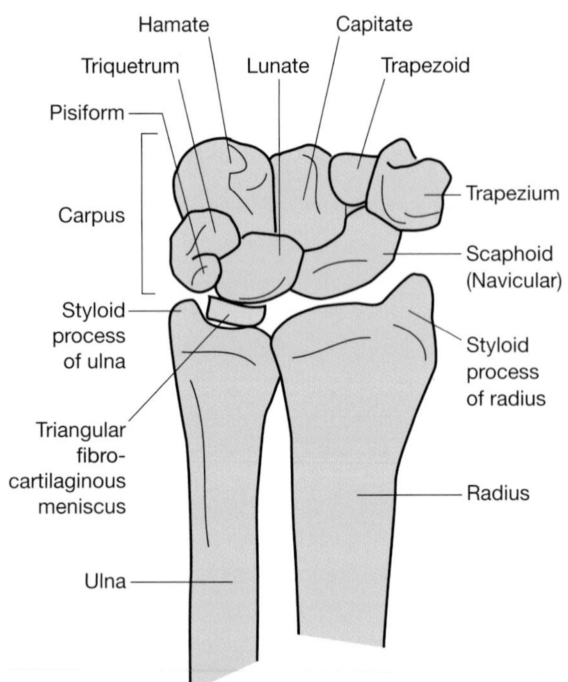

Figure 10.1 The eight small carpal bones of the hand form an "egg," which rests in a shallow dish formed by the distal radius and ulnar meniscus.

simple hinge joints stabilized by collateral ligaments on their medial and lateral aspects.

Movement of the wrist and digits is performed by the flow of the long, sinewy tendons passing from their origins in the forearm across the palmar and dorsal aspects of the wrist. These tendons, along with the major neurovascular structures of the hand, pass through well-defined tunnels or compartments. Two of these tunnels on the palmar side of the wrist are particularly rigid in their cross-sectional dimension. As such, neurovascular structures passing through them are particularly vulnerable to compression injuries should any space-occupying lesion invade the space of this tunnel (i.e., edema from injury or thyroid dysfunction, or adipose tissue due to obesity). These tunnels are so often involved in clinical syndromes that they bear specific mention. They are the carpal tunnel, which contains the median nerve together with the flexor tendons of the digits, and the tunnel of Guyon, which contains the ulnar nerve. Injury to the median nerve presents as paresthesias, atrophy, and loss of sensation to the thenar eminence of the thumb, the index and long fingers, and the radial half of the ring finger. Compression injury of the ulnar nerve will affect the medial aspect of the hand (hypothenar eminence, small finger, and ulnar half of the ring finger), together with the ulnar intrinsic muscles of the hand. This muscular compromise will lead to classic posturing of the digits called the *benediction hand,* referring to the appearance of a priest's hand when giving a blessing (see pp. 282–284, Figure 10.97).

Observation

The examination should begin in the waiting room before the patient is aware of the examiner's observation. Information regarding the degree of the patient's disability, level of functioning, posture, and gait can be observed. The clinician should pay careful attention to the patient's facial expressions with regard to the degree of discomfort the patient is experiencing. The information gathered in this short period can be very useful in creating a total picture of the patient's condition.

Note the manner in which the patient is sitting and how he or she is posturing the upper extremity. Is the arm relaxed at the side or is the patient cradling it for protection? What is the relaxed posture of the hand itself? Note whether the wrist or hand is edematous. Note the shape of the hand and if there are any changes in contour. The patient may have a protuberance secondary to a ganglion, nodule, or bony dislocation. Note any bony deformities. The patient may have a swan neck, boutonniere deformity, or claw fingers. Compare one hand to the other, remembering that the dominant hand may be larger in the normal individual. What is the cosmetic appearance of the hand? Many patients are extremely self-conscious of how their hands look.

How willing is the patient to use the upper extremity? Will he or she allow you to shake their hand? Is the patient able to move the hand in an effortless and coordinated fashion or is he or she stiff and uncoordinated? Is the patient willing to bear weight on an extended wrist? Watch as the patient gets up from the chair to see whether he or she pushes down with the wrist. Pain may be altered by changes in position so watch the patient's facial expression to give you insight into the pain level.

Observe the patient as he or she assumes the standing position. Observe the patient's posture. Pay particular attention to the position of the head, cervical spine, and the thoracic kyphosis. Note the height of the shoulders and their relative positions. Once the patient starts to ambulate, observe whether he or she is willing to swing the arms. Arm swing can be limited by either loss of motion, pain, or neurological damage.

Once the patient is in the examination room, ask him or her to disrobe. Observe the ease with which the patient uses the upper extremities and the rhythm of the movements. Observe for symmetry of bony structures. Note the carrying angle with the upper extremity postured in the anatomical position. Observe the hand on all surfaces. Observe for areas of muscle wasting that may be secondary to peripheral nerve lesions. Inspect for scars, open lesions, abrasions, calluses, color, hair growth patterns, nails, and the presence of any trophic changes. Abnormalities may be secondary to reflex sympathetic dystrophy, shoulder hand syndrome, Raynaud's disease, or peripheral vascular or metabolic disease. Observe the skin. Is the skin smooth with a loss of the creases? Is there an increase in moisture or a decrease in sensibility? Spindlelike fingers can be secondary to systemic lupus erythematosus, long-standing neuropathy, or rheumatoid arthritis. Clubbing and cyanosis of the nails may be secondary to pulmonary disease.

Subjective Examination

The wrist and hand are extremely active structures that are both complicated and delicate. They are very vulnerable to injury. Since they are non-weight-bearing, problems are most commonly related to overuse syndromes, inflammation, and trauma. You should inquire about the nature and location of the patient's complaints as well as their duration and intensity. Note whether the pain travels up to the elbow. The behavior of the pain during the day and night should also be addressed.

You should determine the patient's functional limitations. How much was the patient able to do before the onset of symptoms? Which is the dominant hand? How incapacitated does the patient consider himself or herself to be? Question the patient regarding actual use of the upper extremity. Is the patient able to comb his hair, fasten her bra, fasten buttons, handle small objects, or feed himself? Is this injury traumatic in nature? What was the mechanism of the injury? Does the patient regularly participate in any vigorous sport activity that would stress the wrist or hand? What is the patient's occupation? Does he or she use tools or spend a great deal of time at a computer terminal stressing the wrist and hand repetitively?

If the patient reports a history of trauma, it is important to note the mechanism of injury. The direction of the force, the position of the upper extremity, and the activity the patient was participating in at the time of the injury contribute to your understanding of the resulting problem and help you to better direct your examination. The degree of pain, edema, and disability at the time of the trauma and within the initial 24 hours should be noted. Does the patient have a previous history of the same injury? Does the patient report any clicking, grating, or snapping? This may be due to a stenosing tenosynovitis or to a loose body. Is any grating present? This may be due to osteoarthritis.

The patient's disorder may be related to age, gender, ethnic background, body type, static and dynamic posture, occupation, leisure activities, hobbies, and general activity level. It is important to inquire about any change in daily routine and any unusual activities that the patient has participated in. The location of the symptoms may give you some insight into the etiology of the complaints. The cervical spine and the shoulder can refer pain to the wrist and hand and should be included as part of the examination. The most common nerve roots that refer pain are C6, C7, C8, and T1. (Please refer to Box 2.1, see p. 15 for typical questions for the subjective examination.)

Gentle Palpation

The palpatory examination is started with the patient in the sitting position. You should first examine for areas of localized effusion, discoloration, birthmarks, calluses, open sinuses or drainage, incisional areas, abrasions, bony contours, muscle girth and symmetry, and skin creases. You should not have to use deep pressure to determine areas of tenderness or malalignment. It is important to use firm but gentle pressure, which will enhance your palpatory skills. By having a sound basis of cross-sectional anatomy, you will not need to physically penetrate through several layers of tissue to have a good sense of the underlying structures. Remember that if you increase the patient's pain at this point in the examination, the patient will be very reluctant to allow you to continue and may become more limited in his or her ability to move.

Palpation is most easily performed with the patient in a relaxed position. The sitting position with the extremity supported on a table is preferred for ease of examination of the wrist and hand. Remember that for palpation of all the structures described, the hand is in the anatomical position. While locating the bony landmarks, it is also useful to pay attention to areas of increased or decreased temperature and moisture. This will help you identify areas of acute and chronic inflammation.

Anterior (Palmar) Aspect

Bony Structures

Since thick skin and fascia cover the palm, the bony structures are more difficult to palpate on the anterior surface. The carpal bones are more accessible and easier to identify from the dorsal aspect. Descriptions of their locations are found later in this chapter.

Soft-Tissue Structures

Start your palpation by observing the superficial palmar surface. The skin is thicker than on the dorsal aspect. The skin contains many sweat glands but is free of hair. Observe the creases in both the longitudinal and transverse directions. You will notice that the longitudinal creases are more distinct when the patient opposes the thumb. The transverse creases are more distinct when the patient flexes the metacarpophalangeal joints. Note the absence of the fibro-fatty tissues and how the skin is securely attached to the deep fascia in the area of the skeletal joints forming the creases. They are useful to identify the underlying anatomical structures. At the level of the wrist, you will notice the proximal and then the distal wrist creases. On the lateral side, notice the thenar (radial longitudinal) crease that surrounds the thenar eminence.

Continuing distally, note the proximal palmar (flexion) crease, which begins simultaneously with the thenar crease, just proximal to the head of the second metacarpal. It travels medially across the palm along the middle of the shafts of the third through fifth metacarpals.

The distal palmar (transverse) crease is located on the palmar surface of the heads of the second or third through fifth metacarpals. It becomes more distinct as the patient flexes the metacarpophalangeal joints.

As you continue distally, you will notice the proximal digital creases located at the level of the finger webs. There are no joints under these creases. The metacarpophalangeal joints are about 2 cm proximal to the proximal digital creases.

The proximal and distal interphalangeal creases lie superficial to the proximal and distal interphalangeal joints and deepen as the joints are flexed (Figure 10.2).

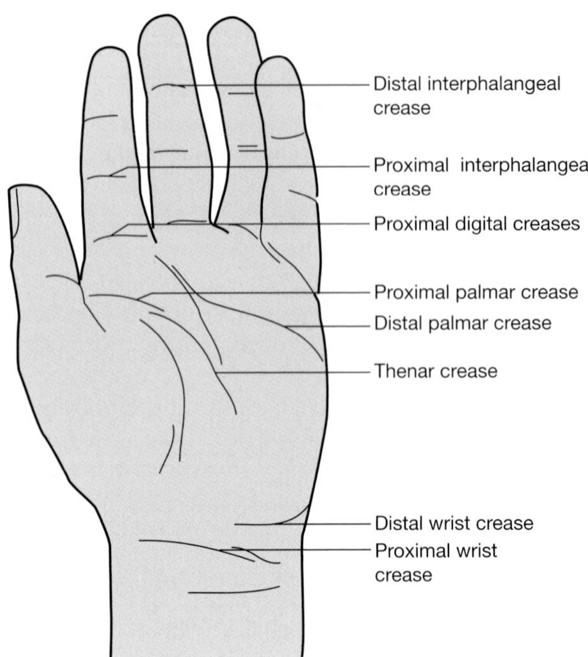

Figure 10.2 Palpation of the palmar surface of the hand.

To enable you to more easily organize the palpation of the deeper soft tissues, the anterior surface of the hand can be divided into three areas: the medial, middle, and lateral compartments. Each compartment is described, from proximal to distal.

Medial (Ulnar) Compartment

Flexor Carpi Ulnaris. Move your fingers to the medial palmar surface and locate the pisiform bone (see description on p. 242, Figure 10.11). The tendon of the flexor carpi ulnaris is palpable proximal to its attachment on the pisiform (Figure 10.3). The tendon becomes more distinct when you resist wrist flexion and ulnar deviation.

Ulnar Artery. The ulnar pulse can be palpated on the medial volar surface of the wrist (Figure 10.4). Press against the distal aspect of the ulna, just proximal to the pisiform, to facilitate palpating the pulse. Remember not to press too hard since the pulse will be obliterated.

Ulnar Nerve. The ulnar nerve passes into the hand lateral to the pisiform, medial and posterior to the ulnar artery, and then under the hook of the hamate. It is not readily palpable in the wrist, but it is at the medial elbow (see p. 206, Figure 9.7).

Hypothenar Eminence. Place your fingers on the pisiform and move distally until you reach the distal palmar crease. You will feel the longitudinal bulk

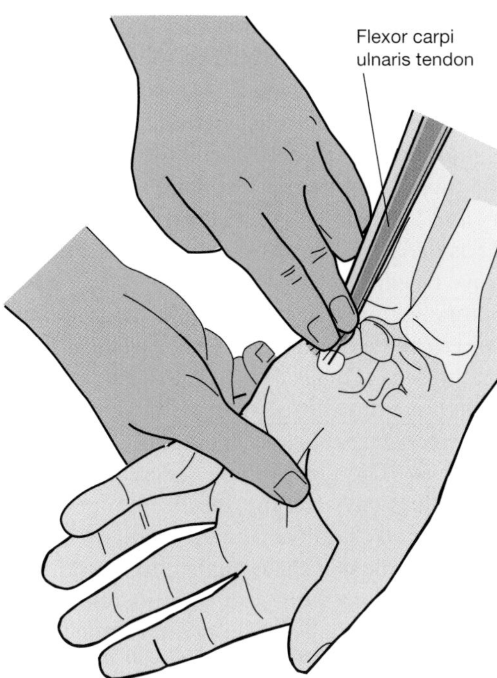

Figure 10.3 Palpation of the flexor carpi ulnaris.

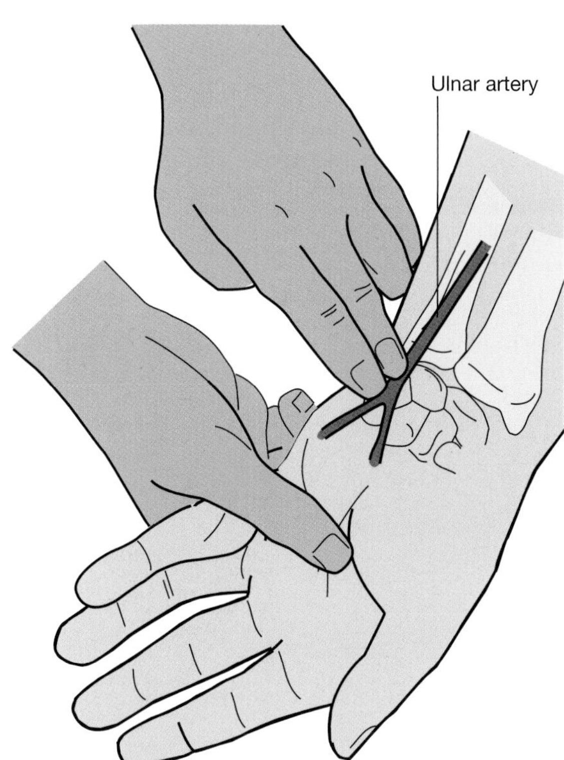

Figure 10.4 Palpation of the ulnar artery.

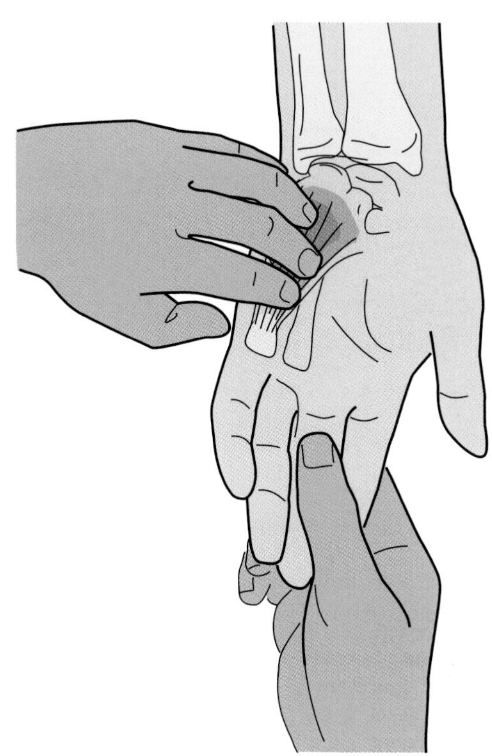

Figure 10.5 Palpation of the hypothenar eminence.

of the muscle bellies of the hypothenar eminence (Figure 10.5). The eminence is composed of the palmaris brevis, abductor digiti minimi, flexor digiti minimi brevis, and the opponens digiti minimi. It is not possible to differentiate between these muscles on palpation. Examine the hypothenar eminence and compare it to the one in the opposite hand for size and symmetry. Atrophy and diminished sensation can be indicative of compression of the ulnar nerve in the elbow in the cubital tunnel or in the canal of Guyon secondary to trauma or from compression from a ganglion. Power grip will be significantly impaired.

Middle Compartment

Palmaris Longus. Continue to move laterally along the anterior surface of the wrist. The long thin tendon in the middle is the palmaris longus. It can be palpated just proximal to its attachment to the anterior distal surface of the flexor retinaculum and the palmar aponeurosis (Figure 10.6). The tendon becomes more distinct when the patient flexes the wrist and approximates the thenar and hypothenar eminences, causing a tensing of the palmar fascia. The palmaris longus is absent in either one or both wrists in approximately 13% of the population. However, its absence does not alter the patient's function (Moore and

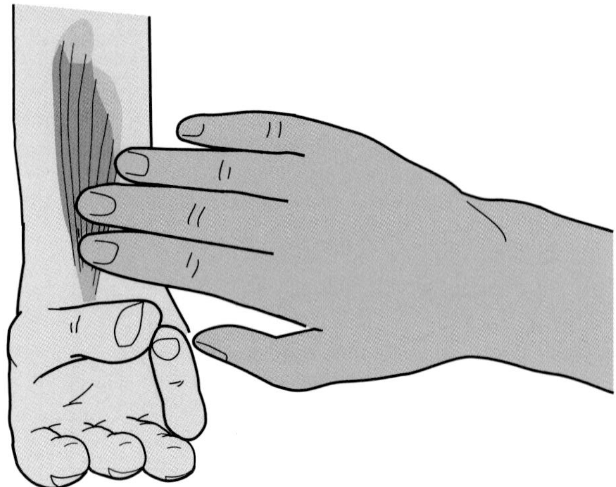

Figure 10.6 Palpation of the palmaris longus.

Dalley, 1999). When the tendon is present, it may be useful as a donor site for two-stage tendon reconstructive surgery. The tendon can be used to help locate the median nerve, which runs just lateral to it at the wrist.

Flexor Digitorum Profundus and Superficialis. The tendons of the flexor digitorum profundus and superficialis travel in a common sheath passing under the flexor retinaculum and deep to the palmar aponeurosis. They then divide, are covered by synovial membrane, and enter into individual osseofibrous digital tunnels. In some individuals, it is possible to palpate the individual tendons as they travel along the palm toward the digits. Ask the patient to flex and extend the fingers and you will feel the tendon become more prominent as the fingers contract into flexion and taut as they move toward extension.

If snapping, "clunking," or grating in the tendon is noted with either flexion or extension, a trigger finger may be present. This is caused by swelling of the tendon, which creates difficulty in gliding under the pulley at the metacarpal head during movement.

Carpal Tunnel. The carpal tunnel is created by the flexor retinaculum covering the anterior concavity of the carpal bones. Its floor is formed medially by the pisiform and the hook of the hamate and laterally by the tubercle of the scaphoid and the tubercle of the trapezium (Figure 10.7). The tunnel allows the flexor tendons of the digits and the median nerve to travel through to the hand. It is extremely significant clinically because of the frequency of compression of the median nerve secondary to edema, fracture, arthritis, cumulative trauma, or repetitive motion injuries. This

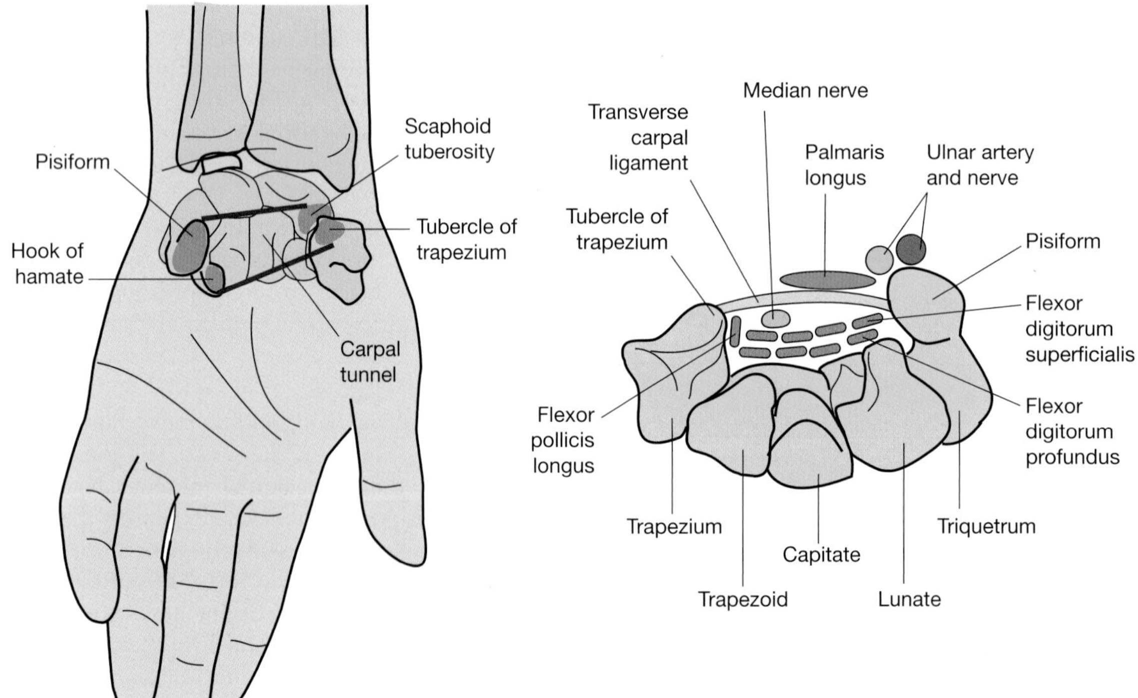

Figure 10.7 The carpal tunnel.

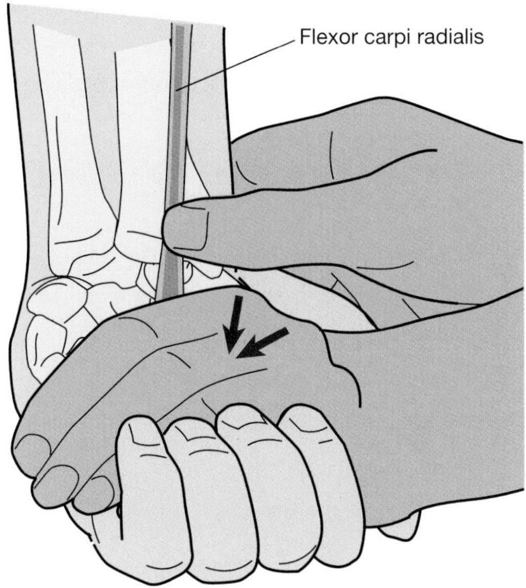

Figure 10.8 Palpation of the flexor carpi radialis.

is referred to as carpal tunnel syndrome. You can confirm the diagnosis with electrodiagnostic testing.

Palmar Aponeurosis. The palmar aponeurosis is a triangular-shaped fascia found in the palm of the hand covering the long finger flexors. It divides into four bands, which join with the fibrous finger sheaths. It is palpable as a resistance to your pressure in the center of the palm while the fingers are in extension. Marked finger flexion at the metacarpophalangeal joints with increased fibrosis of the palmar fascia is indicative of a Dupuytren-like contracture.

Lateral (Radial) Compartment

Flexor Carpi Radialis. If you continue to move laterally from the palmaris longus, the next tendon you will palpate is the flexor carpi radialis (Figure 10.8). The tendon is palpable at the level of the wrist as it passes into the hand and attaches at the base of the second metacarpal. In some individuals, the muscle may be absent. The tendon is made more distinct by providing resistance during wrist flexion and radial deviation.

Radial Artery. The radial pulse can be palpated just lateral to the tendon of the flexor carpi radialis. Press against the radius to facilitate palpating the pulse. Remember not to press too hard or the pulse will be obliterated.

Thenar Eminence. The thenar eminence is comprised of the three short muscles of the thumb: abductor pollicis brevis, flexor pollicis brevis, and opponens pollicis. It is located at the base of the thumb and is a thick, fleshy prominence that is freely movable on palpation. It is demarcated by the thenar crease.

Compare both hands for symmetry, especially paying attention to the size, shape, and feel of the thenar eminence. Note that the dominant side may be noticeably larger, particularly when the individual engages in racquet sports or is a manual laborer. Notice any atrophy. The muscles are innervated by the recurrent branch of the median nerve and may be affected when the individual has carpal tunnel syndrome. The thenar eminence may actually become hollow in advanced stages of the pathology.

Fingers. Observe the bony alignment of the phalanges. They should be symmetrical and straight from both the anterior–posterior and medial–lateral views. The patient may present with a swan neck deformity secondary to a contracture of the intrinsic muscles. This is often seen in patients with rheumatoid arthritis. A boutonniere deformity may be present when the patient ruptures or lacerates the central tendinous slip of the extensor digitorum communis tendon, which allows the lateral bands to migrate volarly. This can occur secondary to trauma. In rheumatoid arthritis, the balance between the flexors and extensors is disturbed, not allowing the central slip to pull properly and letting the lateral bands migrate volarly. Claw fingers can also be present secondary to loss of the intrinsic muscles and a subsequent overactivity of the extrinsic muscles.

Note the presence of any nodules. Heberden's nodes can be found on the dorsal aspect of the distal interphalangeal joint and are associated with osteoarthritis. Bouchard's nodes can be found on the dorsal aspect of the proximal interphalangeal joint and are associated with rheumatoid arthritis.

Examine the finger pads. They are highly innervated and vascularized. The pads are especially susceptible to infection because of their location and use. Note any area of edema, erythema, and warmth. Osier's nodes may be present secondary to subacute bacterial endocarditis.

Medial (Ulnar) Aspect

Bony Structures

Ulna Styloid Process

Place your fingers along the shaft of the ulna (see description on p. 209, Figure 9.16) and follow it distally until you come to the rounded prominence of the ulna styloid process. It is more defined than the radial styloid process. The ulna styloid process is located

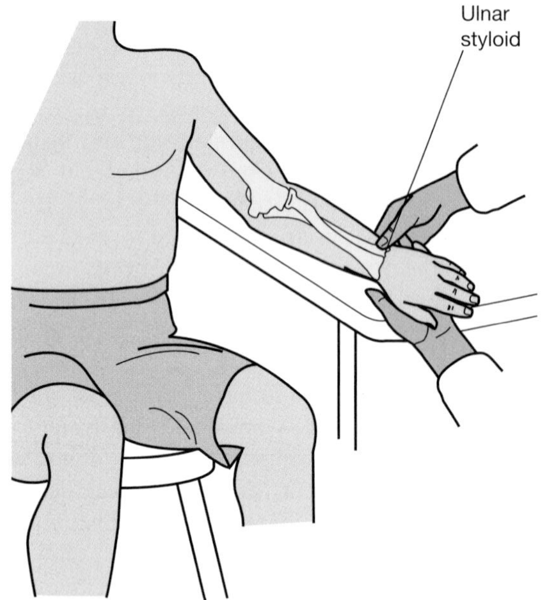

Figure 10.9 Palpation of the ulna styloid process.

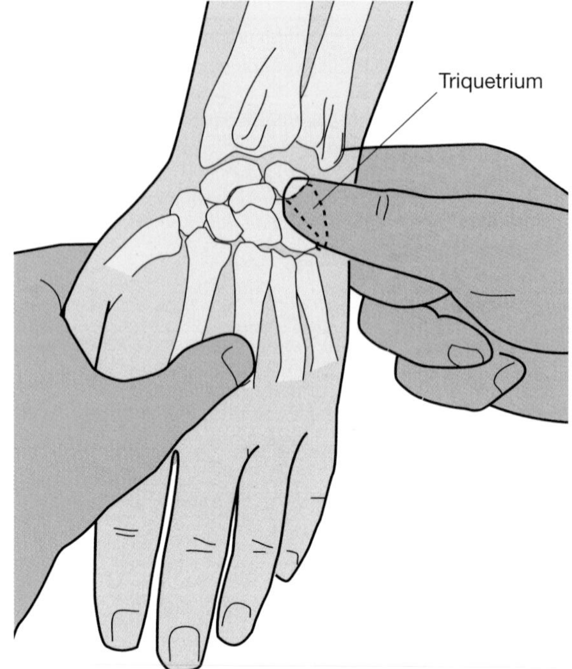

Figure 10.10 Palpation of the triquetrum.

more proximal than its radial counterpart and slightly more posterior (Figure 10.9). The ulna styloid process does not have a direct articulation with the carpal bones.

Triquetrum

Palpate the ulna styloid process and continue to move distally on the medial aspect of the wrist. You will first find the space for the articular meniscus and then feel the rounded surface of the triquetrum. Move the patient's hand into radial deviation and the triquetrum will move medially into your finger (Figure 10.10). The dorsal aspect can also be palpated and will be more prominent as the patient's hand is flexed. The palmar aspect is not palpable since it is covered by the pisiform.

Pisiform

The pisiform is located on the anterior surface of the triquetrum just distal and anterolateral to the ulna styloid process (Figure 10.11). The pisiform serves as the attachment for the flexor carpi ulnaris.

Hamate

The most palpable portion of the hamate is the hook or the hamulus. It is located proximal to the radial border of the fourth metacarpal. An easy way to locate the hook is by placing the interphalangeal joint of your thumb over the pisiform and direct your thumb diagonally toward the patient's web space. The hook will be located under your thumb pad, approximately 2.5 cm distal to the pisiform (Warwick and Williams, 1998) (Figure 10.12). Because the bony structure is deep, you must press into the soft tissue to locate it. Be careful because of the proximity of the ulnar nerve. The hook is often tender to touch. You can palpate the posterior aspect by simultaneously placing your index finger over the dorsal aspect of the hand. The hamate is located proximal to the base of the fourth and fifth metacarpals.

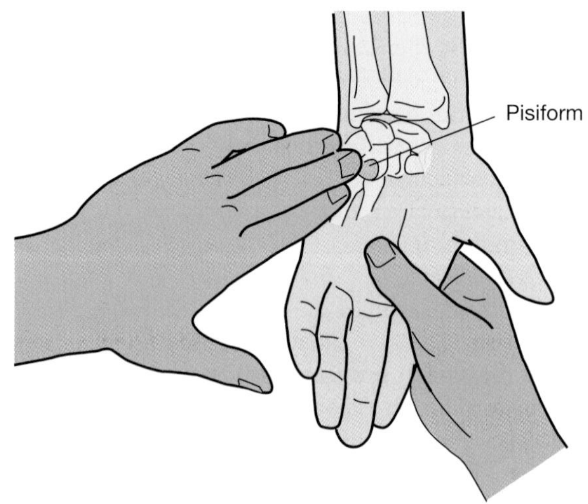

Figure 10.11 Palpation of the pisiform.

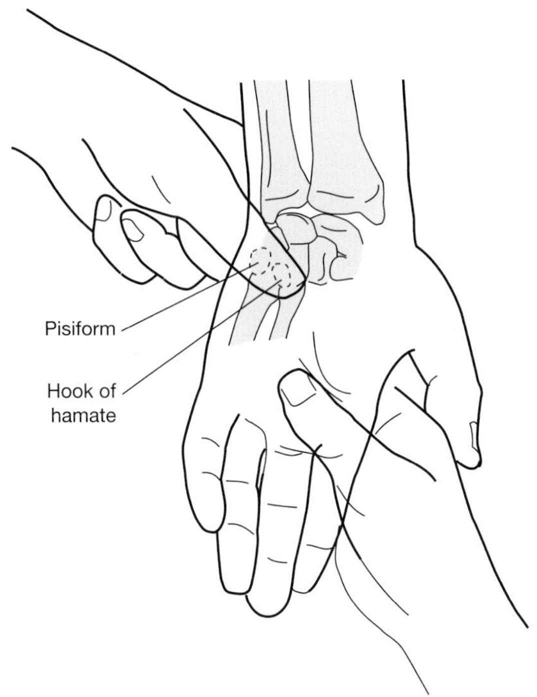

Figure 10.12 Palpation of the hamate.

The hook of the hamate is clinically significant because with the pisiform it forms the canal of Guyon. This is the second most common area of compression neuropathy of the ulnar nerve (see section on "Entrapment Neuropathies" on p. 280, Figure 10.96).

Soft-Tissue Structures

Triangular Fibrocartilaginous Complex

The triangular fibrocartilaginous complex is comprised of the triangular fibrocartilage, the ulnocarpal meniscus, a small recess containing synovium, and the palmar ulnocarpal and ulnolunate ligaments. The triangular cartilage attaches to the radius. The ligaments attach from the cartilage itself to the palmar aspect of the ulnar carpal bones. Therefore, the triangular fibrocartilaginous complex serves to suspend the wrist from the radius (Lichtman, 1988).

To facilitate description, the remainder of the soft-tissue structures is described in the section relating to the anterior surface of the hand.

Lateral (Radial) Aspect

Bony Structures

Radial Styloid Process

Place your fingers along the lateral aspect of the forearm and follow the shaft of the radius distally until you come to the radial styloid process, which is just proximal to the radiocarpal joint (Figure 10.13).

Scaphoid (Navicular)

Allow your fingers to move slightly distal from the radial styloid process and you will notice a small depression. Ask the patient to ulnar deviate the wrist and you will feel your finger being pushed out of the depression by a dome-shaped bone. This is the scaphoid (Figure 10.14). The scaphoid forms the floor of the anatomical snuffbox (see p. 245, Figure 10.17). Tenderness in the area should raise your suspicion. Fractures of the scaphoid can be difficult to diagnose and are commonly overlooked and misdiagnosed as sprains. Since a retrograde vascular supply exists in the scaphoid, nonunion or avascular necrosis (Preiser's disease) can subsequently result.

Trapezium and Trapezoid (Greater and Lesser Multangular)

Continue to move distally from the scaphoid. In the small space between the scaphoid and the base of the first metatarsal, you will find the trapezium and trapezoid (Figure 10.15). It is not possible to clinically differentiate between these two bones and they are commonly referred to as the *trapezii*. The articulation between the trapezii and the first metacarpal, or the first carpometacarpal joint (basal joint), is a saddle joint and allows for increased dexterity of the thumb. It is very commonly affected by degenerative arthritis.

First Metacarpal

Locate the trapezium and the joint line with the first metacarpal. Follow the first metacarpal distally until you reach the metacarpophalangeal joint (Figure 10.16). It is very superficial and easy to locate along its lateral and dorsal aspects. Notice that it is smaller and thicker than the other metacarpals. It has the most mobility of all five metacarpals, allowing for prehension of the thumb. A fracture of the proximal first metacarpal is known as *Bennett's fracture* and may result in an avulsion of the abductor pollicis longus.

Soft-Tissue Structures

Anatomical Snuffbox

Allow your fingers to move slightly distally from the radial styloid process and ask the patient to extend the thumb. You will see a small triangular depression, called the *anatomical snuffbox*. The depression is bordered by the extensor pollicis brevis and abductor

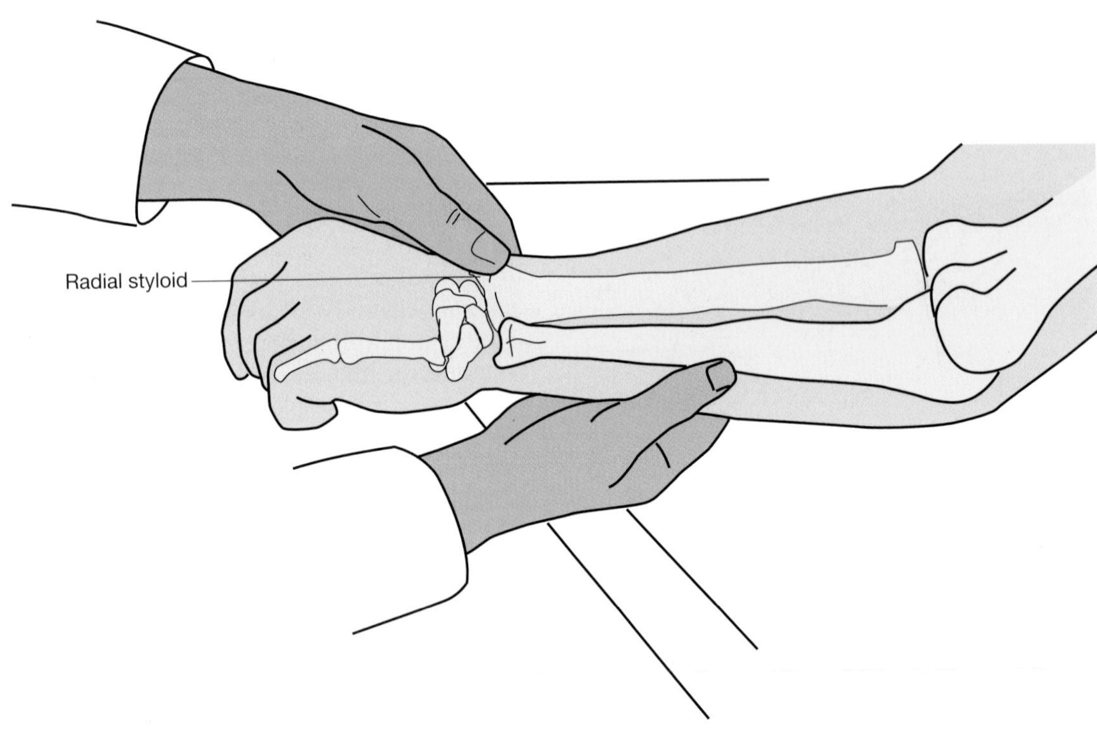

Figure 10.13 Palpation of the radial styloid process.

pollicis longus laterally and the extensor pollicis longus medially. The floor is made up of the scaphoid. The radial pulse can be palpated between the borders (Figure 10.17). If there is tenderness in the snuffbox, you should be suspicious of a fracture of the scaphoid.

Posterior (Dorsal) Aspect

Bony Structures

Dorsal Tubercle of the Radius (Lister's Tubercle). Find the radial styloid process and move medially approximately one-third of the way along the posterior aspect of the radius until you come to a narrow ridge. This is the dorsal tubercle of the radius (Lister's tubercle). It can also be located by finding the indentation between the index and middle fingers and following proximally until you reach the radius (Figure 10.18). It is an important structure since the

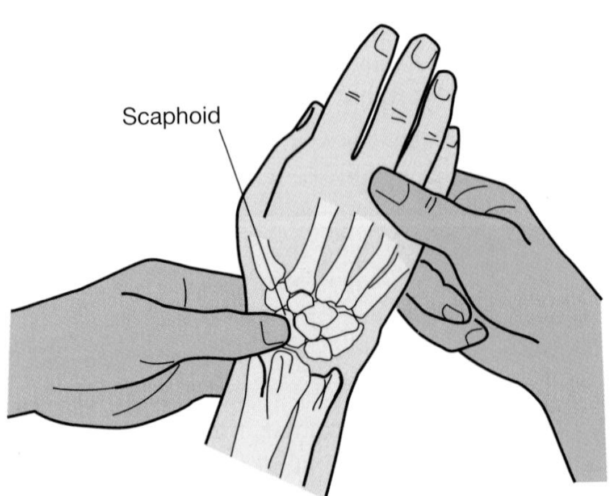

Figure 10.14 Palpation of the scaphoid.

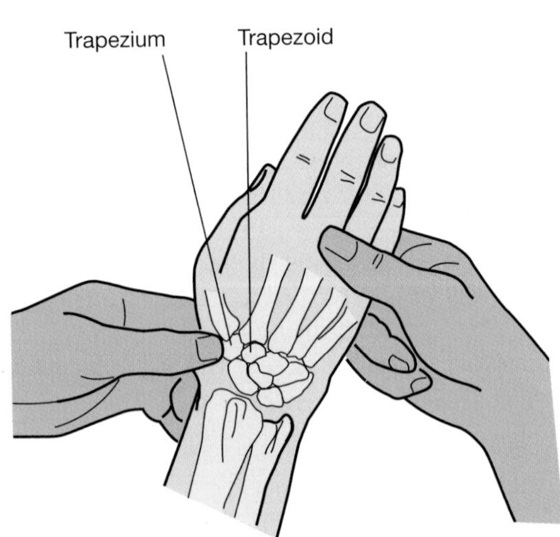

Figure 10.15 Palpation of the trapezium and trapezoid.

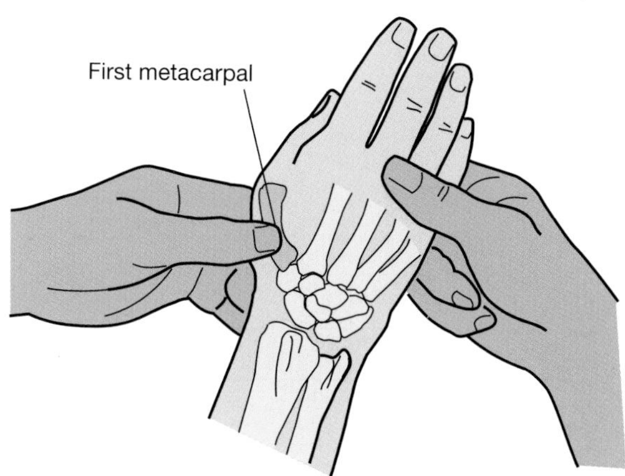

Figure 10.16 Palpation of the first metacarpal.

extensor pollicis longus hooks around it, creating a 45-degree angle as it travels to its attachment at the distal phalanx of the thumb.

Lunate

Keep the patient's wrist in a slightly extended position. Find the dorsal tubercle of the radius and continue slightly distally and medially. You will feel an indentation under your index finger. Flex the patient's wrist and you will feel your finger being pushed out of the indentation by the lunate (Figure 10.19). You can palpate the anterior surface of the lunate by simultaneously placing your thumb in the area between the thenar and hypothenar eminences. The lunate is the most common carpal to dislocate and when it does it can be confused with a ganglion. Tenderness and swelling in the area may be secondary to avascular necrosis or Kienböck's disease.

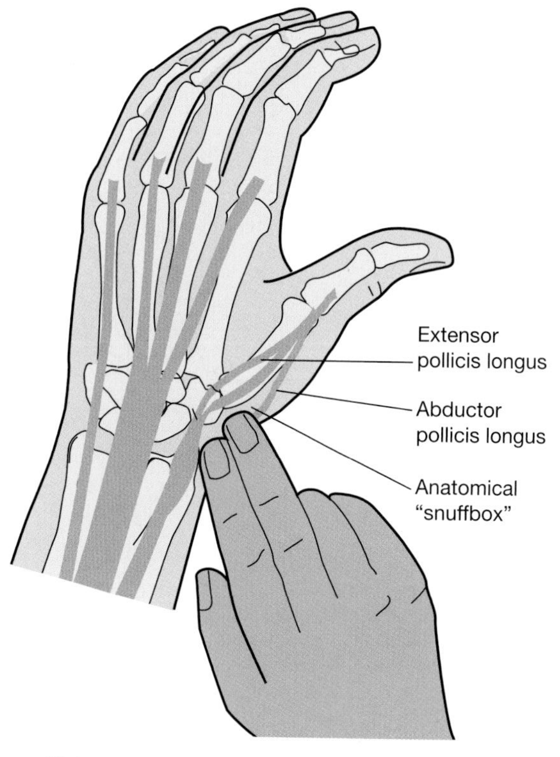

Figure 10.17 Palpation of the anatomical snuffbox.

Capitate

After finding the lunate, you can continue to move distally and you will find the capitate in the space between the lunate and the base of the third metacarpal (Figure 10.20). If the patient's hand is in the neutral or slightly extended position, you will feel a dip under your finger which is the dorsal concavity of the crescent-shaped capitate. As you flex the

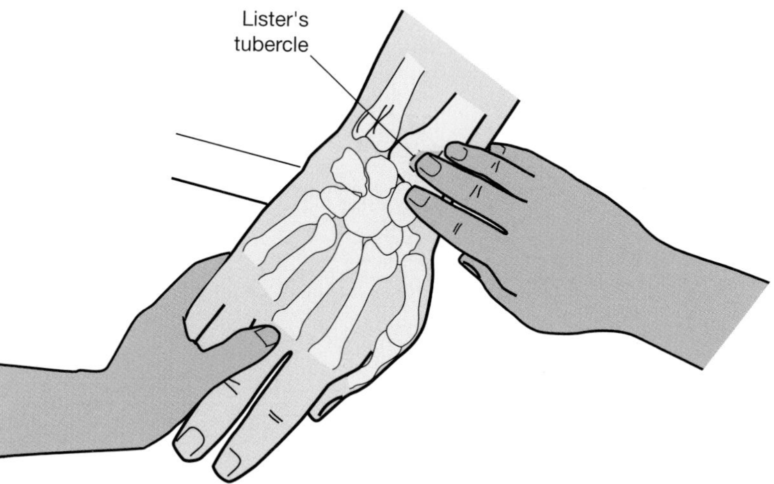

Figure 10.18 Palpation of the dorsal (Lister's) tubercle of the radius.

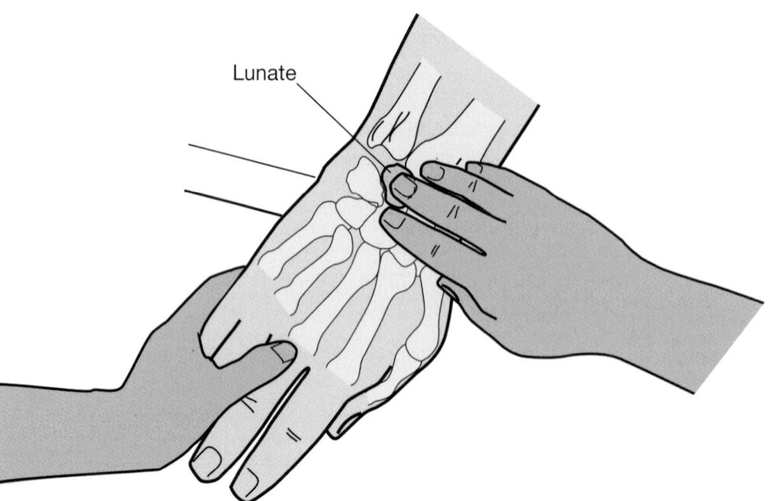

Figure 10.19 Palpation of the lunate.

patient's wrist, the capitate rolls, coming out from under the lunate, filling in the dip, and pushing your finger dorsally.

Metacarpals

The metacarpals are more easily palpated from the dorsal aspect of the hand. Pronate the individual's forearm, rest the palm on your thumb, and palpate the metacarpals using your index and third fingers. Locate the bases of the second through fifth metacarpals just distal to the distal row of carpals. You will notice a flaring of the bones. Trace them distally until you reach the metacarpophalangeal joints (Figure 10.21). You will notice that the fourth and fifth metacarpals are much more mobile than the second and third because of the less rigid attachment at the carpometacarpal joints. This allows for stability on the lateral aspect of the hand and increased mobility on the medial aspect to allow for power grasp.

Metacarpophalangeal Joints

Continue to follow the metacarpals distally until you reach the metacarpophalangeal joints. The "knuckles" are most clearly visualized on the dorsal surface with the patient's fingers flexed. In this position,

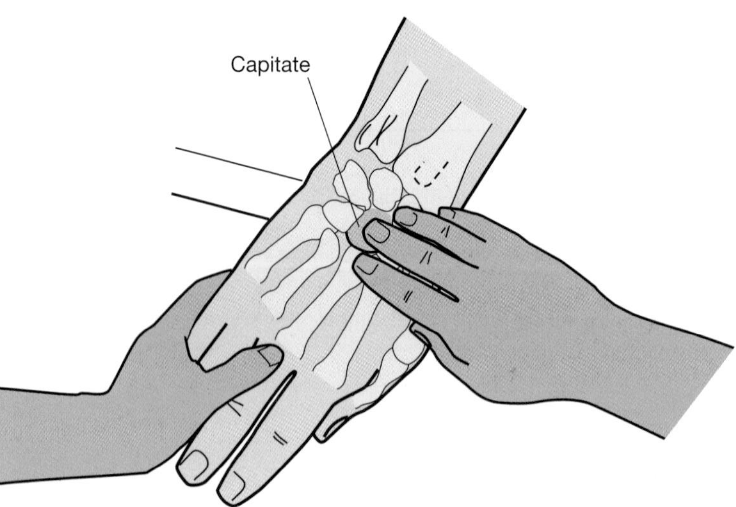

Figure 10.20 Palpation of the capitate.

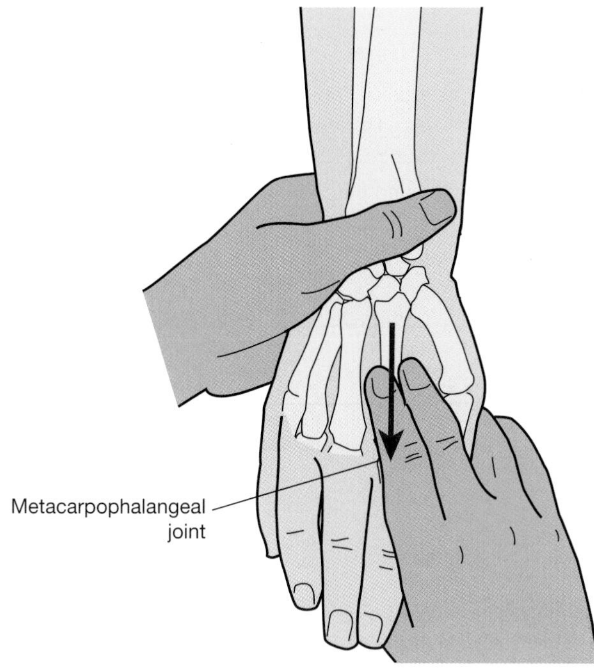

Figure 10.21 Palpation of the metacarpals.

you can more easily visualize and palpate the joint surfaces. The volar aspect of the metacarpophalangeal joints is deceiving since it appears to be more distal than you would expect. Remember that the joints are located deep to the distal palmar crease (Figure 10.22).

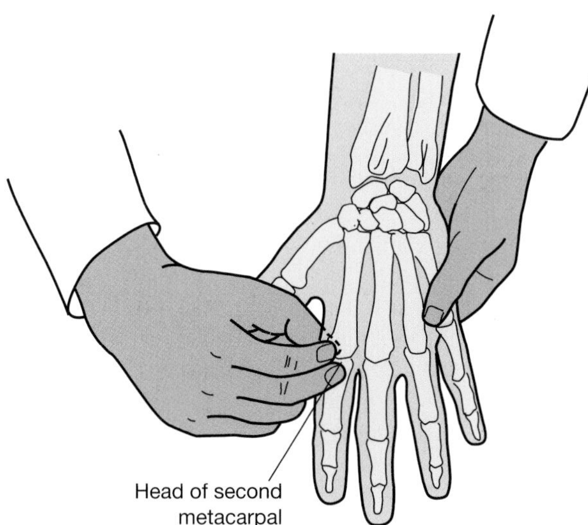

Figure 10.22 Palpation of the metacarpophalangeal joints.

Phalanges and Interphalangeal Joints

The three phalanges of fingers two through five and the two phalanges of the thumb are more easily visualized from the dorsal aspect of the hand. Find the metacarpophalangeal joint and follow the phalanges distally, stopping to palpate the proximal interphalangeal joints and then the distal interphalangeal joints. Note the continuity of the bones and the symmetry of the joints. The interphalangeal joints are common sites for deformities secondary to osteoarthritis and rheumatoid arthritis.

Nails

The fingernails should be smooth and with good coloration. Nail ridges can occur secondary to trauma, avitaminosis, or chronic alcoholism. A direct trauma to the nail can cause bleeding, resulting in a subungual hematoma. Brittle nails with longitudinal ridges can occur secondary to exposure to radiation. Spoon-shaped nails can occur due to Plummer–Vinson syndrome which is secondary to iron deficiency anemia. Psoriasis can cause a scaling deformity of the nails. Congenital absence of the thumbnail may be seen in patients with patella–nail syndrome. This is characterized by a small patella, subluxation of the radial head, and a bony projection from the ilium.

Soft-Tissue Structures

Observe the skin over the dorsum of the hand. Notice that it is much looser than the skin over the palm. This allows for greater mobility of the fingers into flexion. Additional skin is noted over the interphalangeal joints and forms transverse ridging. The extensor tendons are clearly visible on the dorsum of the hand since they are not covered by thick fascia, as on the anterior surface. The individual tendons can be traced as they continue to their distal attachments on the bases of the middle phalanges of fingers two through five. The tendons can be made more distinct by resisting finger extension.

Extensor Retinaculum

The extensor retinaculum is a strong fibrous band located on the dorsal aspect of the wrist. It attaches from the anterior border of the radius to the triquetrum and pisiform bones. There are six tunnels deep to the extensor retinaculum that allow for the passage of the extensor tendons into the hand (Figure 10.23).

To enable you to more easily organize the palpation of the deeper soft tissues, the dorsal surface of the hand is divided into six areas. The individual

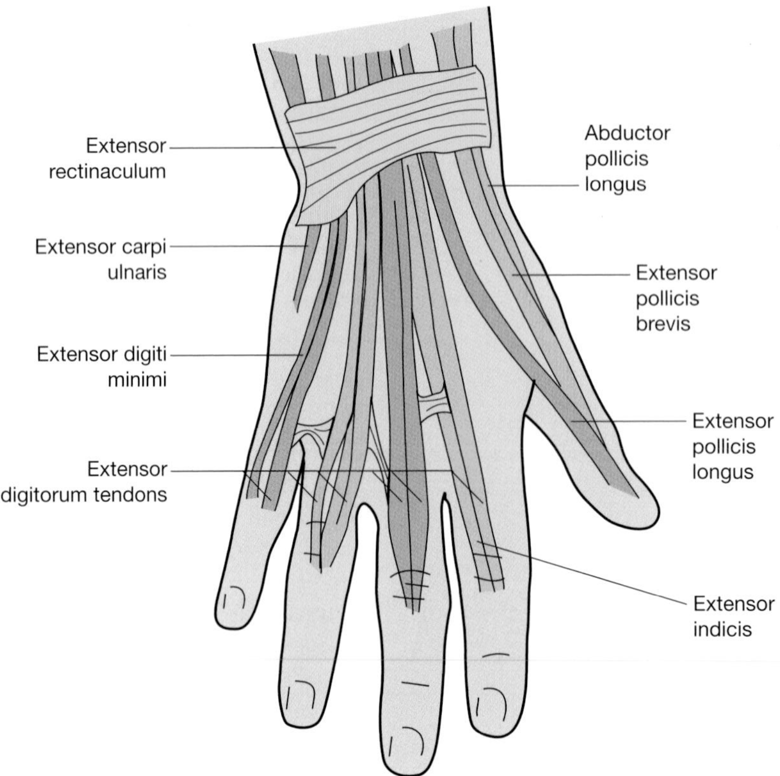

Figure 10.23 Palpation of the extensor retinaculum.

compartments are described, from the lateral to the medial aspect.

Compartment I

The most lateral compartment allows the abductor pollicis longus and extensor pollicis brevis to travel to the thumb (Figure 10.24). These muscles comprise the radial border of the anatomical snuffbox (see pp. 270–274 for full description). The tendons can be made more distinct by resisting thumb extension and abduction.

Tenderness in this area may be indicative of de Quervain's disease, which is a result of stenosing tenosynovitis of the tendon sheath. Differential diagnosis can be done by using Finkelstein's test, which is described in the section on special test of this chapter (see p. 285, Figure 10.99).

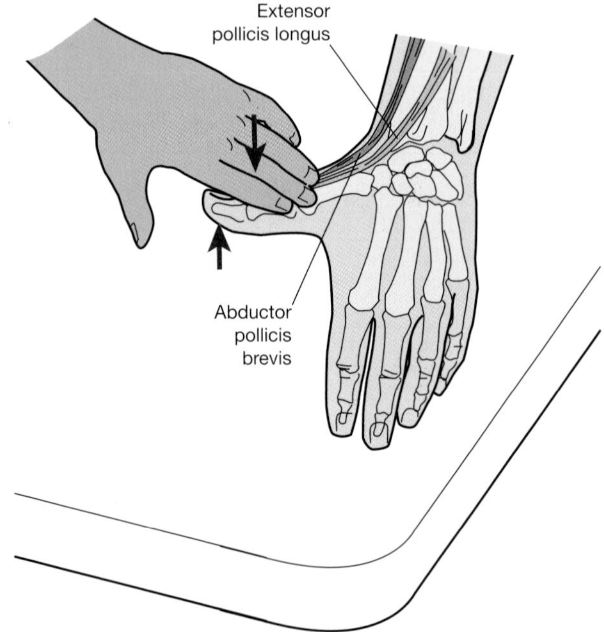

Figure 10.24 Palpation of compartment I.

Compartment II

Continuing into the next most medial compartment, which is located lateral to Lister's tubercle, you will find the extensor carpi radialis longus and the extensor carpi radialis brevis (Figure 10.25). The tendons

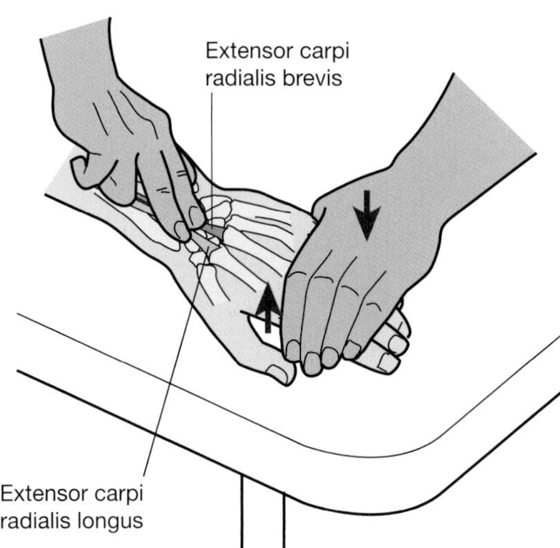

Figure 10.25 Palpation of compartment II.

can be made more distinct by resisting wrist extension and radial deviation.

Compartment III

On the medial aspect of Lister's tubercle, you will find the tendon of the extensor pollicis longus as it wraps around the tubercle (Figure 10.26). This tendon creates the medial border of the anatomical snuffbox (see Figures 10.76 and 10.77).

The tendon travels through a groove on the radius and passes through the extensor retinaculum around the dorsal tubercle of the radius. The tendon has a large degree of angulation, which increases with thumb extension. This tendon can be easily irritated by repetitive use of the thumb. Palpate this tendon for continuity to ensure that it has not been disrupted.

Compartment IV

Compartment IV allows the tendons of the extensor digitorum communis and the extensor indicis to travel to the hand (Figure 10.27). The individual tendons can be traced as they continue to their distal attachments on the bases of the middle and distal phalanges of fingers two through five. It is easiest to locate them in the area between the carpal bones and the metacarpophalangeal joints. The tendons can be made more distinct by resisting finger extension. A rupture or elongation of the terminal portion of the extensor tendon can cause a mallet finger.

Compartment V

As you continue medially, the tendon of the extensor digiti minimi is palpable in a small depression

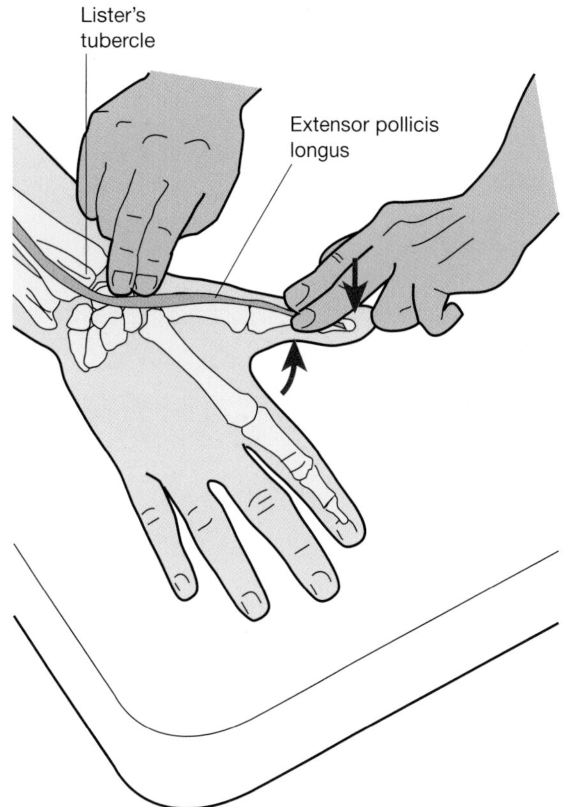

Figure 10.26 Palpation of compartment III.

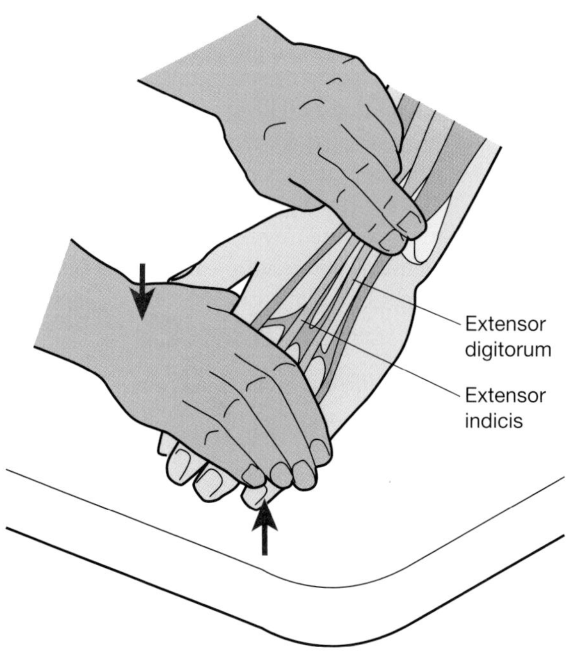

Figure 10.27 Palpation of compartment IV.

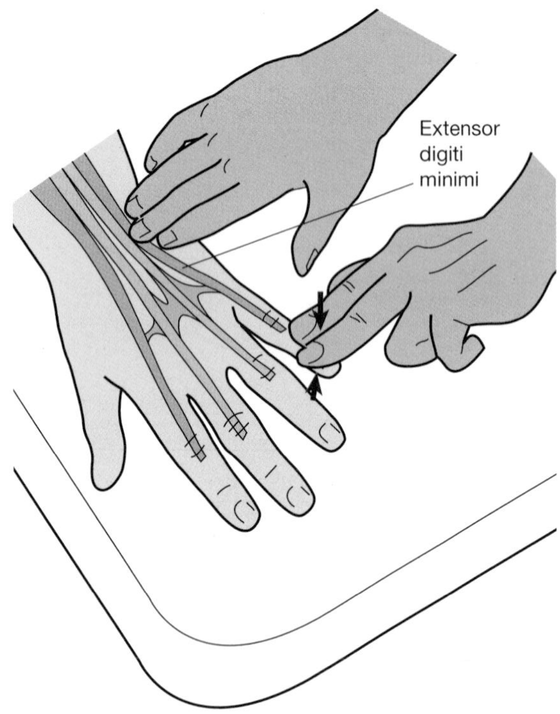

Figure 10.28 Palpation of compartment V.

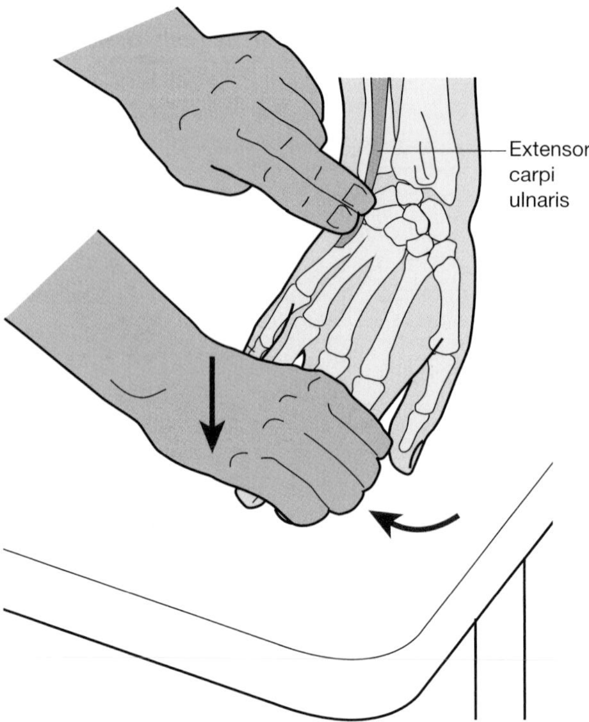

Figure 10.29 Palpation of compartment VI.

located slightly lateral to the ulna styloid process (Figure 10.28). The tendon can be made more distinct by resisting extension of the fifth finger.

Compartment VI

The most medial compartment contains the tendon of the extensor carpi ulnaris. The tendon can be palpated in the groove between the head and the styloid process of the ulna as it passes to its distal attachment at the base of the fifth metacarpal (Figure 10.29). It can be made more distinct by resisting wrist extension and ulnar deviation. The tendon can also be palpated by having the patient ulnar deviate the wrist, which increases the tension of the tendon.

Active Movement Testing

The major movements of the wrist joint are flexion, extension, and ulnar and radial deviation. Pronation and supination of the forearm also must be considered. Movements of the metacarpophalangeal, proximal interphalangeal, and distal interphalangeal joints include flexion and extension. Abduction and adduction also occur at the metacarpophalangeal joints. The thumb movements include flexion, extension, abduction, adduction, and opposition. These should be quick, functional tests designed to clear the joint. If the motion is pain free at the end of the range, you can add an additional overpressure to "clear" the joint. If the patient experiences pain during any of these movements, you should continue to explore whether the etiology of the pain is secondary to contractile or noncontractile structures by using passive and resistive testing.

Quick testing of the movements of the wrist and hand should be performed simultaneously by both upper extremities. The patient should be sitting with the forearms resting on a treatment table. You should face the patient to observe symmetry of movement.

To examine the wrist–hand complex from proximal to distal, start by asking the patient to supinate and pronate the forearm. A full description of this movement is described in Chapter 9 (see pp. 210–211). Have the patient move the arm so that the wrist is positioned at the end of the table with the forearm pronated. Ask the patient to raise the dorsum of the hand toward the ceiling as far as he or she can, to complete wrist extension. Then ask the patient to allow the hand to bend toward the floor as far as possible, to complete wrist flexion. Instruct the patient to move the arm so that the entire hand is supported on the table in the pronated position. Ask the patient to move the hand to the side, allowing the thumb to approximate the radius to complete the motion of radial deviation. Instruct the patient to return to the neutral position, and then move the hand to the opposite side, with the fifth finger approximating the ulna, to complete ulnar deviation. Note that the range of motion should normally be greater for ulnar deviation since there is no direct contact between the carpals and the ulna because of the meniscus.

To quickly assess the movement of the fingers, instruct the patient to make a tight fist. Observe the quality of the movement and whether all of the fingers are working symmetrically. Full range of motion of finger flexion is accomplished if the patient's fingertips can contact the proximal palmar crease. Then instruct the patient to release the grasp and straighten out all the fingers, to accomplish finger extension. You should observe that the fingers are either in a straight line (full extension) or slightly hyperextended. Now ask the patient to spread the fingers apart as far as he or she can, starting with the fingers in the extended position and the forearm pronated. Have the patient return the fingers together and they should all be in contact with each other. This accomplishes finger abduction and adduction.

The last movements to be considered are those of the thumb. Have the patient supinate the forearm and then move the thumb diagonally across the palm as far as he or she can. Full thumb flexion should allow the patient to contact the distal palmar crease at the distal aspect of the hypothenar eminence. Then ask the patient to release flexion and move the thumb laterally away from the palm, increasing the dimension of the web space. This is full thumb extension. Next ask the patient to lift the thumb away from the palm toward the ceiling. This motion is thumb abduction. Ask the patient to release the thumb and return to the palm in contact with the second metacarpal. This is thumb adduction. The last thumb movement to be assessed is opposition. Instruct the patient to contact the fingertips starting with the thumb meeting the fifth finger.

Passive Movement Testing

Passive movement testing can be divided into two areas: physiological movements (cardinal plane), which are the same as the active movements, and mobility testing of the accessory (joint play, component) movements. You can determine whether the noncontractile (inert) elements are causative of the patient's problem by using these tests. These structures (ligaments, joint capsule, fascia, bursa, dura mater, and nerve root) (Cyriax, 1982) are stretched or stressed when the joint is taken to the end of the available range. At the end of each passive physiological movement, you should sense the end feel and determine whether it is normal or pathological. Assess the limitation of movement and see if it fits into a capsular pattern. The capsular pattern of the wrist is equal restriction in all directions (Cyriax, 1982; Kaltenborn, 2011). The capsular pattern of the forearm is equal restriction of pronation and supination, which almost always occurs with significant limitation in the elbow joint (Kaltenborn, 2011). The capsular patterns for the fingers are as follows: the thumb carpometacarpal joint is limited in abduction followed by extension; finger joints have more limitation of flexion than extension (Cyriax, 1982).

Physiological Movements

You will be assessing the amount of motion available in all directions. Each motion is measured from the zero starting position. For the wrist, the radius and the third metacarpal form a straight line with zero degree of flexion and extension. For the fingers, the only resting position described in the literature is for the first carpometacarpal joint. The position is midway between maximal abduction–adduction and flexion–extension (Kaltenborn, 2011).

Supination and Pronation

Supination and pronation are described in Chapter 9 (p. 213).

Wrist Flexion

The best position for measuring wrist flexion is with the patient sitting, with the arm supported on a treatment table. The forearm should be placed such that the radiocarpal joint is located slightly beyond the edge of the supporting surface to allow for freedom of movement at the wrist joint. The forearm should be pronated, the wrist should be in the zero starting position, and the fingers should be relaxed. Hold the patient's forearm to stabilize it. Place your hand under the dorsum of the patient's hand and move the wrist into flexion. The motion may be restricted by tightness in the wrist and finger extensor muscles, the

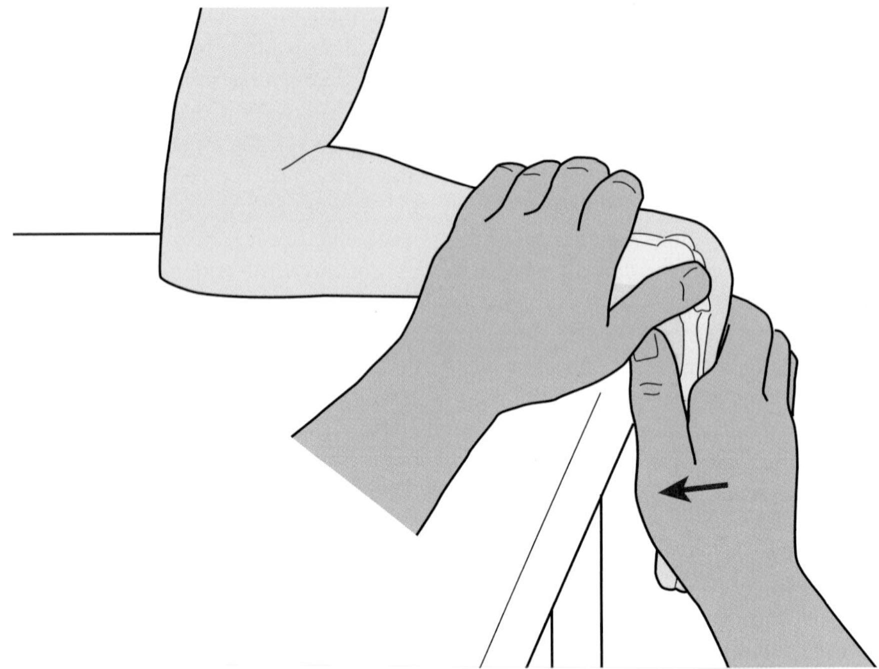

Figure 10.30 Passive movement testing of wrist flexion.

posterior capsule, or the dorsal radiocarpal ligament, producing an abrupt and firm (ligamentous) end feel (Magee, 2008; Kaltenborn, 2011). Normal range of motion is 0–80 degrees (American Academy of Orthopedic Surgeons, 1965) (Figure 10.30).

Wrist Extension

The best position for measuring wrist extension is with the patient sitting, with the arm supported on a treatment table. The forearm should be placed such that the radiocarpal joint is located slightly beyond the edge of the supporting surface to allow for freedom of movement at the wrist joint. The forearm should be pronated, the wrist should be in the zero starting position, and the fingers should be relaxed. Hold the patient's forearm to stabilize it. Place your hand under the palm of the patient's hand and move the wrist into extension. The motion may be restricted by tightness in the wrist and finger flexor muscles, the anterior capsule, or the palmar radiocarpal ligament, producing an abrupt and firm (ligamentous) end feel (Magee, 2008; Kaltenborn, 2011). A hard end feel may be present secondary to bony contact between the radius and the proximal carpals. Normal range of motion is 0–70 degrees (American Academy of Orthopedic Surgeons, 1965) (Figure 10.31).

Radial Deviation

The best position for measuring wrist radial deviation is with the patient sitting, with the arm supported on a treatment table. The forearm should be placed such that the radiocarpal joint is located slightly beyond the edge of the supporting surface to allow for freedom of movement at the wrist joint. The forearm should be pronated, the wrist should be in the zero starting position, and the fingers should be relaxed. Hold the patient's forearm to stabilize it and to prevent the patient from substituting with supination and pronation. Place your hand under the palm of the patient's hand and move the wrist into radial deviation. A hard end feel may be present due to bony contact between the radius and the scaphoid. The motion can be restricted by tension in the ulnar collateral ligament or the ulnar side of the capsule, producing an abrupt and firm (ligamentous) end feel (Magee, 2008; Kaltenborn, 2011). Normal range of motion is 0–20 degrees (American Academy of Orthopedic Surgeons, 1965) (Figure 10.32).

Ulnar Deviation

The best position for measuring wrist ulnar deviation is with the patient sitting, with the arm supported on

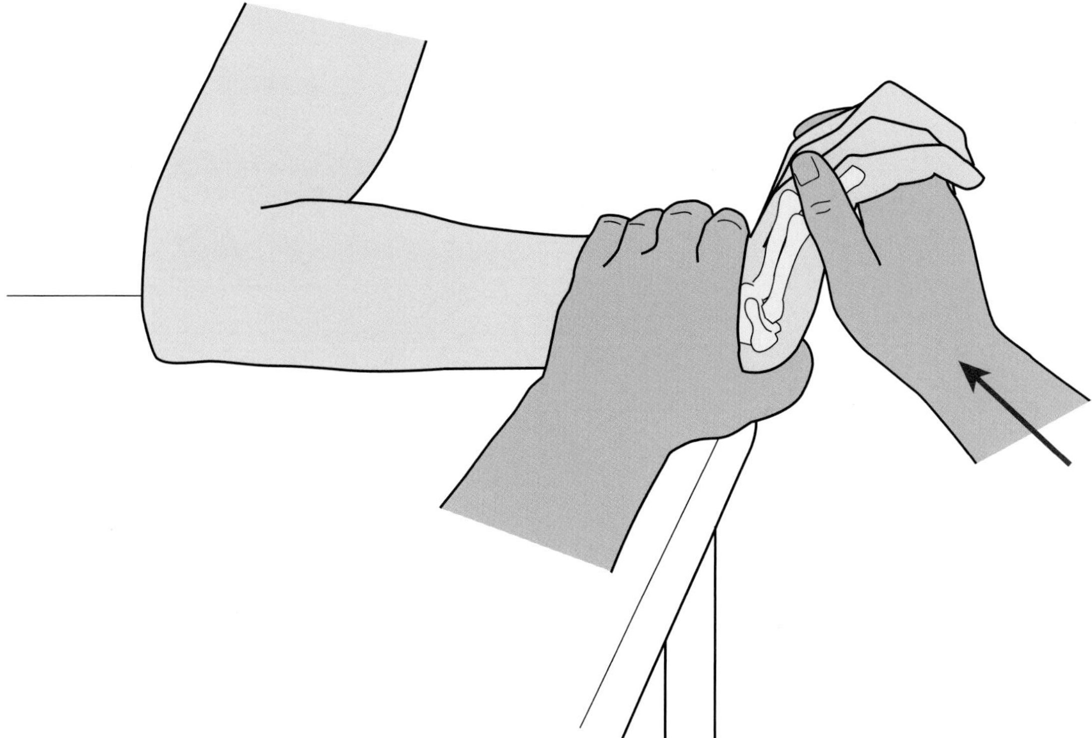

Figure 10.31 Passive movement testing of wrist extension.

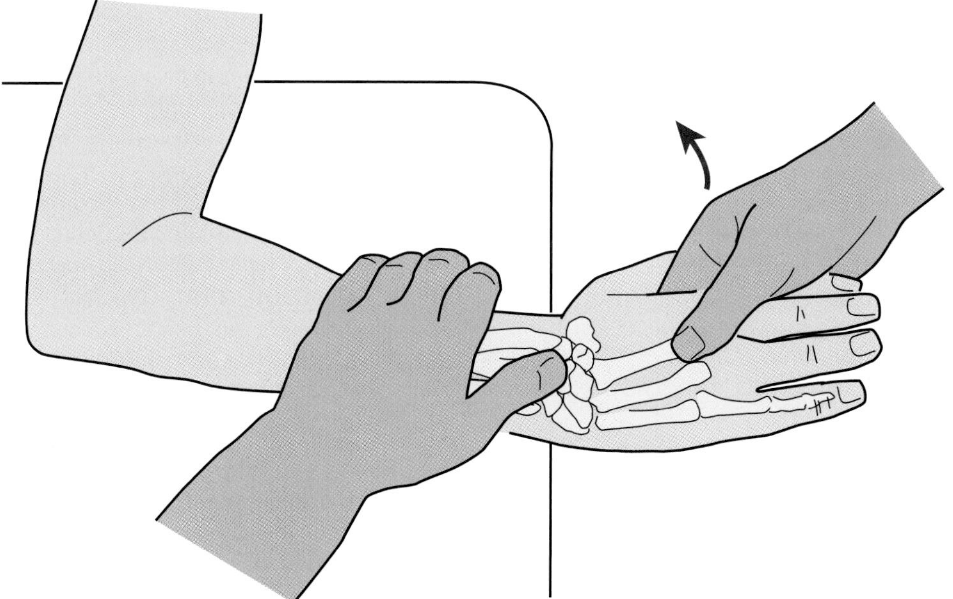

Figure 10.32 Passive movement testing of radial deviation.

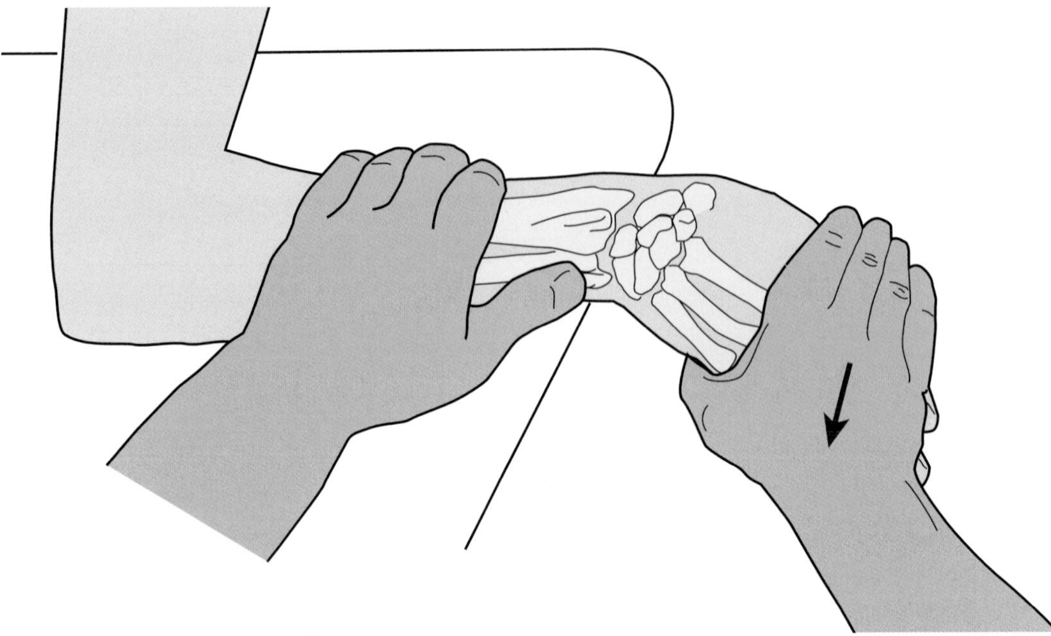

Figure 10.33 Passive movement testing of ulnar deviation.

a treatment table. The forearm should be placed such that the radiocarpal joint is located slightly beyond the edge of the supporting surface to allow for freedom of movement at the wrist joint. The forearm should be pronated, the wrist should be in the zero starting position, and the fingers should be relaxed. Hold the patient's forearm to stabilize it and to prevent the patient from substituting with supination and pronation. Place your hand under the palm of the patient's hand and move the wrist into ulnar deviation. The motion can be restricted by tension in the radial collateral ligament or the radial side of the capsule, producing an abrupt and firm (ligamentous) end feel (Magee, 2008; Kaltenborn, 2011). Normal range of motion is 0–30 degrees (American Academy of Orthopedic Surgeons, 1965) (Figure 10.33).

Fingers

All tests for passive movements of the fingers should be performed with the patient in the sitting position, with the forearm and hand supported on an adjacent treatment table. The examiner should be sitting facing the patient's hand.

Metacarpophalangeal Joint Flexion

The forearm should be positioned midway between pronation and supination with the wrist in the neutral position. The metacarpophalangeal joint should be in the mid position between abduction and adduction. The proximal and distal interphalangeal joints should be comfortably flexed. Avoid the end range of flexion as this will decrease the available range because of tension in the extensor tendons. Place your hand on the metacarpal corresponding to the metacarpophalangeal joint being evaluated. Use your other index finger and thumb to hold the proximal phalanx and move the metacarpophalangeal joint into flexion. The motion can be restricted by tension in the collateral ligaments or the dorsal aspect of the capsule, producing an abrupt and firm (ligamentous) end feel. A hard end feel is possible if contact occurs between the proximal phalanx and the metacarpal (Magee, 2008; Kaltenborn, 2011). Normal range of motion is 0–90 degrees (American Academy of Orthopedic Surgeons, 1965) (Figure 10.34).

Metacarpophalangeal Joint Extension

The forearm should be positioned midway between pronation and supination with the wrist in the neutral position. The metacarpophalangeal joint should be in the mid position between abduction and adduction. The proximal and distal interphalangeal joints should be comfortably flexed. Place your hand on the metacarpal corresponding to the metacarpophalangeal joint being evaluated. Use your other index finger and thumb to hold the proximal phalanx and move the metacarpophalangeal joint into extension.

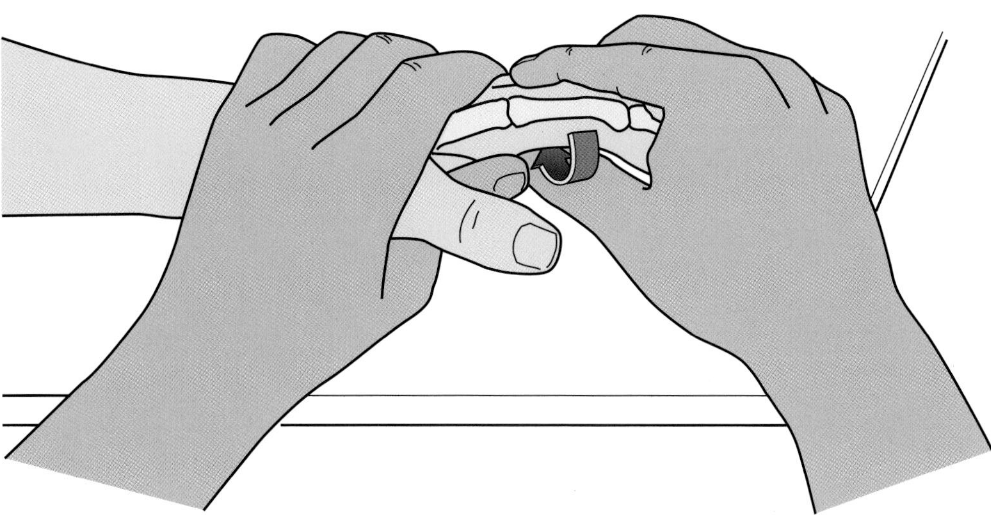

Figure 10.34 Passive movement testing of flexion of the metacarpophalangeal joint.

The motion can be restricted by tension in the volar aspect of the capsule, producing an abrupt and firm (ligamentous) end feel (Magee, 2008; Kaltenborn, 2011). Normal range of motion is 0–45 degrees (American Academy of Orthopedic Surgeons, 1965) (Figure 10.35).

Metacarpophalangeal Abduction and Adduction

The forearm should be fully pronated with the wrist in the neutral position. The metacarpophalangeal joint should be at zero degree of flexion–extension. Use your hand to stabilize the metacarpal to prevent substitution by radial or ulnar deviation. Grasp the finger being examined just proximal to the proximal interphalangeal joint and move it away from the midline for abduction, returning to the midline for adduction. The motion can be restricted by tension in the collateral ligaments of the metacarpophalangeal joints, skin, fascia in the finger web spaces, and the interossei muscles, producing an abrupt and firm (ligamentous) end feel (Magee, 2008; Kaltenborn, 2011). The collateral ligaments of the metacarpophalangeal joints are taut in flexion and relaxed in extension. You will note that the presence of abduction or adduction

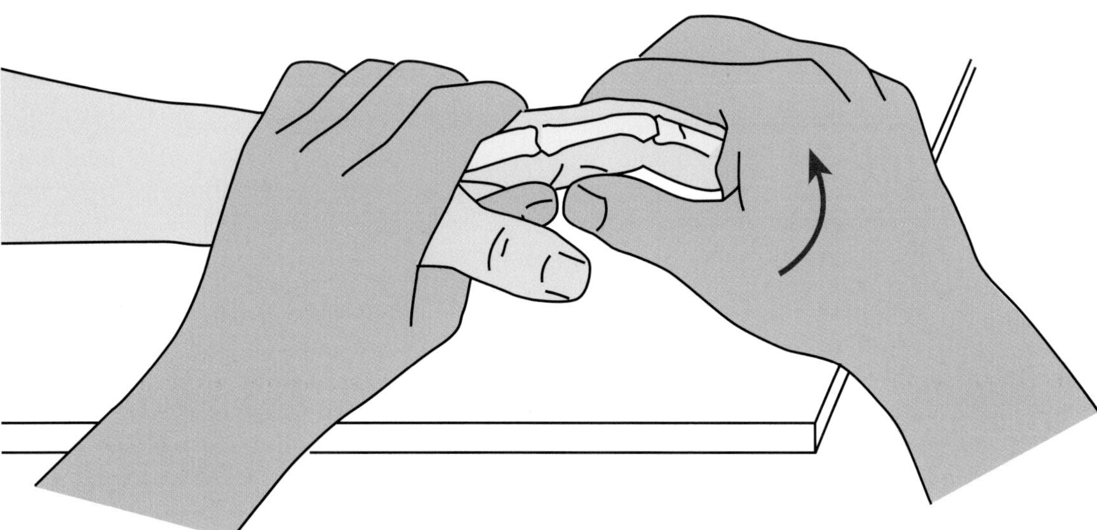

Figure 10.35 Passive movement testing of extension of the metacarpophalangeal joint.

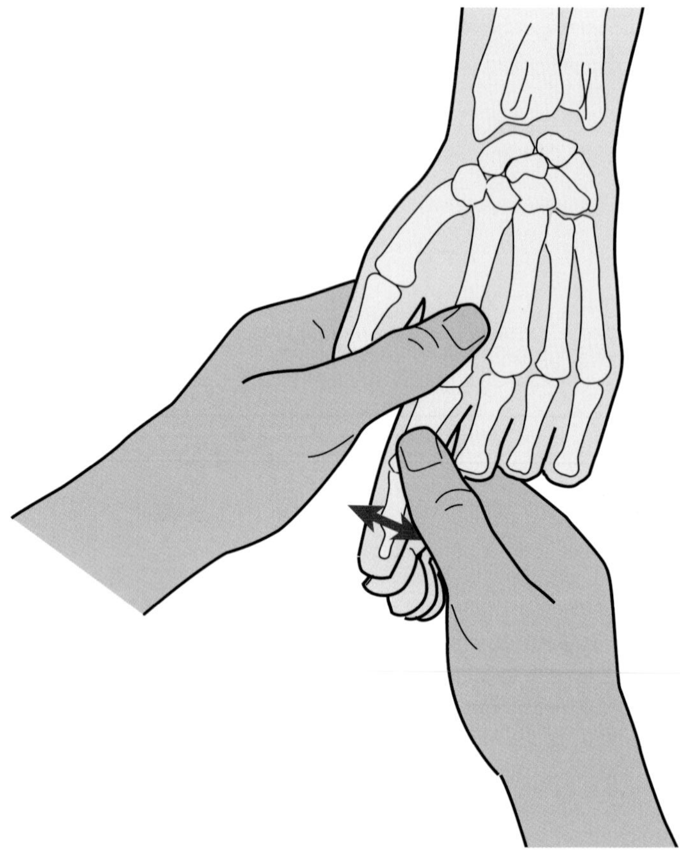

Figure 10.36 Passive movement testing of abduction and adduction of the metacarpophalangeal joint.

of the metacarpophalangeal joint in a flexed position is due to collateral ligament discontinuity or rupture. Normal range of motion is 0–20 degrees (Hoppenfeld, 1976) (Figure 10.36).

Proximal and Distal Interphalangeal Joint Flexion
The forearm should be positioned midway between pronation and supination with the wrist in the neutral position. The metacarpophalangeal joint should be at zero degrees of flexion–extension and abduction–adduction. Place your thumb and index fingers on the proximal phalanx of the finger being examined to stabilize it. Use your other index finger and thumb to hold the middle phalanx and move the proximal interphalangeal joint into flexion. To assess the distal interphalangeal joint, with the hand in the same position, stabilize the middle phalanx and move the distal phalanx into flexion. The motion of the proximal interphalangeal joint can be restricted by contact between the middle and proximal phalanges, producing a hard end feel. A soft end feel is possible secondary to compression of soft tissue on the volar aspect. The motion of the distal interphalangeal joint can be restricted by tension in the dorsal aspect of the capsule or the collateral ligaments, producing an abrupt and firm (ligamentous) end feel (Magee, 2008; Kaltenborn, 2011). Normal range of motion is 0–110 degrees for the proximal interphalangeal joint and 0–65 degrees for the distal interphalangeal joint (Figure 10.37).

Proximal and Distal Interphalangeal Joint Extension
The position and stabilization used for proximal and distal interphalangeal joint extension are the same as those listed for flexion. Grasp the middle phalanx (proximal interphalangeal joint) or the distal phalanx (distal interphalangeal joint) and return the joint to extension. The motion of the proximal and distal interphalangeal joints can be restricted by tension in the volar aspect of the capsule, producing an abrupt and firm (ligamentous) end feel (Magee, 2008; Kaltenborn, 2011). Normal range of motion is zero degree for the proximal interphalangeal joint and 0–20 degrees for the distal interphalangeal joint (Hoppenfeld, 1976) (Figure 10.38).

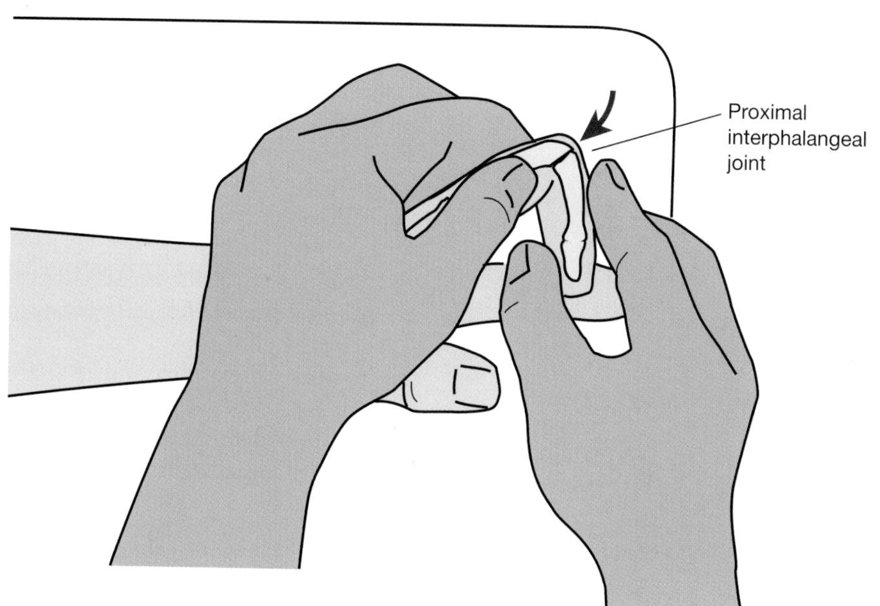

Figure 10.37 Passive movement testing of flexion of the proximal and distal interphalangeal joints.

First Carpometacarpal Abduction and Adduction

The forearm should be positioned midway between pronation and supination with the wrist in the neutral position. The metacarpophalangeal joint should be at zero degrees of flexion–extension and abduction–adduction. The carpometacarpal, metacarpophalangeal, and interphalangeal joints of the thumb should all be at zero degrees. Place your hand around the carpal bones and the second metacarpal to stabilize the hand. Using your other thumb and index finger, grasp the first metacarpal and move the thumb and metacarpal away from the palm, creating abduction. Check adduction by returning the thumb to the palm. Carpometacarpal abduction is restricted

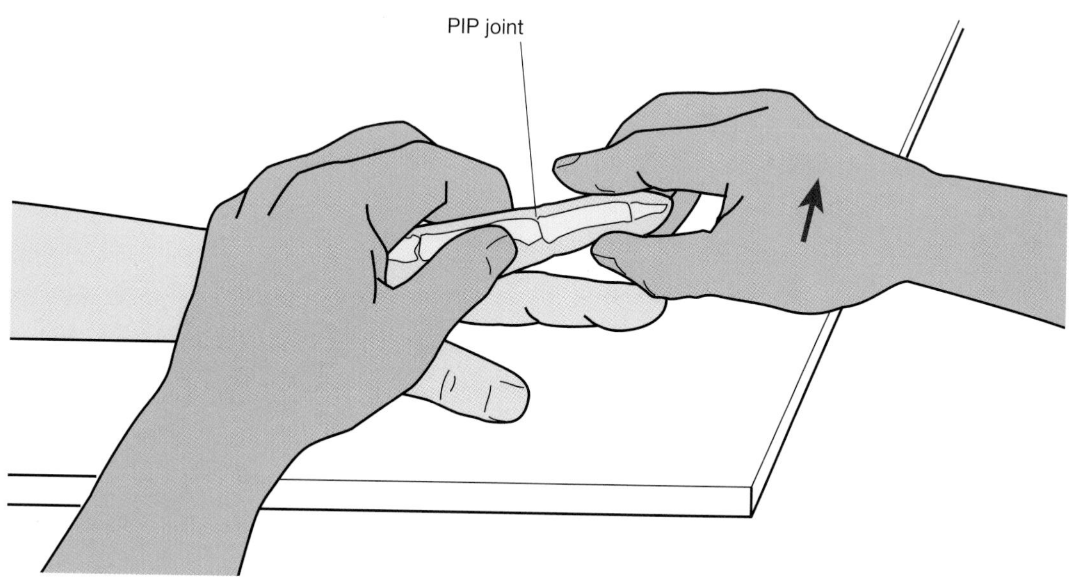

Figure 10.38 Passive movement testing of extension of the proximal and distal interphalangeal joints.

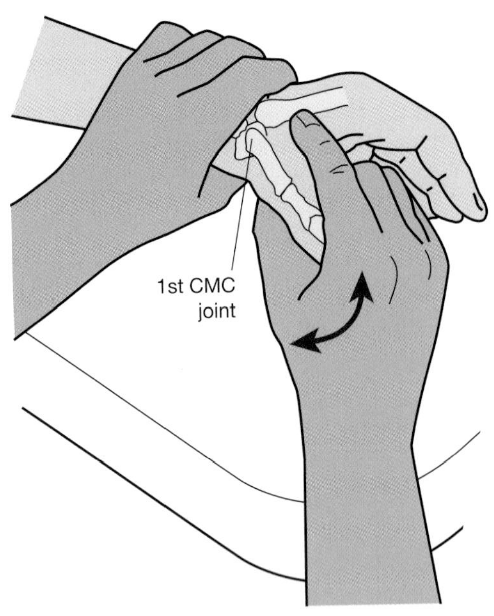

Figure 10.39 Passive movement testing of abduction and adduction of the first carpometacarpal (CMC) joint.

by fascial tension in the web space and tension in the intrinsic muscles, producing an abrupt and firm (ligamentous) end feel (Magee, 2008; Kaltenborn, 2011). Normal range of motion is 0–70 degrees for abduction and zero degree for adduction (American Academy of Orthopedic Surgeons, 1965) (Figure 10.39).

Opposition

The forearm should be positioned in supination with the wrist at zero degrees of flexion–extension and abduction–adduction. The interphalangeal joints of the thumb and fifth finger should be at zero degrees. Using your thumb and index and middle fingers, grasp the fifth metacarpal. Use the same grasp with your other hand on the first metacarpal. Approximate the first and fifth metacarpals (Figure 10.40). Soft-tissue contact of the thenar and hypothenar eminences can produce a soft end feel. Tension in the posterior aspect of the joint capsules or in the extensor muscles can produce an abrupt and firm (ligamentous) end feel (Magee, 2008; Kaltenborn, 2011). Loss of range of motion is determined by measuring the distance between the finger pads of the first and fifth fingers.

Thumb Metacarpophalangeal Flexion

The positions of the patient and examiner for testing thumb metacarpophalangeal flexion are the same as those described in the section on metacarpophalangeal flexion of fingers two through five. Use your thumb and index finger to grasp the first metacarpal and carpometacarpal joint to stabilize them. The movement is accomplished by grasping the proximal phalanx of the thumb and moving it across the palm toward the hypothenar eminence. The motion can be restricted by tension in the collateral ligaments, the dorsal aspect of the capsule, or the extensor pollicis brevis tendon, producing an abrupt and firm

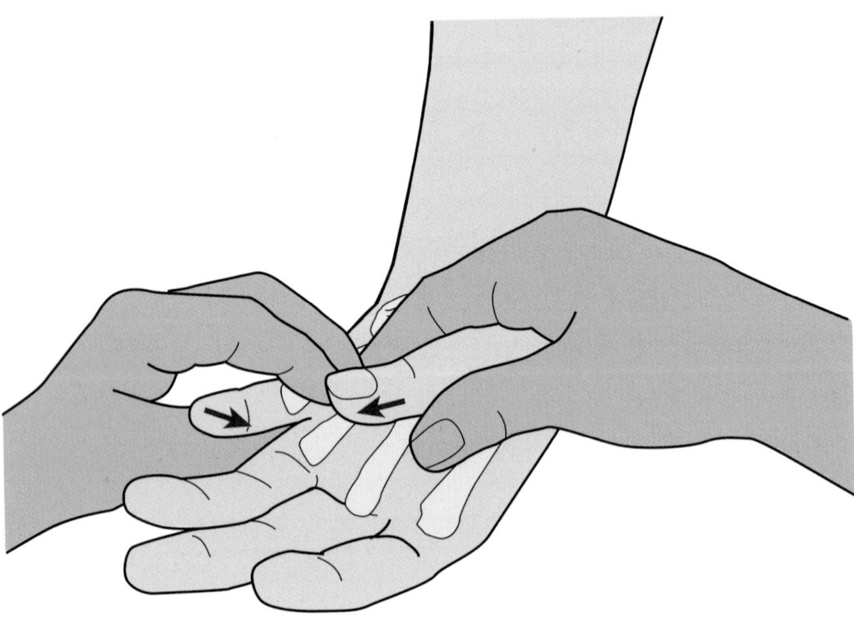

Figure 10.40 Passive movement testing of opposition.

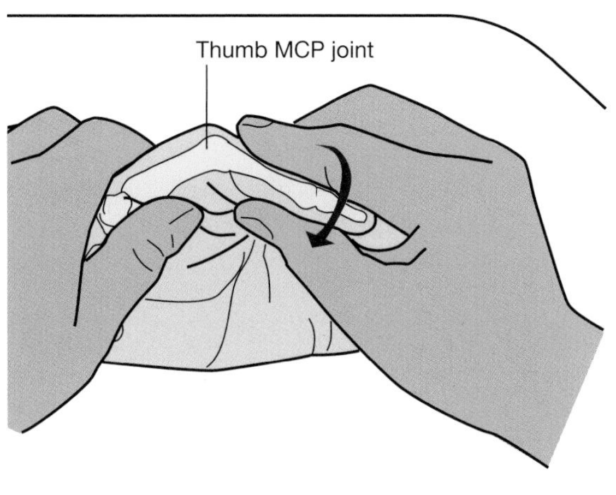

Figure 10.41 Passive movement testing of flexion of the thumb metacarpophalangeal (MCP) joint.

(ligamentous) end feel. A hard end feel is possible if contact occurs between the proximal phalanx and the first metacarpal (Magee, 2008; Kaltenborn, 2011). Normal range of motion is 0–50 degrees (American Academy of Orthopedic Surgeons, 1965) (Figure 10.41).

Thumb Metacarpophalangeal Extension

The positions of the patient and the examiner for thumb metacarpophalangeal extension are the same as those described in the section on metacarpophalangeal extension of fingers two through five. Use your thumb and index finger to grasp the first metacarpal and carpometacarpal joint to stabilize them. The movement is accomplished by the examiner grasping the proximal phalanx of the thumb and moving it laterally away from the palm and opening the web space. The motion can be restricted by tension in the volar aspect of the capsule or the flexor pollicis brevis tendon, producing an abrupt and firm (ligamentous) end feel (Magee, 2008; Kaltenborn, 2011). Normal range of motion is zero degree (American Academy of Orthopedic Surgeons, 1965) (Figure 10.42).

Thumb Interphalangeal Joint Flexion and Extension

The positions of the patient and the examiner and stabilization for thumb interphalangeal flexion and extension are the same as those described in the section on interphalangeal flexion and extension of

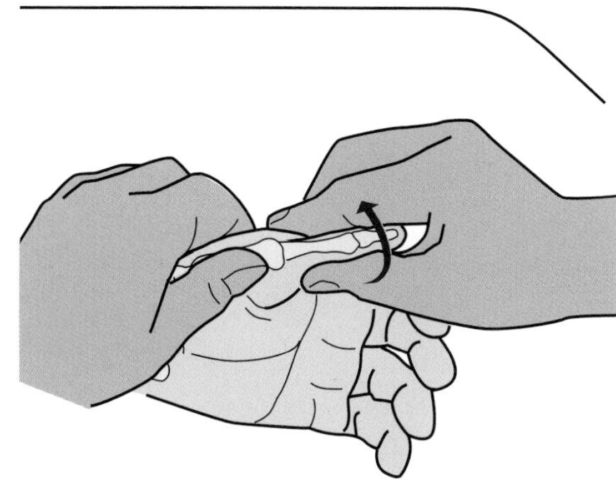

Figure 10.42 Passive movement testing of extension of the thumb metacarpophalangeal joint.

fingers two through five. The end feels and limiting factors are also the same. The normal range of motion for interphalangeal flexion is 0–80 degrees and for interphalangeal extension it is 0–20 degrees (American Academy of Orthopedic Surgeons, 1965) (Figure 10.43).

Mobility Testing of Accessory Movements

Mobility testing of accessory movements will give you information regarding the degree of laxity present in

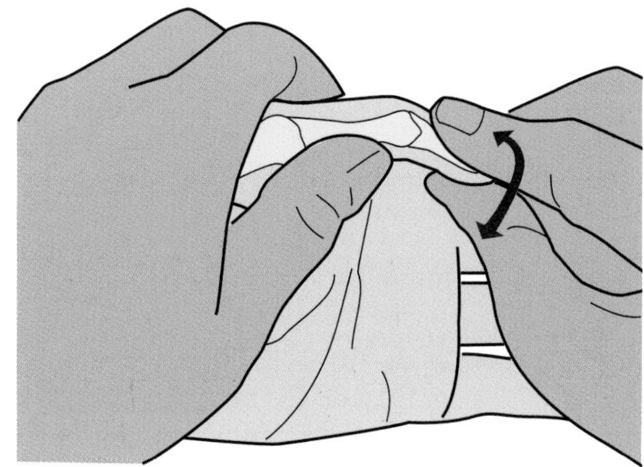

Figure 10.43 Passive movement testing of flexion and extension of the thumb interphalangeal joint.

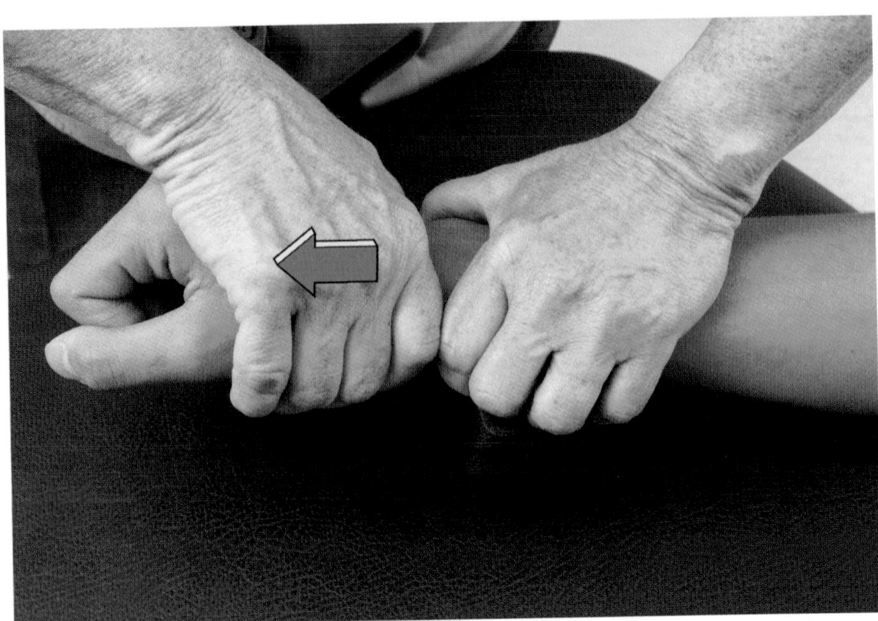

Figure 10.44 Mobility testing of traction of the radiocarpal joint.

the joint. The patient must be totally relaxed and comfortable to allow you to move the joint and obtain the most accurate information. The joint should be placed in the maximal loose packed (resting) position to allow for the greatest degree of joint movement. The resting position of the wrist is as follows: the longitudinal axes of the radius and the third metacarpal form a straight line with slight ulnar deviation (mid position between ulnar and radial deviation). The resting position of the first carpometacarpal joint is with the metacarpal midway between abduction–adduction and flexion–extension. The resting position of the fingers is slight flexion of all joints (plus slight ulnar deviation of the second through fifth metacarpophalangeal joints) (Kaltenborn, 2011).

Ventral and Dorsal Glide of the Radius and Radial Head

Refer to Chapter 9 (pp. 216–217, Figures 9.30 and 9.31) for a full description of these mobility tests.

Traction of the Radiocarpal Joint

Place the patient in the sitting position, with the arm pronated and supported on the treatment table. The wrist should be in the neutral position. Stand so that you are facing the ulnar aspect of the wrist. Stabilize by grasping the dorsal distal aspect of the forearm with your hand. Wrap your other hand around the proximal row of carpals, just distal to the radiocarpal joint. Pull the carpals in a longitudinal direction until you have taken up the slack, producing traction in the radiocarpal joint (Figure 10.44).

Traction of the Midcarpal Joint

Place the patient in the sitting position, with the arm pronated and supported on the treatment table. The wrist should be in the neutral position. Stand so that you are facing the ulnar aspect of the wrist. Stabilize by grasping the dorsal aspect of the proximal carpal row with your hand. Wrap your other hand around the distal row of carpals. Pull the distal row of carpals in a longitudinal direction until you have taken up the slack, producing traction in the midcarpal joint (Figure 10.45).

Individual Carpal Joints

Each of the individual carpal bones can be moved on each other at their specific articulations. Description of these techniques is beyond the scope of this book. The reader should consult a text on mobilization for further details.

Palmar and Dorsal Glide of the Metacarpals

Place the patient in the sitting position, with the forearm pronated and supported on the treatment table.

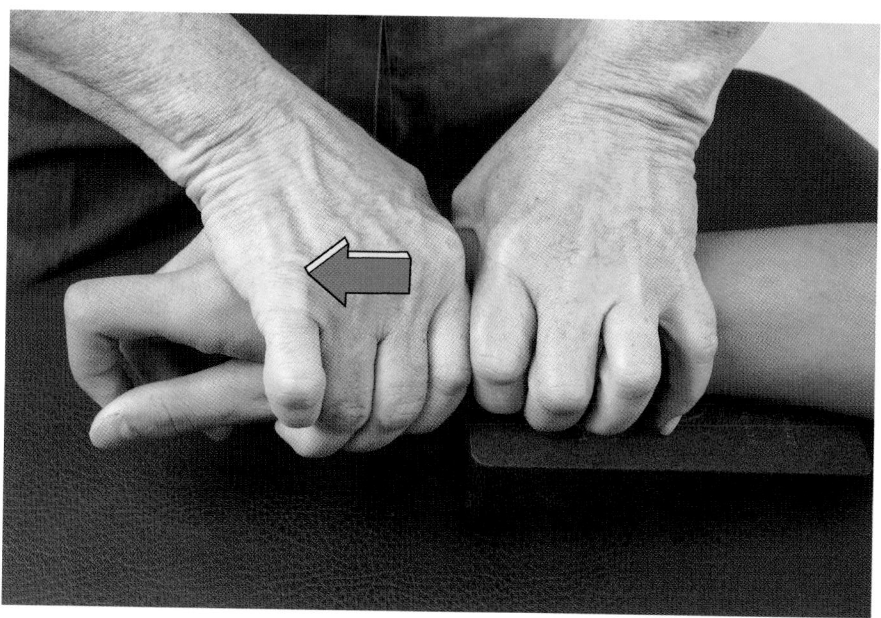

Figure 10.45 Mobility testing of traction of the midcarpal joint.

The wrist should be in the neutral position. Stand so that you are facing the dorsal aspect of the hand. Grasp the third metacarpal with your thumb and then wrap your fingers around the palmar surface. Using the same hold with your other hand, move the second metacarpal first in a dorsal and then a volar direction until all the slack is taken up in each direction. This can be repeated for the fourth and fifth metacarpals (Figure 10.46).

Traction of the Metacarpophalangeal and Proximal and Distal Interphalangeal Joints

Place the patient in a sitting position, with the forearm pronated. Sit facing the patient so that you can hold the ulnar aspect of the patient's hand against your body. Grasp the metacarpal just proximal to the metacarpophalangeal joint to stabilize it. Using your thumb and index finger, grasp the proximal phalanx.

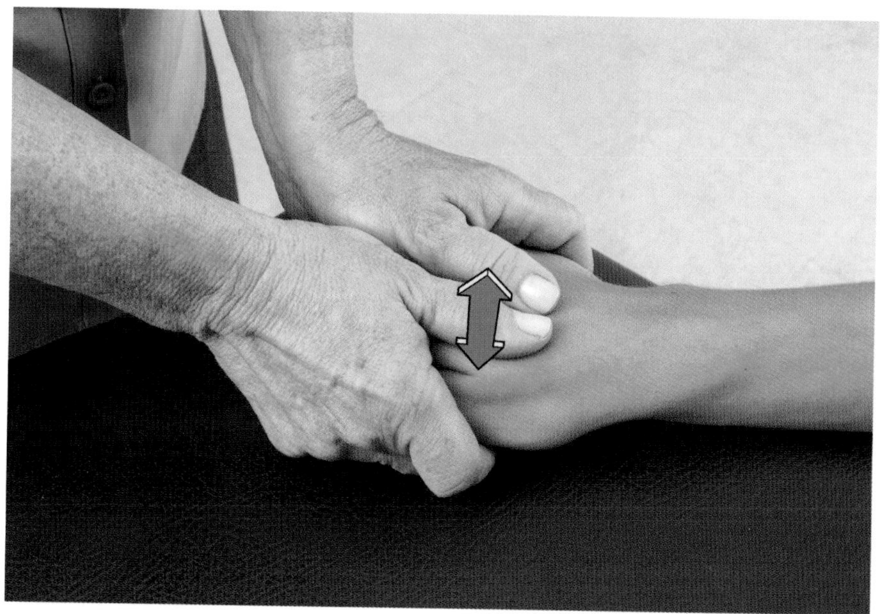

Figure 10.46 Mobility testing of palmar and dorsal glide of the metacarpals.

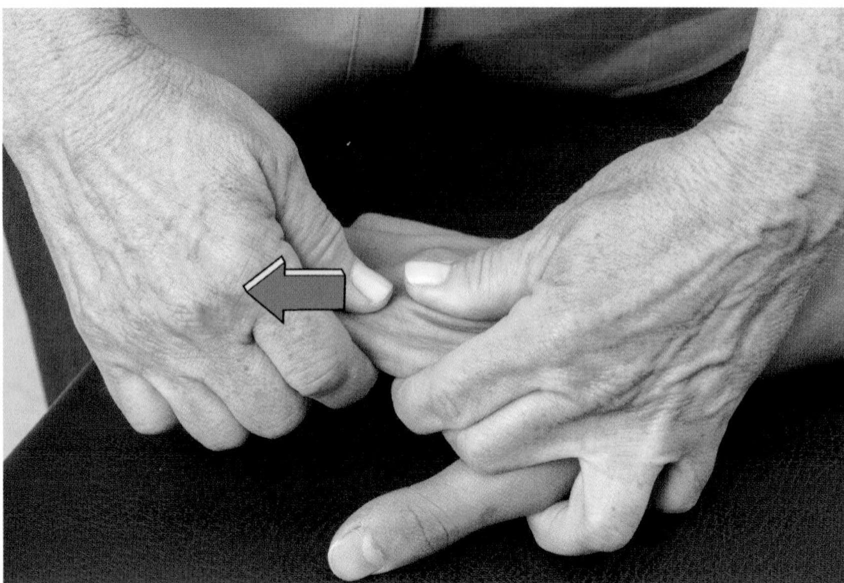

Figure 10.47 Mobility testing of traction of the metacarpophalangeal (shown in diagram) and proximal and distal interphalangeal joints.

Pull in a longitudinal direction until you have taken up the slack, producing traction in the metacarpophalangeal joint. To produce traction in the proximal interphalangeal joint, the stabilization is moved to the proximal phalanx and the middle phalanx is mobilized. To produce traction in the distal interphalangeal joint, the stabilization is moved to the middle phalanx and the distal phalanx is moved (Figure 10.47).

Traction of the First Carpometacarpal Joint

Place the patient in a sitting position, with the forearm midway between supination and pronation. Stand so that you are facing the dorsal aspect of the hand. Using your thumb and index finger, grasp the trapezeii for stabilization. Using the thumb and index finger of your other hand, grasp the proximal aspect of the first metacarpal, just distal to the carpometacarpal joint.

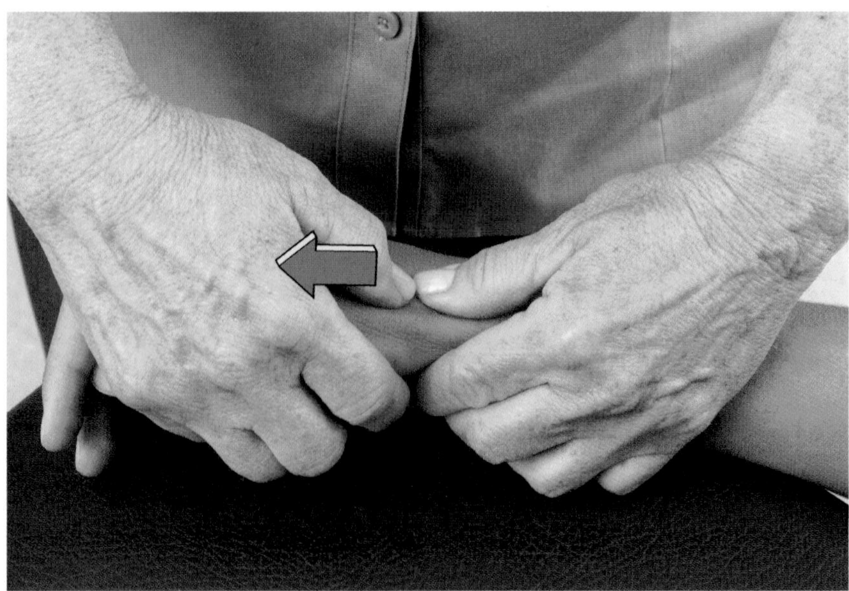

Figure 10.48 Mobility testing of traction of the first carpometacarpal joint.

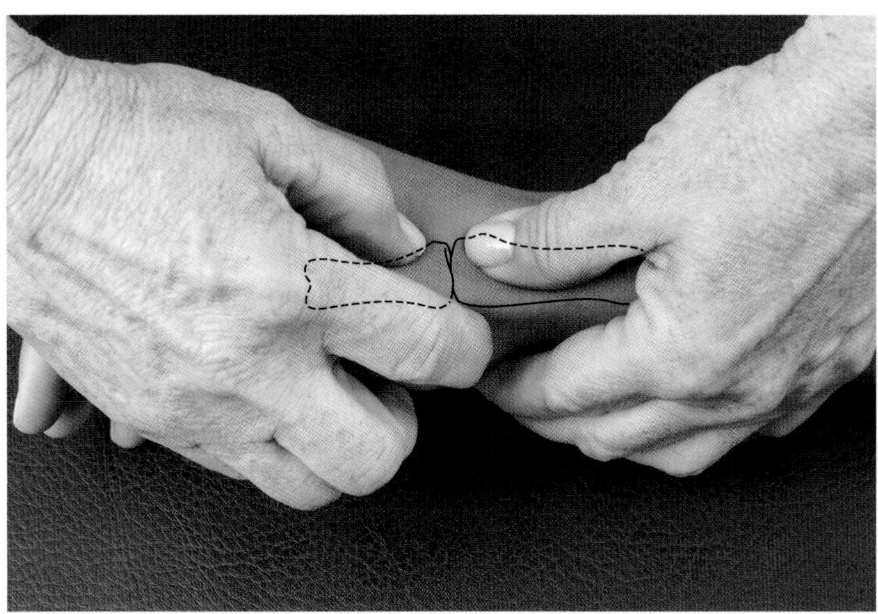

Figure 10.49 Mobility testing of ulnar glide of the first metacarpophalangeal joint.

Pull in a longitudinal direction until you have taken up all the slack, producing traction in the first carpometacarpal joint (Figure 10.48).

Ulnar Glide of the First Metacarpophalangeal Joint

Place the patient in a sitting position, with the forearm midway between supination and pronation. Stand so that you are facing the dorsal aspect of the hand. Using your thumb and index finger, grasp the first metacarpal for stabilization. Using the thumb and index finger of your other hand, grasp the proximal aspect of the proximal phalanx and glide it in an ulnar direction until all of the slack is taken up (Figure 10.49). Rupture of the ulnar collateral ligament of the first metacarpophalangeal joint is known as *gamekeeper's* or *skier's thumb* (Figure 10.50).

Resistive Testing

The Wrist

The primary movements of the wrist are flexion and extension. The wrist is also able to deviate in the radial and ulnar directions because of the attachments of the flexor and extensor muscles of the wrist on the radial and ulnar borders of the hand.

Flexion

The flexors of the wrist are the flexor carpi radialis (Figure 10.51) and flexor carpi ulnaris (Figure 10.52).

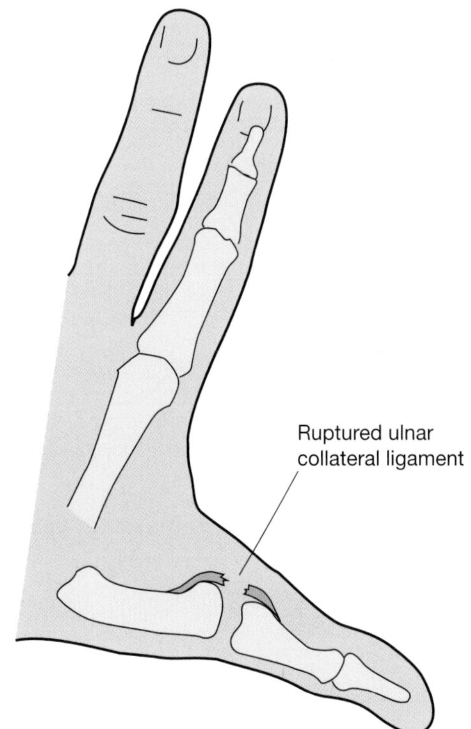

Figure 10.50 Gamekeeper's (skier's) thumb.

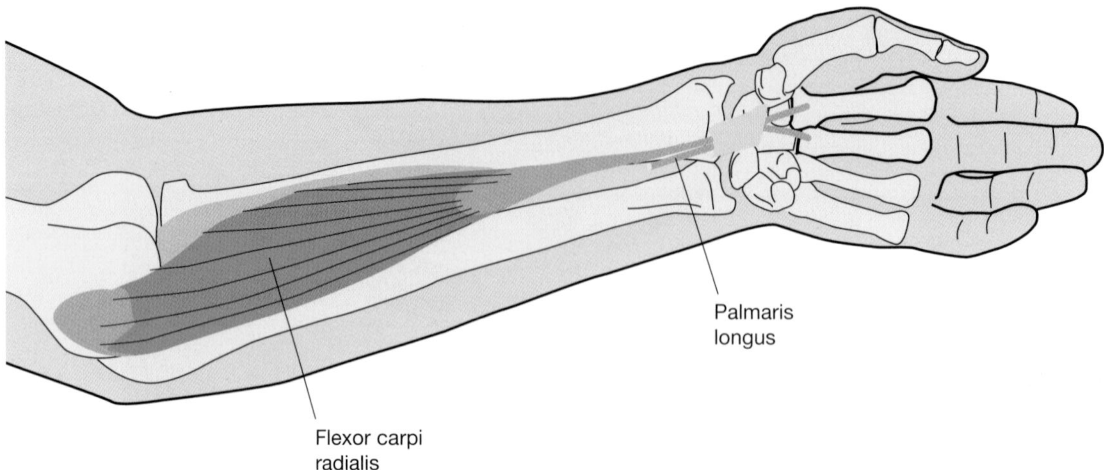

Figure 10.51 The flexor carpi radialis muscle.

They are assisted by the flexor digitorum superficialis and profundus.

- Position of patient: Sitting or supine. The forearm is supinated.
- Resisted test: Support the patient's forearm with one hand and ask the patient to flex the wrist so that the hand moves directly upward, perpendicular to the forearm. If you ask the patient to flex the wrist radially and apply resistance proximal to the thumb, you will isolate the flexor carpi radialis (Figure 10.53). Likewise, if you ask the patient to flex the wrist in an ulnar direction and you apply resistance to the hypothenar eminence, you will isolate the flexor carpi ulnaris muscle (Figure 10.54).

Testing wrist flexion with gravity eliminated is performed by asking the patient to place the hand and forearm on a table with the forearm midway between pronation and supination, and to flex the wrist with the table supporting the weight of the hand and forearm.

Weakness of wrist flexion results in difficulty with feeding oneself and performing personal hygiene.

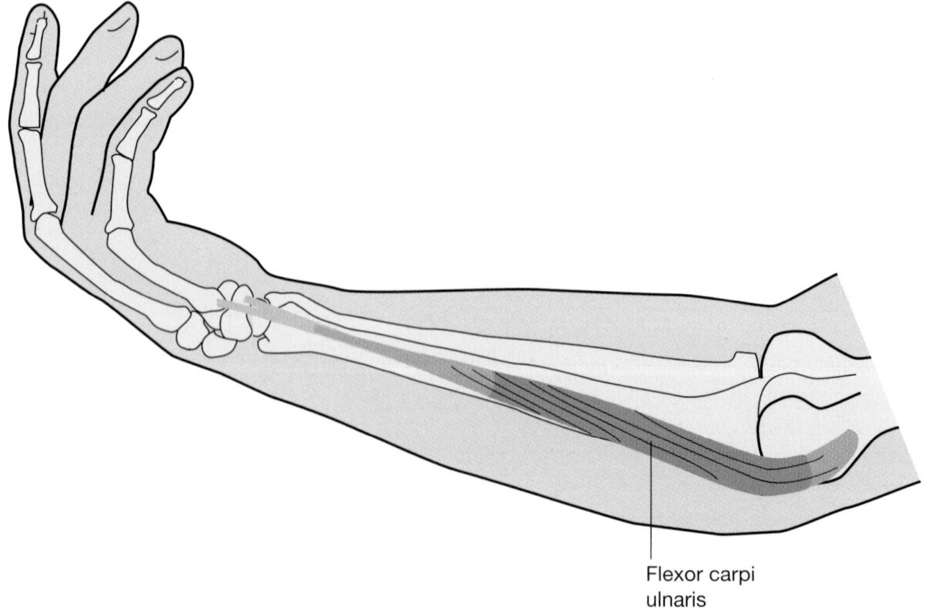

Figure 10.52 The flexor carpi ulnaris muscle.

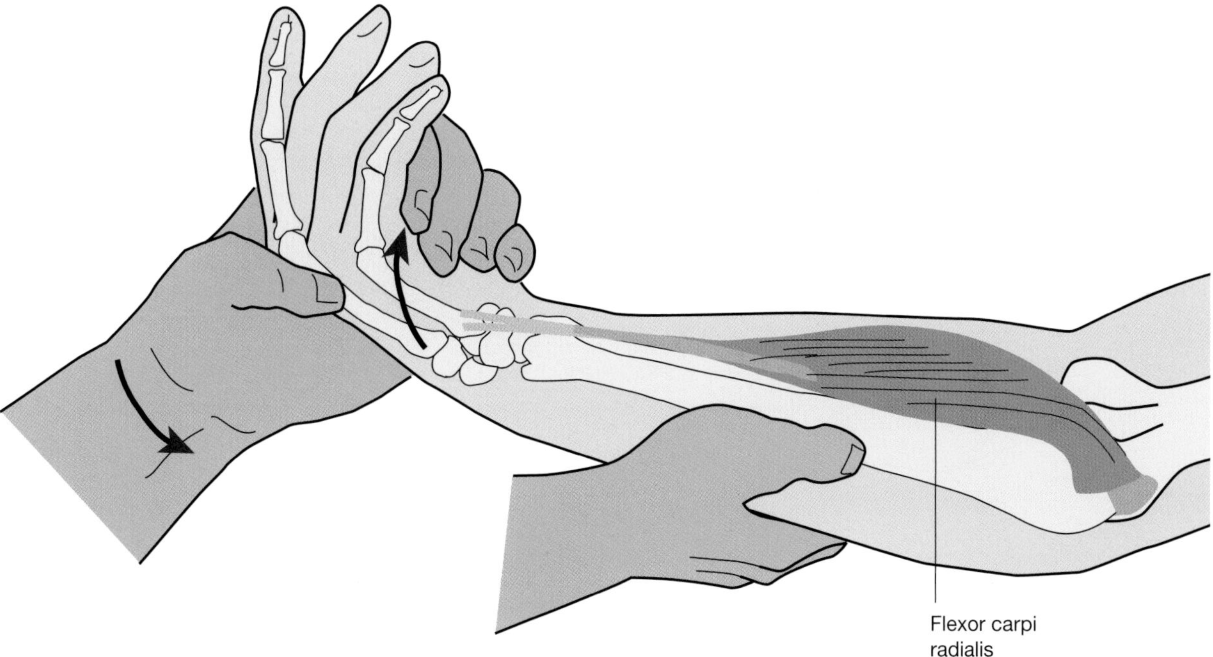

Figure 10.53 Testing wrist flexion, isolating the flexor carpi radialis.

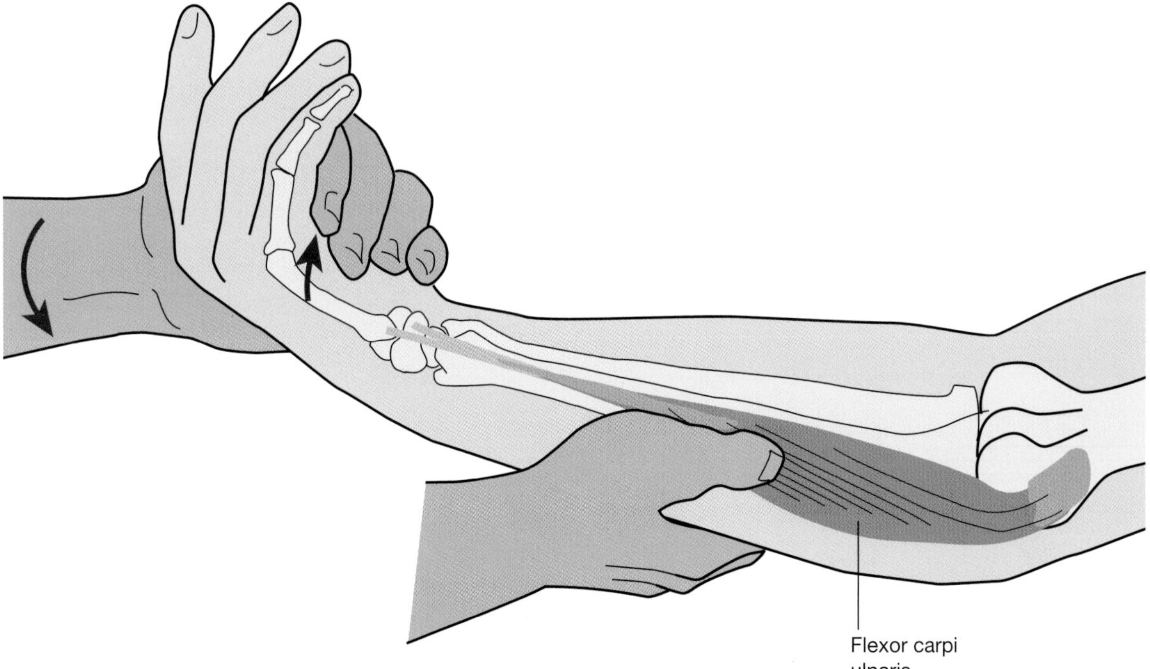

Figure 10.54 Testing wrist flexion while isolating the flexor carpi ulnaris.

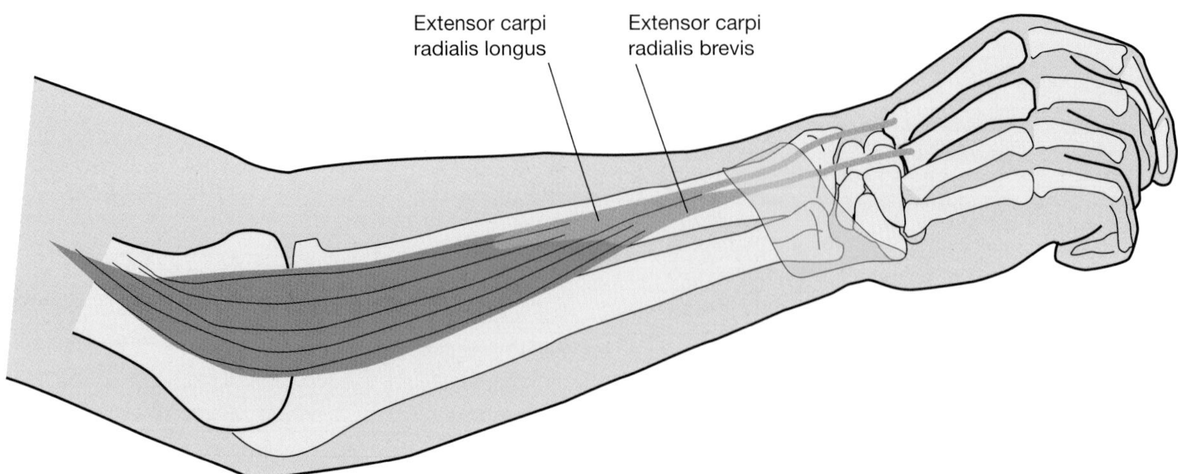

Figure 10.55 The extensor carpi radialis longus and brevis.

Extension

The extensors of the wrist on the radial side are the extensor carpi radialis longus and brevis (Figure 10.55). The extensor of the wrist on the ulnar side is the extensor carpi ulnaris (Figure 10.56). These muscles are assisted by the extensor digitorum, extensor indicis, and extensor digiti minimi.

- Position of patient: Sitting with the elbow slightly flexed.
- Resisted test: Support the patient's pronated forearm on the treatment table and ask the patient to extend the wrist in the line of the forearm while you apply resistance to the dorsum of the hand (Figure 10.57). You can isolate the extensor carpi radialis longus and brevis by applying resistance along the second and third metacarpals. The patient should try to extend the wrist in a radial direction. You can isolate the extensor carpi ulnaris by having the patient extend the wrist in an ulnar direction while applying resistance to the fourth and fifth metacarpals.

Testing wrist extension with gravity eliminated is performed with the patient's forearm in a mid position between pronation and supination and the hand resting on the table. The patient attempts to extend the wrist through the range of motion while the table supports the weight of the hand and forearm.

Painful resisted wrist extension may be due to lateral epicondylitis (see p. 231).

Weakness of wrist extension results in a weakening of the grip due to loss of the tenodesis effect. Extension of the wrist is necessary for the finger flexors to

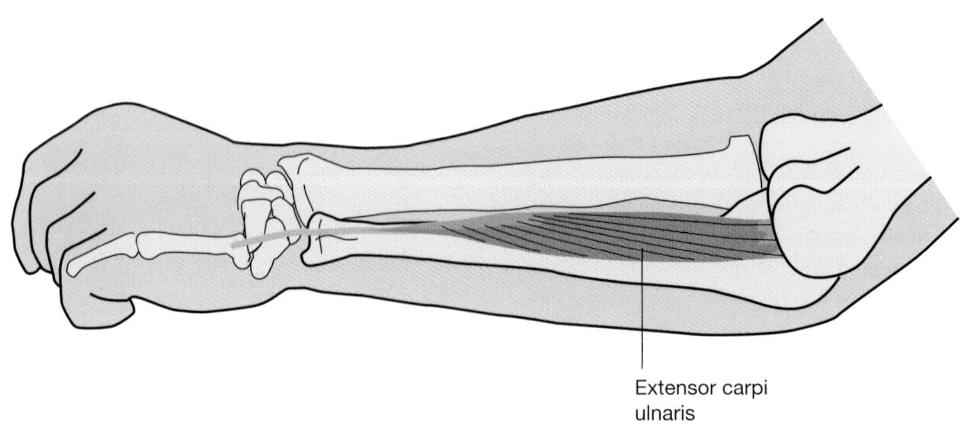

Figure 10.56 The extensor carpi ulnaris.

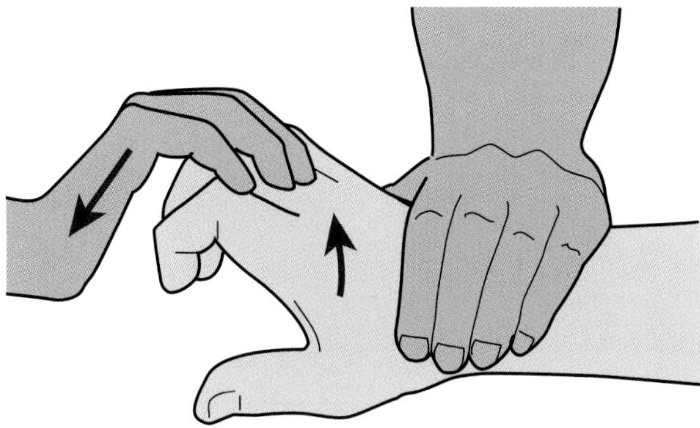

Figure 10.57 Testing wrist extension.

be in a stretched position so that they can function properly. Note that your grip strength is very weak with a fully flexed wrist. Grip strength is maximal at about 20 degrees of wrist extension.

The Hand

Flexion, extension, abduction, and adduction of the second through fifth fingers should be examined. The superficial and deep finger flexors should be tested in isolation.

Special attention should be devoted to the thumb and its movements of flexion, extension, abduction, adduction, and opposition.

Distal Interphalangeal Joint Flexion

The long finger flexor muscle is the flexor digitorum profundus (Figure 10.58). This is the only muscle that flexes the distal interphalangeal joint. It also can flex the wrist and the proximal joints of the fingers. Note that the flexor digitorum profundus to the index and middle fingers is innervated by the median nerve. The flexor digitorum profundus to the ring and fifth fingers is innervated by the ulnar nerve.

- Position of patient: Sitting.
- Resisted test: Test each finger individually by supporting it with one hand. Ask the patient to flex the distal phalanx while you apply resistance on the palmar surface of the finger over the distal finger pad (Figure 10.59).

Pain located in the region of the metacarpophalangeal joint associated with a swelling may be due to tenosynovitis of the flexor tendon, and may cause a "triggering" of the finger. A clicking sensation may be palpated along the flexor tendon where the inflammation exists. The patient may be unable to extend the finger independently due to a ball-and-valve phenomenon (Figure 10.60).

Proximal Interphalangeal Joint Flexion

The flexor digitorum superficialis attaches to the middle phalanx of the finger and flexes the proximal interphalangeal and metacarpophalangeal joints, and the wrist (Figure 10.61). It is assisted by the flexor digitorum profundus.

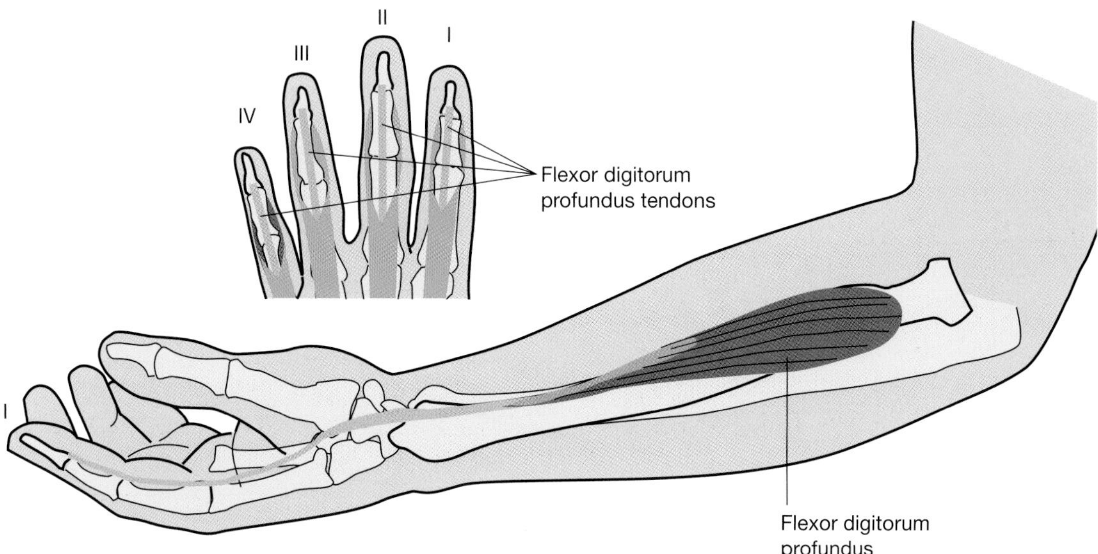

Figure 10.58 The flexor digitorum profundus. Note the innervation to the index and middle fingers is from the median nerve, and that to the ring and little fingers is from the ulnar nerve.

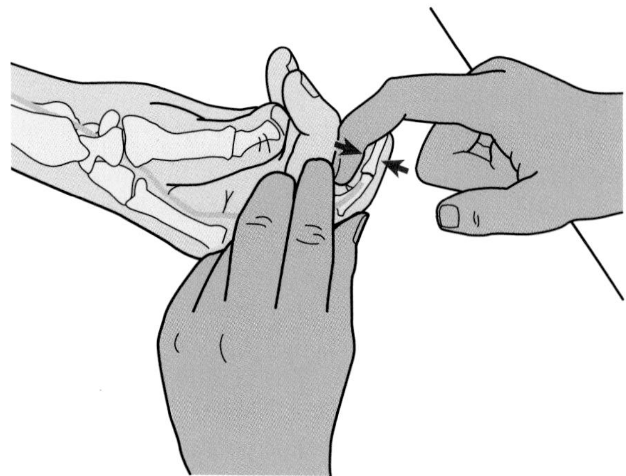

Figure 10.59 Testing distal interphalangeal joint flexion.

- Position of patient: Sitting.
- Resisted test: The goal of the test is to isolate the flexor digitorum superficialis. This can be accomplished by stabilizing the patient's metacarpophalangeal joint with one hand and asking the patient to flex the proximal interphalangeal joint while the distal interphalangeal joint is maintained in extension.

Apply resistance to the palmar aspect of the middle phalanx (Figure 10.62).

This test can also be performed by hyperextending all of the patient's fingers except for the thumb

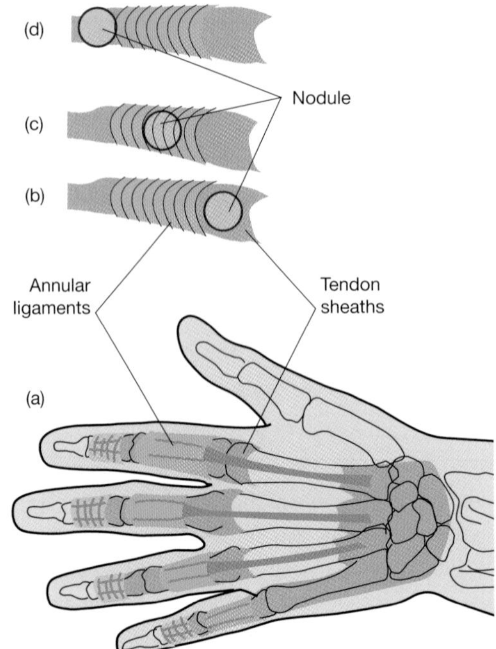

Figure 10.60 Trigger fingers. (a) The anatomy of the flexor tendons within their sheaths and the annular ligaments is shown. (b) A nodular thickening of the tendon sheath passes underneath the ligament during flexion of the finger. (c) The nodule is shown under the annular ligament. (d) After flexion of the finger, re-extension is not possible because the nodule is unable to pass under the annular ligament.

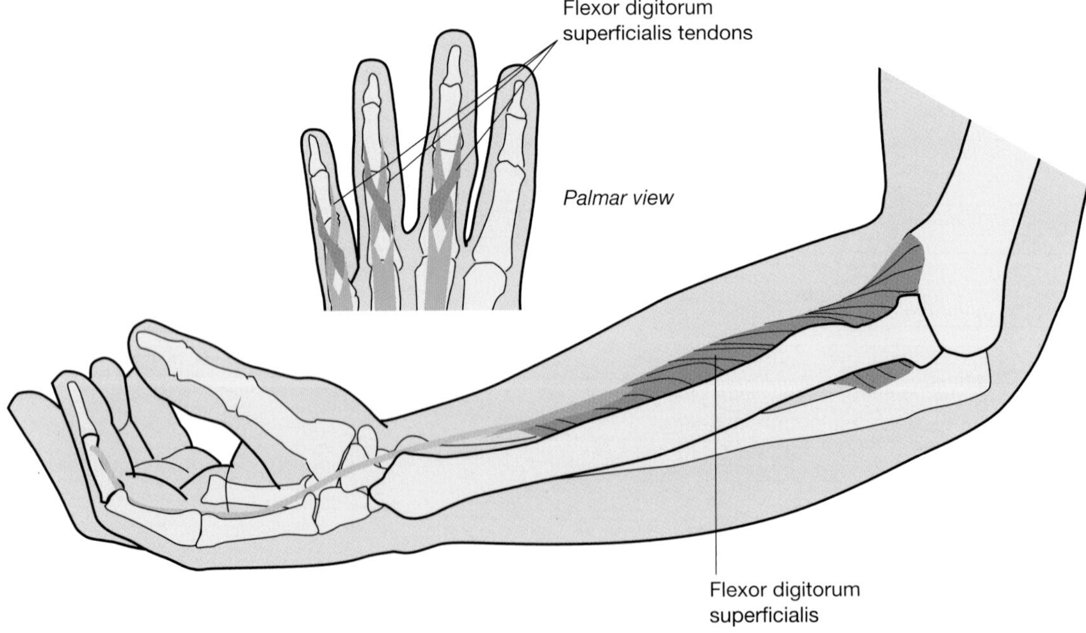

Figure 10.61 The flexor digitorum superficialis muscle. This muscle is innervated by the median nerve only.

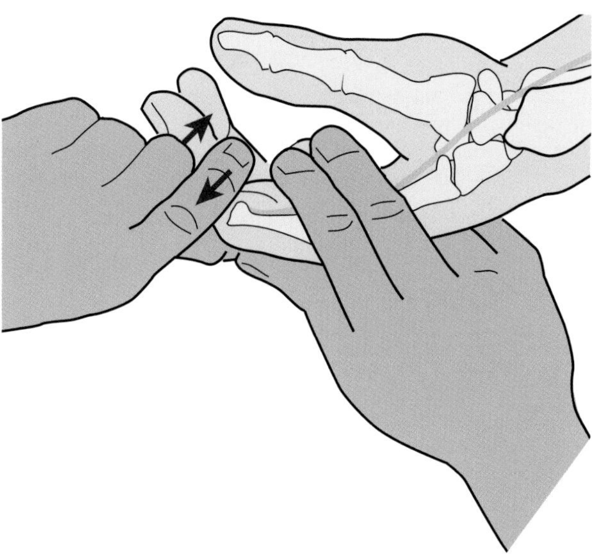

Figure 10.62 Testing flexion of the proximal interphalangeal joint.

and the one being tested. Due to the mechanical disadvantage of the flexor digitorum profundus in this position, only the flexor digitorum superficialis will flex the finger being tested (Figure 10.63).

Weakness of finger flexion results in the inability to grip or carry objects with the fingers.

Finger Extension

The extensors of the metacarpophalangeal joints are the extensor digitorum, extensor indicis, and extensor digiti minimi (Figure 10.64). The interphalangeal

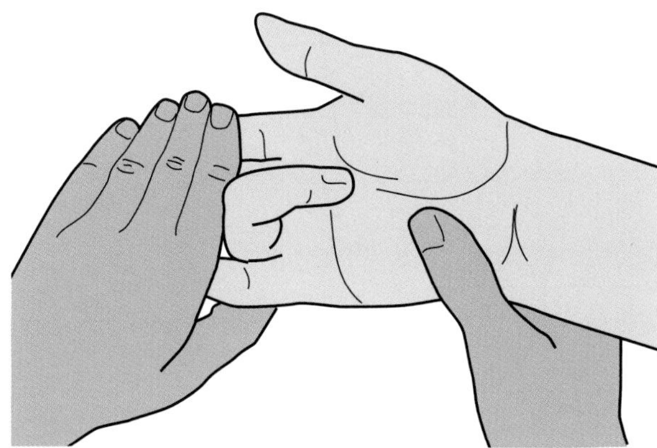

Figure 10.63 Testing flexion of the proximal interphalangeal joint by the flexor digitorum superficialis only.

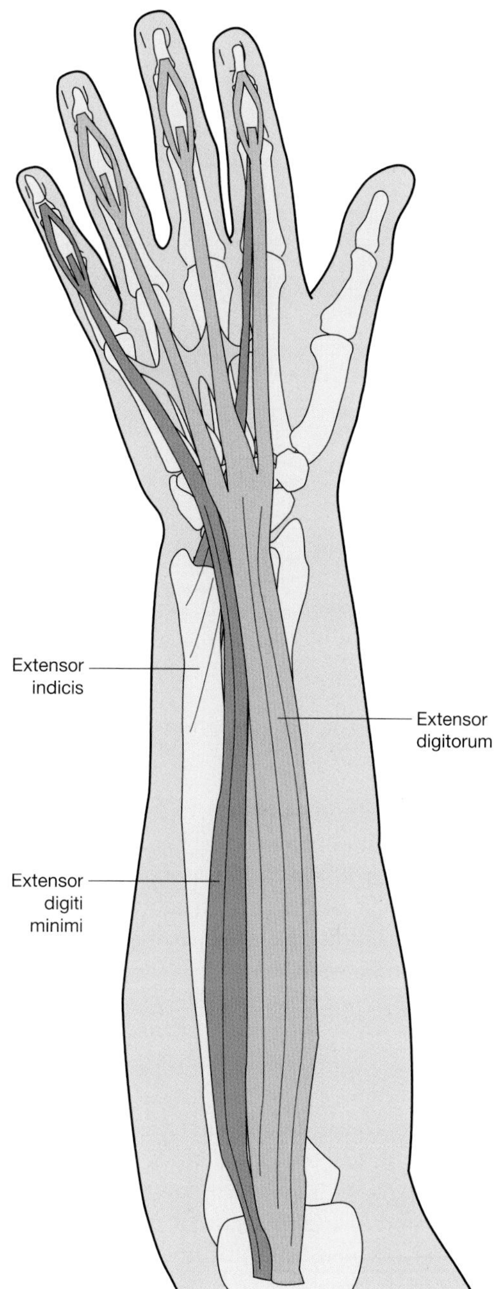

Figure 10.64 The extensor digitorum, extensor indicis, and extensor digiti minimi.

joints are extended with the help of the lumbricals and interossei. The finger extensors also assist in wrist extension.

- Position of patient: Sitting. The pronated forearm is supported on a table.
- Resisted test: Ask the patient to extend the fingers at the metacarpophalangeal joints. Apply

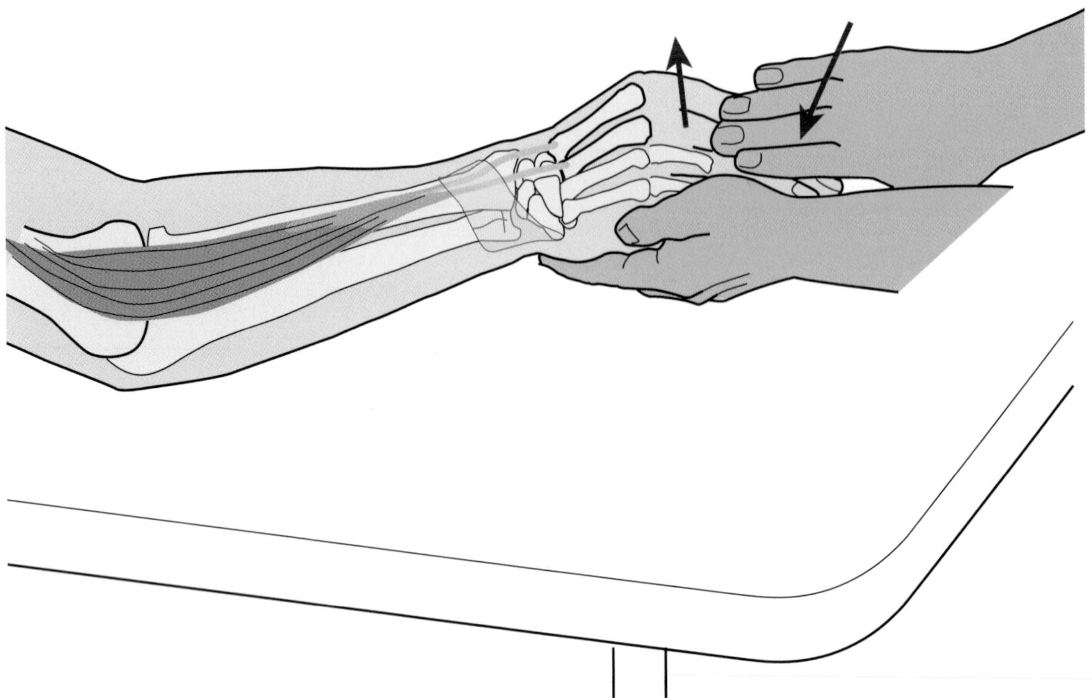

Figure 10.65 Testing metacarpophalangeal joint extension.

resistance with your fingers to the posterior aspect of the proximal phalanges (Figure 10.65).

Weakness of finger extension results in the fingers remaining in a position of flexion at the metacarpophalangeal joints. Relative weakness of wrist flexion may also be noted.

The Interossei

It is said that the interossei function primarily to abduct and adduct the second through fifth digits. The palmar interossei adduct the fingers (Figure 10.66), and the dorsal interossei abduct the fingers (Figure 10.67). Mnemonics for these are "PAD" and "DAB." Abduction and adduction of the digitis provides little functional advantage other than providing for a variety of handgrip sizes. A very important function of the interossei is to flex and rotate the proximal phalanx of the finger. Note that when closing your hand, the four fingers point toward the scaphoid tubercle (Figure 10.68). This occurs because of the coordinated function of the interossei. Likewise, the rotation of the fingers as they extend also requires precise function of these muscles. Weakness or contracture of the interossei will prevent normal hand function. The rotational alignment of the

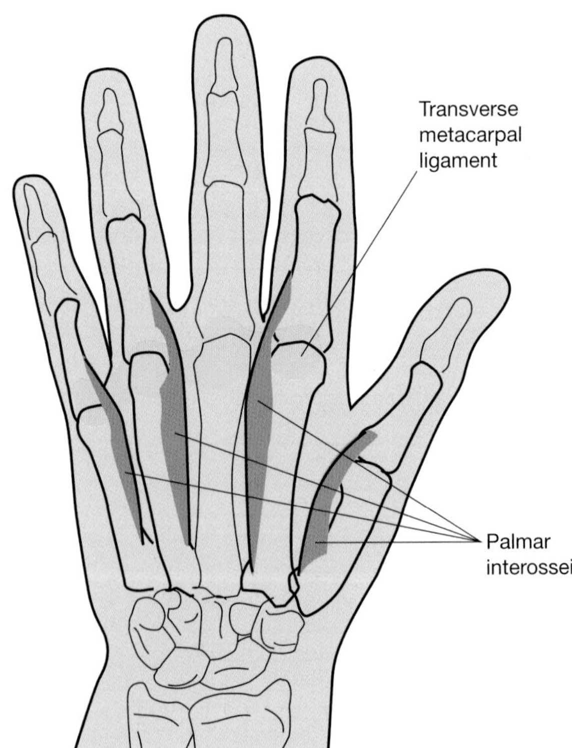

Figure 10.66 The palmar interossei.

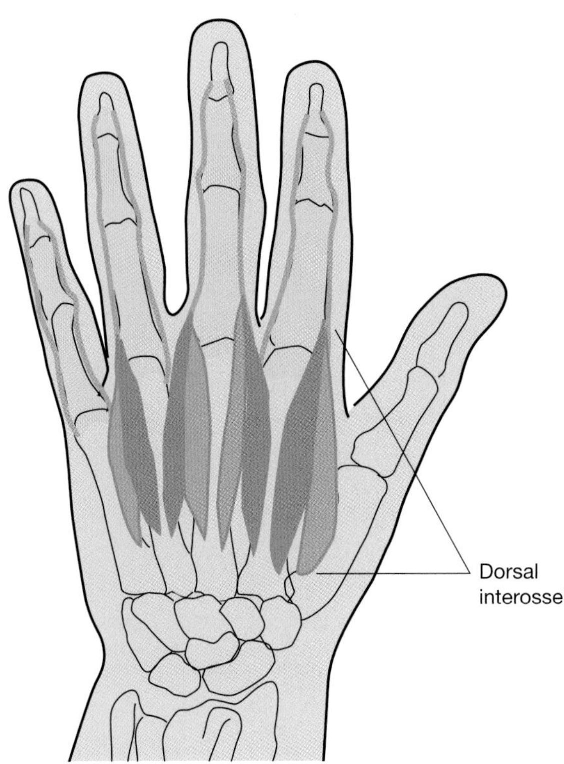

Figure 10.67 The dorsal interossei.

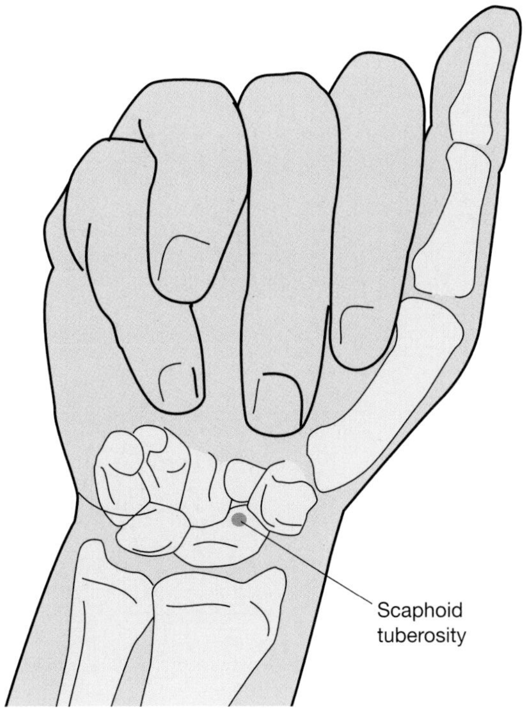

Figure 10.69 Malrotation due to a fracture of the fourth proximal phalanx results in overlapping of the fingers with flexion.

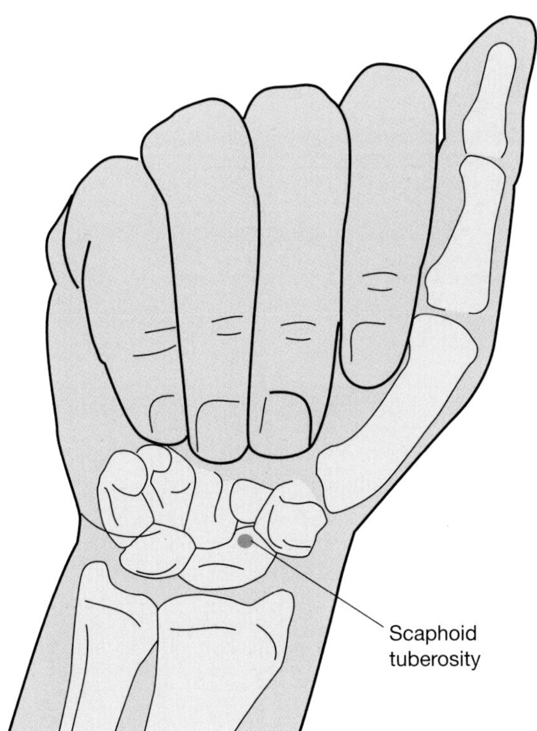

Figure 10.68 The normal hand in a flexed posture shows all four fingers pointing toward the scaphoid tubercle.

metacarpals and proximal phalanges following a fracture is extremely important for preservation of normal function of the associated interossei muscles. Malalignment due to a fracture can result in overlapping of the fingers as the patient closes his or her fist (Figure 10.69).

- Position of patient: Sitting. The forearm is pronated.
- Resisted test: The palmar interossei are tested by attempting to abduct the fingers as the patient squeezes the fingers into adduction (Figures 10.70a–10.70d). The dorsal interossei are tested by asking the patient to spread the fingers apart as you attempt to adduct them one on the other (Figures 10.71a–10.71d).

The Thumb

Flexion

The flexors of the thumb are the flexor pollicis longus and flexor pollicis brevis (Figures 10.72 and 10.73). The flexor pollicis longus also assists in wrist flexion.

- Position of patient: Sitting. The forearm is supinated and the hand is in a relaxed posture.

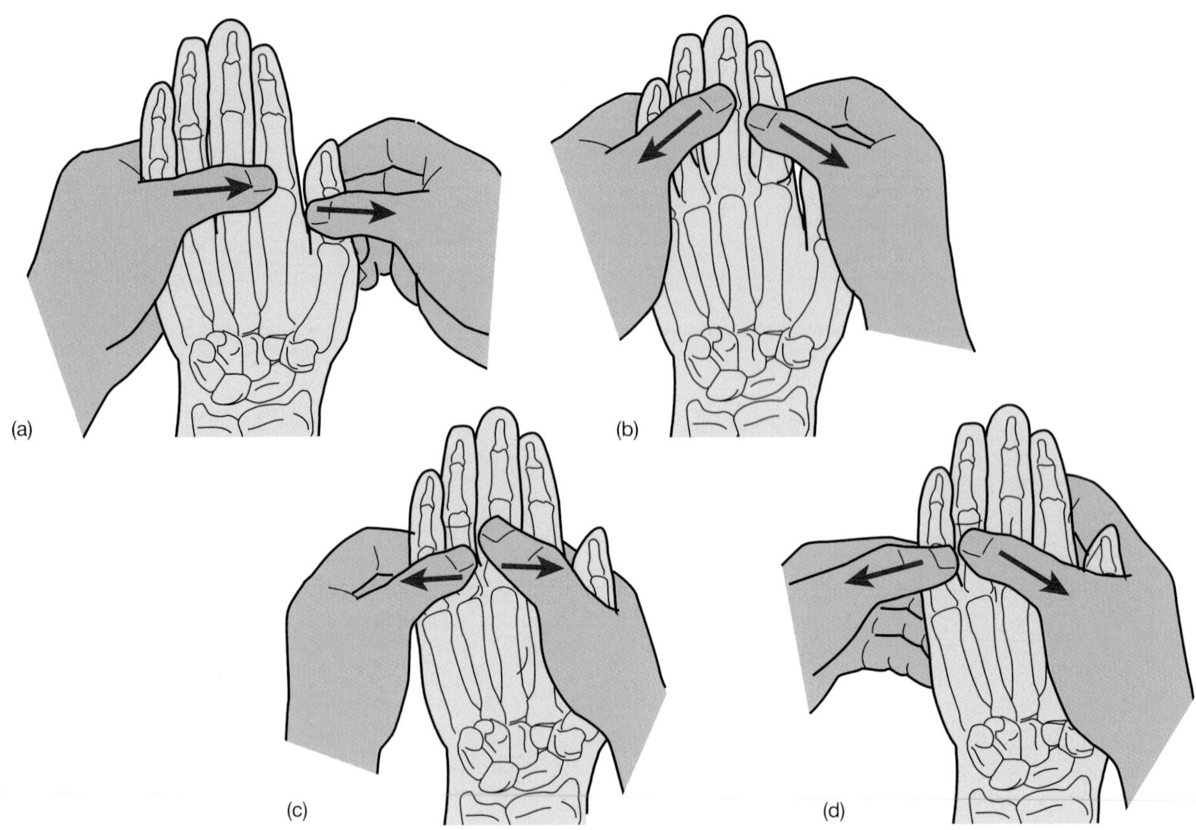

Figure 10.70 Testing adduction of the fingers.

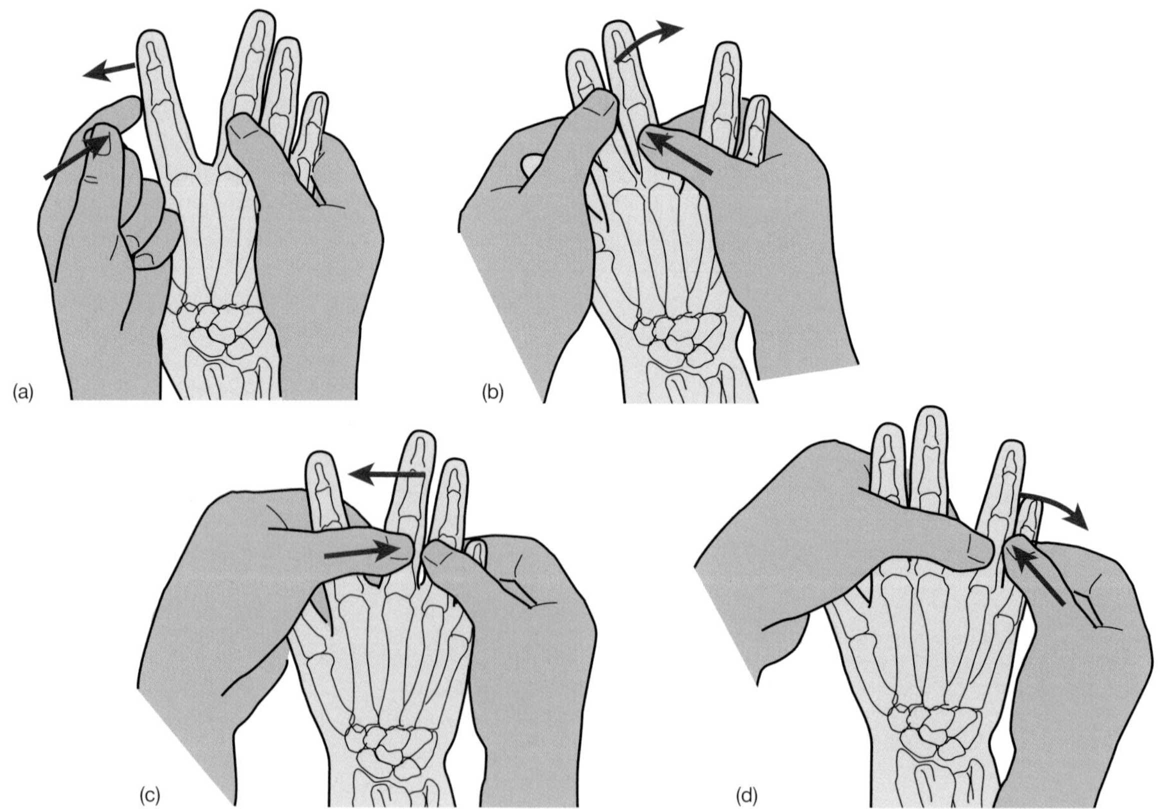

Figure 10.71 Testing abduction of the fingers.

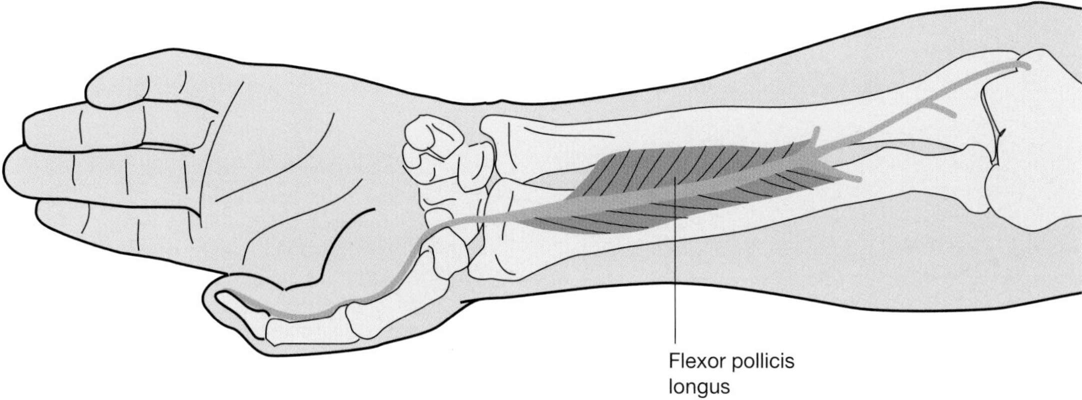

Figure 10.72 The flexor pollicis longus muscle.

- Resisted test: The flexor pollicis longus is tested by supporting the patient's thumb on the palmar surface as the patient attempts to flex the interphalangeal joint (Figure 10.74). The flexor pollicis brevis is tested by applying pressure to the proximal phalanx of the thumb on the palmar surface while the patient attempts to flex the thumb, keeping the interphalangeal joint extended (Figure 10.75).

Painful resisted thumb flexion may be due to tenosynovitis.

Weakness of the short thumb flexor will result in a weakened grip. Weakness of the long thumb flexor will result in difficulty holding a pencil or small objects.

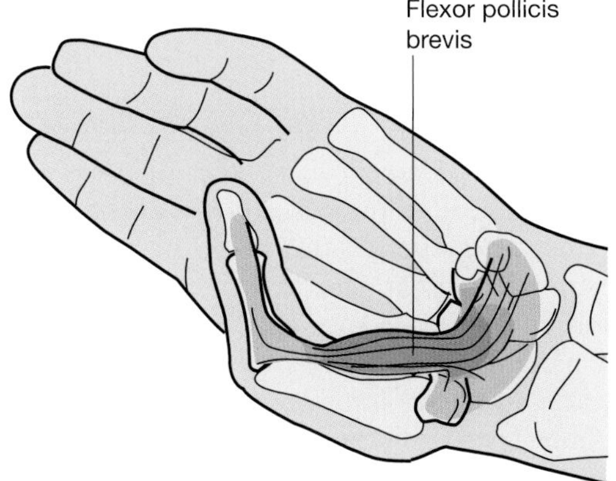

Figure 10.73 The flexor pollicis brevis muscle. This muscle has innervation to the superficial head from the median nerve and the deep head from the ulnar nerve.

Extension

The extensors of the thumb are the extensor pollicis longus and extensor pollicis brevis (Figures 10.76 and 10.77).

- Position of patient: Sitting. The forearm is supinated and the wrist is in neutral.
- Resisted test: The patient's hand is supported with your hand and you resist thumb movement away from the index finger in the plane of the palm, first proximally over the proximal phalanx, to test the extensor pollicis brevis and then distally, over the distal phalanx to test the extensor pollicis longus (Figures 10.78 and 10.79).

Painful extension of the thumb may result from tenosynovitis at the wrist where the extensor pollicis brevis crosses the radial styloid process. This is called de Quervain's syndrome. Associated tenosynovitis in the abductor pollicis longus muscle may also be noted (see special test for de Quervain's syndrome on p. 285, Figure 10.99).

Weakness of thumb extension results in a flexion deformity of the thumb.

Abduction

The abductors of the thumb are the abductor pollicis longus, innervated by the radial nerve (Figure 10.80), and the abductor pollicis brevis, innervated by the median nerve (Figure 10.81).

- Position of patient: Sitting. The forearm is supinated and the wrist is in neutral.
- Resisted test: The abductor pollicis longus is tested by resisting first metacarpal abduction with your hand, putting pressure on the palmar aspect of the first metacarpal as the patient attempts to elevate the thumb in a plane perpendicular to the hand.

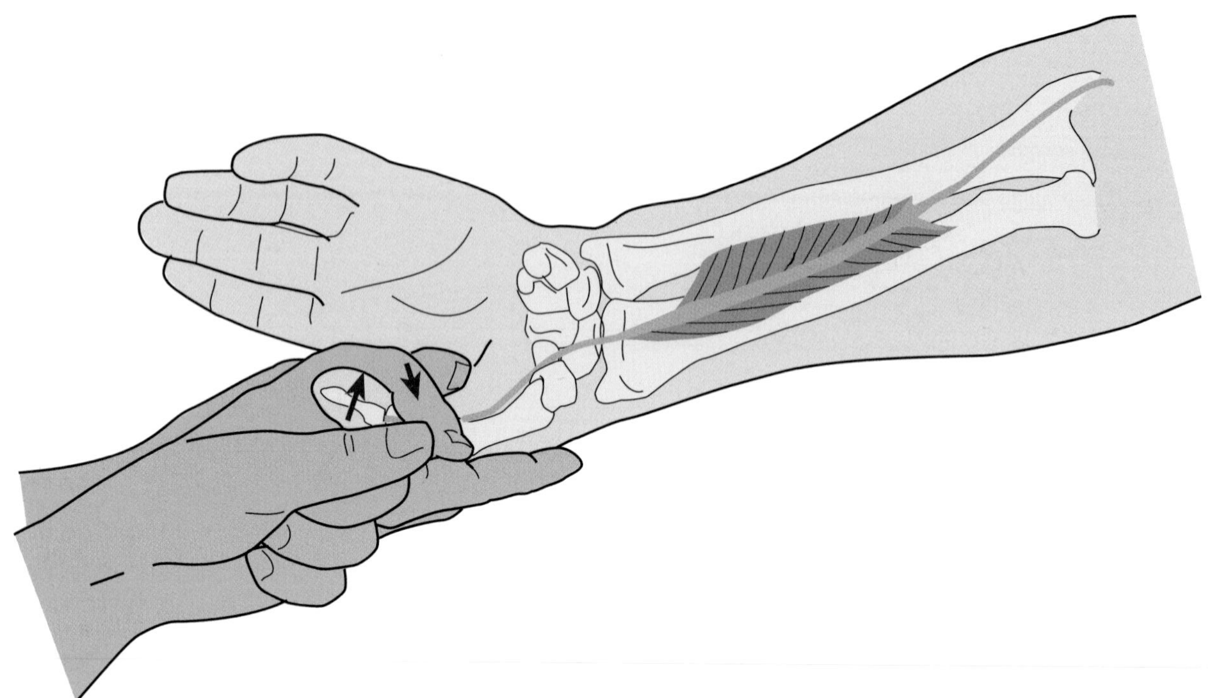

Figure 10.74 Testing flexion of the interphalangeal joint of the thumb.

Support the hand and wrist from underneath with your other hand (Figure 10.82). Testing the abductor pollicis brevis is accomplished by applying pressure to the radial aspect of the proximal phalanx of the thumb as the patient attempts to abduct the thumb in a plane perpendicular to the hand (Figure 10.83).

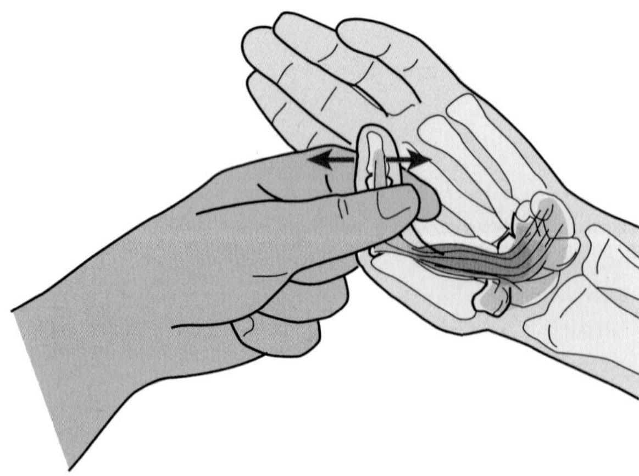

Figure 10.75 Testing flexion of the metacarpophalangeal joint of the thumb.

Painful abduction of the first metacarpal can be due to de Quervain's syndrome affecting the tendon of the abductor pollicis longus as it crosses the radial styloid process (see the special test for de Quervain's syndrome on p. 285, Figure 10.99).

Weakness of thumb abduction results in the patient's inability to grasp a large object, as the thumb cannot be moved away from the hand. Weakness of the abductor pollicis brevis is seen in advanced cases of carpal tunnel syndrome.

Adduction

Thumb adduction is accomplished by the adductor pollicis muscle (Figure 10.84). This muscle is assisted by the deep head of the flexor pollicis brevis. Both of these muscles are innervated by the ulnar nerve.

- Position of patient: Sitting.
- Resisted test: Place your index and long fingers in the patient's first web space. Ask the patient to press your fingers into his or her palm with the thumb. Try to pull the patient's thumb upward into abduction in a plane perpendicular to his or her palm (Figure 10.85).

Weakness of thumb adduction prevents the patient from making a strong clenched fist.

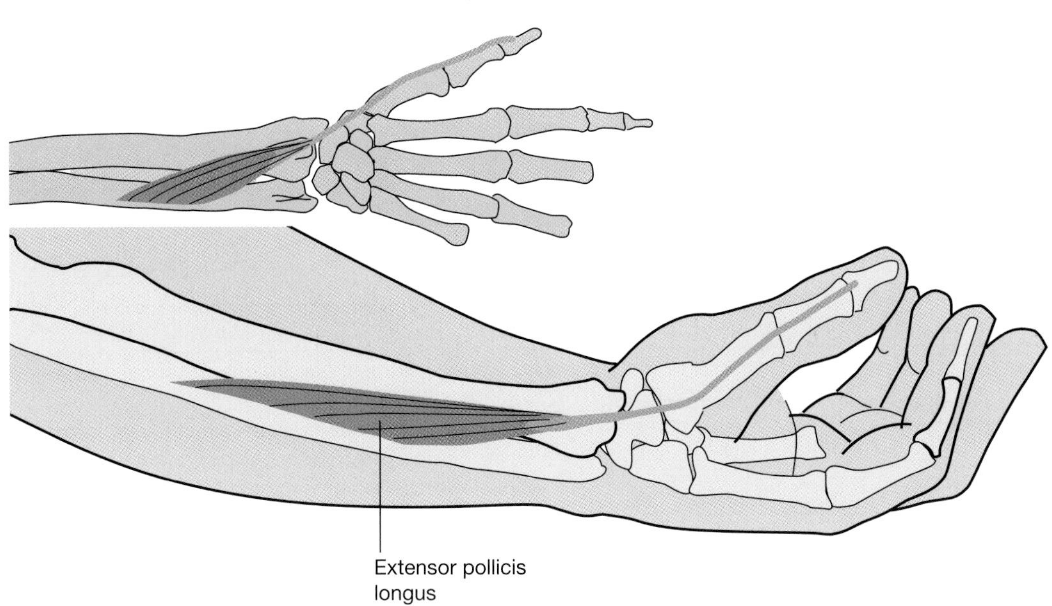

Figure 10.76 The extensor pollicis longus.

To test for Froment's sign, ask the patient to hold a piece of paper between the thumb and the radial aspect of the index finger. Try to pull the paper away from the patient and if the adductor pollicis is weak, the patient will flex the thumb interphalangeal joint as a compensatory measure as he or she attempts to compensate with the flexor pollicis longus for a weak adductor pollicis (Figure 10.86).

Opposition of the Thumb and Fifth Finger

The muscles responsible for opposition are the opponens pollicis and opponens digiti minimi

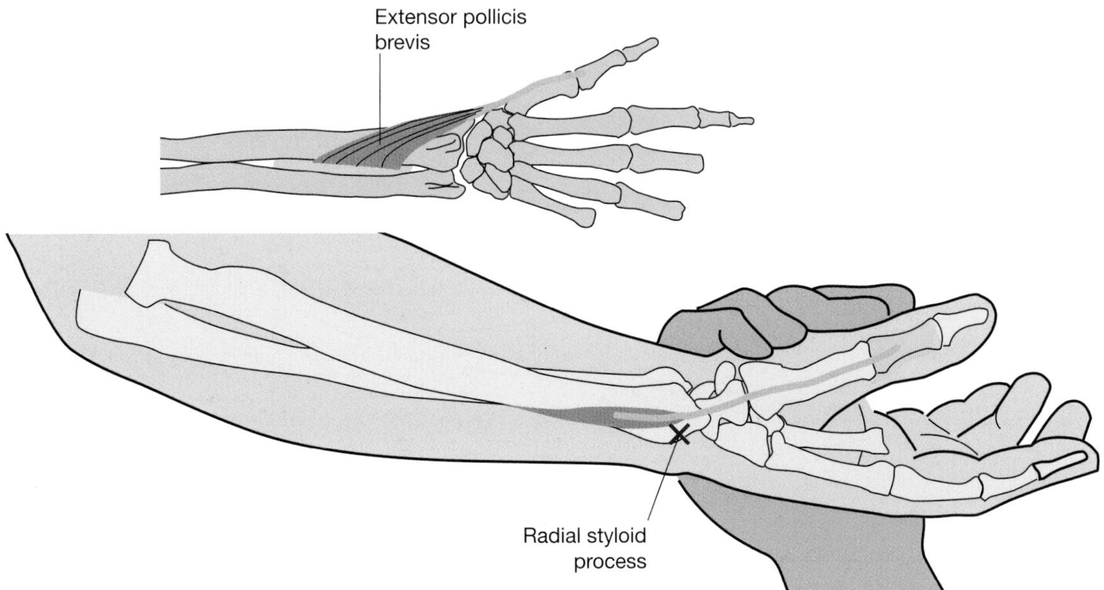

Figure 10.77 The extensor pollicis brevis. Note that the tendon rides over the radial styloid process, and this is a common site of tenosynovitis, also known as de Quervain's syndrome.

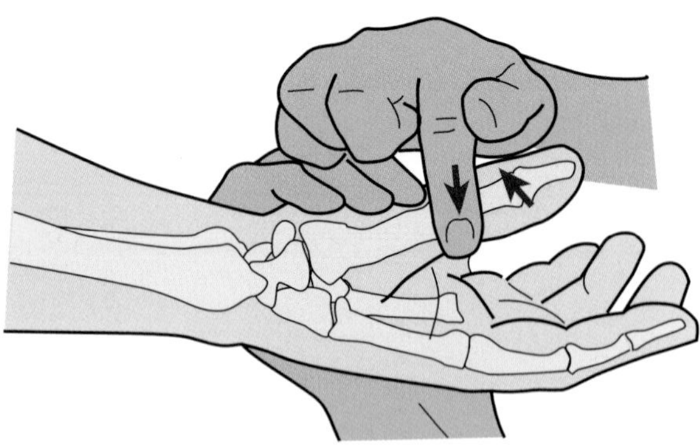

Figure 10.78 Testing extension of the metacarpophalangeal joint of the thumb.

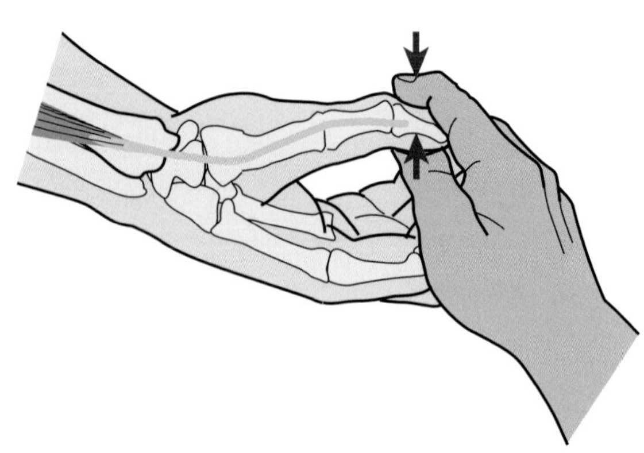

Figure 10.79 Testing extension of the interphalangeal joint of the thumb. The extensor pollicis brevis also extends the metacarpophalangeal and carpometacarpal joints of the thumb.

(Figure 10.87). They are innervated by the median and ulnar nerves, respectively.

- Position of patient: Sitting.
- Resisted test: The patient attempts to bring the palmar surfaces of the tips of the thumb and fifth finger together. Apply resistance against the anterior aspect of the first and fifth metacarpals so as to pry them apart (Figure 10.88). The muscles can be tested separately to note their individual strengths. Note that the patient can attempt to flex the thumb with the flexor pollicis longus and brevis in the plane of the palm. Opposition occurs with the thumb away from the palm.

Weakness of opposition of the thumb and fifth finger results in the inability to hold a pencil and grasp objects firmly.

Neurological Examination

Motor

The innervation and spinal levels of the muscles that function across the wrist and hand are outlined in Table 10.1.

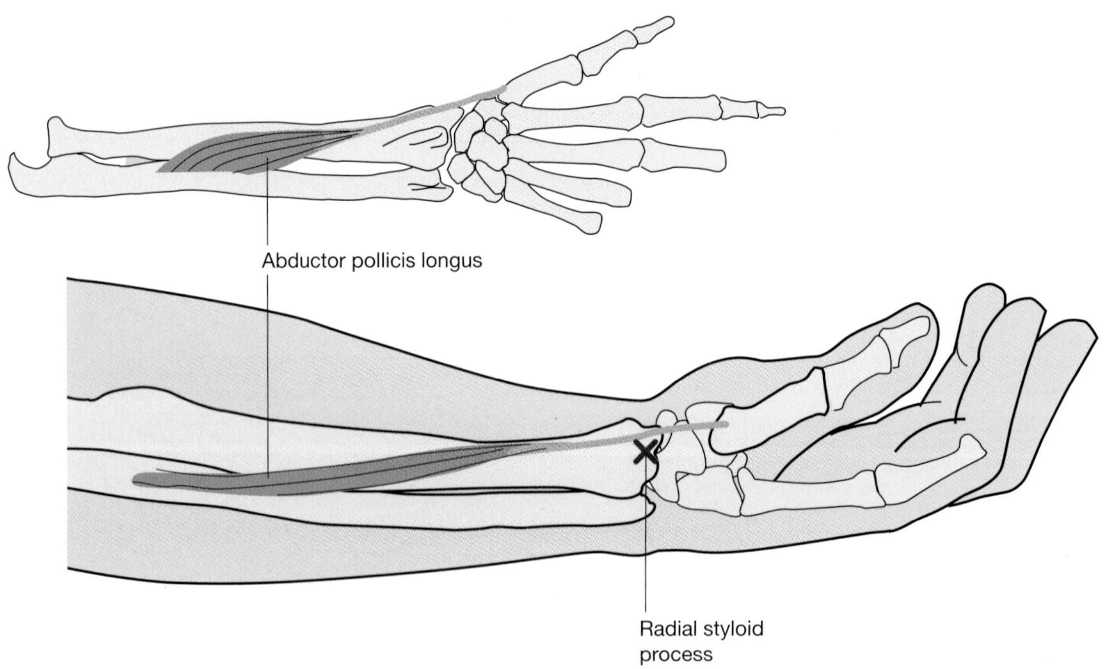

Figure 10.80 The abductor pollicis longus. Note that the tendon rides over the radial styloid process and is often affected by tenosynovitis in de Quervain's syndrome.

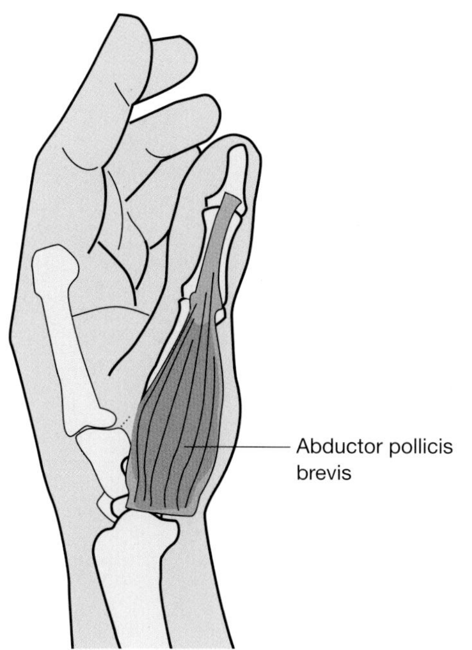

Figure 10.81 The abductor pollicis brevis.

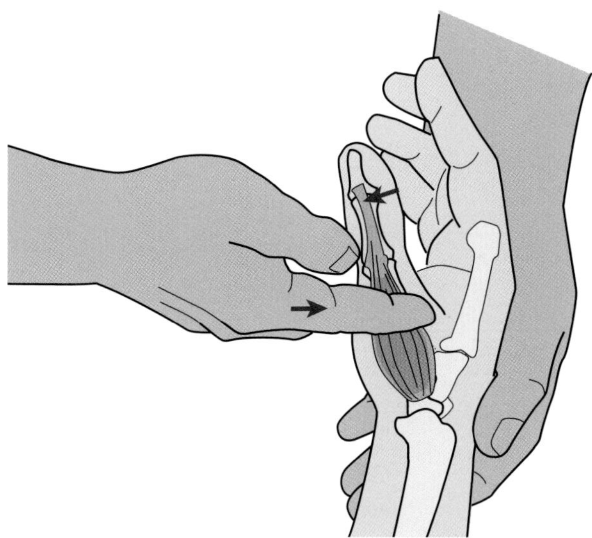

Figure 10.83 Testing abduction of the metacarpophalangeal joint of the thumb. The abductor pollicis brevis is weak in patients with carpal tunnel syndrome.

Sensation

Light touch and pinprick sensation should be checked in the wrist and hand after the motor examination. The dermatomes for the hand are C6, C7, and C8 (Figure 10.89). Peripheral nerves and their distributions in the wrist and hand are shown in Figures 10.90 and 10.91. Note the key sensory areas for the C6, C7, and C8 dermatomes.

Entrapment Neuropathies

Median Nerve

Entrapment of the median nerve within the carpal tunnel is extremely common (Figure 10.92). A variety of primary conditions are associated with carpal tunnel syndrome (Table 10.2). The definitive diagnosis of carpal tunnel syndrome is made with electrodiagnostic studies. Pain or numbness of the thumb, index and

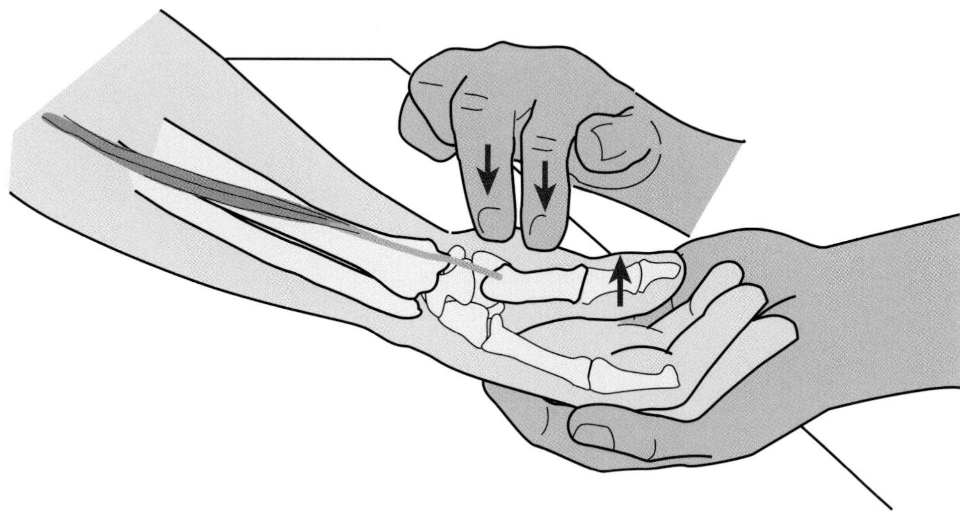

Figure 10.82 Testing abduction of the carpometacarpal joint of the thumb.

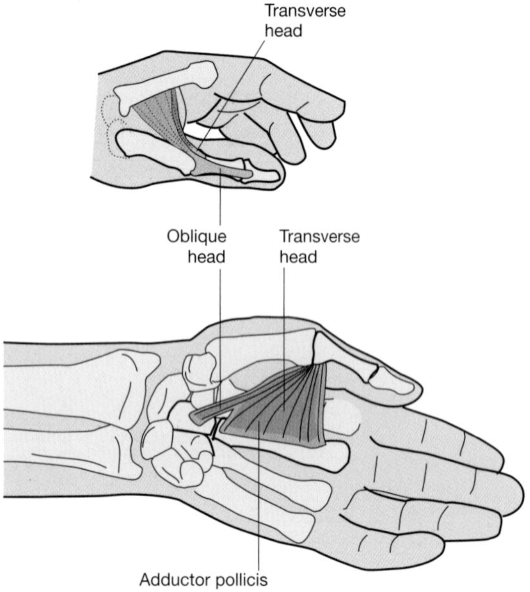

Figure 10.84 The adductor pollicis.

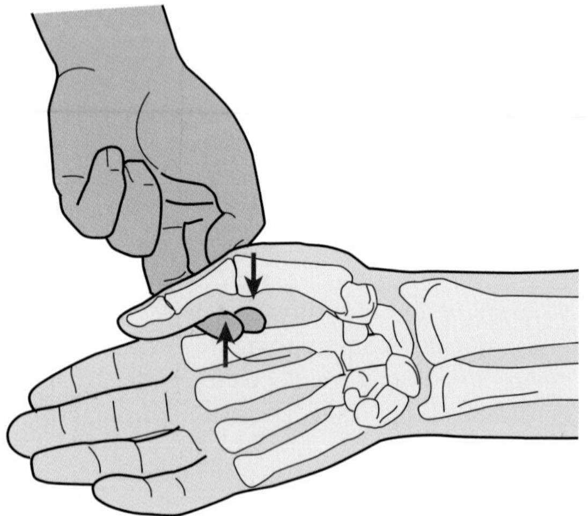

Figure 10.85 Testing adduction of the thumb.

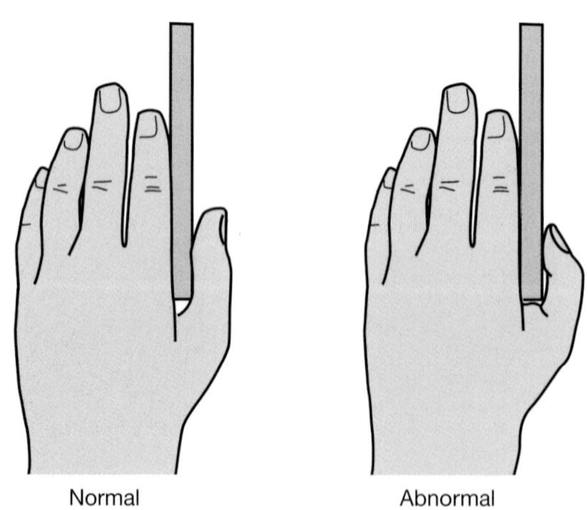

Figure 10.86 Froment's sign. The patient will flex the interphalangeal joint of the thumb to compensate for weakness of the adductor pollicis seen in ulnar nerve injury.

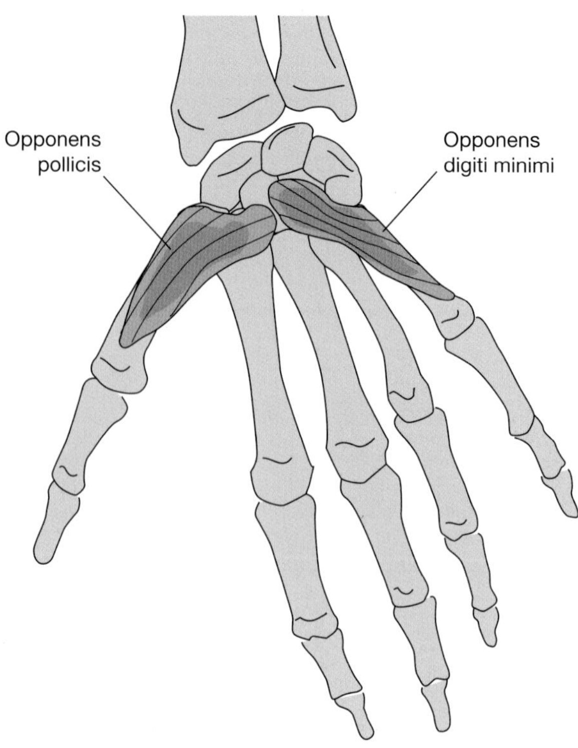

Figure 10.87 The opponens pollicis and the opponens digiti minimi muscles.

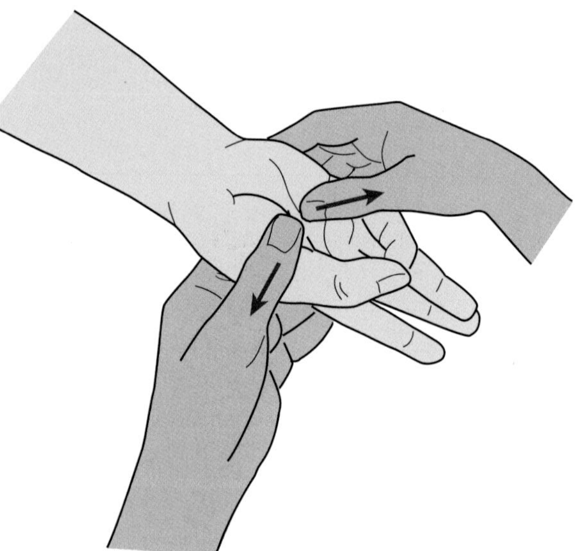

Figure 10.88 Testing opposition of the thumb and fifth finger.

Table 10.1 Muscle, Innervation, and Root Levels of the Hand and Wrist

Movement	Muscles	Innervation	Root Levels
Flexion of wrist	Flexor carpi radialis	Median	C6, C7
	Flexor carpi ulnaris	Ulnar	C8, T1
Extension of wrist	Extensor carpi radialis longus	Radial	C6, C7 (radial)
	Extensor carpi radialis brevis	Posterior interosseous (radial)	C6, C7, C8
	Extensor carpi ulnaris	Posterior interosseous (radial)	
Flexion of fingers	Flexor digitorum profundus	Anterior interosseous profundus (median): lateral two digits	C8, T1
	Flexor digitorum sublimis	Ulnar: medial two digits median	C8, T1
	Lumbricals	First and second: median Third and fourth: ulnar (deep terminal branch)	C7, C8, T1
	Interossei	Ulnar (deep terminal branch)	C7, C8, T1
	Flexor digiti minimi	Ulnar (deep terminal branch) little finger	C8, T1 C8, T1 C8, T1
Extension of fingers	Extensor digitorum communis	Posterior interosseous (radial)	C6, C7, C8
	Extensor indicis (second finger)	Posterior interosseous (radial)	C7, C8
	Extensor digiti minimi (little finger)	Posterior interosseous (radial)	C6, C7, C8
Abduction of fingers (with fingers extended)	Dorsal interossei	Ulnar (deep terminal branch)	C8, T1
	Abductor digiti minimi (little finger)	Ulnar (deep terminal branch)	C8, T1
Adduction of fingers (with fingers extended)	Palmar interossei	Ulnar (deep terminal branch)	C8, T1
Flexion of thumb	Flexor pollicis brevis	Superficial head: median (lateral terminal branch)	C8, T1
	Flexor pollicis longus	Deep head: ulnar	C8, T1
	Opponens pollicis	Anterior interosseous (median) Median (lateral terminal branch)	C8, T1 C8, T1
Extension of thumb	Extensor pollicis longus	Posterior interosseous (radial)	C6, C7, C8
	Extensor pollicis brevis	Posterior interosseous (radial)	C6, C7
	Abductor pollicis longus	Posterior interosseous (radial)	C6, C7
Abduction of thumb	Abductor pollicis longus	Posterior interosseous (radial)	C6, C7
	Abductor pollicis brevis	Median (lateral terminal branch)	C6, C7, C8
Adduction of thumb	Adductor pollicis	Ulnar (deep terminal branch)	C8, T1
Opposition of thumb and little finger	Opponens pollicis	Median (lateral terminal branch)	C8, T1
	Flexor pollicis brevis	Superficial head: median (lateral terminal branch)	C8, T1
	Abductor pollicis brevis	Median (lateral terminal branch)	C6, C7, C8
	Opponens digiti minimi	Ulnar (deep terminal branch)	C8, T1

middle fingers, as well as thenar atrophy may be noted in the patient with carpal tunnel syndrome.

Various tests have been used to diagnose carpal tunnel syndrome on physical examination. They include Tinel's test, the tourniquet test, and Phalen's test.

Tinel's Test

This test is performed by tapping over the median nerve, which is located just medial to the flexor carpi radialis tendon at the most proximal aspect of the palm (Figure 10.93). The test result is positive when the patient reports pain or tingling in the first three digits (https://www.youtube.com/watch?v=2wNGyEPdv_M).

Tourniquet Test

This test attempts to exacerbate the median neuropathy in the carpal tunnel by causing temporary ischemia. A blood pressure cuff is inflated proximal to the elbow, about where you would take measurements for systolic pressure. The test result is positive if the patient notes numbness or tingling in the

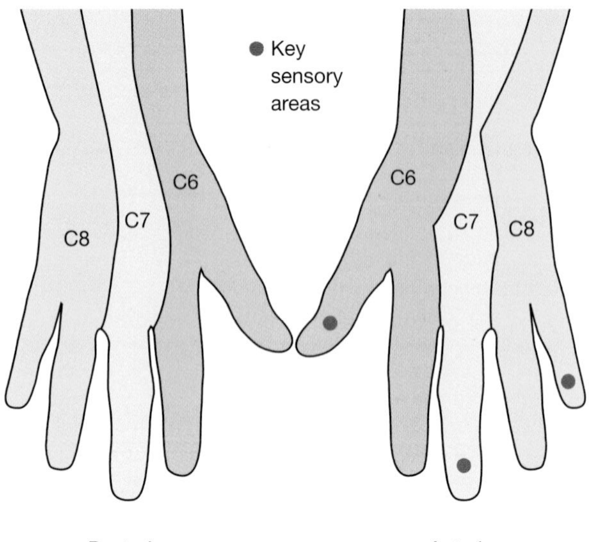

Figure 10.89 The dermatomes of the hand and wrist. Note the key sensory areas for C6, C7, and C8 at the interphalangeal joints of the thumb and the long and fifth fingers, respectively.

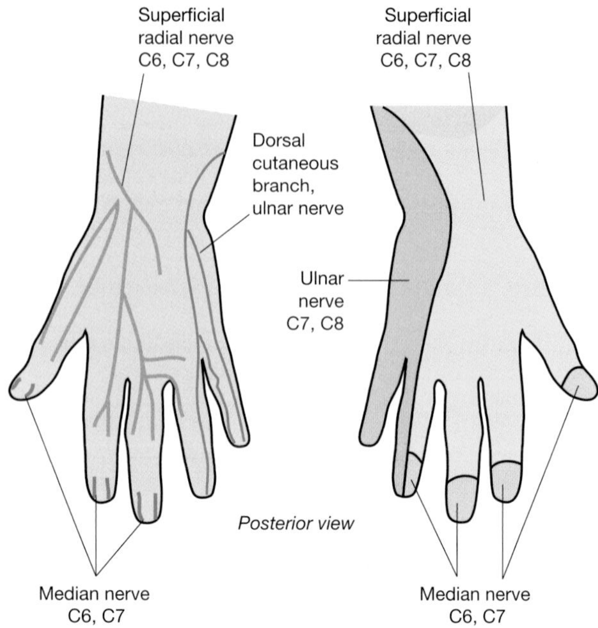

Figure 10.91 The posterior view of the wrist and hand shows the peripheral nerves and their respective territories.

distribution of the median nerve within 60 seconds. This test produces a high rate of false-positive results.

Phalen's Test

This test makes use of the fact that the carpal tunnel narrows in a position of increased wrist flexion. The patient is asked to flex both of the wrists against one another. The test result is positive if the patient notes paresthesias or numbness in the thumb, index, or middle fingers after holding this position for 60 seconds or less (Figure 10.94). This test has the fewest false-negative results (https://www.youtube.com/watch?v=952eYGo19gE).

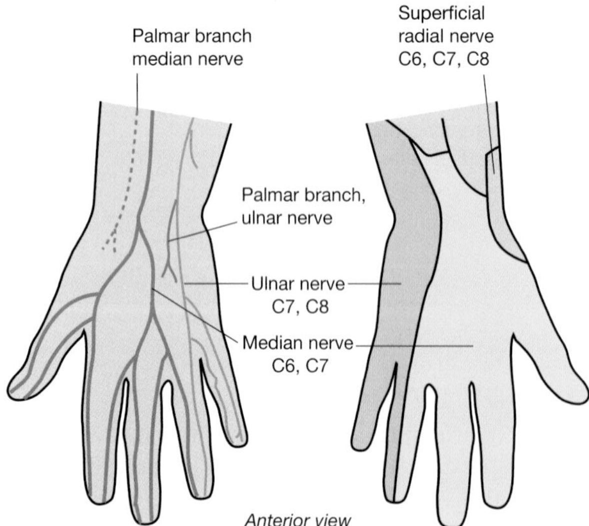

Figure 10.90 The anterior view of the wrist and hand shows the peripheral nerves and their respective territories.

Ulnar Nerve

The ulnar nerve gives off a dorsal cutaneous branch approximately 8 cm proximal to the wrist (Figure 10.95). This branch has no motor function.

The ulnar nerve continues into the wrist through Guyon's canal (Figure 10.96). There are two motor branches of the ulnar nerve in the hand and one sensory branch to the palmar aspect of the medial hand.

Dorsal Cutaneous Ulnar Nerve Entrapment

This sensory branch of the ulnar nerve may be injured by a fracture of the ulna, a ganglion cyst, or an ulnar artery aneurysm. Loss of sensation on the dorsal medial aspect of the hand will be noted. Hand function will otherwise be normal.

Ulnar Nerve Compression at Guyon's Canal

Compression of the ulnar nerve in Guyon's canal (see Figure 10.96) most often results from a ganglion, but can also occur with rheumatoid arthritis or trauma. The findings on examination include weakness of the ulnar-innervated intrinsic hand muscles, which

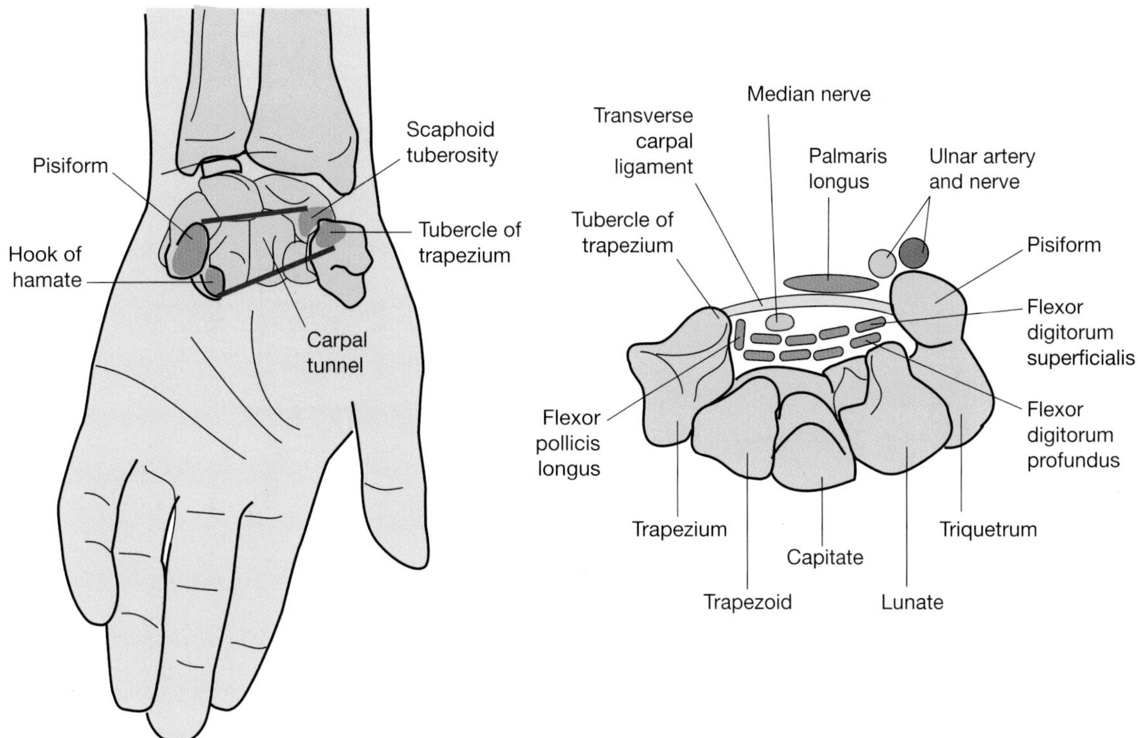

Figure 10.92 The carpal tunnel and its contents. The roof of the tunnel is formed by the transverse carpal ligament. The flexor tendons of all five fingers and the flexor carpi radialis are located within the carpal tunnel, along with the median nerve. Note that the tunnel is located at the proximal palm and not under the creases of the wrist.

include the interossei and the medial two lumbricals. If the superficial sensory branch to the fourth and fifth digits is involved, decreased sensation will be noted on the palmar aspect of these fingers. A characteristic posture of the hand known as a benediction deformity (Figure 10.97) results from ulnar nerve damage at Guyon's canal, affecting both the hypothenar and intrinsic muscles.

Damage to the median and ulnar nerves at the wrist, which occurs most commonly with trauma, results in a deformity known as a *claw hand* (Figure 10.98). This is also referred to as an *intrinsic minus hand.*

Table 10.2 Disorders Associated with Carpal Tunnel Syndrome

Trauma
Wrist fracture (Colles' fracture, scaphoid fracture, etc.)
Wrist contusion or hematoma
Endocrine disorders
Hypothyroidism
Pregnancy
Diabetes mellitus
Menopause
Obesity
Inflammation
Tenosynovitis
Others
Gout, inflammatory arthritides
Ganglion cysts
Osteoarthritis of the carpal bones
Generalized edema from any cause

Special Tests

Finkelstein's Test (de Quervain's Syndrome)

This test is used to diagnose tenosynovitis of the first dorsal compartment of the wrist, which contains the tendons of the abductor pollicis longus and extensor pollicis brevis muscles (Figure 10.99). Pain and swelling are usually present over the radial styloid process. A ganglion cyst may be noted. Finkelstein's test is performed by having the patient place the thumb inside the closed fist. Take the patient's hand and deviate the hand and wrist in the ulnar direction

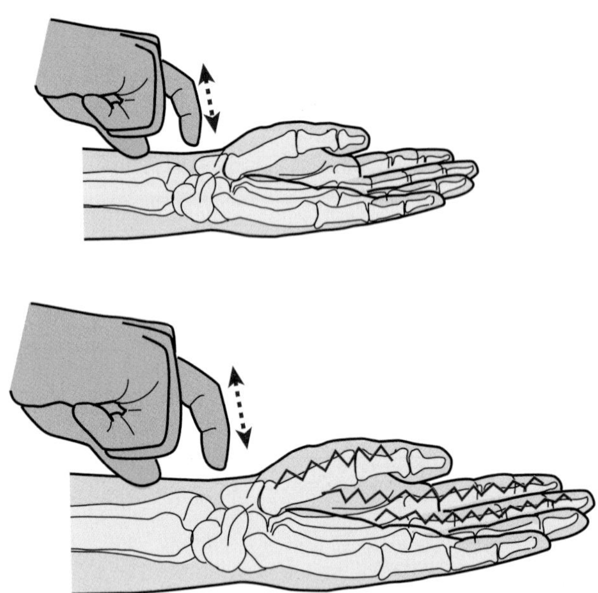

Figure 10.93 Testing Tinel's sign at the wrist for carpal tunnel syndrome.

to stretch the tendons of the first extensor compartment. Pain over the radial styloid process is pathognomonic of de Quervain's syndrome. Arthritis of the first carpometacarpal joint will also sometimes cause pain with the maneuver.

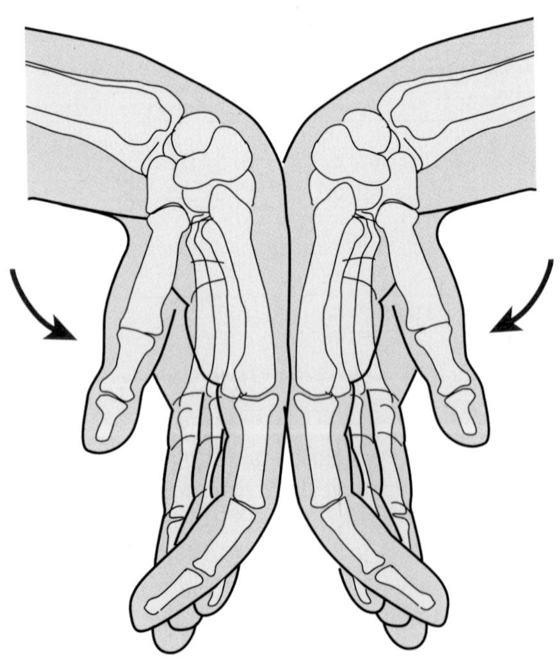

Figure 10.94 Phalen's test. This position is held for at least 60 seconds.

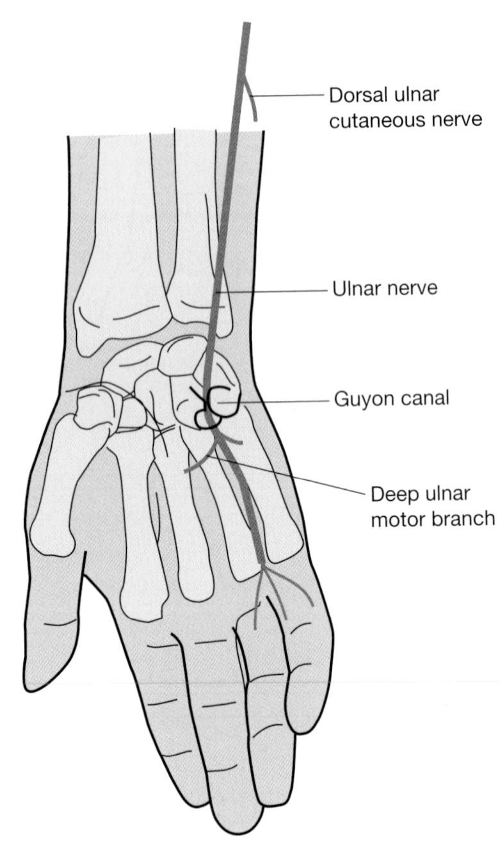

Figure 10.95 The ulnar nerve and its branches.

Tenosynovitis of the hand and wrist is encountered frequently. Tenderness to palpation is noted in characteristic locations (Figure 10.100). Passively stretching the involved muscle will also produce pain (https://www.youtube.com/watch?v=Z6P7uQSBuSo).

Tests for Flexibility and Stability of the Joint

Bunnell-Littler Test (Intrinsic Muscles Versus Contracture)

This test is useful in determining the cause of restricted flexion of the proximal interphalangeal joints of the fingers (Figure 10.101). A limitation in flexion at these joints may be caused by tightness of the intrinsic muscles (interossei and lumbricals) or secondary to contracture of the joint capsule. The purpose of the test is to put the finger in a position of relaxation of the intrinsic muscles by flexing the metacarpophalangeal joint. Attempt to flex the proximal interphalangeal joint (Figure 10.102). If the joint can be flexed, the difficulty in flexion with the metacarpophalangeal joint extended is due to

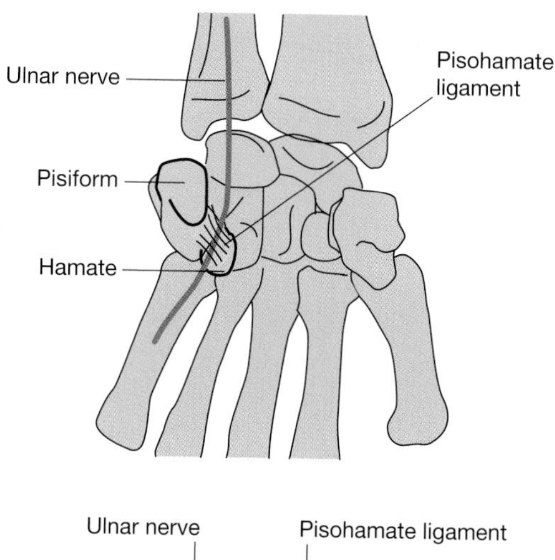

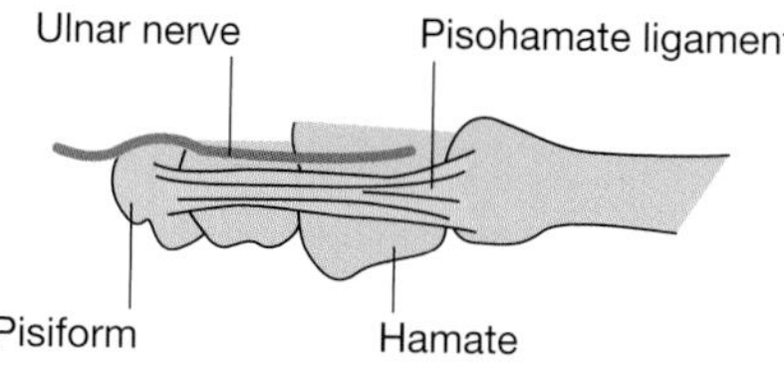

Figure 10.96 The anatomy of Guyon's canal. The ulnar nerve enters the wrist through this canal. It gives off a superficial sensory branch and a deep motor branch. Three types of lesions are possible at Guyon's canal. The trunk may be affected, the sensory branch may be affected, or the deep motor branch may be affected. These lesions can occur simultaneously. Injury to the ulnar nerve at Guyon's canal can result from pressure due to crutch walking, pressure from bicycle handlebars, or a pneumatic drill.

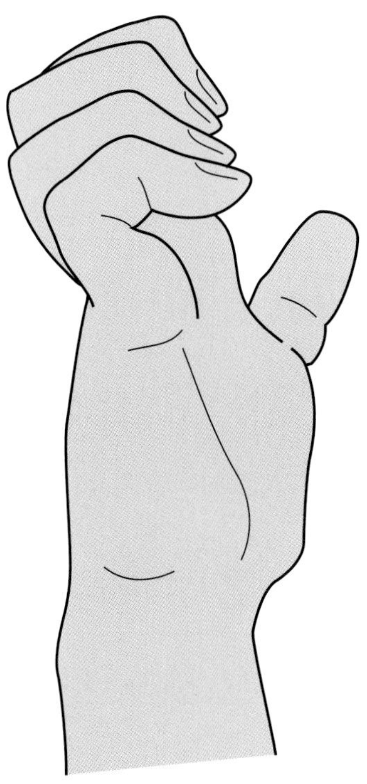

Figure 10.98 The claw hand deformity results from loss of intrinsic muscles with overactivity of the extensor digitorum, causing hyperextension of the metacarpophalangeal joints. This is most often caused by combined damage to the median and ulnar nerves at the wrist.

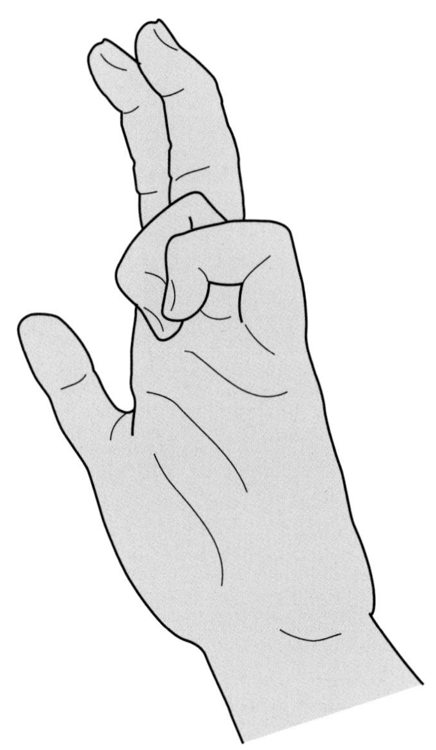

Figure 10.97 The benediction hand deformity results from damage to the ulnar nerve. There is wasting of the interosseous muscles, the hypothenar muscles, and the two medial lumbrical muscles.

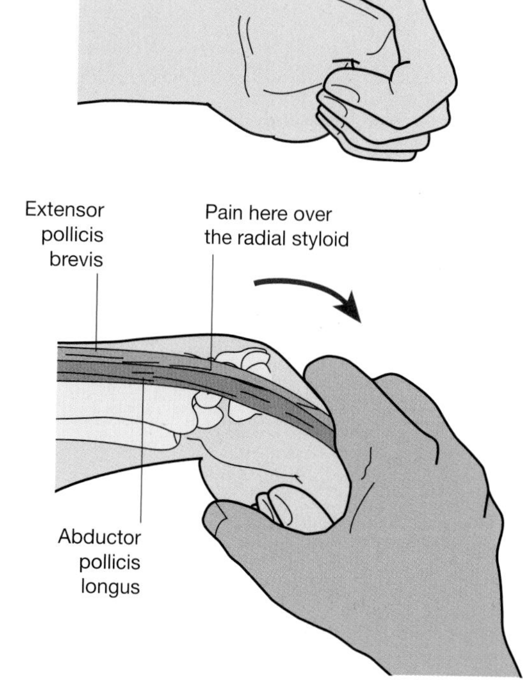

Figure 10.99 Finkelstein's test is used to diagnose tenosynovitis of the first dorsal compartment of the wrist, which includes the extensor pollicis brevis and abductor pollicis longus muscles.

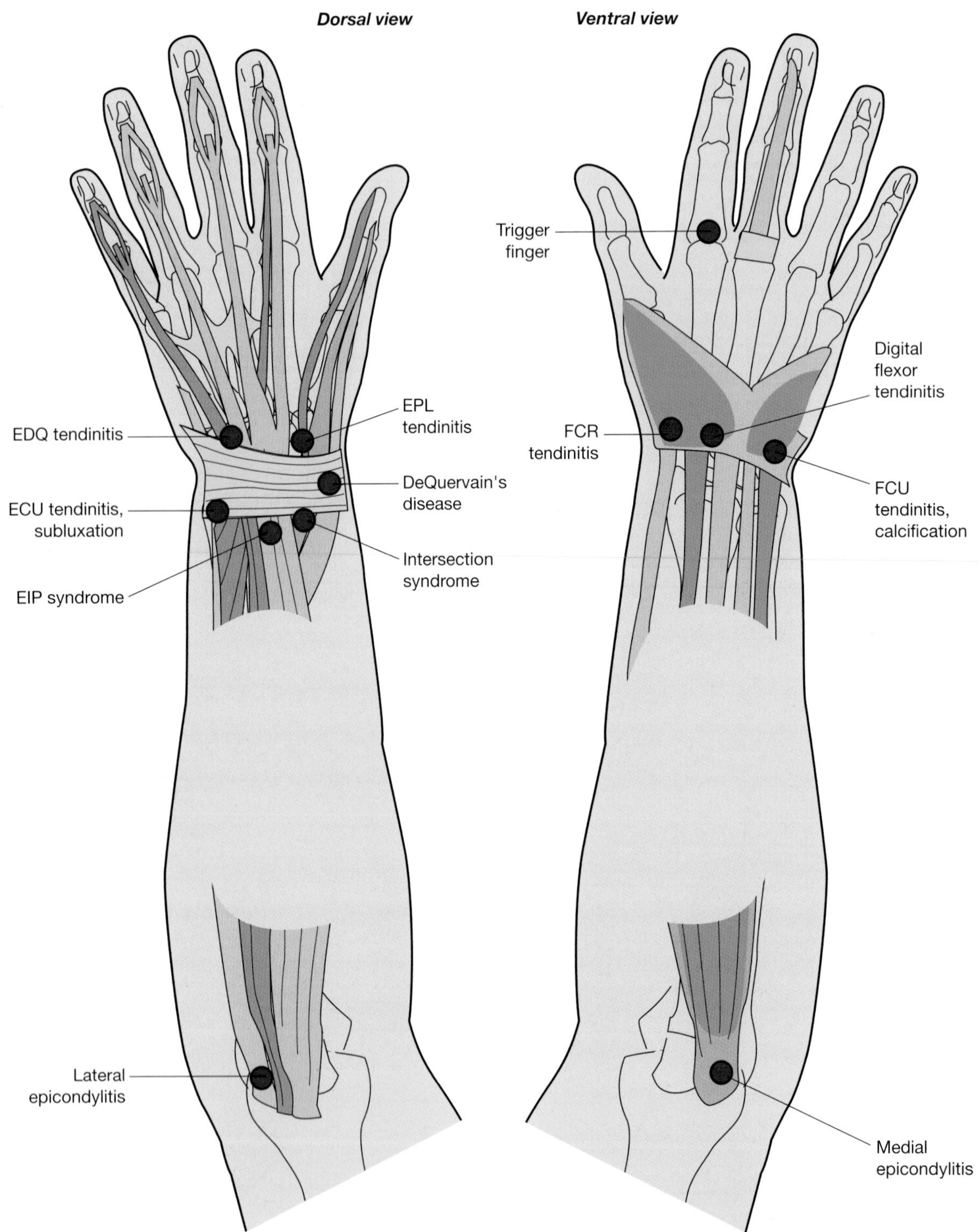

Figure 10.100 Common locations for tendinitis of the hand and wrist are shown posteriorly (left) and anteriorly (right).

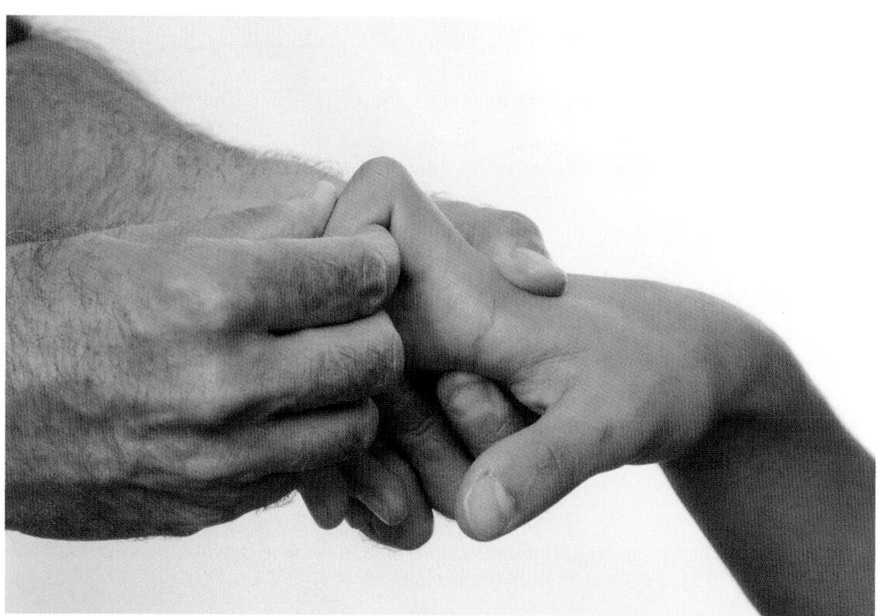

Figure 10.101 The Bunnell-Littler test. Put the metacarpophalangeal joint in slight extension and attempt to flex the proximal interphalangeal joint. If you are unable to do so, there is either a joint capsular contracture or tightness of the intrinsic muscles.

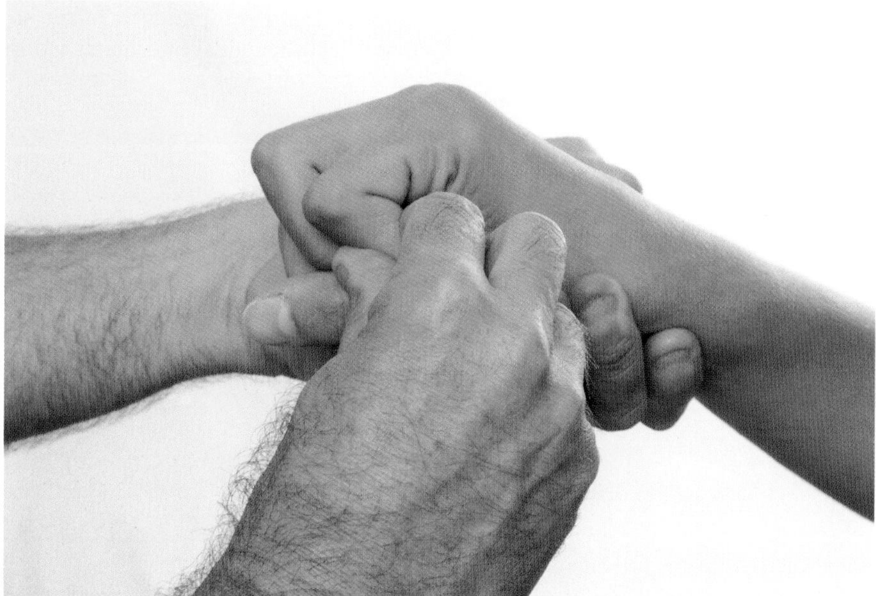

Figure 10.102 Placing the metacarpophalangeal joint in flexion relaxes the intrinsic muscles. If you are now able to flex the proximal interphalangeal joint, the intrinsic muscles are tight.

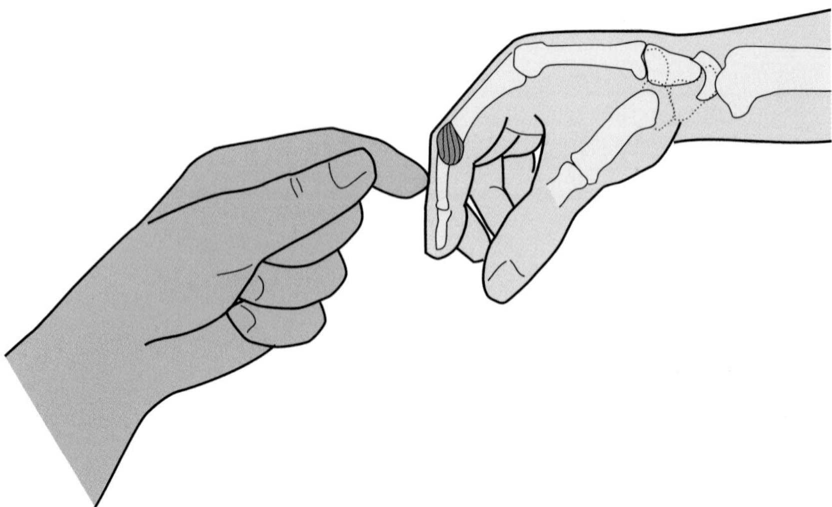

Figure 10.103 If you are unable to flex the proximal interphalangeal joint, even with the intrinsic muscles in a relaxed position, there is a joint capsular contracture of the proximal interphalangeal joint.

tightness of the intrinsic muscles. If a joint contracture is present, relaxing the intrinsic muscles will have no effect on the restricted mobility of the proximal interphalangeal joint and you will be unable to flex this joint in any position of the finger (Figure 10.103) (https://www.youtube.com/watch?v=dZ1QAxTpf0M).

Retinacular Test

The retinacular test is used to determine the cause of the patient's inability to flex the distal interphalangeal joint. This inability may be caused by either joint contracture or tightness of the retinacular ligaments. Hold the patient's finger so that the proximal interphalangeal and metacarpophalangeal joints

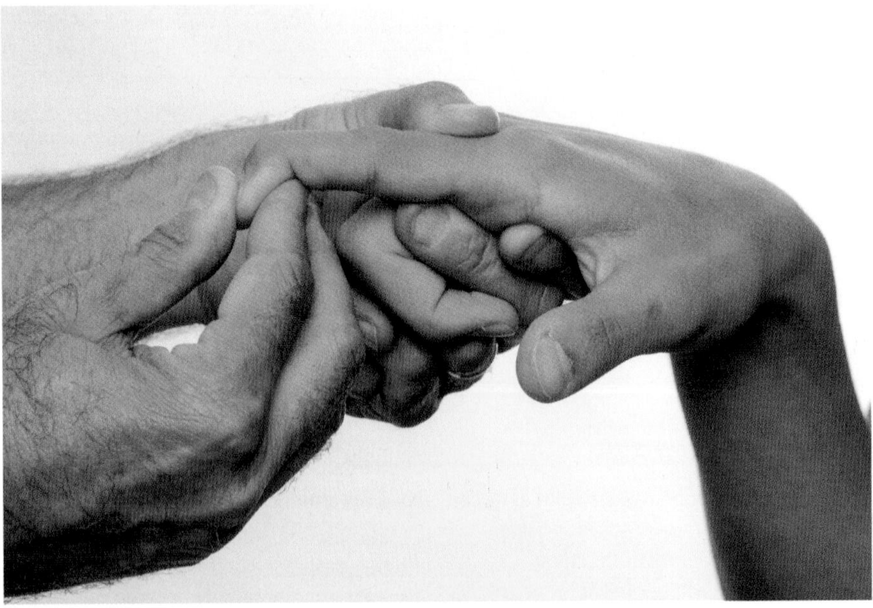

Figure 10.104 Test for retinacular ligament tightness. Attempt to flex the distal interphalangeal joint (DIP) with the proximal interphalangeal (PIP) and metacarpophalangeal (MCP) joints in neutral.

are in neutral position. Now support the finger and attempt to flex the distal interphalangeal joint (Figure 10.104). If the distal interphalangeal joint does not flex, perform the retinacular test by initially flexing the proximal interphalangeal joint to relax the retinacular ligaments (Figure 10.105). Now try to flex the distal interphalangeal joint with the ligaments relaxed. If the distal interphalangeal joint still does not flex, there is a contracture of the distal interphalangeal joint (https://www.youtube.com/watch?v=guUz5nkYlkQ).

Scaphoid–Lunate Dissociation (Watson's) Test

This test is used to diagnose abnormal separation of the lunate and scaphoid bones (Figure 10.106). The normal separation should be less than 2 mm (Watson, 1988).

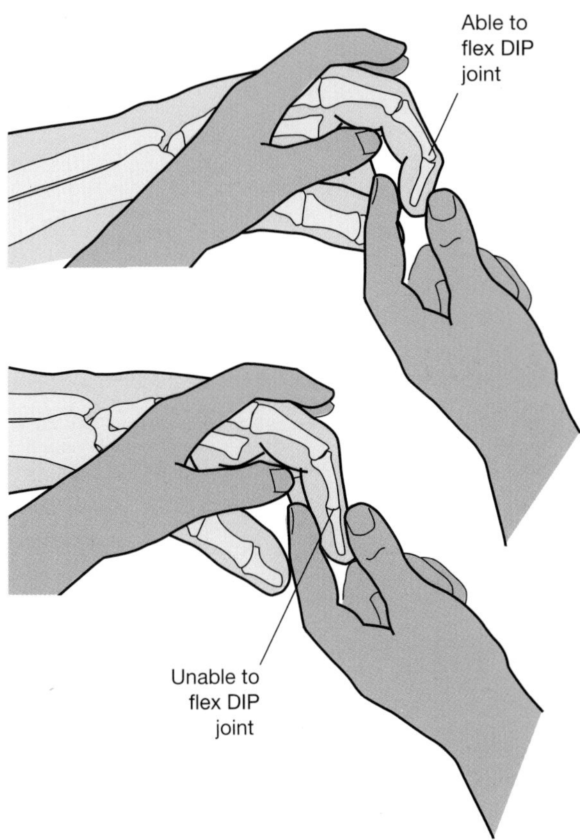

Figure 10.105 Testing for retinacular ligament tightness is performed by first relaxing the proximal interphalangeal joint into flexion. If you can now flex the distal interphalangeal joint, the retinacular ligaments are tight. If the proximal interphalangeal joint is flexed and you still cannot flex the distal interphalangeal joint (DIP), there is a contracture at the distal interphalangeal joint.

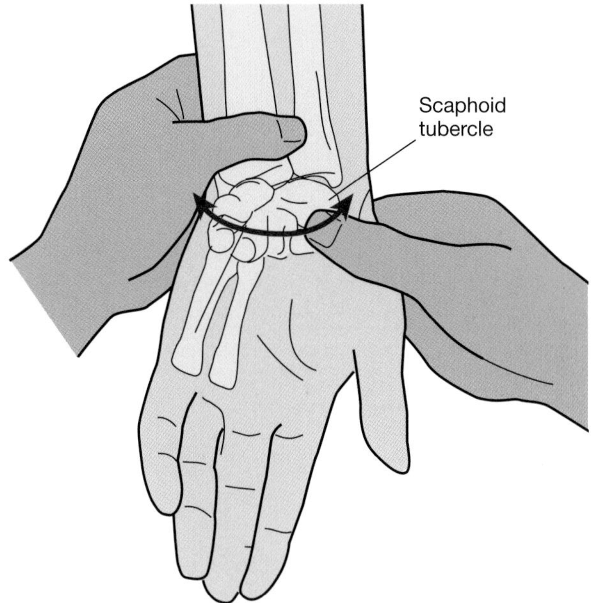

Figure 10.106 Watson's test for scaphoid–lunate dissociation. The scaphoid tubercle is palpated with the thumb and the wrist is passively moved from ulnar to radial deviation with your other hand. The presence of pain, crepitus, or occasionally an audible click reflects a positive test result.

Increased separation due to a fracture displacement causes disruption of the wrist and can lead to arthritis. This test result is difficult to interpret. Stabilize the patient's radius with one hand while your thumb presses against the scaphoid tubercle. Take the patient's hand and passively glide the wrist in an ulnar-to-radial direction. The test result is positive if the patient complains of pain or if you note crepitus or an audible click. Ulnar deviation of the wrist brings the tubercle of the scaphoid out from behind the radius (https://www.youtube.com/watch?v=FTIbOdQV164).

Allen's Test

This test is used to check the patency of the radial and ulnar arteries at the level of the wrist (Figure 10.107). The patient is first asked to open and close the hand firmly several times. The hand is then squeezed very tightly to prevent any further arterial flow into the hand. Place one thumb over the radial artery and the other thumb over the ulnar artery at the wrist and press firmly. Now ask the patient to open the hand while you maintain pressure over both arteries. Remove your thumb from one of the arteries and watch for the hand to turn red. This indicates

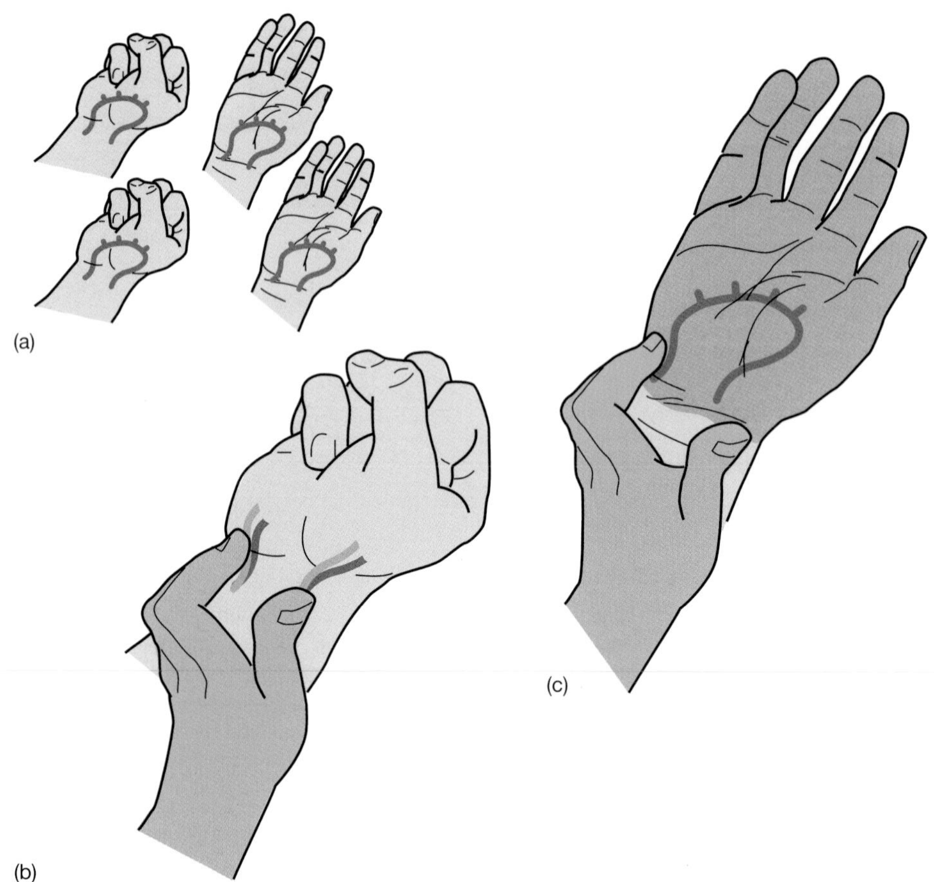

Figure 10.107 Allen's test is used to evaluate the patency of the radial and ulnar arteries at the wrist. (a) The hand is opened and closed rapidly and firmly. (b) Both arteries are compressed as the patient maintains a closed fist. (c) Release pressure over one of the arteries as the patient opens the hand and observe for flushing of the hand. Normal color should return to the entire hand.

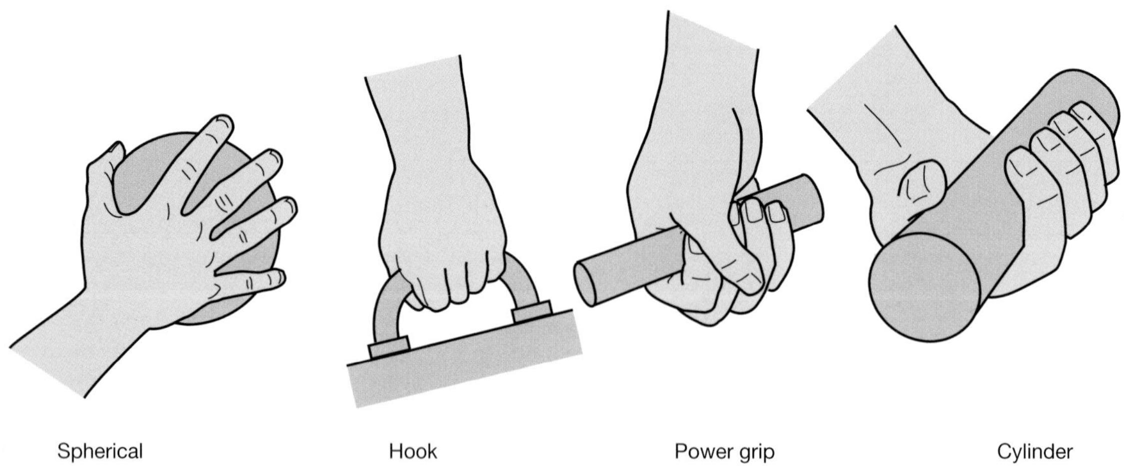

Figure 10.108 Types of power grips include the spherical, hook, fist, and cylinder grips.

normal circulation of that artery. Repeat the test, releasing pressure from the other artery. Check both arteries and both hands for comparison (https://www.youtube.com/watch?v=gdgomN6TsuE).

Grip and Pinch Evaluation

Different types of power grips and pinches are shown in Figures 10.108 and 10.109. Observe the patient's ability to posture the fingers and hand as illustrated.

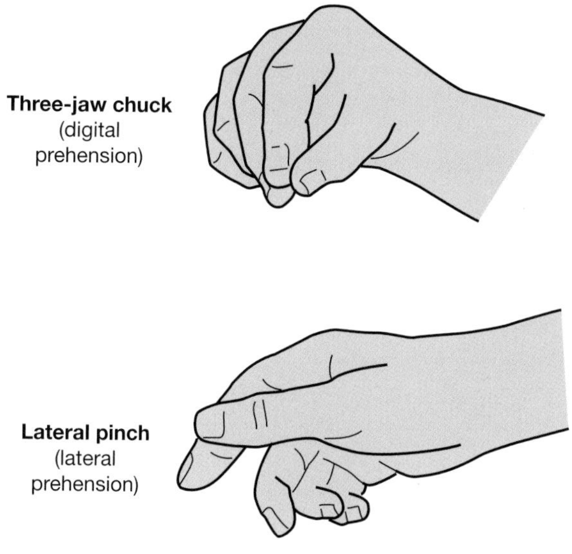

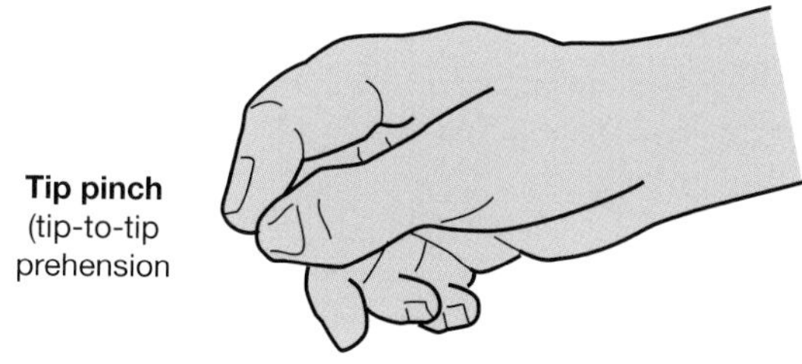

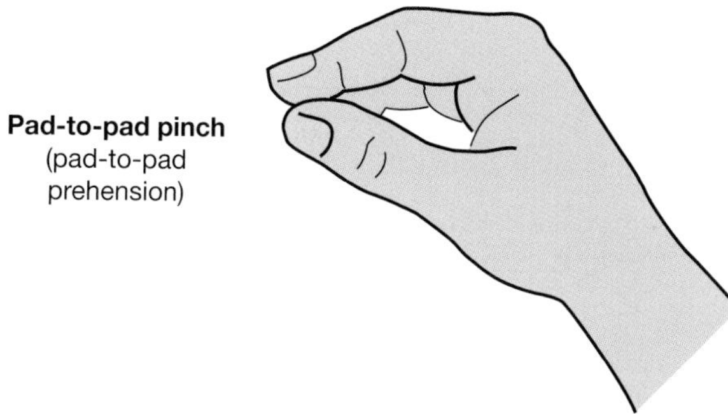

Figure 10.109 Various types of pinches.

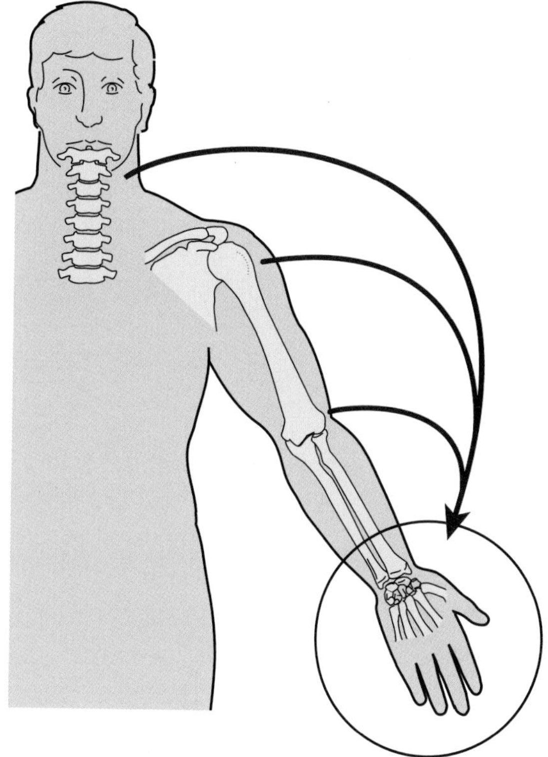

Figure 10.110 Pain may be referred to the hand and wrist from the neck, shoulder, or elbow.

Referred Pain Patterns

The patient may complain of wrist and hand pain and in fact have pathology in the neck, shoulder, or elbow (Figure 10.110). Any disease process affecting the sixth, seventh, or eighth cervical nerves or the first thoracic nerve will affect the function of the hand. Damage to the brachial plexus or peripheral nerves higher up in the arm will also affect hand function. Shoulder or elbow joint pathology may also refer pain to the hand.

Radiological Views

Radiological views of the hand and wrist are shown in Figures 10.111 and 10.112.

U = Ulna
R = Radius
S = Scaphoid
M = Metacarpals
P = Phalanges
W = Wrist joint
CMC = First carpometacarpal joint

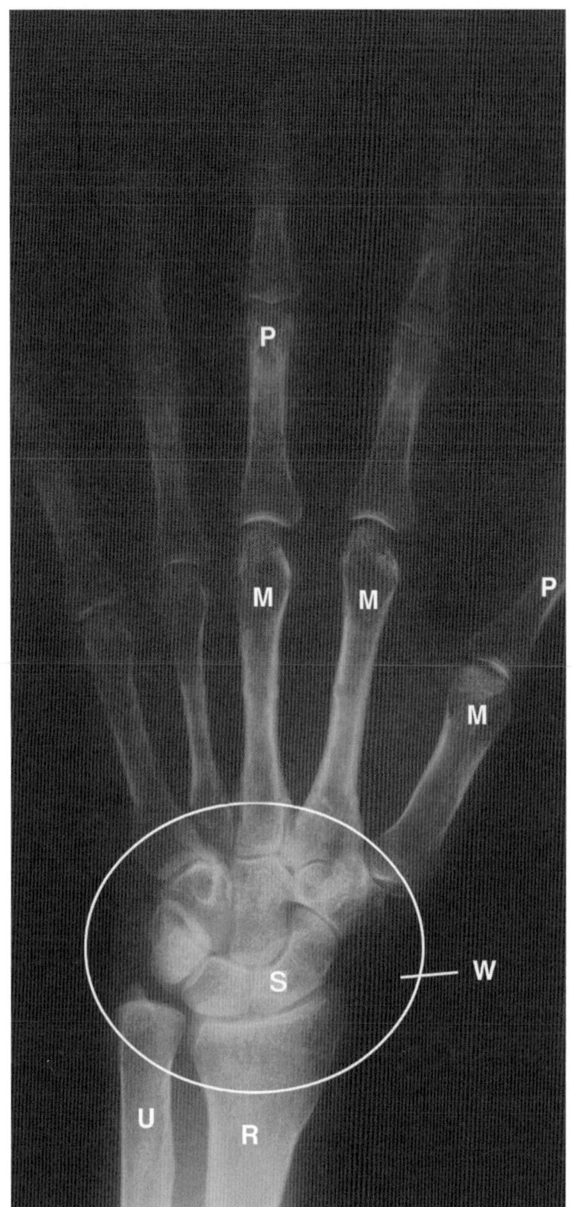

Figure 10.111 Anteroposterior view of the wrist and hand.

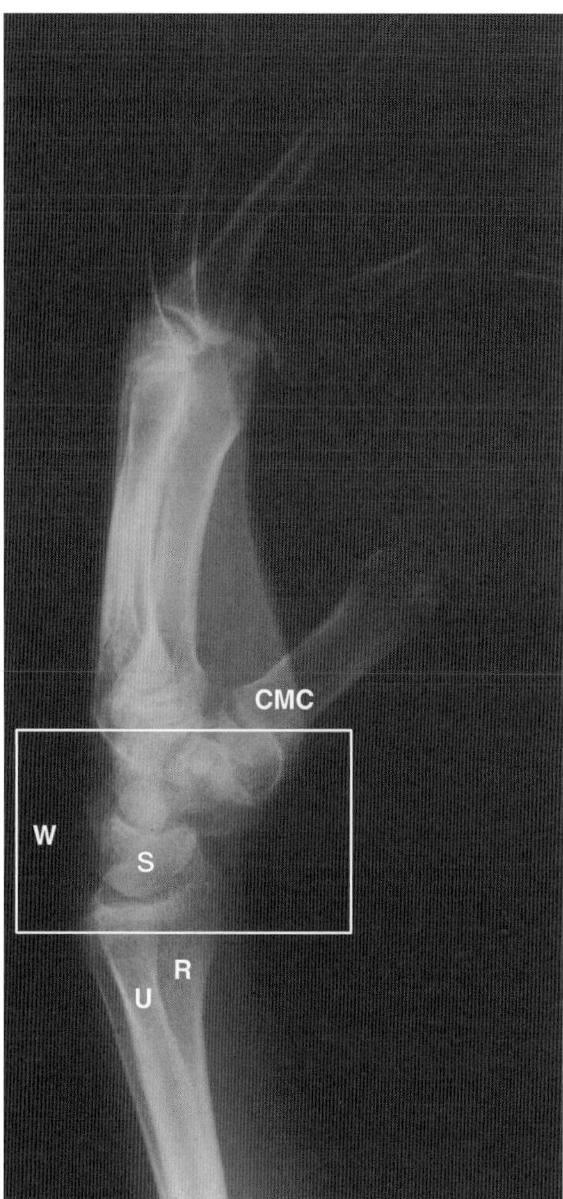

Figure 10.112 Lateral view of the wrist and hand.

PARADIGM FOR CARPAL TUNNEL SYNDROME

A 45-year-old female office worker presents with complaints of "pins and needles" in her dominant right hand. She states that she has been having pain in her neck, upper arm, and thumb.

Her symptoms seem to be aggravated by typing for long periods of time at her word processor. She is often awakened during the night by pain in her hand. She can find relief by shaking her hand or holding it under warm water. She recalls no injuries to either her hand or neck, and has no difficulty rotating her head when driving. She has recently been told that she has an "underactive thyroid" and has had a 20-pound weight gain. The remainder of her medical history is unremarkable.

On physical examination, the patient is a slightly obese woman in no apparent distress. She has full range of motion of her cervical spine and upper extremity joints without pain. There are no symptoms produced with vertical compression applied to the head and neck. She has diminished light touch in the distal palmar aspects of the thumb, index, and long fingers. She has positive Tinel's and Phalen's tests. X-rays of the cervical spine and hand are reported as showing no pathology. Electrodiagnostic studies (electromyography (EMC) and nerve conduction) demonstrate no motor deficits in the upper extremity, but confirm increased latency of the signal across the wrist.

This paradigm is consistent with distal rather than proximal nerve injury because of:

A history of repetitive hand/wrist movements
No history of trauma to the neck
History of a possible contributory collateral medical condition
Symptoms suggestive of compromised circulation to the nerve (see Table 10.2)

CHAPTER 11

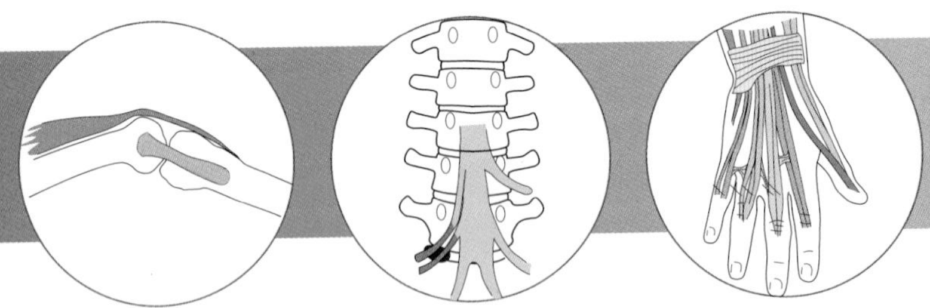

The Hip

FURTHER INFORMATION

Please refer to Chapter 2 for an overview of the sequence of a physical examination. For purposes of length and to avoid having to repeat anatomy more than once, the palpation section appears directly after the section on subjective examination and before any section on testing, rather than at the end of each chapter. The order in which the examination is performed should be based on your experience and personal preference as well as the presentation of the patient.

Functional Anatomy

The hip is a large, deep ball-and-socket articulation. As such, it is quite stable, while permitting a significant range of motion. To achieve stability, the hip relies on a combination of ligamentous and articular (i.e., acetabular, labrum) structures. The primary ligaments of the hips are the capsular Y ligament and the intra-articular ligamentum teres. Aside from the modest vascular supply the ligamentum provides to the femoral head, the ligamentum teres provides relatively little stability to the hip joint. The capsular Y ligament is, on the other hand, a significant stabilizer for the hip joint. It is important for its ability to shorten and tighten with extension and internal rotation, a fact found to be useful in the reduction of certain fractures. Since the hip is offset laterally from the midline of the body, unassisted it provides little stability to the torso during unilateral stance. During gait, the body's center of gravity is normally medial to the supporting limb. As such, ligamentous structures of the hip are insufficient to stabilize the body during the unilateral support phase of gait. For stability during gait, the body is critically dependent upon the muscles proximal to the hip joint.

The muscles providing medial–lateral stability are the glutei (minimus, medius, and maximus) and the iliotibial band (ITB) (with the tensor fasciae latae). These muscles and tissues lie lateral to the hip joint. In general, the hip can be visualized as a fulcrum on which the pelvis and torso are supported (Figure 11.1). The medial aspect of the fulcrum experiences the downward force of the body's weight (merging at a point in space 1 cm anterior to the first sacral segment in the midline of the body). The other side of the fulcrum is counterbalanced by the muscular contraction effort of the abductor muscles. The ratio of the relative lengths over which these two opposing forces work is 2:1. Hence, the glutei must be capable of exerting two times the body weight of contractile effort during unilateral stance in order to maintain the pelvis at equilibrium. A corollary of this is that during unilateral support, the hip will experience a total of three times body weight of compressive load (body weight + [2 × body weight] muscular contractile force across the hip joint). This is a sixfold increase

Musculoskeletal Examination, Fourth Edition. Jeffrey M. Gross, Joseph Fetto and Elaine Rosen.

Companion website: www.wiley.com/go/musculoskeletalexam

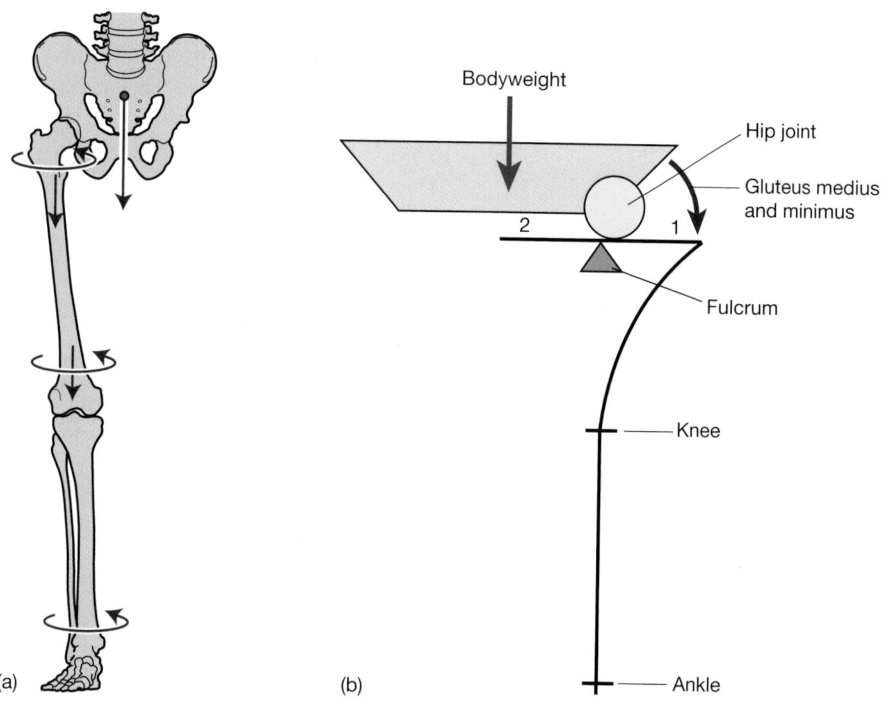

Figure 11.1 (a) The classic Koch model depicts the hip as a fulcrum of uneven lengths. Stability against the inward rotation of the pelvis during unilateral stance is provided dynamically by the abductor musculature (gluteus medius, gluteus minimus). (b) During unilateral support, the body's center of gravity creates a compression and varus moment deforming force at the hip, knee, and ankle of the supporting limb.

over the force experienced by the hip during bilateral stance.

The glutei are supplemented by the ITB, which is a broad fibrous sheath extending from the iliac crest of the pelvis to its attachment at the distal end of the femur and on across to the anterolateral aspect of the knee joint. As such, it functions as a tension band and has the important task of converting what would otherwise be a potentially unsustainable tensile load into a moderate and well-tolerated compression load along the lateral femoral cortex (Figures 11.2 and 11.3). The importance of these soft-tissue structures for proper hip function can be greatly appreciated when they are compromised by either pain, injury, or neurological impairment. The result will be a severely compromised and dysfunctional pattern of gait. The most dramatic demonstration of the importance of the ITB soft tissues as stabilizers of the hip can be seen when one compares the functional capacities of subjects who have had a below-knee amputation with those of subjects who have had an above-knee amputation. The below-knee amputee, with the benefit of modern technology, can function with as little as 10% energy inefficiency as compared to a normal, intact individual. In fact, it is possible for a below-knee amputee with a properly fitted prosthesis to run 100 m in 11 seconds. The below-knee amputee also is able to easily sustain unilateral stance on the amputated extremity. The above-knee amputee, however, experiences at least 40% energy deficiency in function as compared to normal individuals. The above-knee amputee is also unable to stand unilaterally on the amputated limb without leaning toward the affected side. This inability to stand erect without listing is termed a *positive Trendelenburg* sign. In the amputee, this is directly due to the loss of the static stabilizing function of the ITB due to compromise of the ITB insertion with above-knee amputation. The loss of the static stabilizing effect of the ITB places too great a functional demand on the remaining muscular soft tissues (gluteus medium, gluteus minimus, hip capsule) to efficiently stabilize the pelvis during unilateral support stance.

Observation

The examination should begin in the waiting room before the patient is aware of the examiner's observation. Information regarding the degree of the patient's

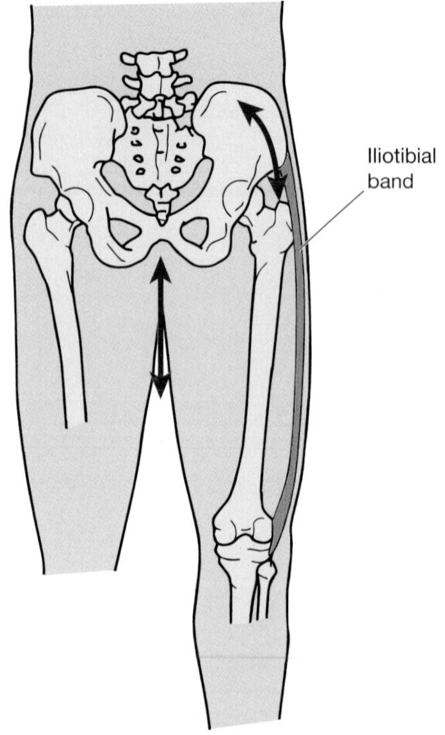

Figure 11.2 A more complete model of hip mechanics includes the ITB. This inelastic structure extends from the lateral iliac crest to the distal part of the femur and on across the knee joint to the tubercle of Gerdy on the anterolateral aspect of the tibia. As such, the ITB acts as a static stabilizer of the hip during the unilateral stance phase of gait. As a tension band, it protects the femur from excessive medial bending deformation. It therefore converts what would otherwise be potentially damaging tension loads on the lateral femur into well-tolerated compression stresses.

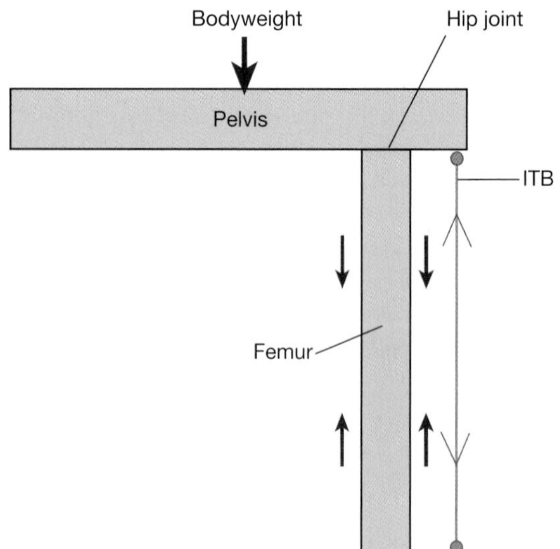

Figure 11.3 This is a mechanical model of the situation depicted in Figure 11.2.

disability, level of functioning, posture, and gait can be observed. The clinician should pay careful attention to the patient's facial expressions with regard to the degree of discomfort the patient is experiencing. The information gathered in this short period can be very useful in creating a total picture of the patient's condition.

Note the manner in which the patient is sitting in the waiting room. If the patient is sitting reclined posteriorly, he or she may have decreased range of motion in hip flexion. If the patient is leaning to one side, this may be due to pain in the ischial tuberosity secondary to bursitis, sacroiliac dysfunction, or radiating pain from the low back. Pain may be altered by changes in position, so watch the patient's facial expression to give you insight into their pain level.

Observe the patient as he or she assumes the standing position. How difficult is it to go from flexion to extension? Can the patient evenly distribute weight between both lower extremities? Once the patient starts to ambulate, a brief gait analysis should be initiated. Note any gait deviations and whether the patient requires or is using an assistive device. Details and implications of gait deviations are discussed in Chapter 14.

Subjective Examination

The hip is an extremely stable joint. Therefore, complaints and dysfunctions are usually limited to problems relating to trauma or deterioration. You should inquire about the nature and location of the complaints and their duration and intensity. The course of the pain during the day and night should be addressed. This will give you information regarding how the pain responds to changes in position, activity, and swelling.

The patient's disorder may be related to age, gender, ethnic background, body type, static and dynamic posture, occupation, leisure activities, hobbies, and general activity level. It is important to inquire about any change in daily routine and any unusual activities that the patient has participated in. If an incident occurred, the details of the mechanism of injury are important to help direct your examination.

The location of the symptoms may give you some insight into the etiology of the complaints. Pain that is located over the anterior and lateral aspects of the thigh may be referred from LI or L2. Pain into the knee may be referred from L4 or L5 or from the hip joint. The patient may complain about pain over the lateral or posterior aspect of the greater trochanter, which may be indicative of trochanteric bursitis or piriformis syndrome. (Please refer to Box 2.1, see p. 15 for typical questions for the subjective examination.)

Gentle Palpation

The palpatory examination is started with the patient in the supine position. You should first examine for areas of localized effusion, discoloration, birthmarks, open sinuses or drainage, incisional areas, bony contours, muscle girth and symmetry, and skinfolds. You should not have to use deep pressure to determine areas of tenderness or malalignment. It is important to use firm but gentle pressure, which will enhance your palpatory skills. If you have a sound basis of cross-sectional anatomy, you will not need to physically penetrate through several layers of tissue to have a good sense of the underlying structures. Remember that if you increase the patient's pain at this point in the examination, the patient will be very reluctant to allow you to continue, or may become more limited in his or her ability to move.

Palpation is most easily performed with the patient in a relaxed position. Although palpation can be performed standing, the supine, side-lying, or prone positions are preferred for stability and ease of examination.

Anterior Aspect—The Patient Is Positioned in Supine

Bony Structures

Iliac Crest

The iliac crest is superficial, very prominent, and easy to palpate. Place your extended hands so that the index fingers are at the waist. Allow your hands to press medially and rest on the superior aspect of the iliac crests. Iliac crests that are uneven in height may be due to a leg length difference, a pelvic obliquity, a bony anomaly, or a sacroiliac dysfunction (Figure 11.4).

Iliac Tubercle

The iliac tubercle is the widest portion of the iliac crest. After you have located the crest, palpate anteriorly and medially along the outer lip. You will find the widest portion approximately 3 in. from the top of the crest (Figure 11.5).

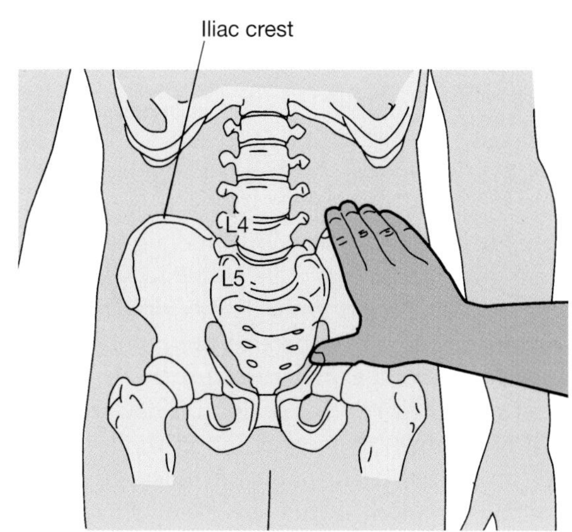

Figure 11.4 Palpation of the iliac crest.

Anterior Superior Iliac Spines

Place your hands on the iliac crests and allow your thumbs to reach anteriorly and inferiorly on a diagonal toward the pubic ramus. The most prominent protuberance is the anterior superior iliac spine. Place your thumb pads in a superior orientation so that they can roll under the anterior superior iliac spines for the most accurate determination of position. This area is

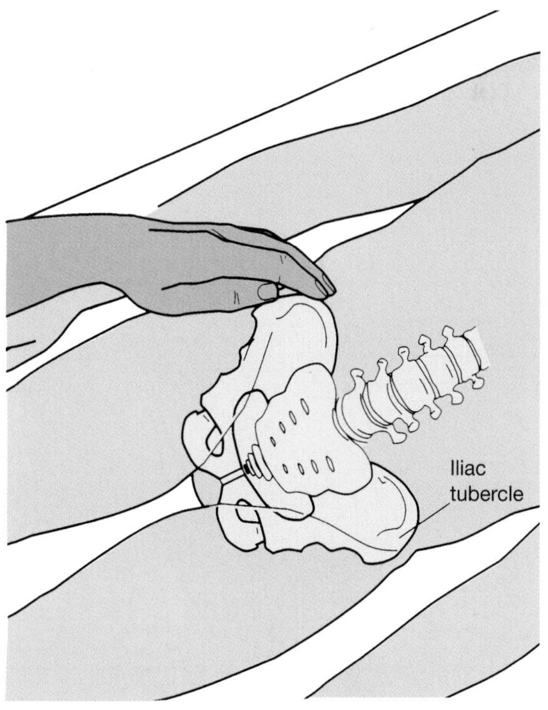

Figure 11.5 Palpation of the iliac tubercle.

normally superficial but can be obscured in an obese patient. Differences in height may be due to an iliac rotation or shear (Figure 11.6).

Pubic Tubercles

Place your hands so that your middle fingers are on the umbilicus and allow your palms to rest over the abdomen. The heel of your hands will be in contact with the superior aspect of the pubic tubercles. Then move your finger pads directly over the tubercles to determine their relative position. They are located medial to the inguinal crease and at the level of the greater trochanters. The pubic tubercles are normally tender to palpation. If they are asymmetrical either in height or in an anterior posterior dimension, there may be a subluxation or dislocation or a sacroiliac dysfunction (Figure 11.7).

Greater Trochanters

Place your hands on the iliac crests and palpate distally along the lateral aspect of the pelvis until you reach a small plateau. Allow your extended hands to rest on top of the greater trochanters to determine their height. They are located at the same level as the pubic tubercles. The superior and posterior aspects of

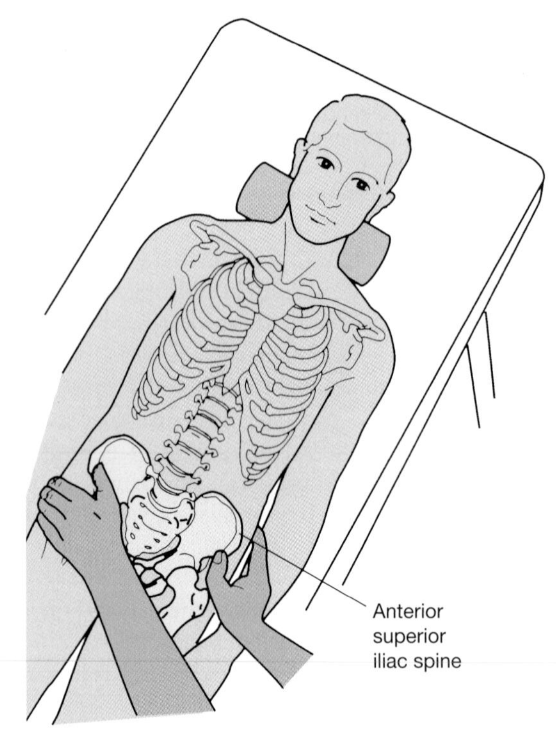

Figure 11.6 Palpation of the anterior superior iliac spines.

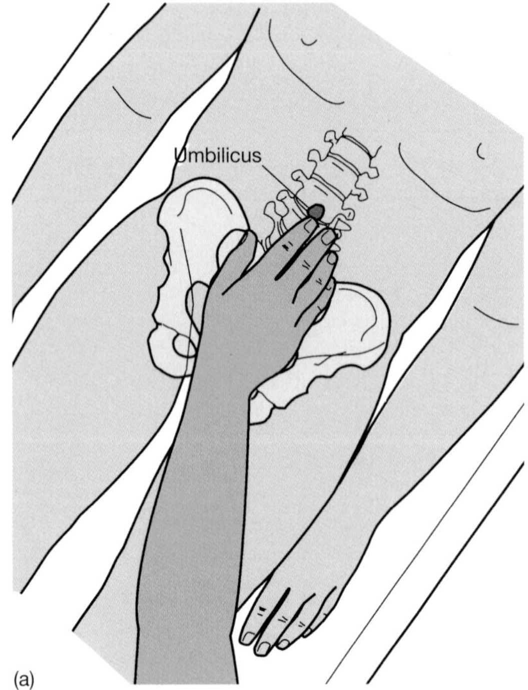

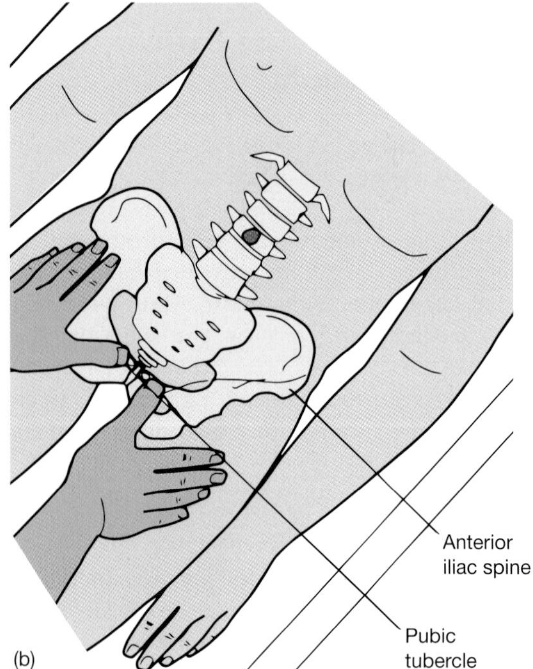

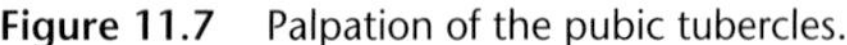

Figure 11.7 Palpation of the pubic tubercles.

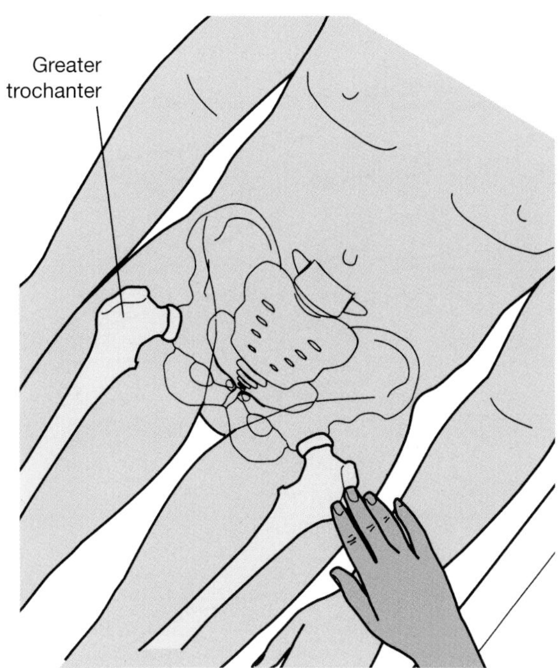

Figure 11.8 Palpation of the greater trochanters.

the greater trochanters are superficial and easily palpable. The anterior and lateral aspects are covered by the attachments of the gluteus medius and tensor fasciae latae, making the bony prominence more difficult to locate. You can confirm your hand placement by having the patient medially and laterally rotate the lower extremity. A difference in height may be secondary to a malalignment following a hip fracture, a congenitally dislocated hip, or a congenital anomaly. If the patient is examined in a weight-bearing position, a height difference could be secondary to a leg length difference. If tenderness is noted in this area, the patient may have a trochanteric bursitis or a piriformis syndrome (Figure 11.8).

Soft-Tissue Structures

Femoral Triangle

The femoral triangle is located in the area directly caudal to the crease of the groin. The base of the triangle is formed by the inguinal ligament. The lateral border is the medial aspect of the sartorius and the medial border is the adductor longus. The floor is trough like and is comprised of the iliacus, psoas major, adductor longus, and pectineus. The femoral vessels are located superficial to the floor and consist of the femoral artery, vein, and nerve and some lymph nodes. The tissues can be most easily accessed by placing the patient's lower extremity in a position of flexion, abduction, and external rotation (Figure 11.9).

Inguinal Ligament

The inguinal ligament attaches to the anterior superior iliac spines and the pubic tubercles and is found under the inguinal crease of the groin. This ligament feels cordlike as you run your fingers across it. If a bulge is found, the patient may have an inguinal hernia (Figure 11.10).

Femoral Artery

The femoral pulse can most easily be detected at the midway point between the pubic tubercles and the anterior superior iliac spines. This is a valuable pulse to assess and is normally strong. If a weak pulse is detected, occlusion of the aorta or the iliac arteries should be considered (Figure 11.11). If the patient is obese, a hand-over-hand technique may be useful.

Femoral Vein

The femoral vein is located medial to the femoral artery at the base of the femoral triangle. It is not easily palpable in the normal individual. This area may be inspected for enlarged lymph nodes, which may indicate an infection or systemic disease (Figure 11.12).

Femoral Nerve

The femoral nerve is located on the lateral aspect of the femoral artery. This very important structure is not normally palpable.

Sartorius Muscle

The sartorius muscle can be visualized by asking the patient to flex, abduct, and laterally rotate the hip and to flex the knee. It is most easily palpable at the proximal anteromedial aspect of the thigh (Figure 11.13). It is the longest muscle in the body.

Adductor Longus Muscle

The adductor longus muscle can be visualized by asking the patient to abduct the lower extremity and then resist adduction. The tendon is palpable at the proximal medial aspect of the thigh inferior to the pubic symphysis. The adductor longus muscle may be injured during athletic activities (e.g., soccer) (Figure 11.14).

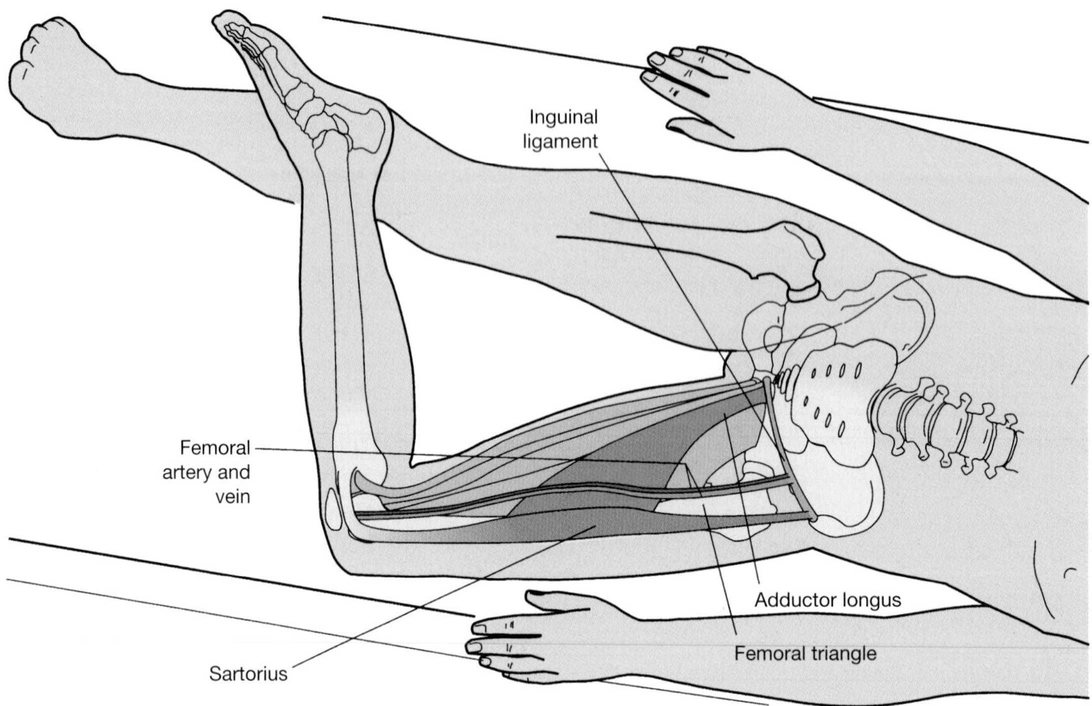

Figure 11.9 The femoral triangle.

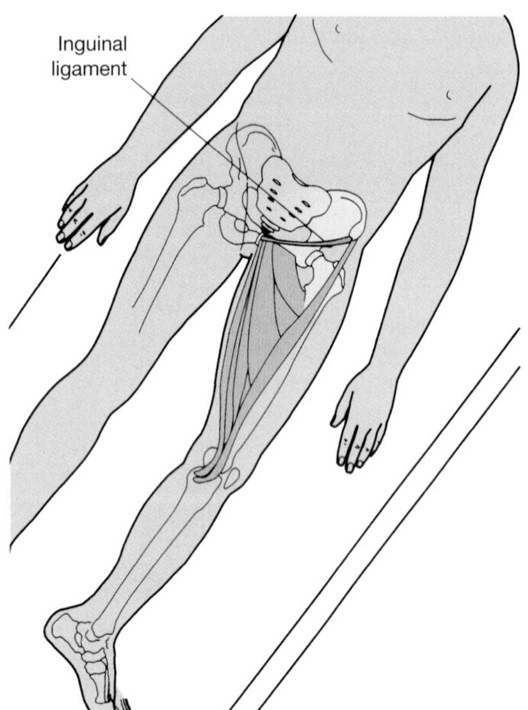

Figure 11.10 The inguinal ligament.

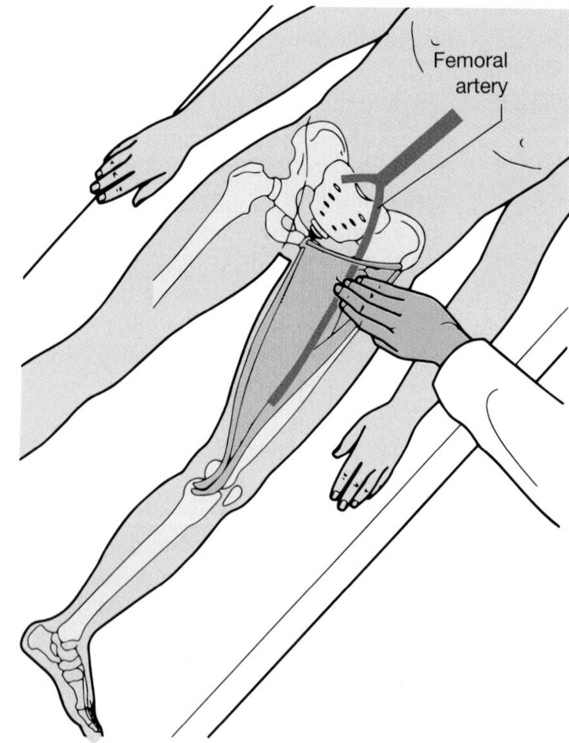

Figure 11.11 Palpation of the femoral pulse.

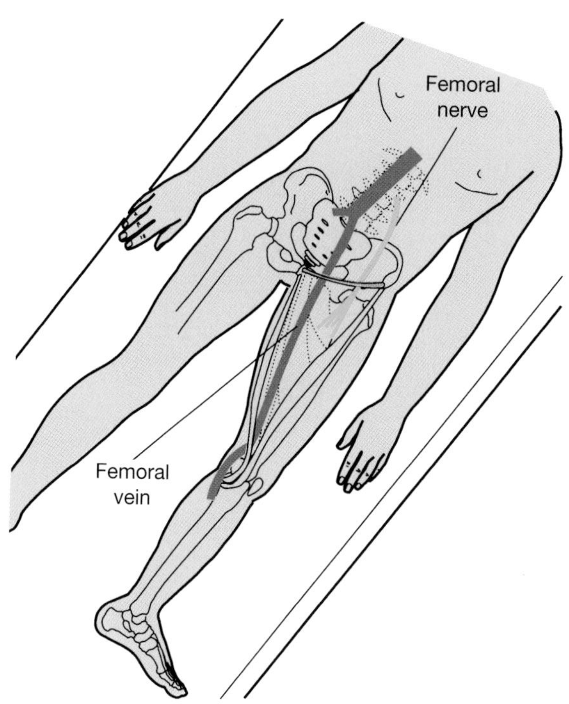

Figure 11.12 Femoral vein and nerve.

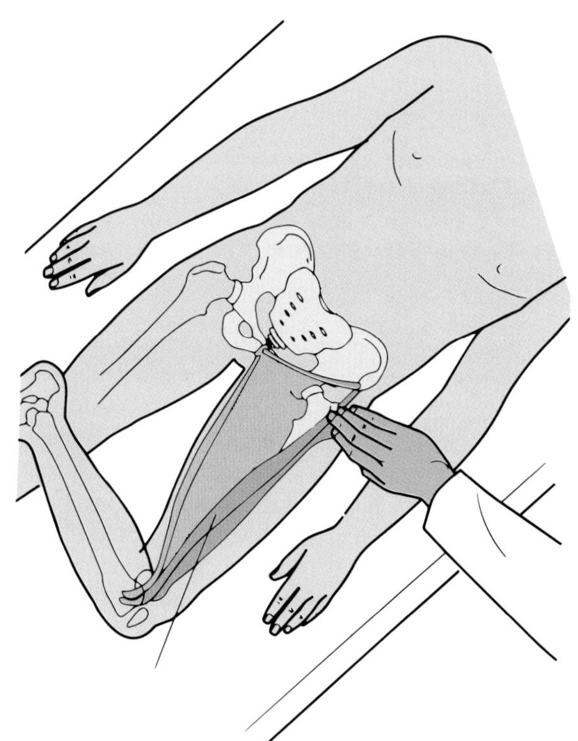

Figure 11.13 Palpation of the sartorius muscle.

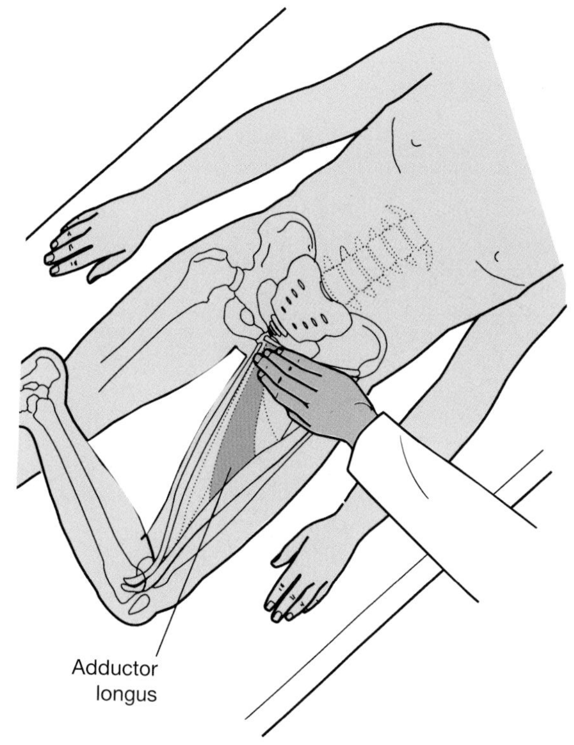

Figure 11.14 Palpation of the adductor longus muscle.

Posterior Aspect—The Patient Is Positioned in Prone

Bony Structures

Posterior Superior Iliac Spines

The posterior superior iliac spines can be found by placing your extended hands over the superior aspect of the iliac crests and allowing your thumbs to reach on a diagonal in an inferior medial direction until they contact the bony prominences. Have your thumbs roll toward a cranial orientation to more accurately determine the position of the posterior superior iliac spines. Many individuals have dimpling, which makes the location more obvious. However, you should be careful because not everyone has dimpling and if it is present, it may not coincide with the actual location of the posterior superior iliac spines. With your fingers on the posterior superior iliac spines, if you move your thumbs at a medial and superior angle of approximately 30 degrees, you will come in contact with the posterior arch of L5. If you move your thumbs medially in a caudad and inferior angle of approximately 30 degrees, you will come in contact with the base of the sacrum. If you are having difficulty, you can also

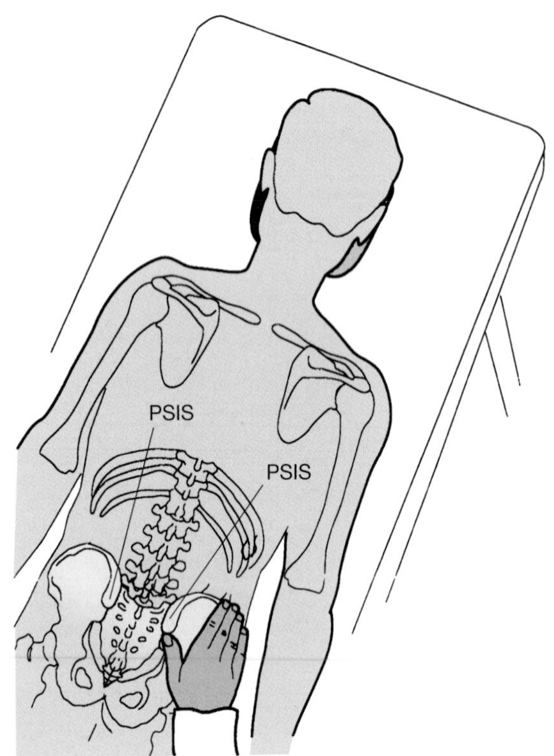

Figure 11.15 Palpation of the posterior superior iliac spines.

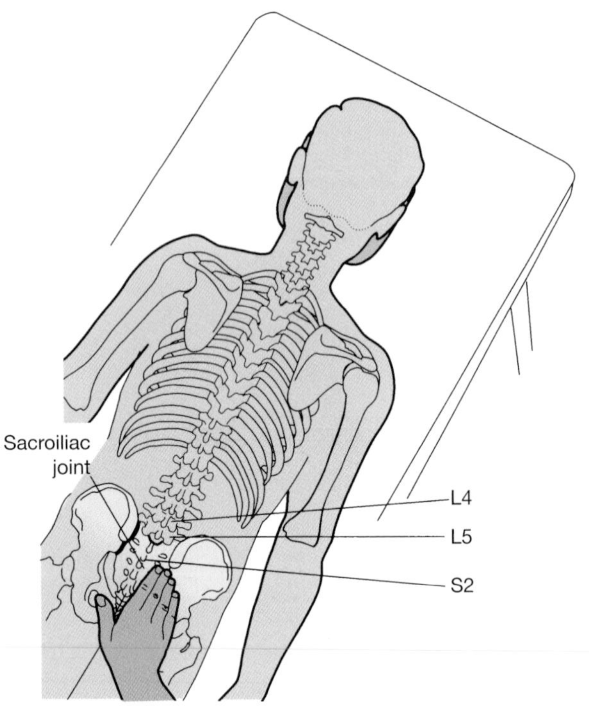

Figure 11.16 Palpation of the sacroiliac joint.

locate the posterior superior iliac spines by following the iliac crests posteriorly until you arrive at the spines (Figure 11.15).

Sacroiliac Joint

The actual joint line of the sacroiliac joint is not palpable because it is covered by the posterior aspect of the innominate bone. You can get a sense of its location by allowing your thumb to drop medially from the posterior superior iliac spine. The sacroiliac joint is located deep to this overhang at approximately the second sacral level (Figure 11.16).

Ischial Tuberosity

You can place your thumbs under the middle portion of the gluteal folds at approximately the level of the greater trochanters. Allow your thumbs to face superiorly and gently probe through the gluteus maximus until your thumbs are resting under the ischial tuberosity. Some people find it easier to perform this palpation with the patient in the side-lying position with the hip flexed; with this position, the ischial tuberosity is more accessible because the gluteus maximus is pulled up, reducing the muscular cover. If this area is tender to palpation, it may be indicative of an inflammation of the ischial bursa (Figure 11.17).

Side-Lying Position

Soft-Tissue Structures

Piriformis Muscle

The piriformis muscle is located between the anterior inferior aspect of the sacrum and the greater trochanter. This muscle is very deep and is normally not palpable. However, if the muscle is in spasm, a cordlike structure can be detected under your fingers as you palpate the length of the muscle (Figure 11.18). The piriformis is able to influence the alignment of the sacrum by pulling it anteriorly by virtue of its attachment. The sciatic nerve runs either under, over, or through the muscle belly. Compression of the nerve can occur when the muscle is in spasm.

Sciatic Nerve

The sciatic nerve is most easily accessed with the patient in the side-lying position, which allows the

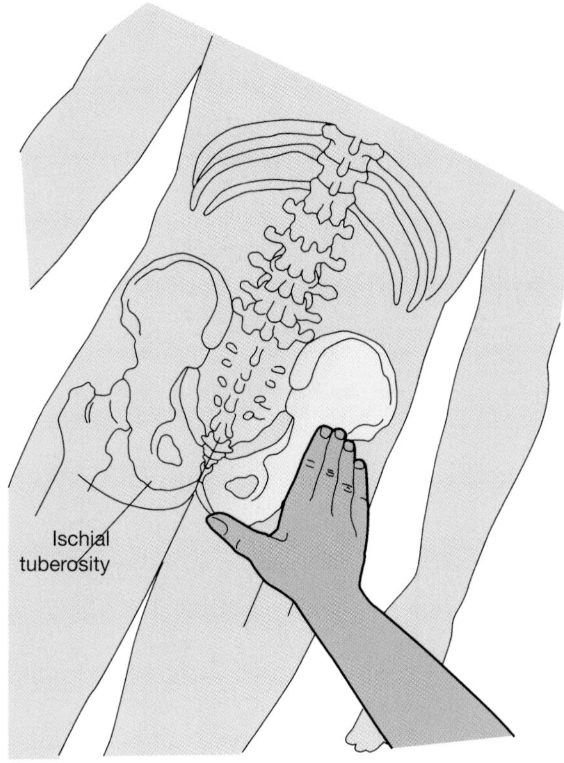

Figure 11.17 Palpation of the ischial tuberosity.

nerve to have less muscle cover since the gluteus maximus is flattened. Locate the mid position between the ischial tuberosity and greater trochanter. The sciatic nerve emerges from the internal pelvis, exiting via the greater sciatic notch and foramen under, over or through the piriformis muscle. You may be able to roll

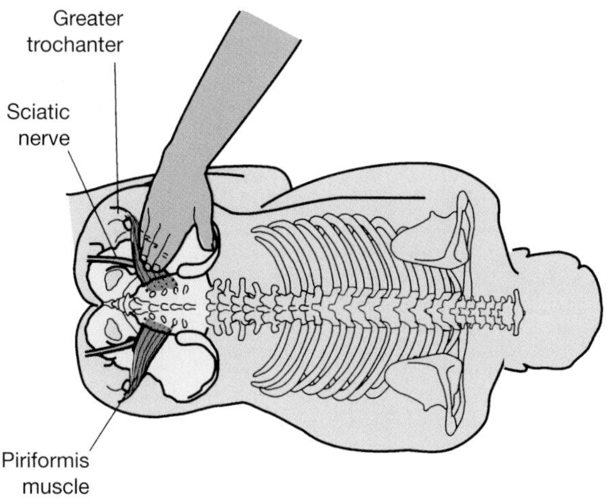

Figure 11.18 Palpation of the piriformis muscle.

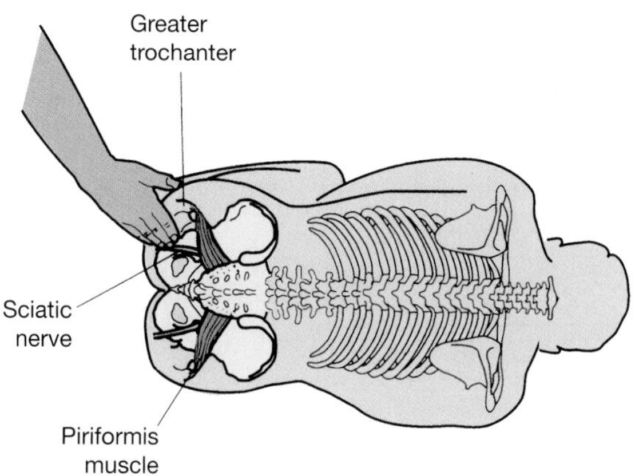

Figure 11.19 Palpation of the sciatic nerve.

the nerve under your fingers if you take up the soft-tissue slack. Tenderness in this area can be due to an irritation of the sciatic nerve secondary to lumbar disc disease or piriformis spasm (Figure 11.19).

Trigger Points

Most muscles about the hip can develop myofascial dysfunction and have trigger points within them. Common trigger point locations for the gluteus maximus, gluteus medius, piriformis, tensor fascia latae, and iliopsoas muscles are illustrated in Figures 11.20, 11.21, 11.22, 11.23, and 11.24.

While myofascial dysfunction can result in a sciatica-like pain syndrome, it should be noted that true sciatic nerve damage is associated with sensory loss, muscle weakness, or loss of reflexes. These findings do not occur in myofascial pain syndromes.

Active Movement Testing

You should have the patient perform the following movements: flexion and extension around the frontal axis, abduction and adduction around the sagittal axis, and medial and lateral rotation around the longitudinal axis. These should be quick, functional tests designed to clear the joint. If the motion is pain free at the end of the range, you can add an additional overpressure to "clear" the joint. If the patient experiences pain during any of these movements, you should continue to explore whether the etiology of the pain is secondary to contractile or noncontractile structures by using passive and resistive tests.

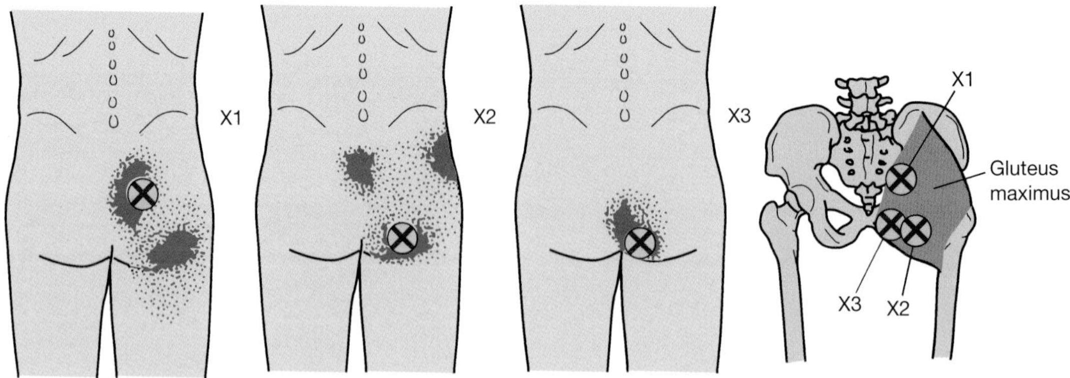

Figure 11.20 Trigger points (XI, X2, X3) in the gluteus maximus muscle. The referred pain patterns are noted by the dark and stippled areas. (Adapted with permission from Travell and Rinzler, 1952.)

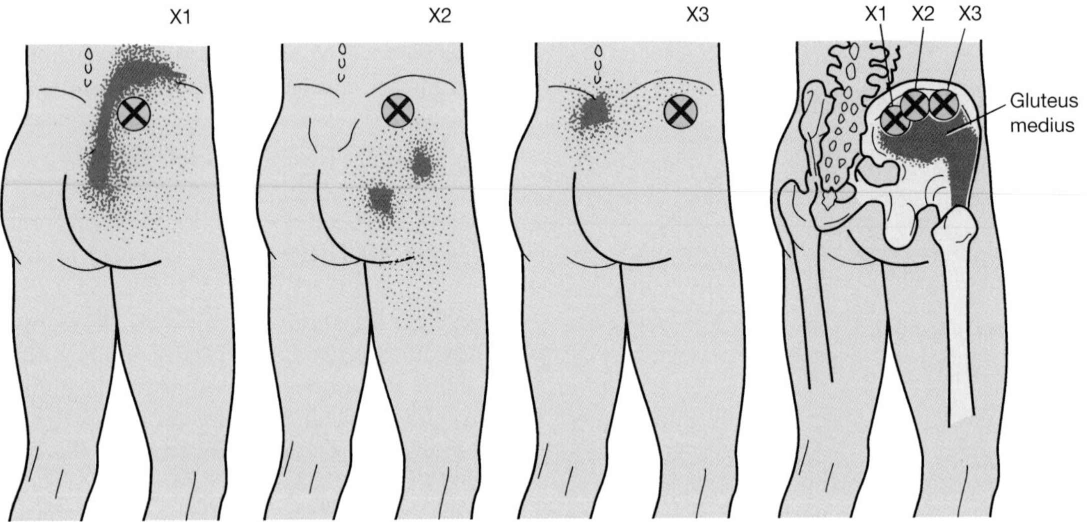

Figure 11.21 Trigger points (XI, X2, X3) in the gluteus medius muscle. The referred pain patterns are noted by the dark and stippled areas. (Adapted with permission from Travell and Rinzler, 1952.)

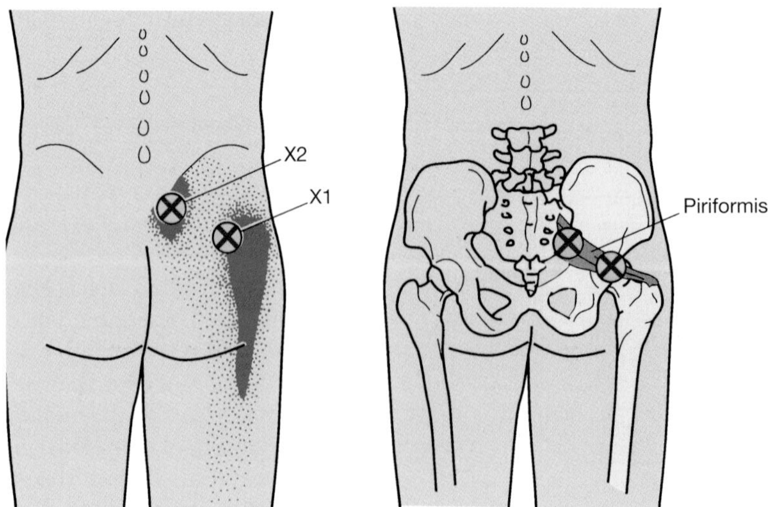

Figure 11.22 Trigger points (X1, X2) in the piriformis muscle. The referred pain patterns are noted by the dark and stippled areas. (Adapted with permission from Travell and Rinzler, 1952.)

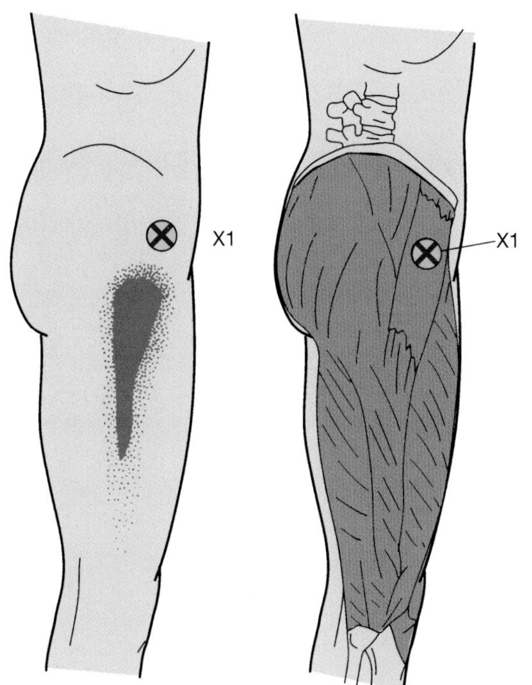

Figure 11.23 A trigger point, X1, in the tensor fascia latae muscle. The referred pain pattern is noted by the dark and stippled areas. (Adapted with permission from Travell and Rinzler, 1952.)

Flexion

The patient, in the supine position, is instructed to bend the hip and bring the knee toward the chest as far as he or she can without causing a posterior pelvic rotation (Figure 11.25).

Extension

The patient, in the supine position, is instructed to return the lower extremity to the table (Figure 11.26).

Abduction

The patient, in the supine position, is instructed to bring the lower extremity out to the side as far as possible without creating an obliquity of the pelvis (Figure 11.27).

Adduction

The patient, in the supine position, is instructed to return the lower extremity to the midline from the abducted position (Figure 11.28).

Medial (Internal) Rotation

The patient, in the supine position, is instructed to roll the extended lower extremity inward without lifting the buttock off the table (Figure 11.29).

Lateral (External) Rotation

The patient, in the supine position, is instructed to roll the lower extremity outward (Figure 11.30).

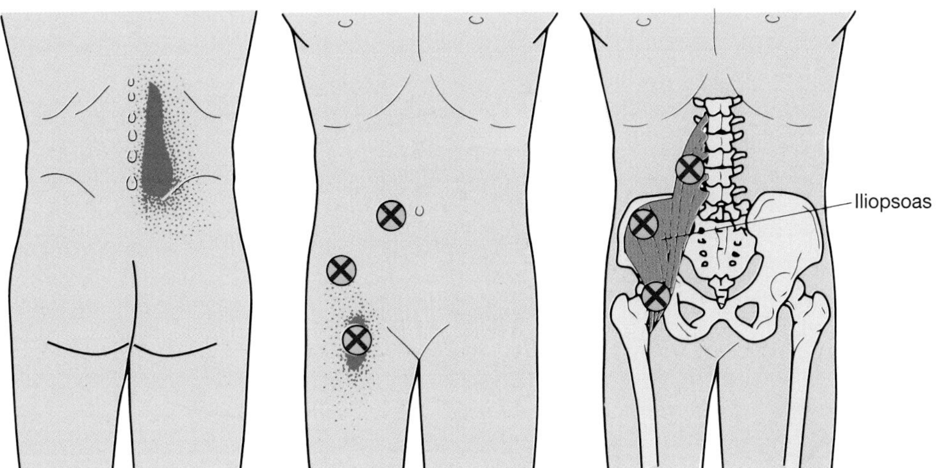

Figure 11.24 Trigger points in the iliacus and psoas muscles. The referred pain patterns are noted by the dark and stippled areas. Note that pain can be felt both anteriorly and along the lumbar spine. (Adapted with permission from Travell and Rinzler, 1952.)

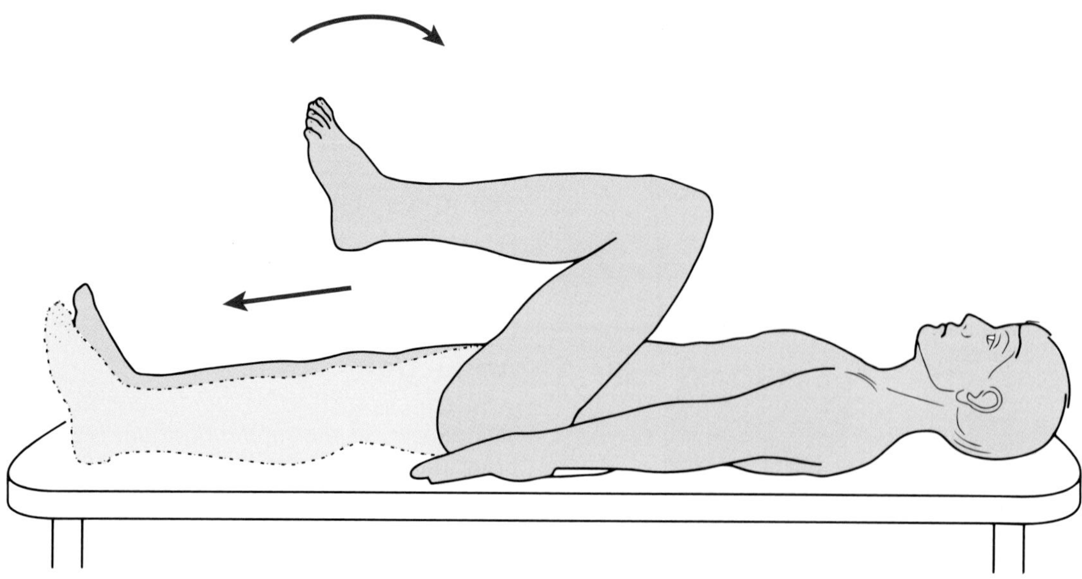

Figure 11.25 Active movement testing of flexion.

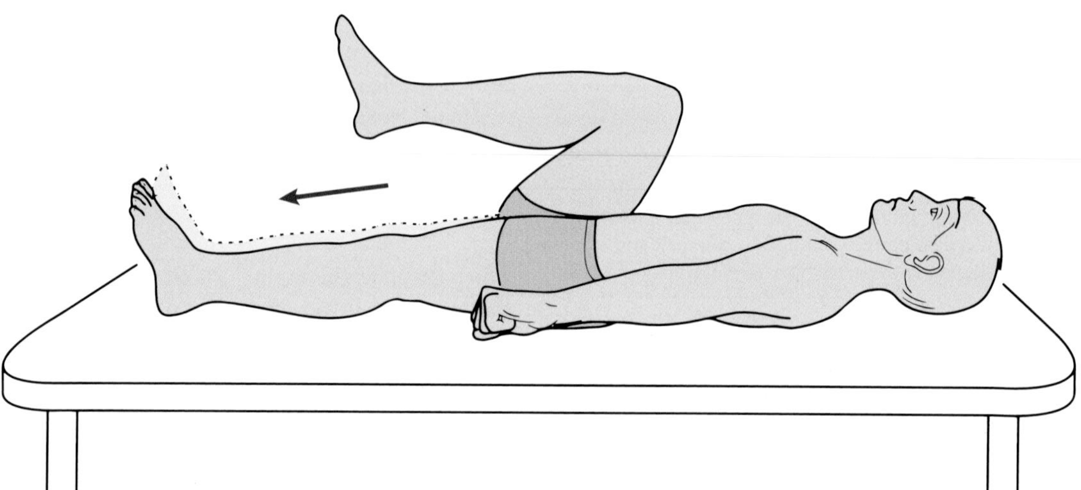

Figure 11.26 Active movement testing of extension.

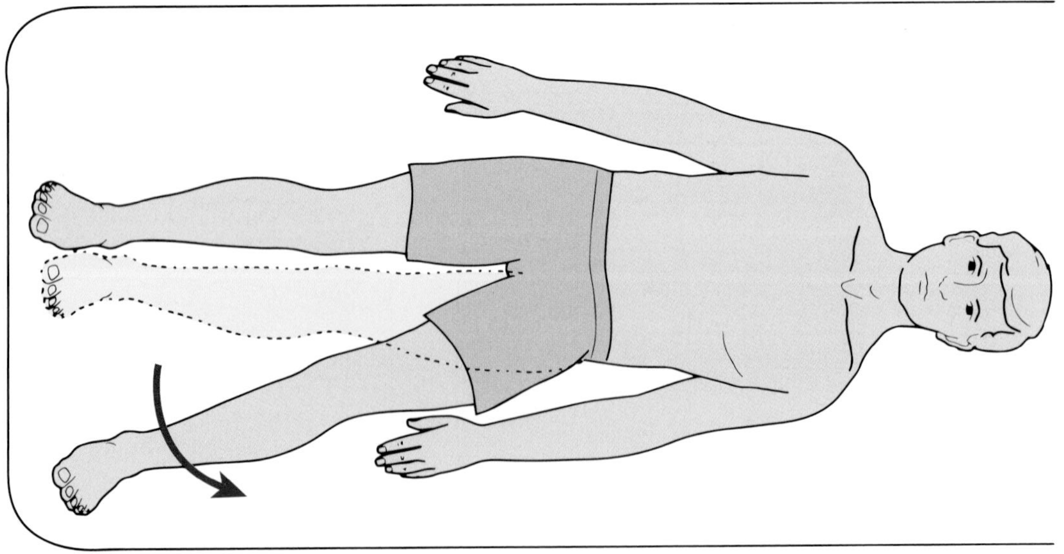

Figure 11.27 Active movement testing of abduction.

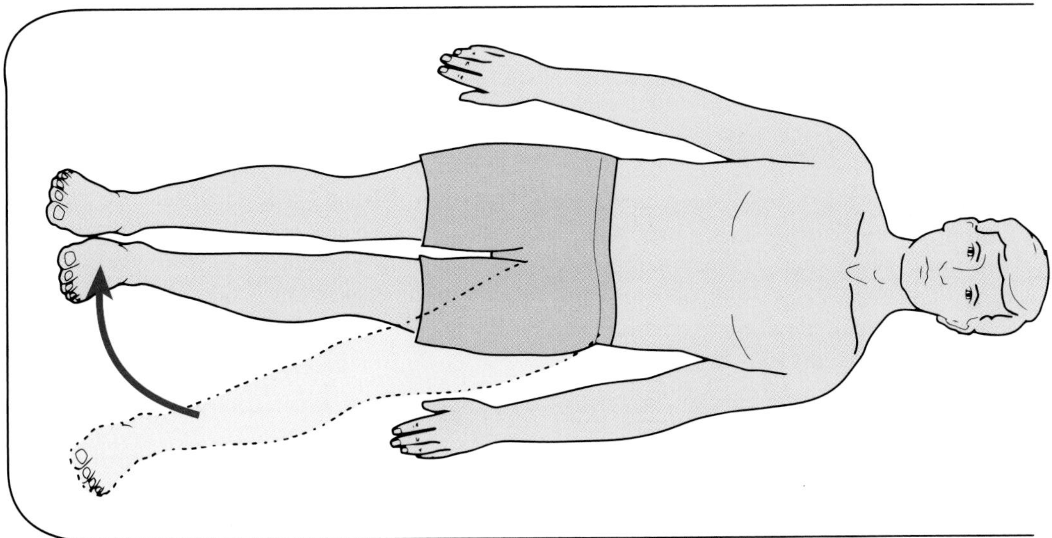

Figure 11.28 Active movement testing of adduction.

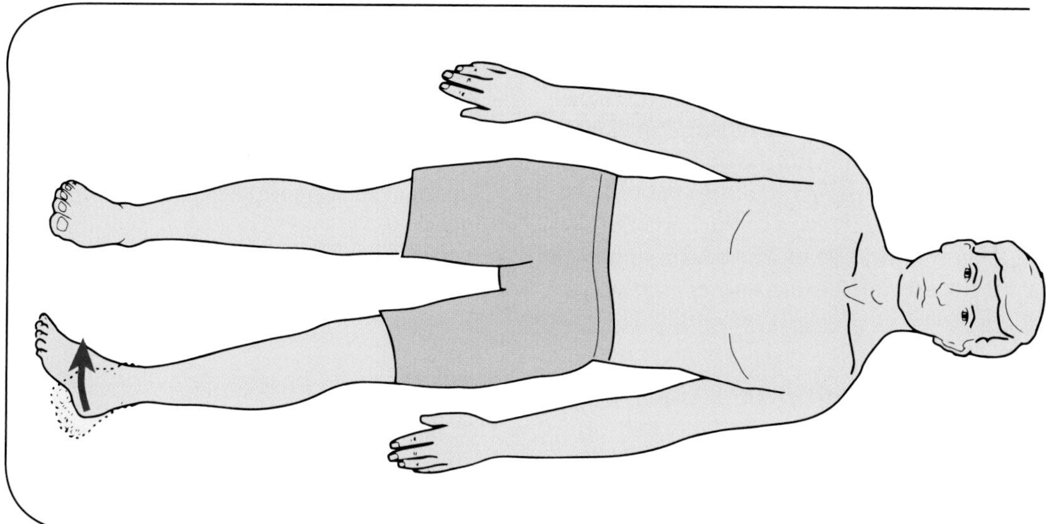

Figure 11.29 Active movement testing of medial (internal) rotation.

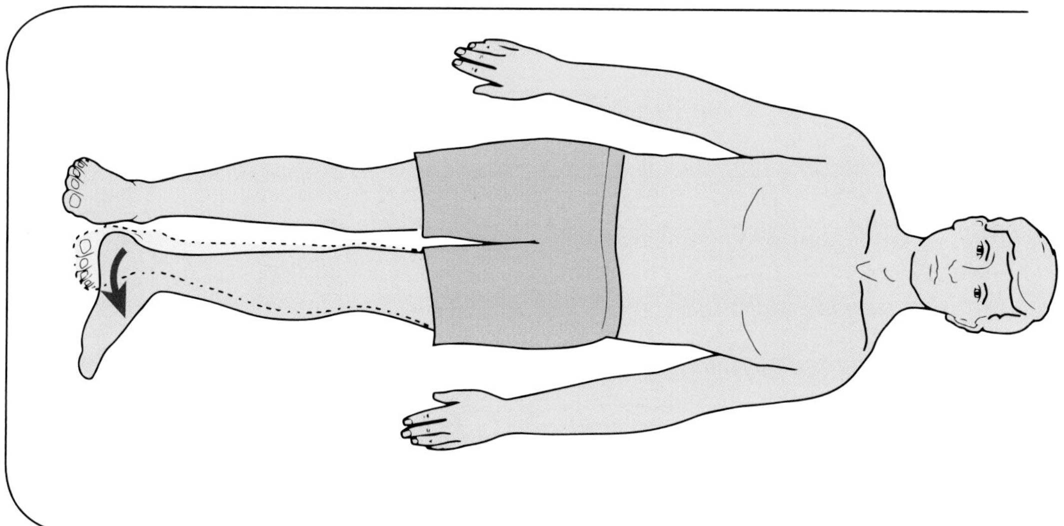

Figure 11.30 Active movement testing of lateral (external) rotation.

Passive Movement Testing

Passive movement testing can be divided into two areas: physiological movements (cardinal plane), which are the same as the active movements, and mobility testing of the accessory (joint play, component) movements. You can determine whether the noncontractile (inert) elements can be incriminated by using these tests. These structures (ligaments, joint capsule, fascia, bursa, dura mater, and nerve root) (Cyriax, 1982) are stretched or stressed when the joint is taken to the end of the available range. At the end of each passive physiological movement, you should sense the end feel and determine whether it is normal or pathological. Assess the limitation of movement and see if it fits into a capsular pattern. The capsular pattern of the hip is medial rotation, extension from zero degree, abduction, and lateral rotation (Kaltenborn, 2011). If you find that the patient has limited motion, experiences pain during hip flexion with the knee extended or with the knee flexed, and presents with a noncapsular pattern, you should consider that the patient has the sign of the buttock (Cyriax, 1982). This is indicative of a serious lesion such as neoplasm, fracture of the sacrum, or ischiorectal abscess.

Physiological Movements

Assess the amount of motion available in all directions. Each motion is measured from the anatomical starting position which is zero degrees of flexion–extension, abduction–adduction, and medial–lateral rotation. Patients will substitute for tightness in the joint or surrounding muscles with trunk or pelvic movement. Therefore, it is important to monitor where the movement is taking place while stabilizing the pelvis.

Flexion

The patient is placed in a supine position with the hip in the anatomical position. Place your hand over the patient's knee and ankle and create flexion in the hip and knee joint. Increased motion (substitution) can be achieved by posteriorly tilting the pelvis; therefore, stabilization of the pelvis is important for the accurate determination of hip movement. Hip flexion is normally blocked by the approximation of the anterior part of the thigh and the abdomen. If the patient is obese, range of motion can be limited by early contact with the abdominal area. The normal end feel is considered to be soft (tissue approximation) (Magee, 2008; Kaltenborn, 2011). Normal range of motion is 0–120 degrees (Figure 11.31) (American Academy of Orthopedic Surgeons, 1965).

Extension

The patient is placed prone with the hip in the anatomical position. The knee must be extended to put the rectus femoris on slack so that it does not

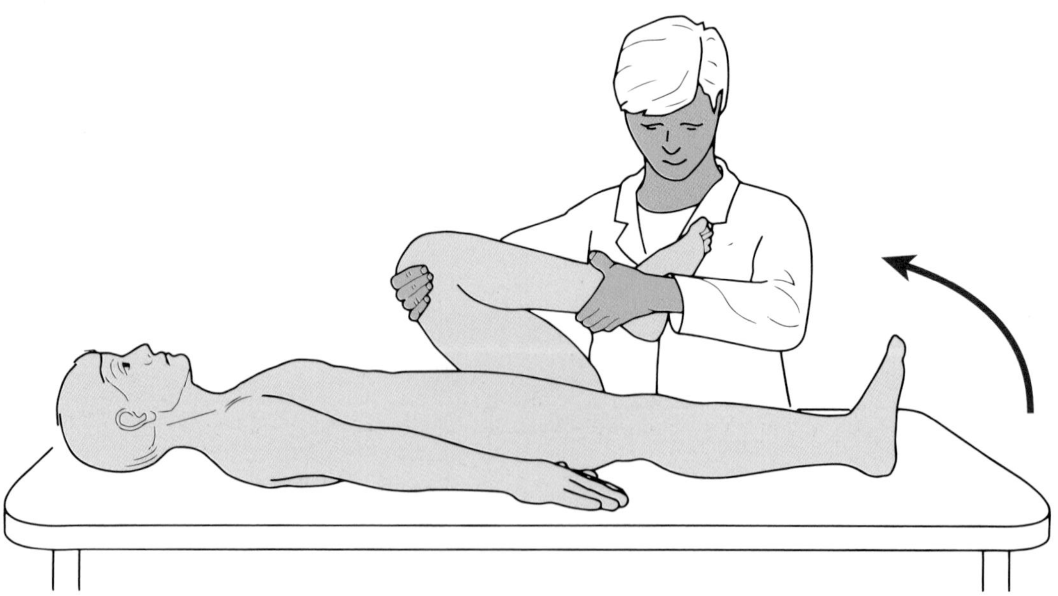

Figure 11.31 Passive movement testing of flexion.

decrease the available range. Place your hand under the anterior distal aspect of the thigh and lift the lower extremity toward the ceiling. Increased motion (substitution) can be created by increasing the lumbar lordosis and by anterior tilting of the pelvis. Stabilization of the pelvis is important to obtain accurate measurements. The normal end feel is firm (ligamentous) due to tension from the anterior capsular ligaments (Magee, 2008; Kaltenborn, 2011). Tight anterior muscles can also contribute to the limitation of motion. Normal range of motion is 0–30 degrees (Figure 11.32) (American Academy of Orthopedic Surgeons, 1965).

Abduction

The patient is placed supine with the hip in the anatomical position. Place your hand on the medial distal aspect of the leg and move the lower extremity laterally. Increased motion (substitution) can be created by laterally rotating the lower extremity and hiking the pelvis. Stabilization of the pelvis is important to obtain accurate measurements. Normal end feel is firm (ligamentous) due to tension from the medial capsular ligaments (Magee, 2008; Kaltenborn, 2011). Motion can also be limited by tightness in the adductor muscles. Normal range of motion is 0–45 degrees (Figure 11.33) (American Academy of Orthopedic Surgeons, 1965).

Adduction

Place the patient supine with the hip in the anatomical position. Abduct the contralateral hip to allow enough room for movement. Place your hand on the lateral distal aspect of the leg and move the lower extremity medially. Increased motion (substitution) can be created by laterally tilting the pelvis. Stabilization of the pelvis is important to obtain accurate measurements. Normal end feel is firm (ligamentous) due to tension from the lateral capsule and superior band of the iliofemoral ligament. Motion can also be limited by tightness in the abductor muscles. Normal range of motion is 0–30 degrees (Magee, 2008; Kaltenborn, 2011) (Figure 11.34) (American Academy of Orthopedic Surgeons, 1965).

Medial (Internal) Rotation

Medial rotation can be assessed with the hip in either flexion or extension. To assess movement with the hip in extension, place the patient prone with the hip in the anatomical position and the knee flexed to 90 degrees. Place your hand on the medial distal aspect of

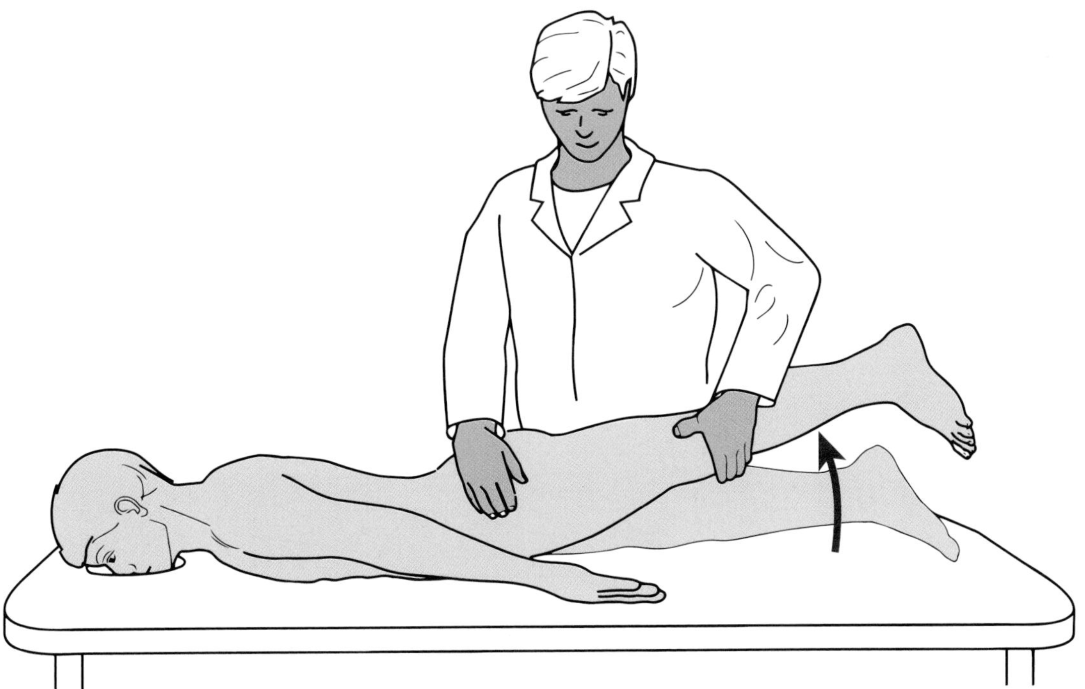

Figure 11.32 Passive movement testing of extension.

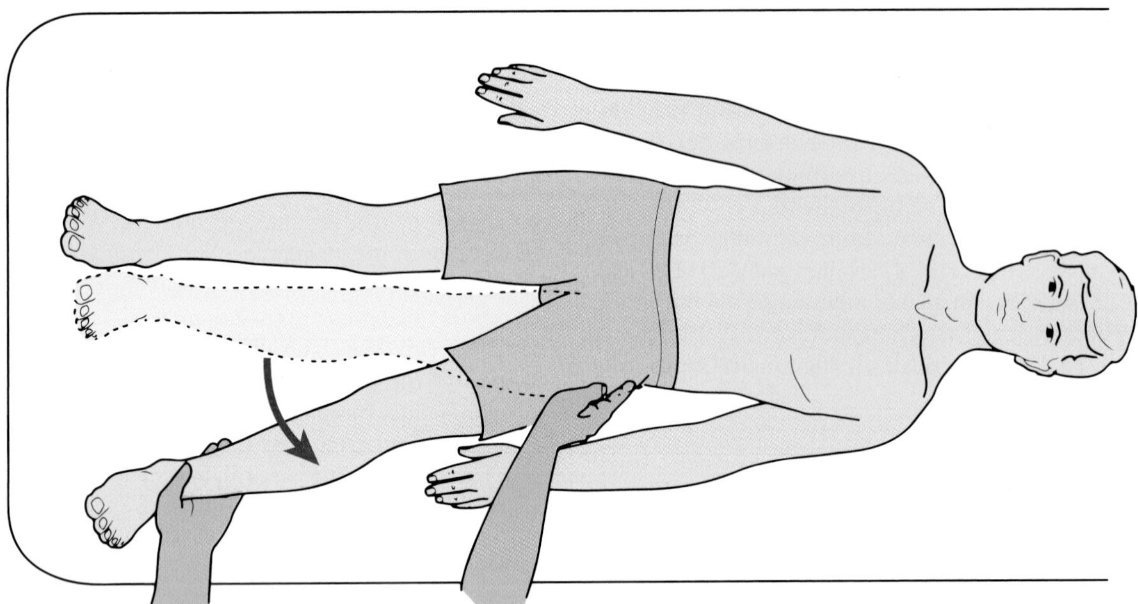

Figure 11.33 Passive movement testing of abduction.

the leg and rotate the leg outward. Increased motion (substitution) can be created by rotating the pelvis. Stabilization of the pelvis is important for accurate measurement. Motion can also be limited by tightness in the external rotator muscles. The normal end feel is firm (ligamentous) due to tension from the posterior capsule and the ischiofemoral ligament (Magee, 2008; Kaltenborn, 2011) (Figure 11.35).

To assess medial rotation with the hip in flexion, have the patient sit with the hip and knee flexed to 90 degrees. Place your hand on the medial distal aspect of the leg and rotate the leg outward. Increased motion

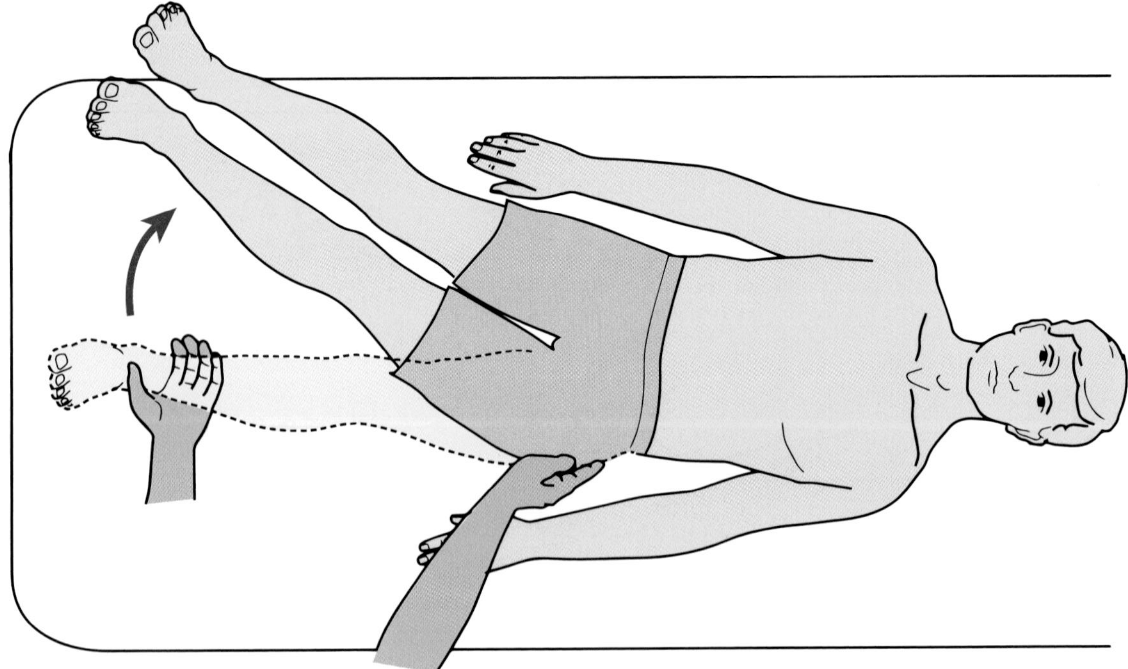

Figure 11.34 Passive movement testing of adduction.

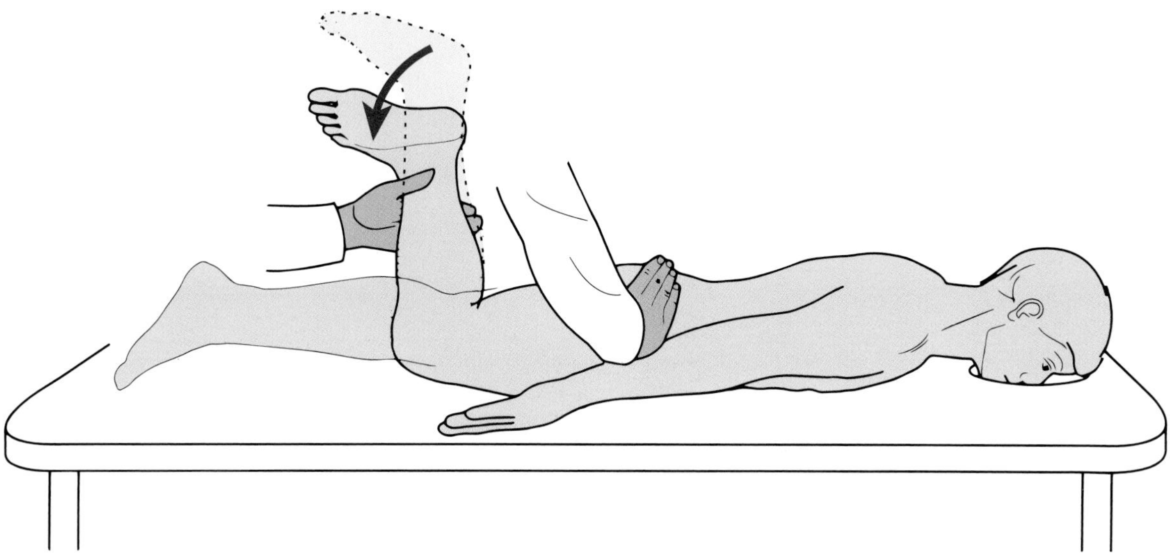

Figure 11.35 Passive movement testing of medial (internal) rotation with the hip extended.

(substitution) can be created by rotating the pelvis and laterally flexing the spine. Stabilization of the pelvis is important for accurate measurement. The normal end feel is firm (ligamentous) due to tension from the posterior capsule and the ischiofemoral ligament (Magee, 2008; Kaltenborn, 2011). Motion can also be limited by tightness in the external rotator muscles. Normal range of motion is 0–5 degrees (Figure 11.36) (American Academy of Orthopedic Surgeons, 1965).

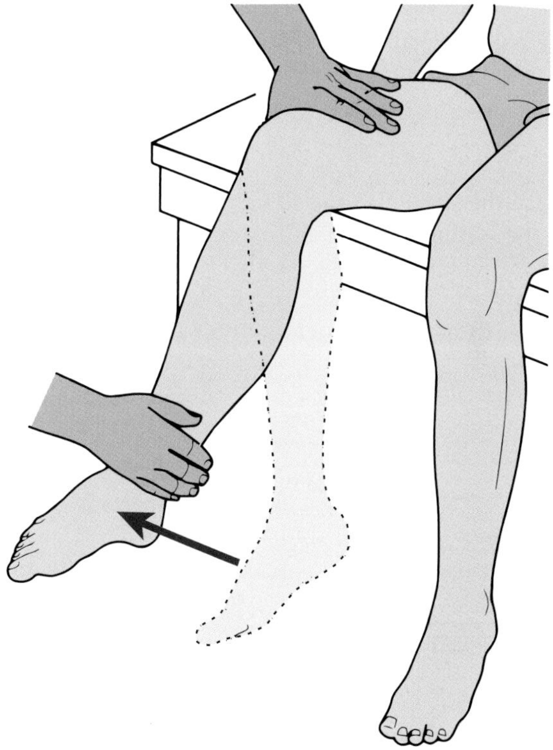

Figure 11.36 Passive movement testing of medial (internal) rotation with the hip flexed.

Lateral (External) Rotation

Lateral rotation is performed in flexion and extension using the same positions as for medial rotation. Place your hand on the lateral distal aspect of the leg and rotate the leg inward. Increased motion (substitution) can be created by further abducting the hip and laterally flexing the spine. Stabilization of the pelvis is important for accurate measurement. The normal end feel is firm (ligamentous) due to tension in the anterior capsule and iliofemoral and pubofemoral ligaments. Motion can also be limited by tightness in the medial rotator muscles. Normal range of motion is 0–45 degrees (Magee, 2008; Kaltenborn, 2011) (Figure 11.37) (American Academy of Orthopedic Surgeons, 1965).

Mobility Testing of Accessory Movements

Mobility testing of accessory movements will give you information about the degree of laxity present in the joint. The patient must be totally relaxed and comfortable to allow you to move the joint and obtain the most accurate information. The joint should be placed in the maximal loose packed (resting) position to allow for the greatest degree of joint movement.

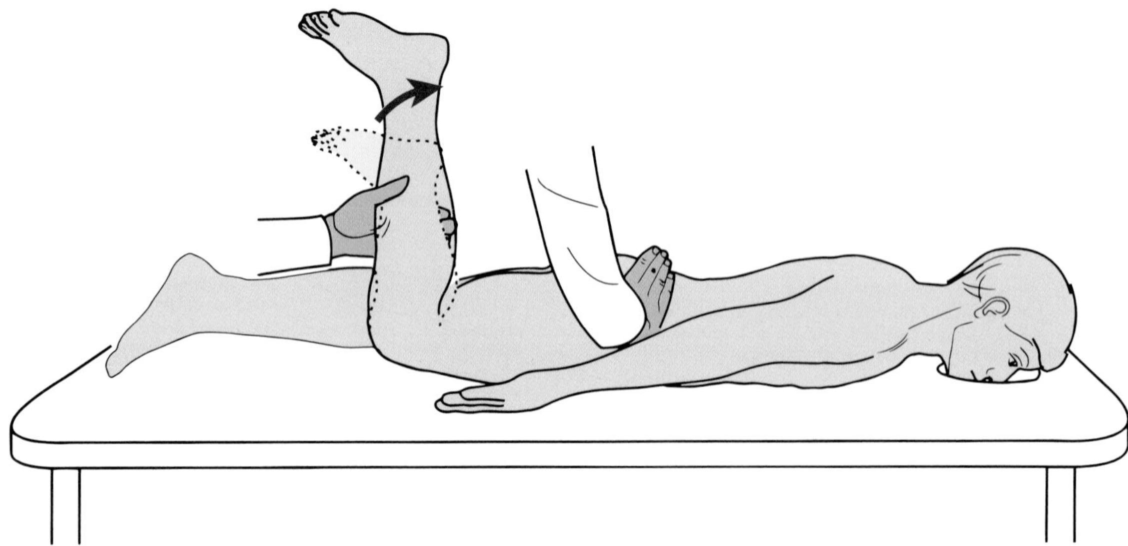

Figure 11.37 Passive movement testing of lateral (external) rotation with the hip extended.

The resting position of the hip is 30 degrees of flexion, 30 degrees of abduction, and a slight lateral rotation (Kaltenborn, 2011).

Traction (Longitudinal Distraction)

Place the patient in the supine position with the hip in the resting position and the knee in flexion. Stand on the side of the table so that your body is turned toward the patient. The pelvis should be stabilized, either with an additional pair of hands or a strap, so that all the movement takes place at the hip joint. Place your hands on the medial and lateral inferior aspects of the thigh. Pull along the axis of the femur in a longitudinal direction until the slack is taken up. This technique provides an inferior separation of the femoral head from the acetabulum (Figure 11.38). This technique can also be performed with the knee in extension. You would place your hands around the patient's malleoli and pull in the same direction as previously described (https://www.youtube.com/watch?v=zhtK9YZpRBw).

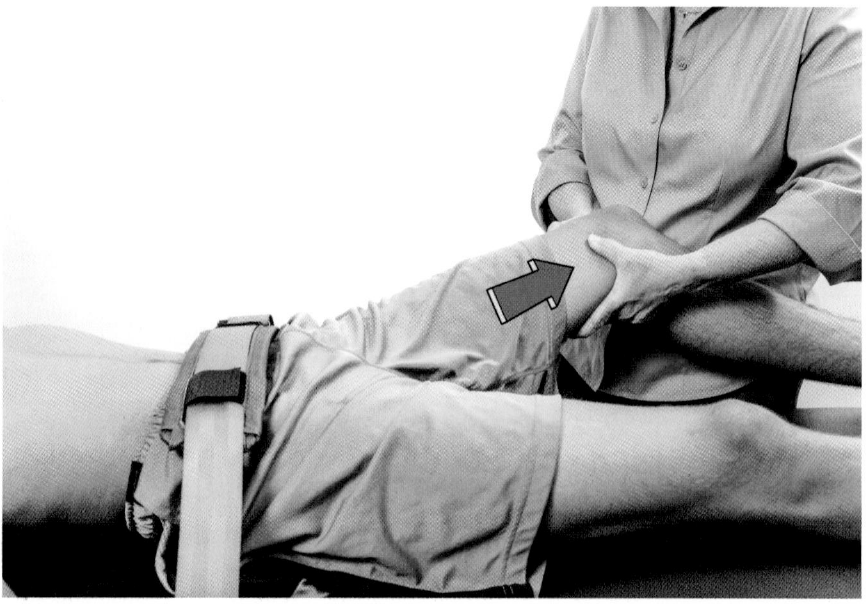

Figure 11.38 Mobility testing of hip traction (longitudinal distraction).

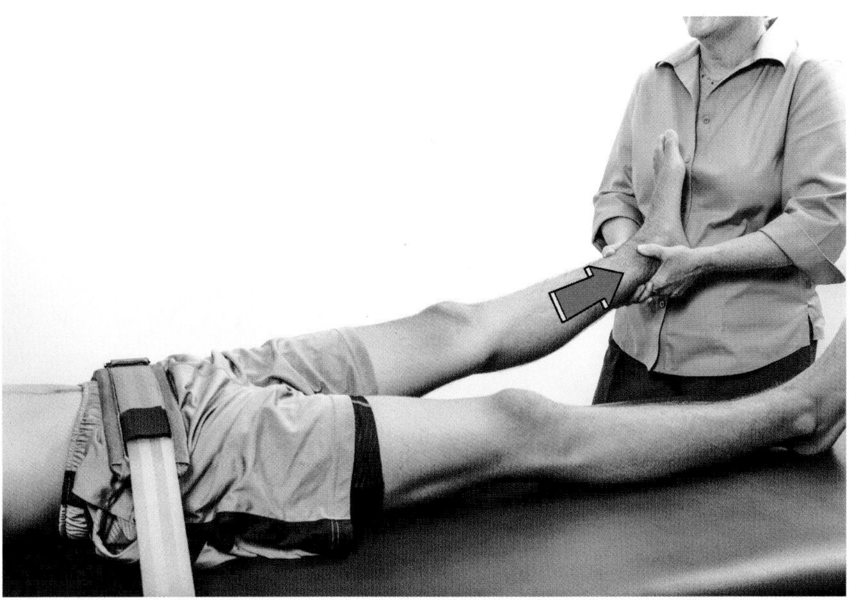

Figure 11.39 Mobility testing of hip distraction through the knee.

Recognize that additional stress is placed on the knee joint. This technique should not be used with patients who have increased laxity in the knee (Figure 11.39).

Lateral Distraction or Glide

Place the patient in the supine position with the hip in the resting position and the knee in flexion. Stand on the side of the table so that your body is turned toward the side of the patient. The pelvis should be stabilized so that all the movement takes place at the hip joint. Place your hands on the proximal medial aspect of the thigh as close to the inguinal crease as possible. Pull laterally at a 90-degree angle from the femur until the slack is taken up. A strap can be used both to stabilize the pelvis and to assist in the lateral pull. This movement will separate the femoral head from the acetabulum (Figure 11.40) (https://www.youtube.com/watch?v=g0CTLfKdwqg).

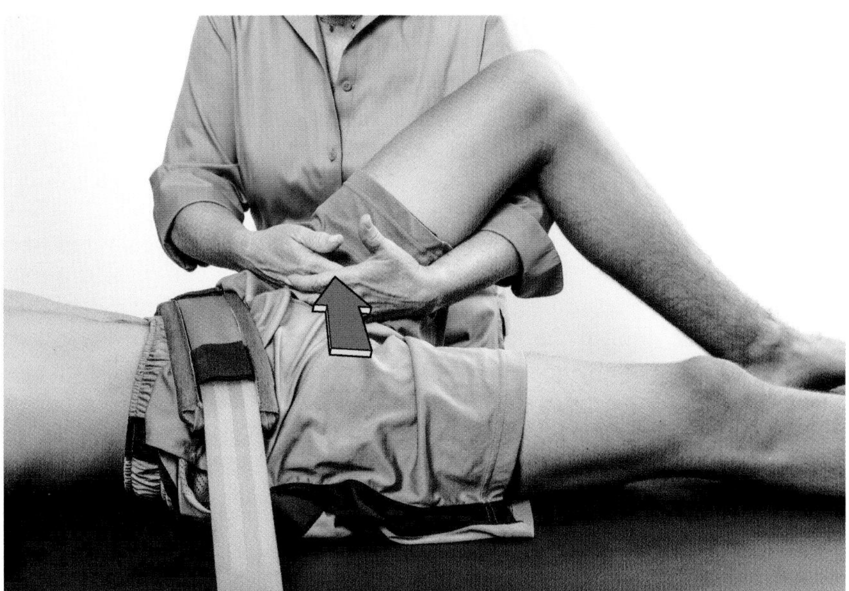

Figure 11.40 Mobility testing of lateral distraction (glide).

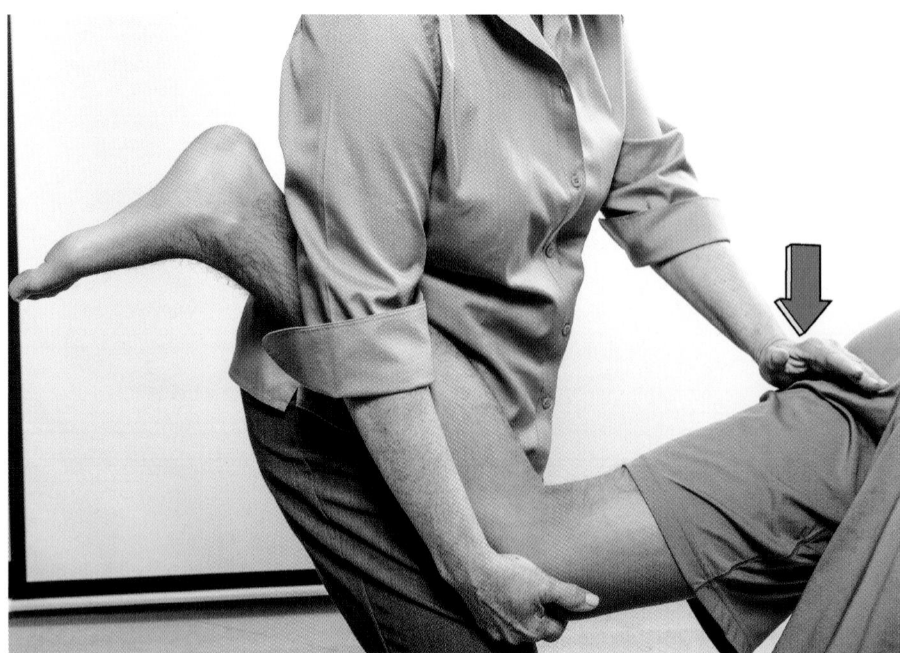

Figure 11.41 Mobility testing of ventral glide of the femoral head.

Ventral Glide of the Femoral Head

Place the patient in the prone position so that the pelvis is resting on the table and the remainder of the lower extremity is unsupported. Stand at the end of the table so that your body is turned toward the medial side of the patient's thigh. The pelvis is stabilized by the treatment table. Place your hands so that you support the lower extremity by holding the distal part of the thigh and allowing the knee to flex. Your other hand should be at the proximal posterior aspect of the thigh as close to the gluteal crease as possible. Push anteriorly with your proximal hand until the slack is taken up. This movement will create an anterior glide of the femoral head (Figure 11.41).

Resistive Testing

There are six motions of the hip to be examined: flexion, extension, abduction, adduction, external (lateral) rotation, and internal (medial) rotation. Although a single action is usually ascribed to each muscle in the hip region, it should be remembered that most of the muscles perform more than one action simultaneously. The position of the leg at the time of muscle contraction is an important determinant of the muscle's function. For example, the adductor longus muscle is a hip flexor up to 50 degrees of hip flexion. Beyond 50 degrees of hip flexion, the adductor longus functions as an extensor. This is an example of inversion of muscular action.

Flexion

The most powerful flexors of the hips are the psoas and the iliacus, which share a common tendon (Figure 11.42). The iliopsoas is assisted by the rectus femoris, sartorius, and tensor fascia latae, which cross both the hip and the knee joints.

- Position of patient: Sitting upright with knees bent over the edge of the table, with hands holding onto the edge of the table for support and to prevent substitution.
- Resisted test: Ask the patient to raise the thigh off the table while you resist this movement by applying pressure downward on the thigh just above the knee (Figure 11.43).

Testing hip flexion with gravity eliminated is performed with the patient in a side-lying position (Figure 11.44). The upper part of the leg is elevated slightly, and the patient is asked to flex the hip.

Inguinal pain during resisted hip flexion may be due to iliopsoas bursitis or abdominal pathology.

Weakness of hip flexion results in difficulty getting out of a chair, walking up an incline, and climbing stairs.

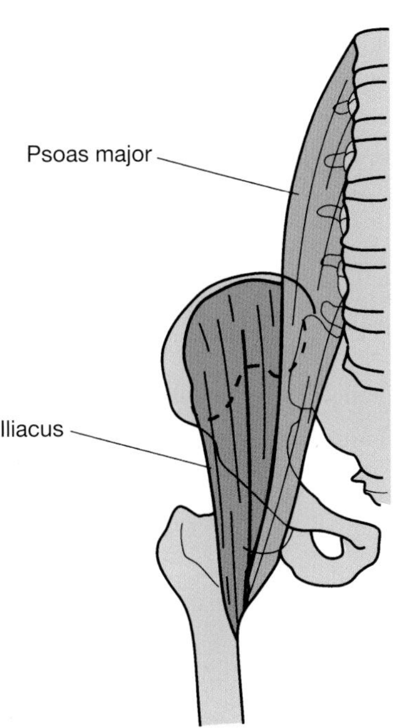

Figure 11.42 The flexors of the hip.

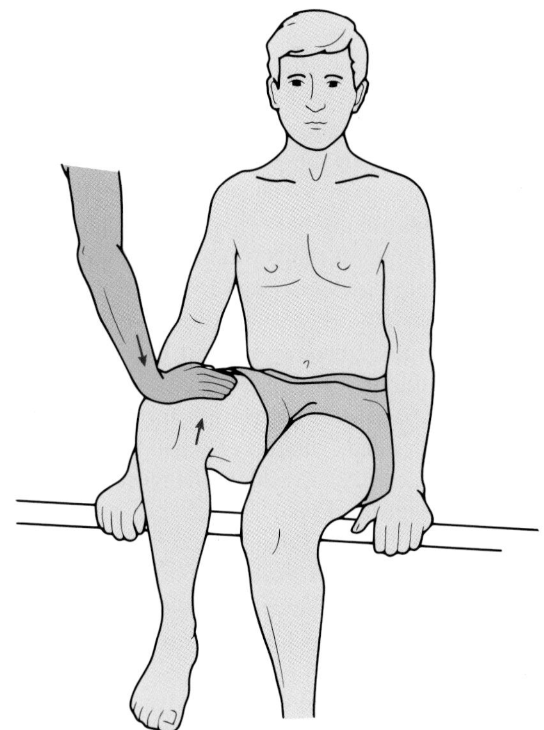

Figure 11.43 Testing hip flexion.

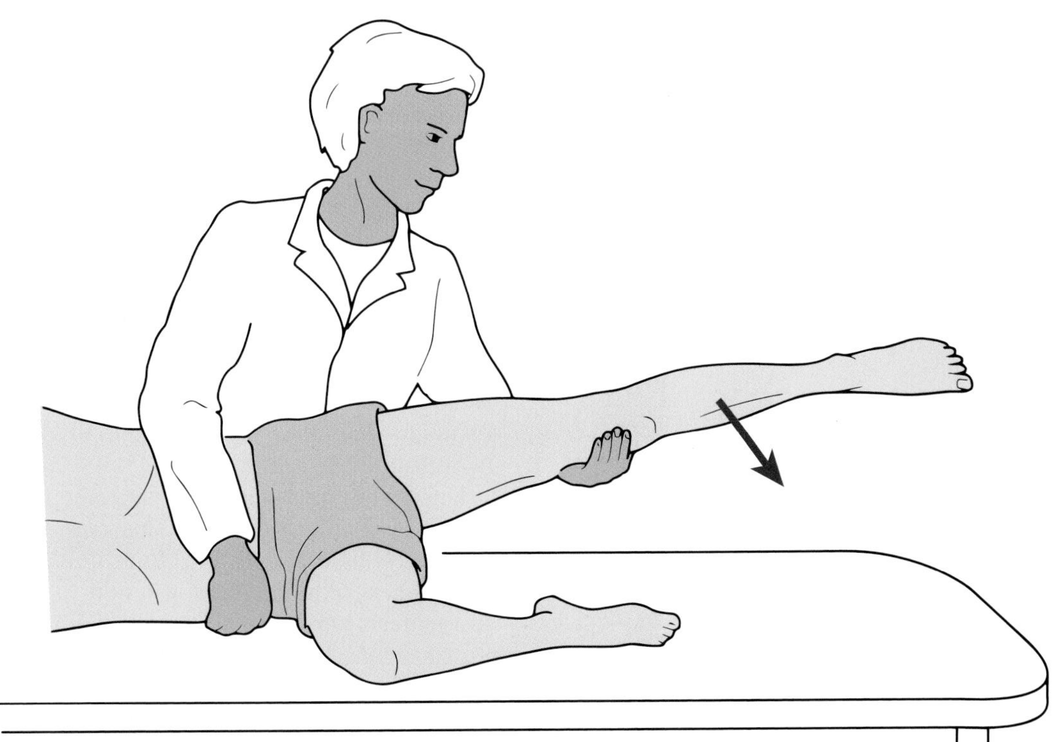

Figure 11.44 Testing hip flexion with gravity eliminated.

Extension

The extensors of the hip are the glutei and hamstrings (Figure 11.45). The gluteal muscles attach to the femur and ITB (gluteus maximus only), and the hamstrings attach to the proximal part of the tibia. The gluteus maximus is the strongest of all the hip extensors. The strength of the hamstrings in hip extension is dependent on the position of the knee. With the knee flexed, the hamstrings are at a disadvantage and are relatively weaker. As the knee is extended, the hamstrings are stretched more and become stronger extensors of the hip.

- Position of patient: Lying prone on the table with the knee extended. The test can also be performed with the knee flexed to isolate the gluteus maximus (Figure 11.46).
- Resisted test: Stabilize the pelvis with one hand with downward pressure, and apply downward resistance above the knee posteriorly on the thigh. Ask the patient to elevate the leg and thigh off the table.

Testing hip extension with gravity eliminated is performed by having the patient lie on the opposite side with the hip flexed and the knee extended (Figure 11.47). Elevate the upper part of the leg (test leg), which is flexed at the hip, and support the weight of the leg as the patient attempts to extend the hip toward you. The gluteus maximus is isolated by performing this test with the patient's knee flexed (Figure 11.46).

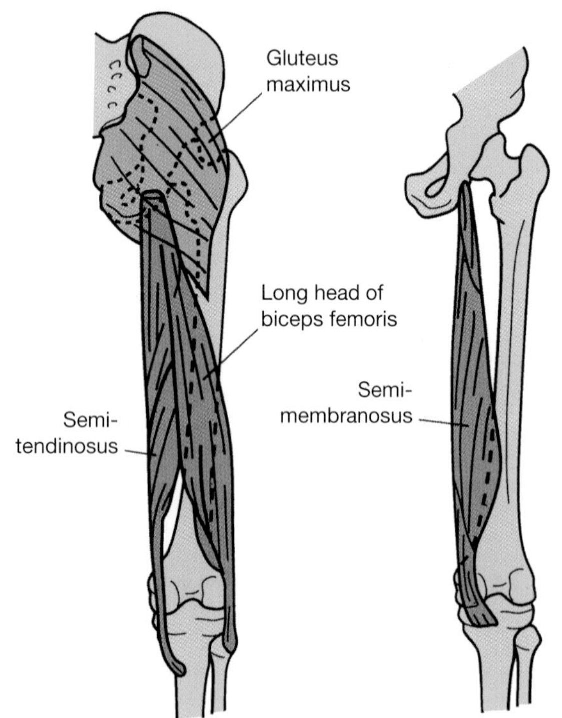

Figure 11.45 The extensors of the hip.

Painful resisted hip extension can be due to spasm of the gluteus maximus or hamstring muscles. Pain can also be caused by ischial bursitis at the ischial tuberosity. Pain may be referred to the hip extensors from spondylolisthesis or a herniated lumbosacral disc.

Weakness of the hip extensors results in difficulty with ambulation and return to erect posture. Stair climbing and walking up an incline are also restricted.

Abduction

The main abductor muscle is the gluteus medius. It is assisted by the gluteus maximus and piriformis (Figure 11.48). The efficiency of the gluteus medius muscle is increased because of the presence of the femoral neck. The more lateral attachment of the muscle increases its resultant torque (Figure 11.49). The primary function of the hip abductors, rather than moving the thigh away from the midline, is to prevent the pelvis from adducting on the thigh (dropping) during unilateral stance.

- Position of patient: Lying on the side with the lower leg slightly flexed at the hip and the knee. The upper leg is in neutral position at the hip and extended at the knee (Figure 11.50).
- Resisted test: Stabilize the pelvis with one hand to prevent the patient from rolling forward or backward. As the patient attempts to elevate the leg from the table, put downward pressure on the inferior distal aspect of the leg.

Testing abduction with gravity eliminated is performed by having the patient lie supine with the knees extended (Figure 11.51). The patient tries to move the leg into abduction so as to separate the legs. Be careful not to allow the patient to externally rotate the hip (substitution).

Lateral hip pain during resisted abduction can be due to trochanteric bursitis. This can result from an excessively tight gluteus medius or minimus.

Weakness of hip abduction results in an abnormal gait pattern, known as a *Trendelenburg gait*.

Adduction

The strongest hip adductor is the adductor magnus (Figure 11.52). Along with the adductor longus,

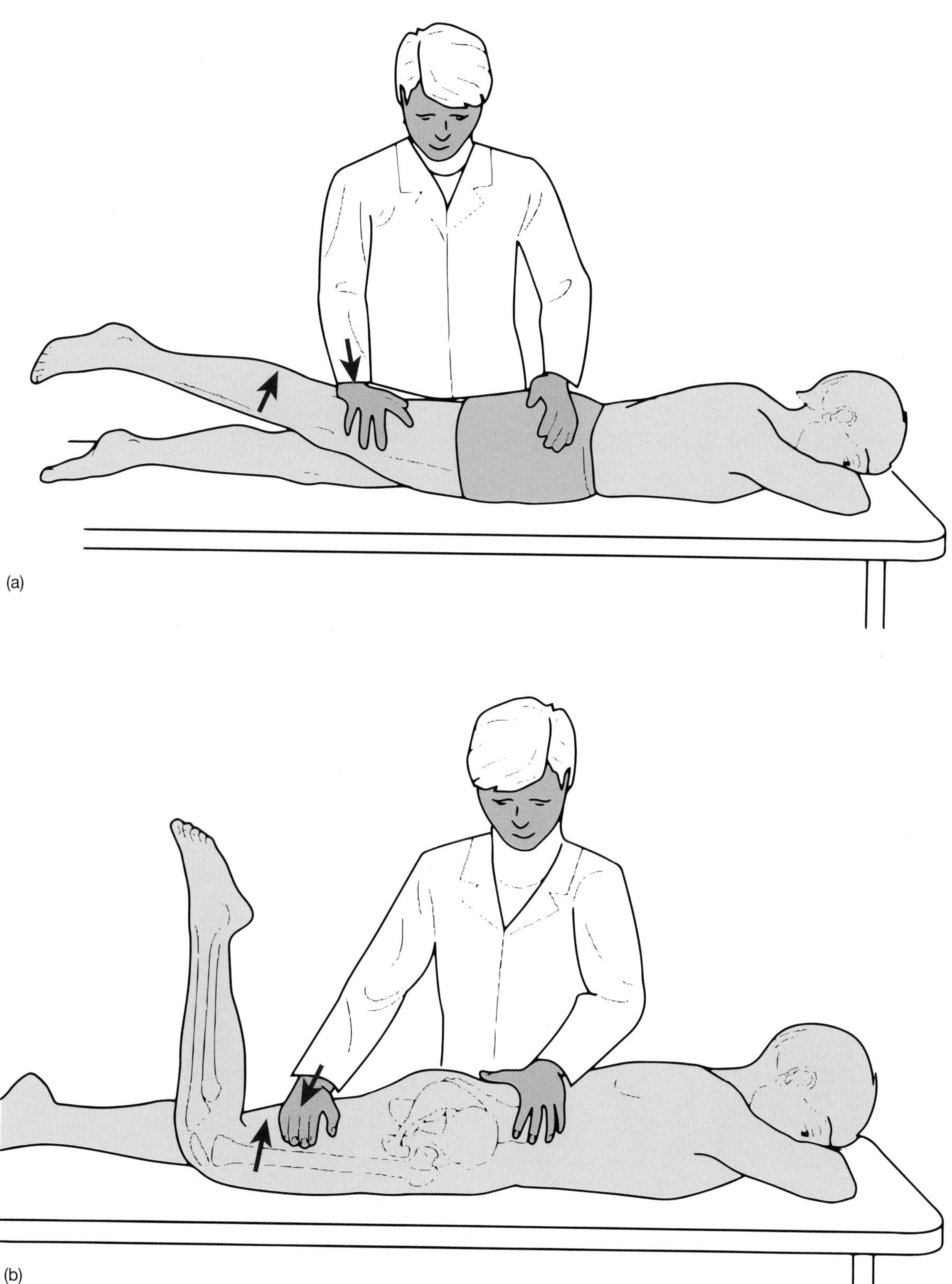

Figure 11.46 (a) Testing hip extension, (b) Isolating the gluteus maximus by testing hip extension with the knee flexed.

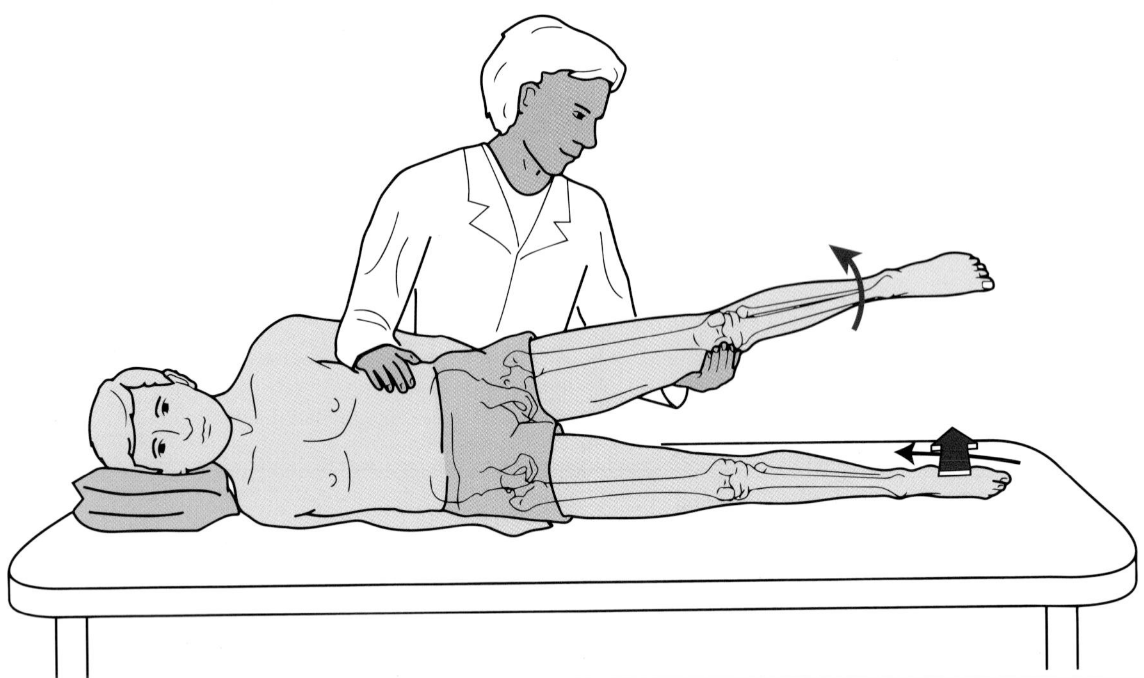

Figure 11.47 Testing hip extension with gravity eliminated.

adductor brevis, and gracilis, the adductor muscles also function to stabilize the pelvis. The hamstrings, gluteus maximus, pectineus, and some of the short rotators also assist in adduction. The hip adductors prevent the lower extremity from sliding into abduction during ambulation (Figure 11.53).

- Position of patient: Lying on the side, with the spine, hip, and knee in neutral position (Figure 11.54).

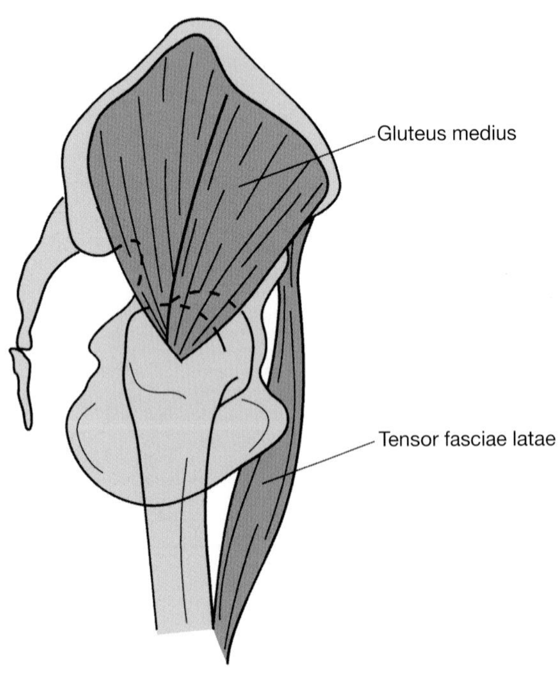

Figure 11.48 The abductors of the hip.

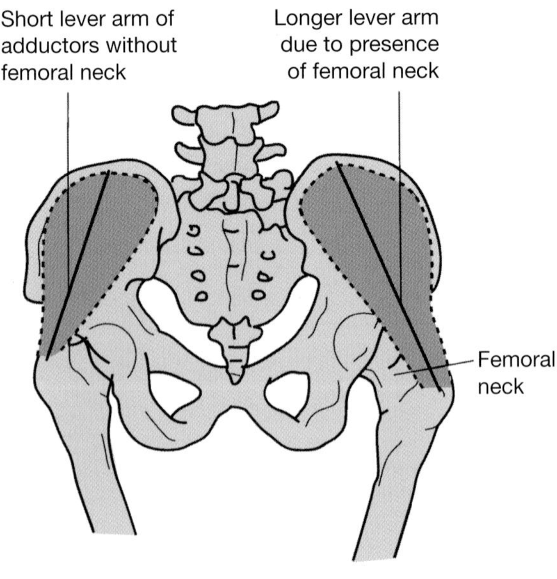

Figure 11.49 The presence of the femoral neck increases the efficiency of the hip abductors.

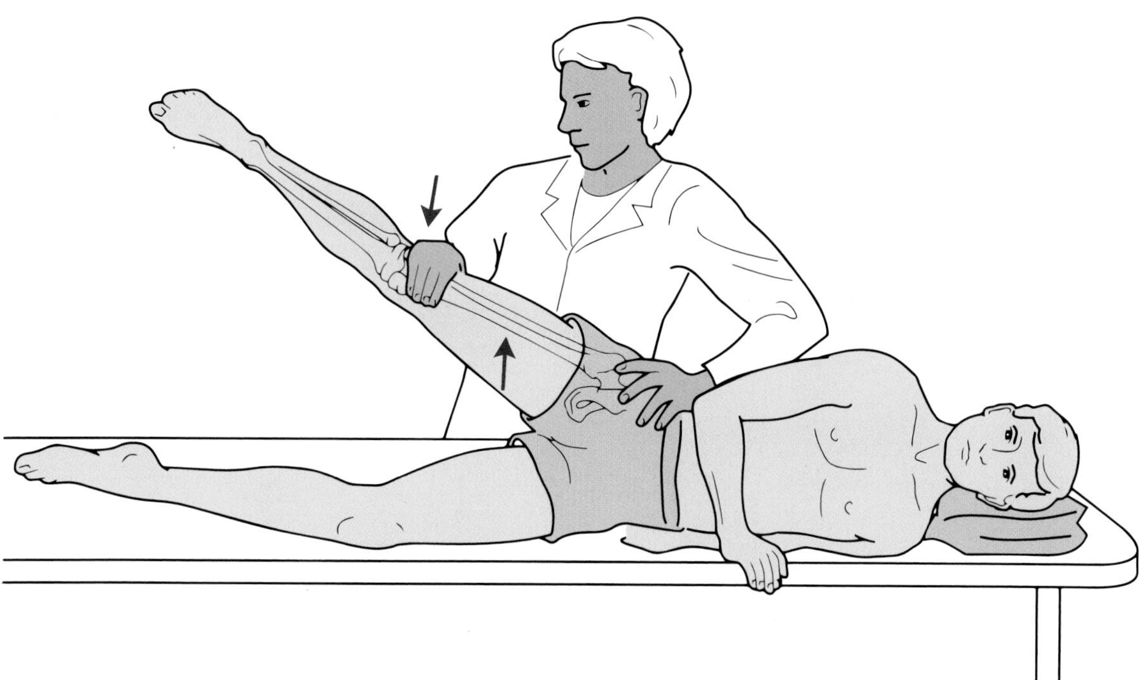

Figure 11.50 Testing hip abduction.

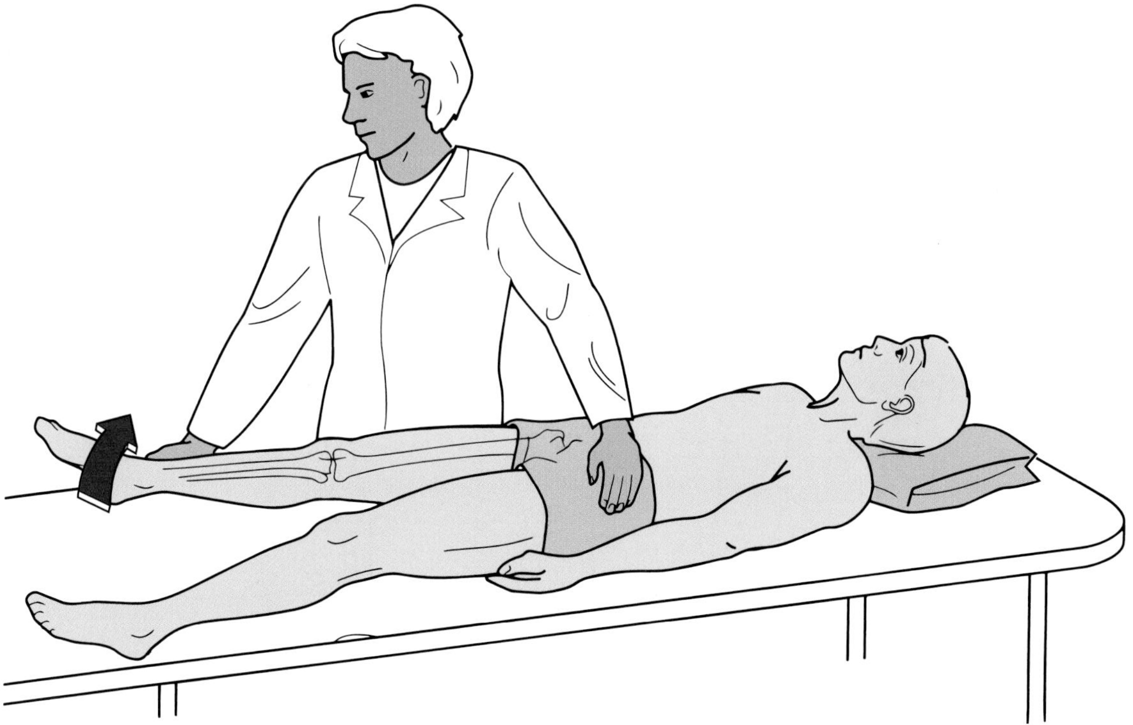

Figure 11.51 Testing hip abduction with gravity eliminated.

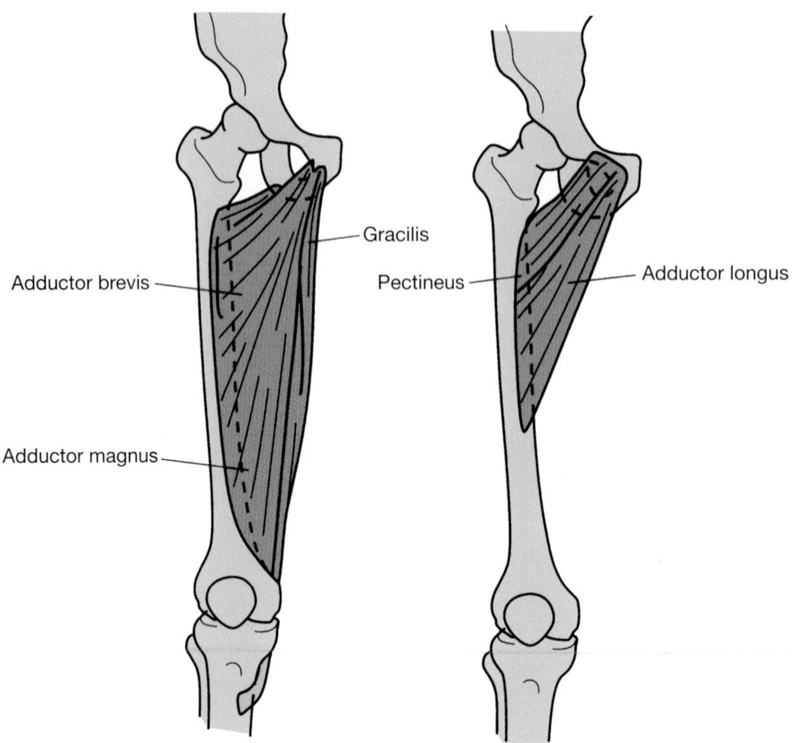

Figure 11.52 The adductors of the hip.

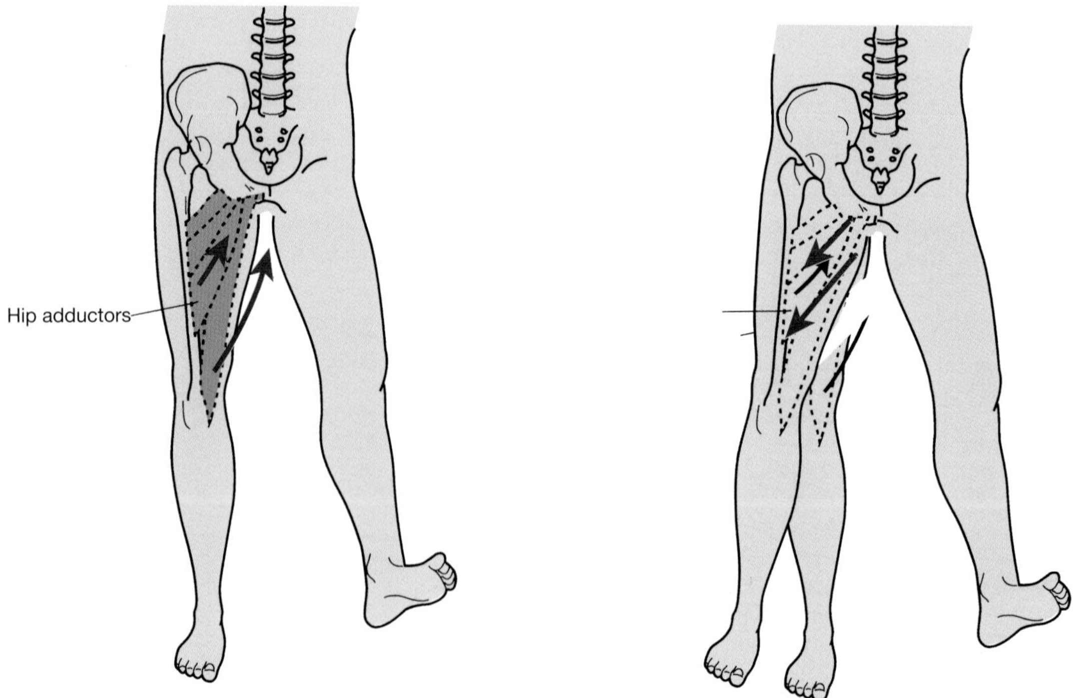

Figure 11.53 During the stance phase of gait, there is a tendency for the weight-bearing limb to slide into abduction. Powerful hip adductors prevent this from occurring, especially during running.

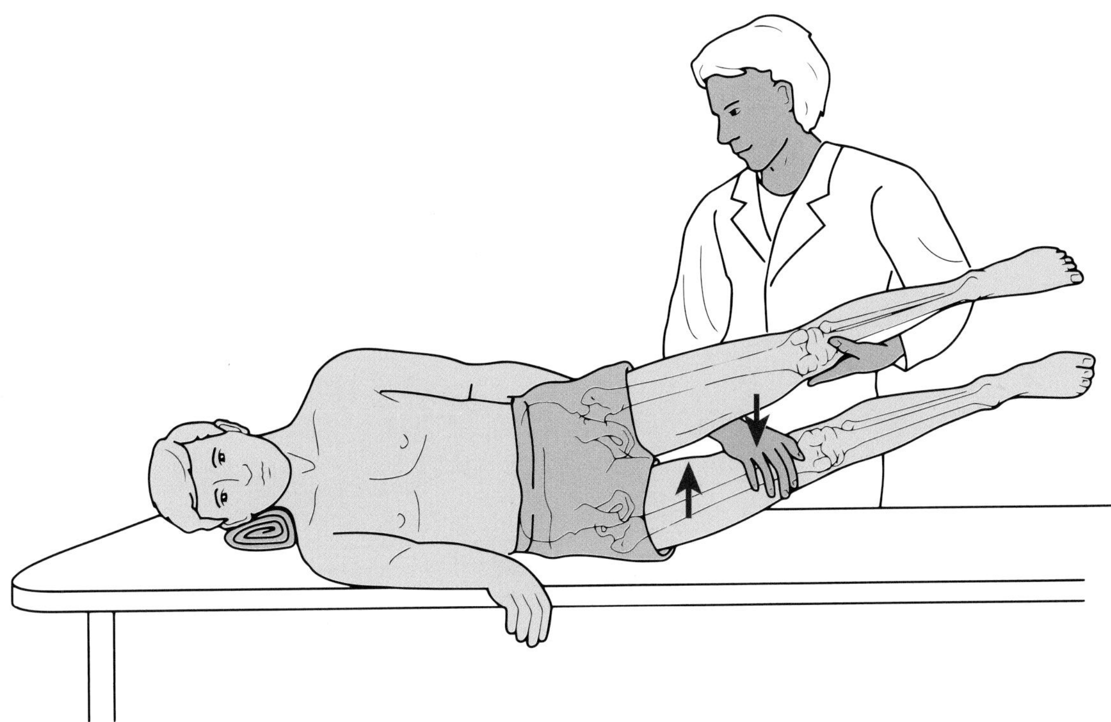

Figure 11.54 Testing hip adduction.

- Resisted test: Lift the upper leg and support it with one hand while pressing down on the lower limb just above the knee with the other hand. Ask the patient to raise the lower extremity off the examining table against your resistance.

Testing hip adduction with gravity eliminated is performed with the patient lying supine (Figure 11.55). The hip is passively or actively abducted, and the patient attempts to bring the limb back toward the midline.

Painful resisted adduction can be due to tendinitis or a tear in the adductor longus, which is the most commonly "pulled groin muscle." Pain in the region of the pubic ramus can be due to osteitis pubis. Pain below the knee can be due to a pes anserinus bursitis irritated by the contracting gracilis muscle at its distal attachment.

External (Lateral) Rotation

The external rotators of the hip include the piriformis, obturator internus, obturator externus, and the two gemelli. The quadratus femoris and pectineus also assist in external rotation (Figure 11.56).

- Position of patient: Sitting with both knees flexed over the edge of the table (Figure 11.57).
- Resisted test: Hold the patient's leg at the medial aspect above the ankle. The patient then attempts to rotate the leg upward so as to reach the opposite knee.

Testing external rotation with gravity eliminated is performed with the patient lying supine with the knee and hip in neutral position (Figure 11.58). The patient attempts to rotate the lower extremity away from the midline so that the lateral malleolus is in contact with the table.

Painful resisted external rotation can be caused by dysfunction in the piriformis muscle. This can be confirmed by performing the piriformis test.

Piriformis Test

This test is used to isolate the piriformis muscle in external rotation of the hip (Figure 11.59).

- Position of patient: Lying supine with the affected hip and knee flexed.
- Resisted test: Push the patient's thigh and knee into adduction and then ask the patient to push them back toward your chest.

A complaint of pain on attempted external rotation in this position against resistance is considered a positive finding on the piriformis test. This maneuver may

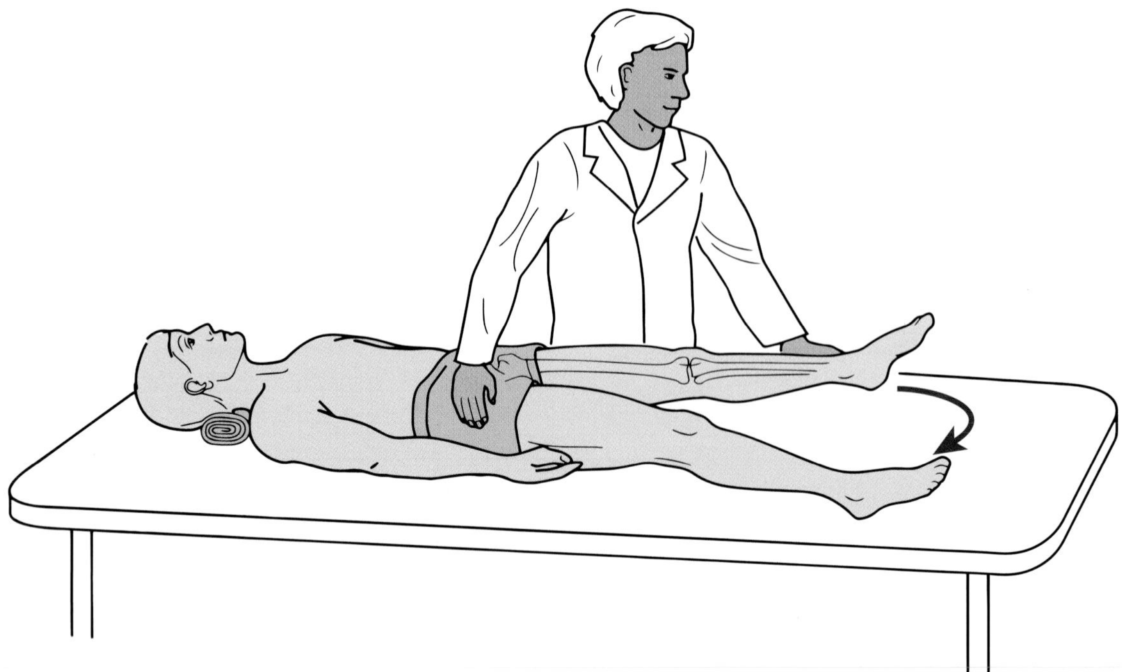

Figure 11.55 Testing hip adduction with gravity eliminated.

elicit tingling or pain in the distribution of the sciatic nerve due to its proximity to the piriformis muscle.

Internal (Medial) Rotation

The internal rotators of the hip are less than half as strong as the external rotators. The gluteus medius, gluteus minimus, and tensor fasciae latae are the primary internal rotators of the hip (Figure 11.60).

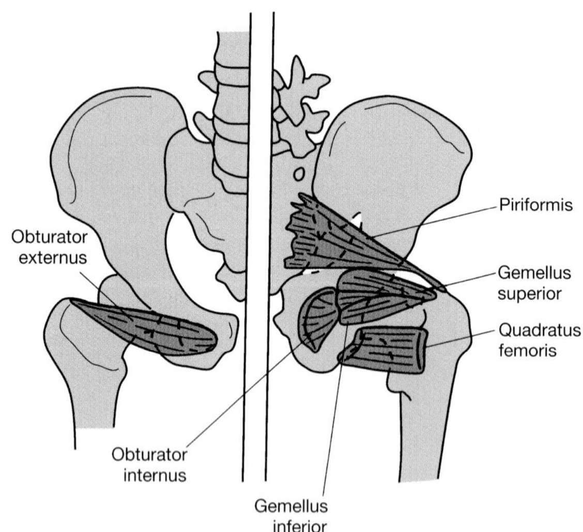

Figure 11.56 The lateral (external) rotators of the hip.

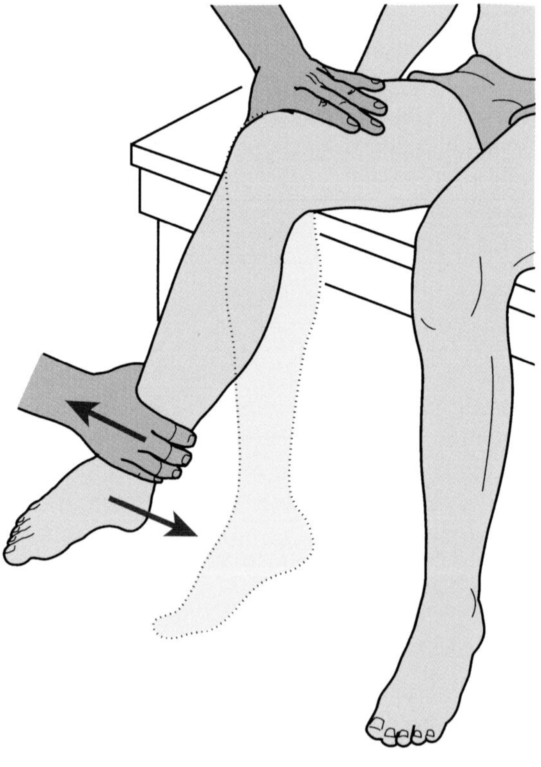

Figure 11.57 Testing hip lateral (external) rotation.

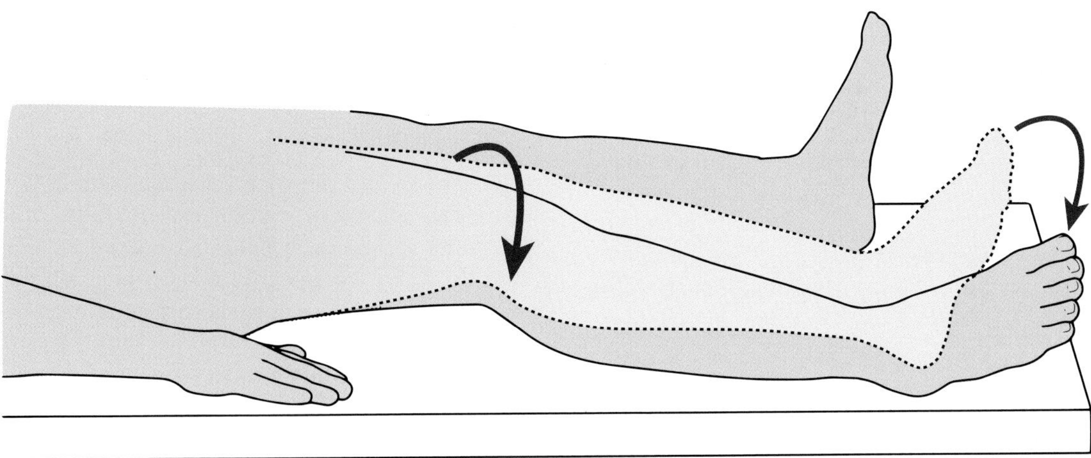

Figure 11.58 Testing hip lateral (external) rotation with gravity eliminated.

Accessory muscles include the semitendinosus and semimembranosus.

- Position of patient: Sitting at the edge of the table with the knees bent over the table (Figure 11.61).
- Resisted test: Place your hand on the distal lateral aspect of the leg proximal to the ankle. The patient attempts to rotate the leg laterally away from the opposite leg.

Testing internal rotation with gravity eliminated is performed with the patient lying supine with the hip and knee in neutral position (Figure 11.62). The patient then attempts to roll the lower extremity inward so as to bring the medial aspect of the foot in contact with the table.

Painful resisted internal rotation can be seen in arthritic conditions of the hip.

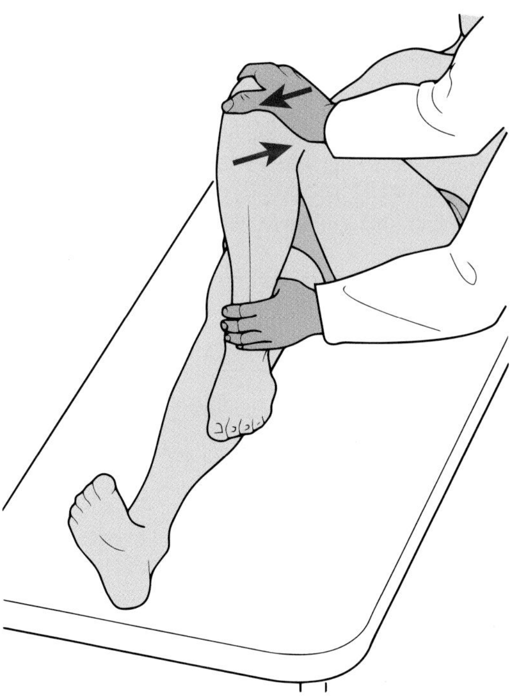

Figure 11.59 The piriformis test isolates this muscle as a cause of buttock pain. Reproduction of symptoms of sciatica, such as tingling or radiating pain down the posterolateral aspect of the thigh and leg, confirms the diagnosis of piriformis syndrome.

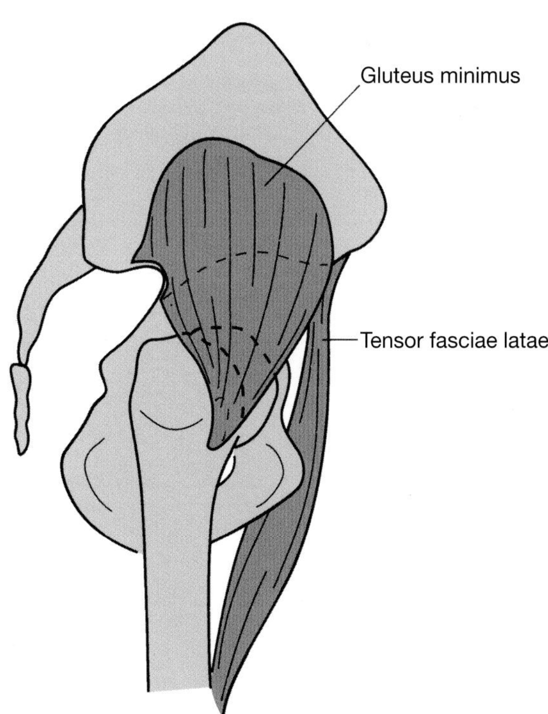

Figure 11.60 The medial (internal) rotators of the hip.

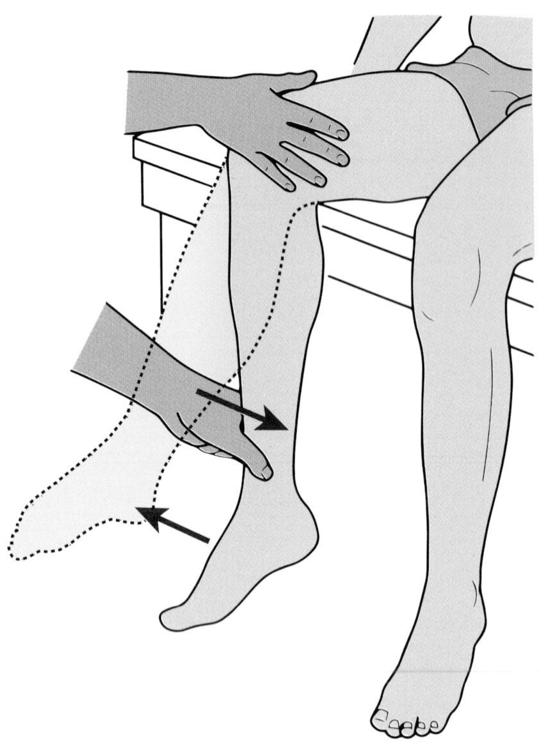

Figure 11.61 Testing hip medial (internal) rotation.

Neurological Examination

Motor

The innervation and spinal levels of the muscles that function across the hip joint are listed in Table 11.1 (p. 325).

Reflexes

There are no reflexes that can be elicited at the hip.

Sensation

Light touch and pinprick sensation should be examined following the motor examination. The dermatomes for the anterolateral aspect of the hip are LI and L2. Refer to Figure 11.63 for the exact locations of the key sensory areas in these dermatomes. We have intentionally included dermatome drawings from *different* sources in this text to emphasize that patients as well as anatomists vary significantly with respect to sensory nerve root innervation of the extremities. The peripheral nerves providing sensation in the hip region are shown in Figure 11.64.

The lateral femoral cutaneous nerve (Figure 11.65) is of clinical significance, as it may be compressed at the waist, where it crosses the inguinal ligament. Pain, numbness, or tingling in the proximal lateral aspect of the thigh may be due to compression of this nerve. This is called *meralgia paresthetica.*

Many common abnormal gait patterns result from dysfunction in the muscles about the hip. These abnormal gait patterns are described in Chapter 14.

Referred Pain Patterns

Pain in the hip and groin region can result from urogenital or abdominal organ disease. For example, resisted hip flexion or external rotation may be painful in patients with appendicitis.

Dysfunction of the knee or diseases of the distal part of the femur can also radiate pain to the hip.

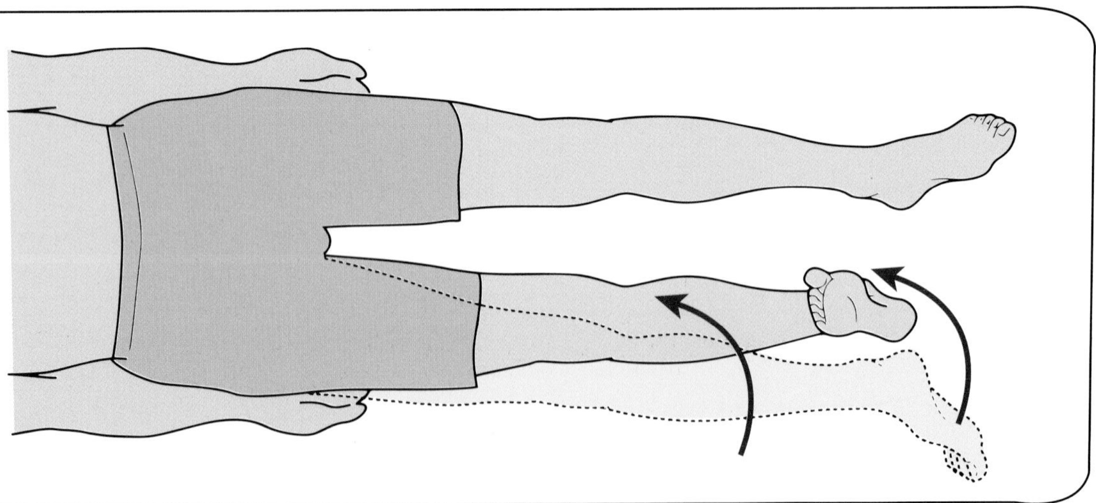

Figure 11.62 Testing hip medial (internal) rotation with gravity eliminated.

Table 11.1 Muscle, Innervation, and Root Levels of the Hip

Movement	Muscles	Innervation	Root Levels
Flexion of hip	Psoas	L1–L3	L1–L3
	Iliacus	Femoral	L2, L3
	Rectus femoris	Femoral	L2–L4
	Sartorius	Femoral	L2, L3
	Pectineus	Femoral	L2, L3
	Adductor longus	Obturator	L2, L3
	Adductor brevis	Obturator	L2–L4
	Gracilis	Obturator	L2, L3
Extension of hip	Biceps femoris	Sciatic	L5, S1, S2
	Semimembranosus	Sciatic	L5, S1
	Semitendinosus	Sciatic	L5, S1,S2
	Gluteus maximus	Inferior gluteal	L5, S1,S2
	Gluteus medius (posterior)	Superior gluteal	L4, L5, S1
	Adductor magnus	Obturator and sciatic	L3, L4
Abduction of hip	Tensor fascia latae	Superior gluteal	L4, L5, S1
	Gluteus medius	Superior gluteal	L4, L5, S1
	Gluteus minimus	Superior gluteal	L4, L5, S1
	Gluteus maximus	Inferior gluteal	L5, S1,S2
	Sartorius	Femoral	L2, L3
Adduction of hip	Adductor magnus	Obturator and sciatic	L3, L4
	Adductor longus	Obturator	L2, L3
	Adductor brevis	Obturator	L2–L4
	Gracilis	Obturator	L2, L3
	Pectineus	Femoral	L2, L3
Internal (medial) rotation of the hip	Adductor longus	Obturator	L2, L3
	Adductor brevis	Obturator	L2–L4
	Adductor magnus	Obturator and sciatic	L3, L4
	Gluteus medius (anterior)	Superior gluteal	L4, L5, S1
	Gluteus minimus (anterior)	Superior gluteal	L4, L5, S1
	Tensor fasciae latae	Superior gluteal	L4, L5, S1
	Pectineus	Femoral	L2, L3
	Gracilis	Obturator	12, L3
External (lateral) rotation of hip	Gluteus maximus	Inferior gluteal	L5, S1,S2
	Obturator internus	Nerve (N) to obturator internus	L5, S1,S2
	Obturator externus	Obturator	L3, L4
	Quadratus femoris	N to quadratus femoris	L4, L5, S1
	Piriformis	L5, S1,S2	L5, S1,S2
	Gemellus superior	N to obturator internus	L5, S1,S2
	Gemellus inferior	N to quadratus femoris	L4, L5, S1
	Sartorius	Femoral	L2, L3
	Gluteus medius (posterior)	Superior gluteal	L4, L5, S1

An LI or L2 radiculopathy and sacroiliac joint dysfunction can also refer pain to the hip.

Special Tests

Flexibility Tests

Thomas Test and Modified Thomas Test

The original Thomas test was used to rule out a hip flexion contracture (Figures 11.66a and 11.66b). The test is performed with the patient lying supine on the examining table. One knee is brought to the patient's chest and held there. Make sure the lower region of the lumbar spine remains flat on the table. In the presence of a hip flexion contracture, the extended leg will bend at the knee and the thigh will raise from the table.

The Thomas test has been modified to ensure that the lumbar spine is stabilized. The patient is asked to sit on the end of the treatment table. The patient

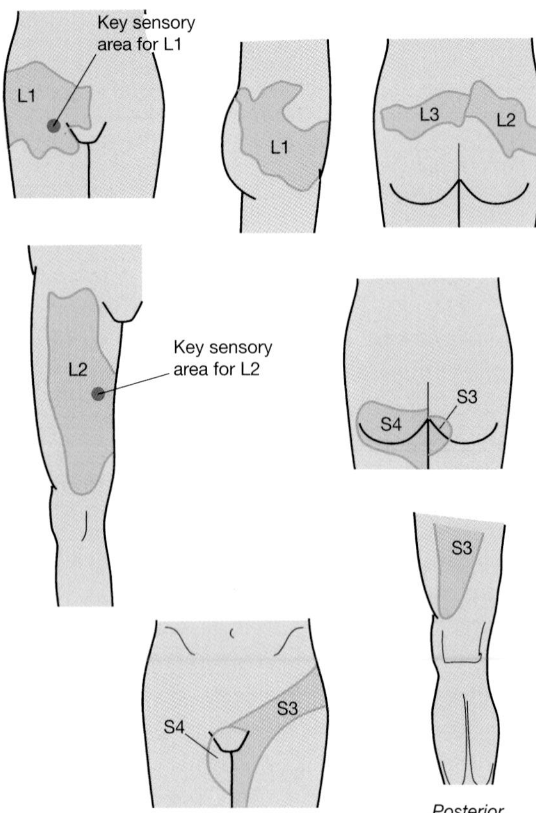

Figure 11.63 The dermatomes of the hip. Note the key areas for testing sensation in the L1 and L2 dermatomes.

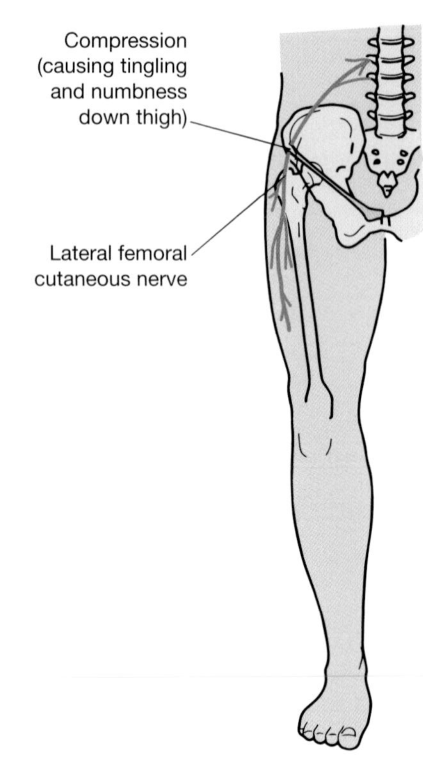

Figure 11.65 The lateral femoral cutaneous nerve (L2, L3) is a purely sensory nerve that can be compressed under the inguinal ligament at the anterior superior iliac spine, causing meralgia paresthetica.

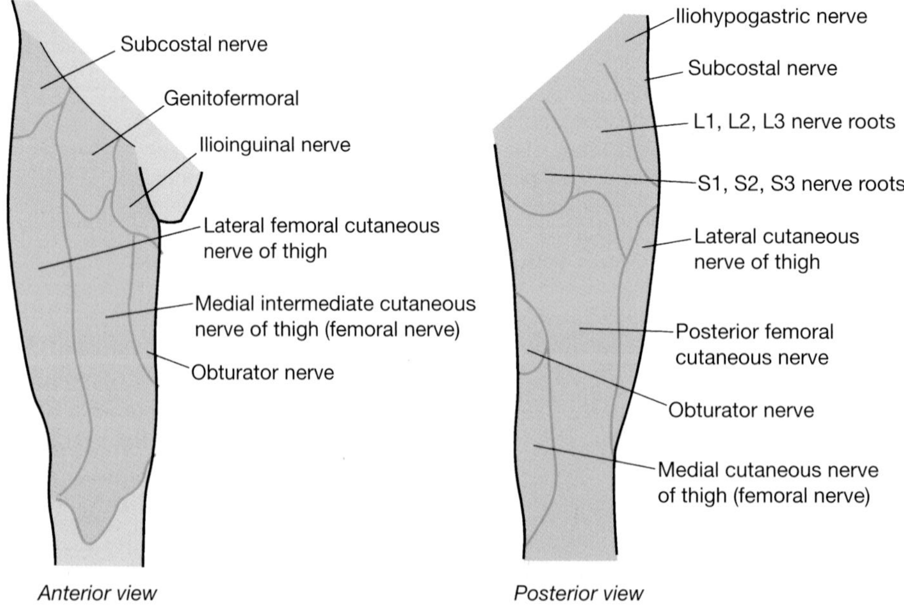

Figure 11.64 The peripheral nerves and their sensory territories.

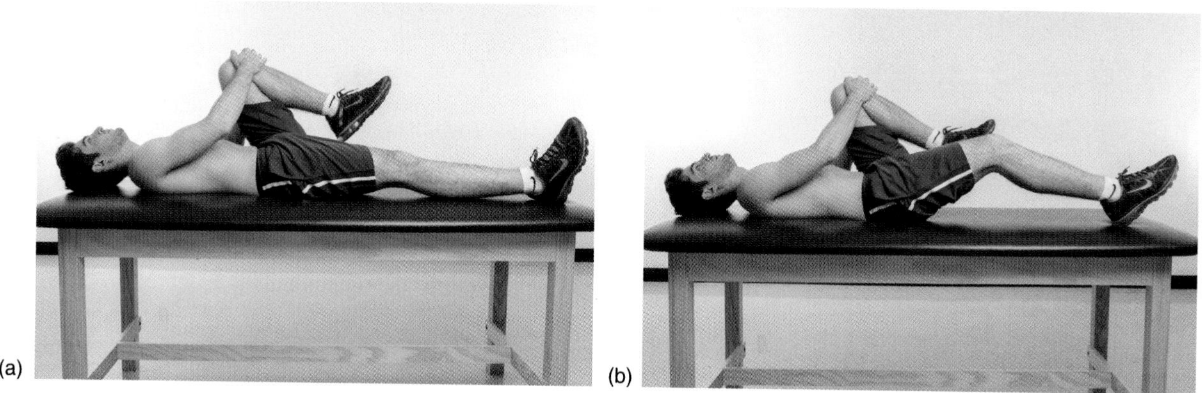

Figure 11.66 Thomas test (a). Normal (b). Note that the patient's knee elevates from the examination table due to a right hip flexion contracture.

then holds both legs while lying back into supine. To ensure proper lumbar alignment, the patient performs a pelvis tilt while holding both legs in maximal flexion. The leg being tested is allowed to drop down. If the iliopsoas has a normal length the thigh should be parallel to the table. To test the rectus femoris the examiner places pressure over the hip into extension and the amount of knee extension is observed. If the rectus is tight then the amount of knee extension will increase. This can also be addressed by putting pressure on the leg to increase knee flexion and if there is tightness then the hip will flex. ITB flexibility can also be tested by performing the test in abduction. Maintain pelvic stability. There should be 20 degrees of adduction present if there is normal flexibility (Dutton, 2012) (https://www.youtube.com/watch?v=q4MFh4aFmfM).

Ober's Test

This test is used to assess tightness of the ITB (Figure 11.67). The patient is placed in a position so as

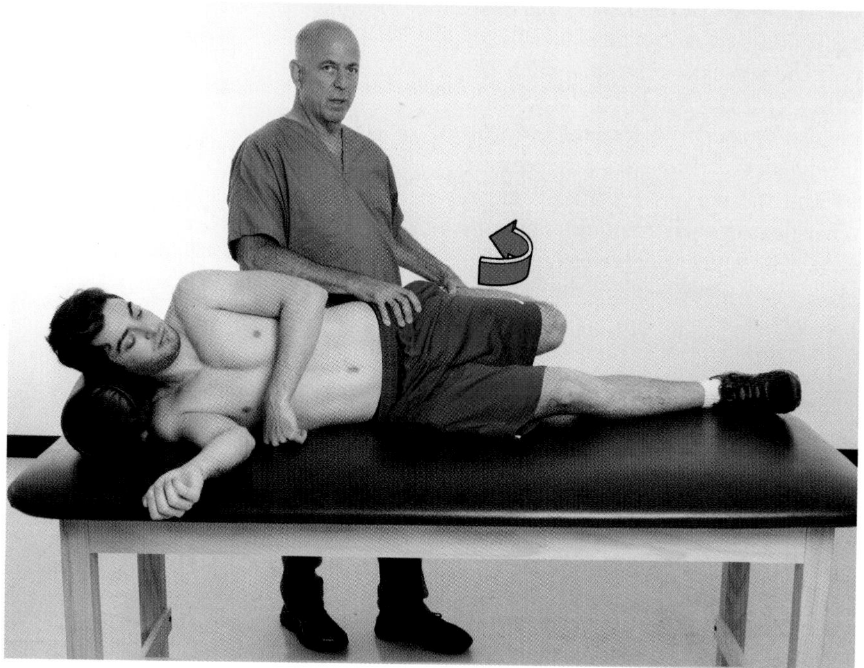

Figure 11.67 Ober's test. The test is performed with the knee in flexion. Extend the hip passively so that the tensor fascia latae (TFL) crosses the greater trochanter of the femur. The test result is positive when the knee fails to drop downward due to excessive tightness of the ITB.

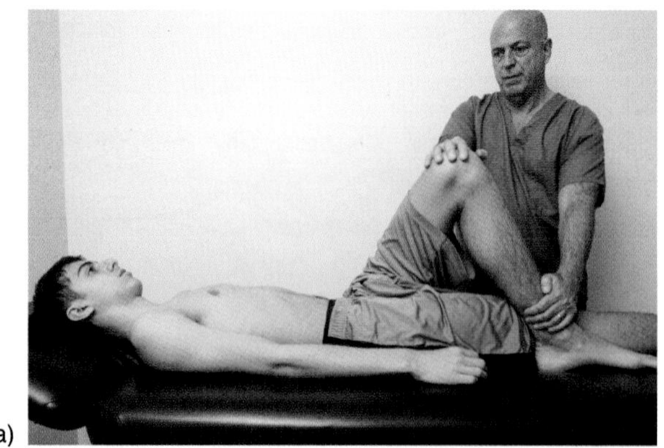

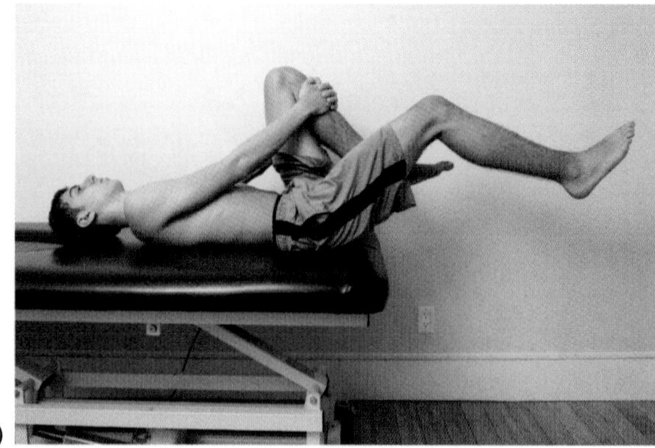

Figure 11.68 (a) Piriformis flexibility test. (b) Abnormal Ely test. Positive finding for rectus femoris tightness is when the thigh elevates and the hip flexes.

to stretch the ITB. The patient lies on the unaffected side. The lower leg is flexed at the hip and knee. The upper leg (test leg) is flexed at the knee and extended at the hip while being lifted in the air by the examiner. The ITB is tight and the test is abnormal when the knee cannot be lowered to the table. If the test is performed with the knee in extension, you may pick up a less obvious contracture of the ITB.

Ely's Test

This test is used to test the flexibility of the rectus femoris. The patient is placed in the side lying position with the test leg up. The examiner passively flexes the patient's knee. If the rectus is restricted then the ipsilateral hip will flex and the pelvis will anteriorly rotate. This test can also be used to determine involvement in the L2–L3–L4 nerve roots. To differentiate between the rectus and the nerve root involvement, relax some of the knee flexion and extend the patient's hip. See Chapter 6, p. 130 femoral nerve stretch, Figure 6.62 (Peeler)

Piriformis Test

This test was described previously in the Resistive Testing section (see pp. 313–314, Figure 11.59).

Piriformis Flexibility Test

The patient is in the supine position with their hip flexed to 60 degrees. Fully adduct the patient's hip followed by internal then external rotation. The normal range should be 45 degrees in either direction. Tightness in internal rotation is due to the superior fibers. Tightness in external rotation is due to tightness in the inferior fibers (Figure 11.68a) (Dutton, 2012).

Trendelenburg's Test

This test is used to determine whether pelvic stability can be maintained by the hip abductor muscles (Figure 11.69). The patient stands on the test leg and raises the other leg off the ground. Normally, the

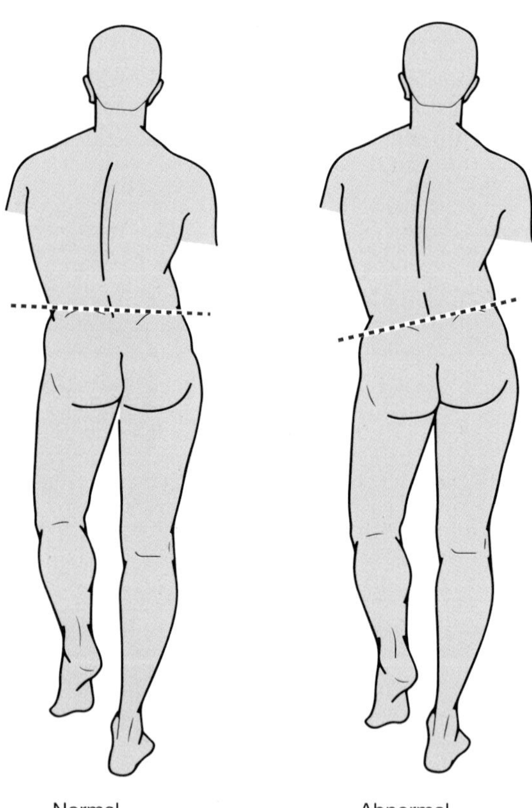

Figure 11.69 Trendelenburg's test (a). Normally, the pelvis on the nonweight-bearing side elevates. (b) Positive finding due to left abductor weakness. Note that the pelvis is dropped on the nonweight-bearing side.

pelvis should tilt upward on the nonweight-bearing side. The test finding is abnormal if the pelvis drops on the nonweight-bearing side (https://www.youtube.com/watch?v=TY-G4ErruUA&index=12&list=PL82F410F7D965AFCD).

Patrick's (Fabere) Test

This test is performed to assess possible dysfunction of the hip and sacroiliac joint (Figure 11.70). The patient is supine with the hip flexed, abducted, and externally rotated. The patient is asked to place the lateral malleolus of the test leg above the knee of the extended, unaffected leg. The test result is positive if this maneuver causes pain for the patient. The test may be amplified by your pressing downward on the test knee. Pain with downward pressure indicates a sacroiliac joint problem, as the joint is compressed in this position. https://www.youtube.com/watch?v=o61MNLZmloc

Sign of the Buttock

This test is performed to determine if there is serious hip pathology (neoplasm, fracture, infection). The patient is in the supine position. Passively assess straight leg raising. If it is limited, assess the range of hip flexion with the knee flexed. If this is also restricted and the patient presents with a noncapsular pattern, the test is considered to be positive (Cyriax, 1982).

Alignment Tests

Test for True Leg Length

This test should be performed if you think the patient has unequal leg length, which may be noted on inspection and during observation of gait. A true leg length discrepancy is always noted when the patient stands with both feet on the floor. The knee of the longer leg will be flexed, or the pelvis will be dropped on the short side. A valgus deformity of the knee or ankle may also be noted. To measure leg length accurately, it is important to make sure that the patient is lying on a flat, hard surface. Both legs should be placed in the same position with regard to abduction and adduction from the midline. Measurement is taken from the anterior superior iliac spine to the distal medial malleolus on the same side (Figure 11.71). This is then compared to the opposite side.

The true leg length discrepancy is due to shortening of either the tibia or the femur. If the patient lies supine with both knees flexed and the feet flat on the table, you can observe whether the knees are at the same height. If the knee is lower on the short side, the difference in leg length is due to a shortened tibia. If the knee extends further on the long side than the other, the shortening is due to a difference in the

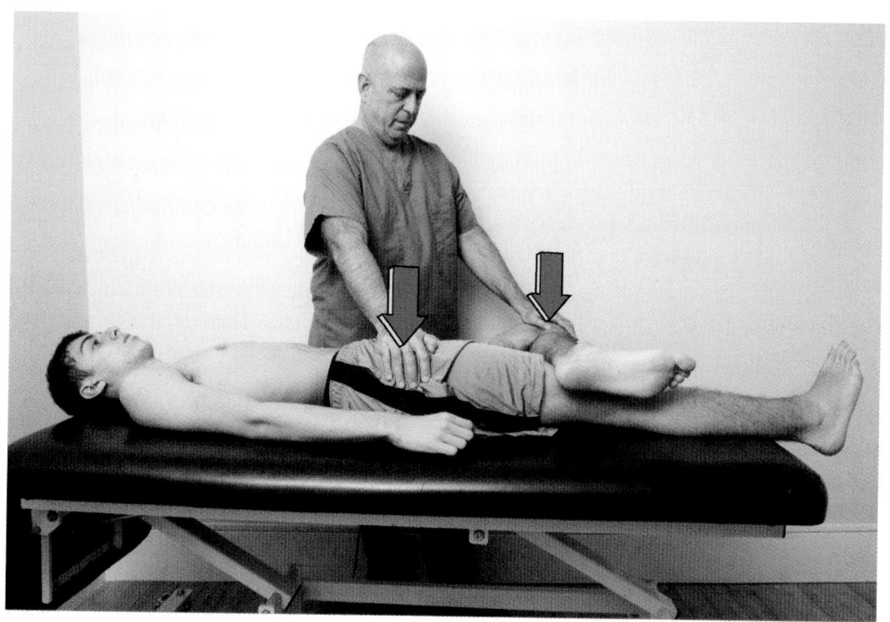

Figure 11.70 Patrick's (Fabere) test. By applying pressure to the pelvis and the knee, you can elicit sacroiliac joint dysfunction as you compress the joint.

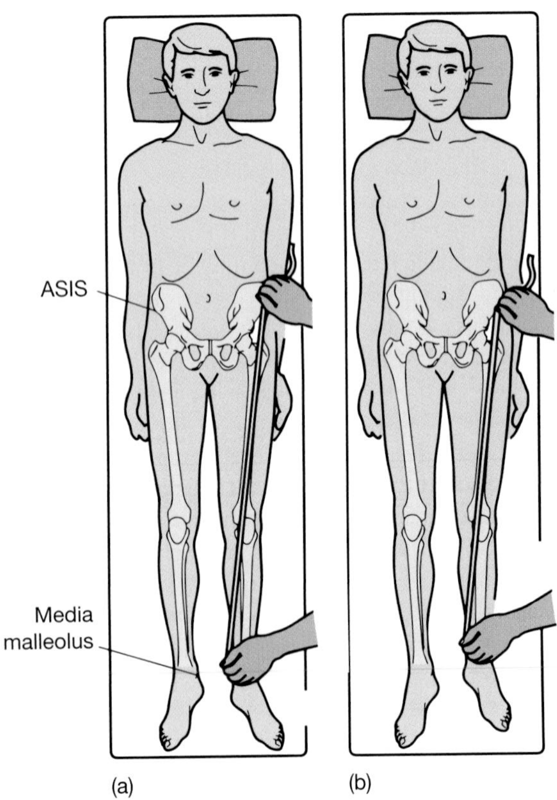

Figure 11.71 (a) True leg length is measured from the anterior superior iliac spine to the medial malleolus. (b) A leg length discrepancy is illustrated.

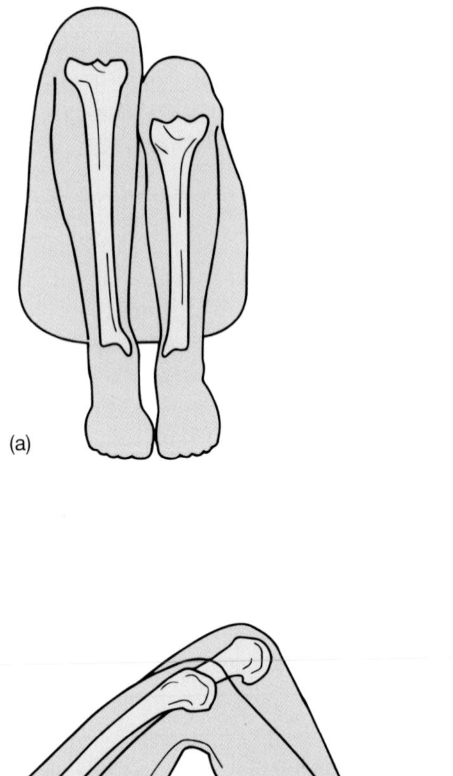

Figure 11.72 (a) The tibia is shorter on the patient's left. (b) The femur is shorter on the right.

femoral length (Figure 11.72). More precise measurements can be made from radiographs.

Apparent Leg Length Discrepancy

This test should be performed after true leg length discrepancy is ruled out. Apparent leg length discrepancy may be due to a flexion or adduction deformity of the hip joint, a tilting of the pelvis, or a sacroiliac dysfunction.

The test is performed with the patient supine, lying as flat as possible on the table. Attempt to have both legs oriented symmetrically. Measure from the umbilicus to the medial malleolus on both sides. A difference in measurement signifies a difference of apparent leg length (Figure 11.73) (https://www.youtube.com/watch?v=Lo87BX7QUhA).

Craig Test

This test is used to measure the degree of femoral anteversion. The femoral head and neck are not perpendicular to the condyles of the femur. The angle that the head and neck of the femur make with the perpendicular to the condyles is called the *angle of anteversion* (Figure 11.74). This angle decreases from about 30 degrees in the infant to about 10–15 degrees in the adult. A patient with femoral anteversion of more than 15 degrees may be noted to have excessive toeing-in. Freedom of internal rotation on passive range of motion would also be noted, with relative restriction of external rotation. Observation of the knees may reveal medially placed patellae, also referred to as *squinting patellae*.

To perform the test for approximation of anteversion of the femur, the patient is placed in the prone position and the test knee is flexed to 90 degrees (Figure 11.75). Examine the greater trochanter and palpate it as you rotate the hip medially and laterally. With the trochanter being palpated in

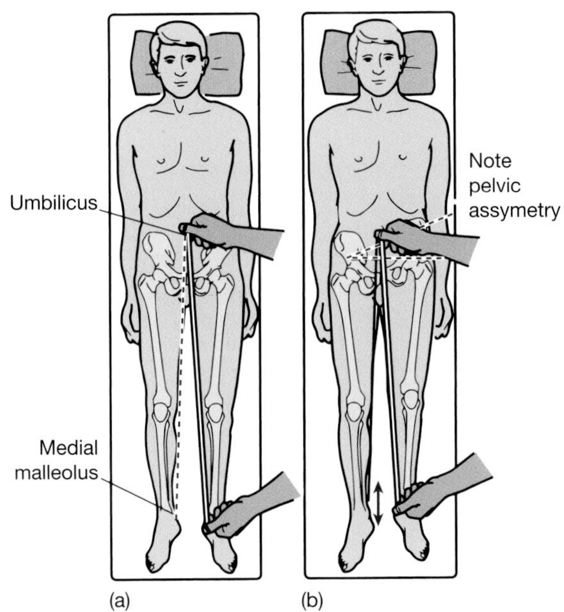

Figure 11.73 (a) Apparent leg length is measured from the umbilicus to the medial malleolus. (b) Here, the difference in apparent leg length is due to an asymmetrical pelvis.

its most lateral position, the angle of anteversion can be measured between the leg and the vertical. More precise measurements can be made from radiographs.

Tests for Integrity of the Hip Joint for Degenerative Joint Disease (DJD) or Labral Tear

Hip Scour (Quadrant) Test

The patient is in the supine position with the tested leg in flexion and the foot resting on the table. The examiner passively flexes the hip and brings the leg into adduction facing the opposite shoulder. (Figure 11.76a) The examiner compresses the joint along the shaft of the femur. This assesses the inner part of the quadrant. The examiner then completes an arc of motion moving from flexion and adduction to flexion and abduction. This assesses the outer quadrant. The femur is maintained in the mid position of rotation throughout the arc of motion. The normal finding is a smooth, painless arc. If there is resistance, apprehension or glitching this may indicate hip pathology (Maitland, 2014a; Magee, 2008; Dutton, 2012) (https://www.youtube.com/watch?v=TY-G4ErruUA&list=PL82F410F7D965AFCD&index=12).

Test for Anterior Labral Tear (FADDIR Test)

The patient is in the supine position. Place the hip into full flexion, lateral rotation, and abduction.

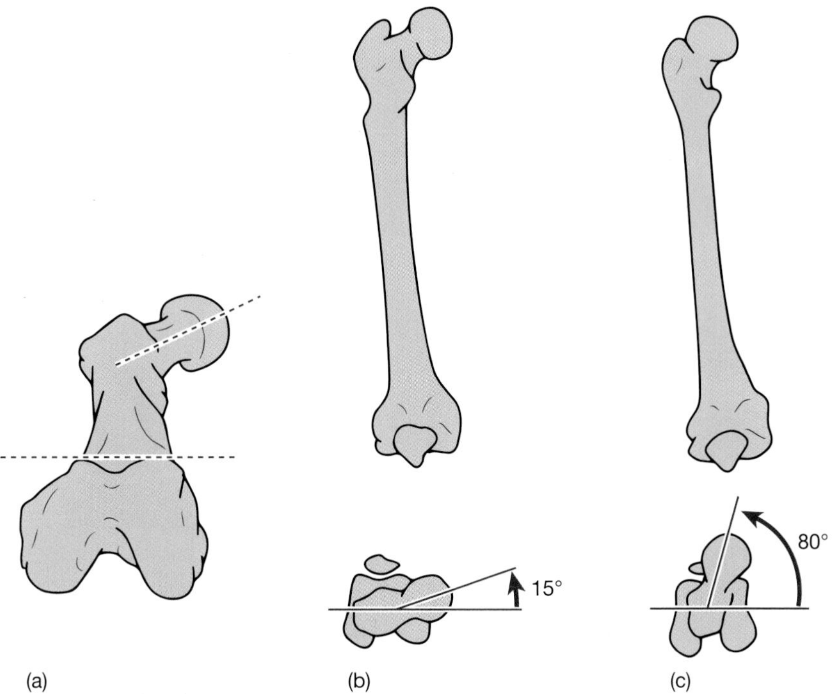

Figure 11.74 (a) The angle of femoral anteversion. (b) Normal angle. (c) Excessive angle.

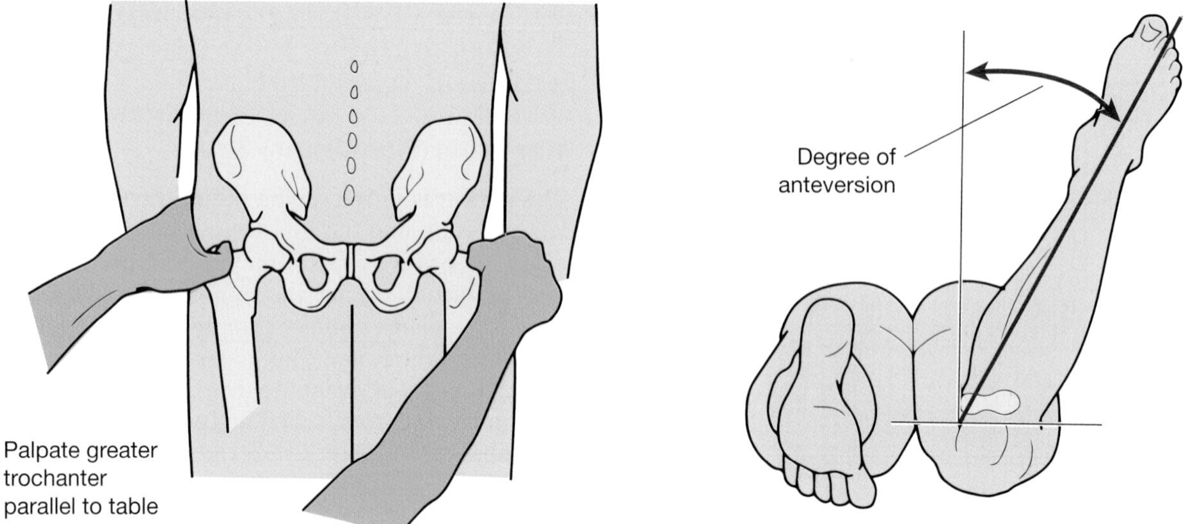

Figure 11.75 Craig test. To measure the angle of femoral anteversion, first palpate the greater trochanter and rotate the leg so that the trochanter is parallel to the examination table. Now note the angle formed by the leg and the vertical.

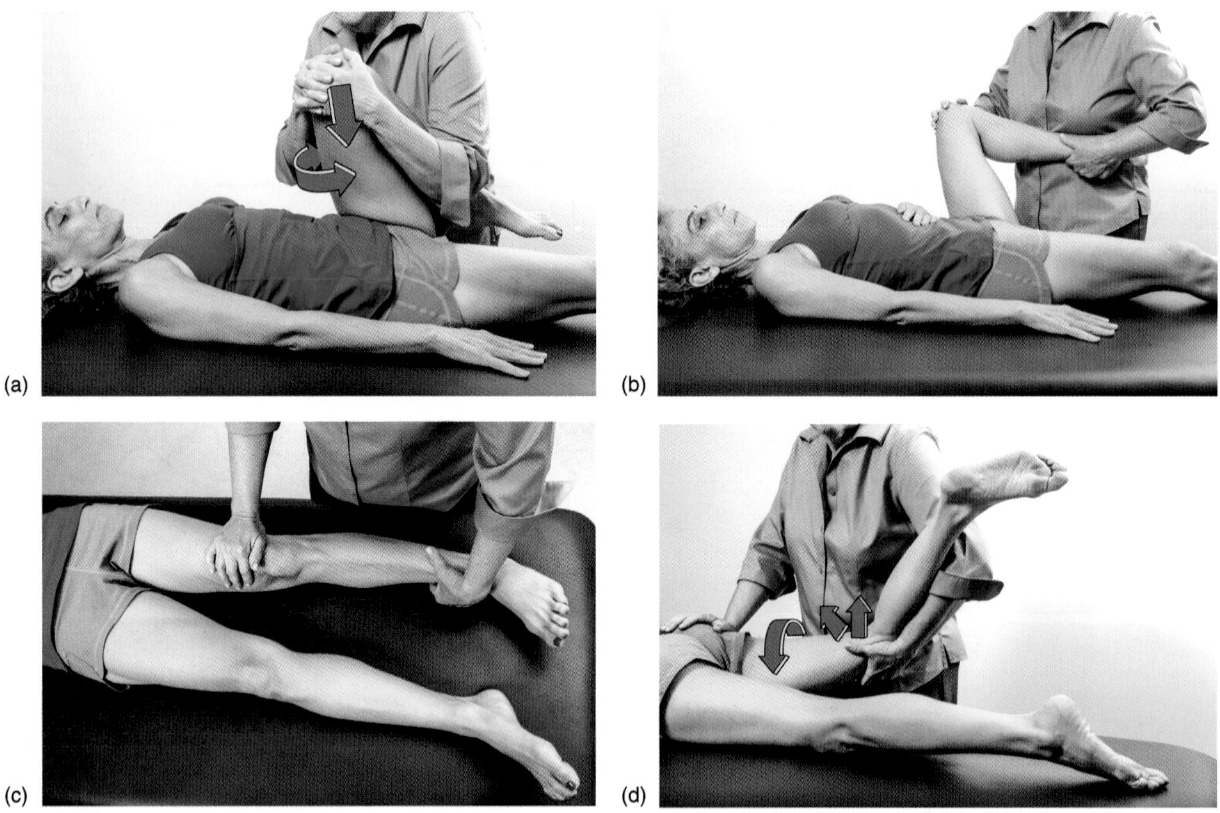

Figure 11.76 (a) Scour test. (b, c) Anterior acetabular labral test. (b) Starting position. (c) Ending position. (d) Posterior acetabular labral test.

(Figures 11.76b and 11.76c) The hip is then moved into extension, adduction, and medial rotation. A positive finding is pain with or without a click. This could indicate an anterior–superior impingement, anterior labral tear or iliopsoas tendinitis (Magee, 2008) (https://www.youtube.com/watch?v=XA1VSK5NBCk).

Posterior Labral Tear

The patient is in the prone position. Place the leg just short of full extension. Stabilize the pelvis. Apply an external rotation, abduction, and extension force. (Figure 11.76d). A positive finding is pain, apprehension or reproduction of the patient's symptoms (Groh and Herrera, 2009) (https://www.youtube.com/watch?v=8wNqjBnhgDs).

Radiological Views

Radiological views of the hip are shown in Figures 11.77, 11.78, and 11.79.

A = Iliac crest
B = Lumbar spine
C = Symphysis pubis
D = Sacroiliac joint
E = Sacrum
F = Femoral head
G = Greater trochanter of femur
I = Ischium
L = Lesser trochanter of femur

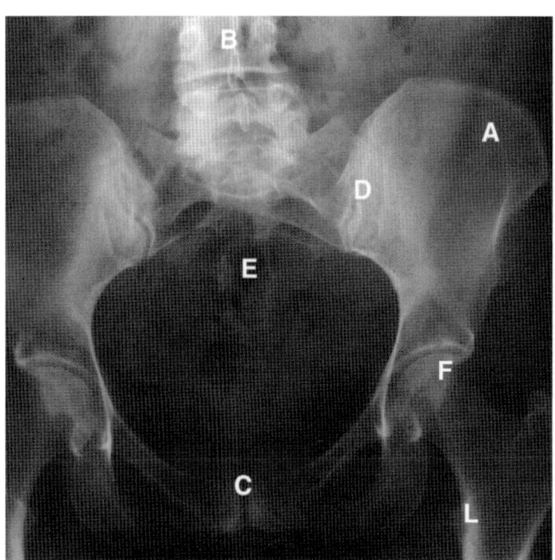

Figure 11.77 Anteroposterior view of the pelvis.

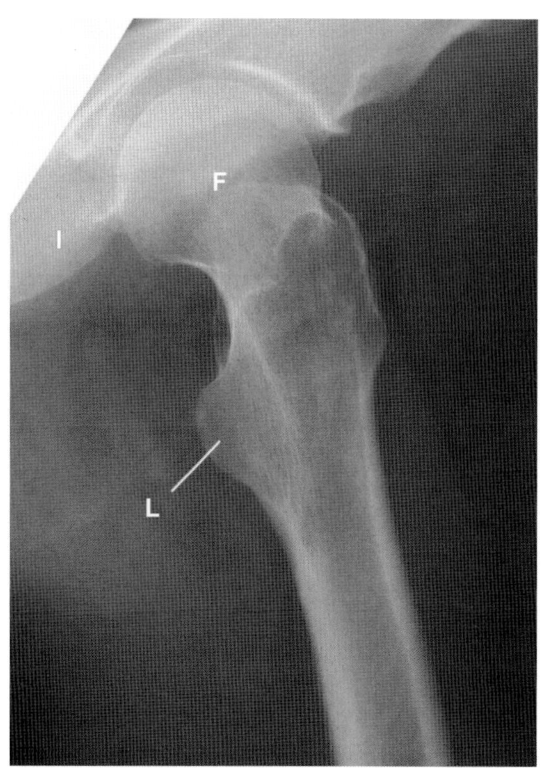

Figure 11.78 "Frog-lateral" view of the hip, with the hip in 45 degrees of flexion and maximum external rotation.

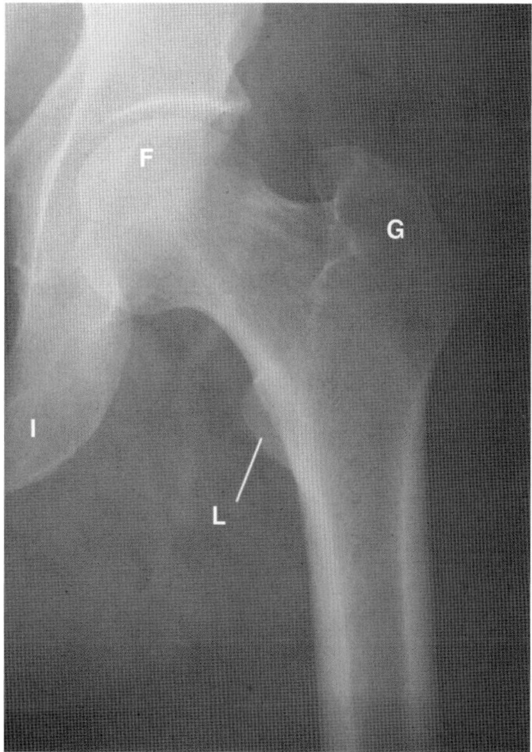

Figure 11.79 Anteroposterior view of the hip joint.

SAMPLE EXAMINATION

History: 30-year-old female recreational hiker returns after a recent 30-mile trek with a complaint of left groin pain, aggravated by weight bearing. No radiology evaluation performed at this time.

Physical Examination: Well-developed, well-nourished female, limping with a cane in the right upper extremity. She complains of pain transitioning from sit to stand. She has full range of motion of the hips, except for moderate limitation due to pain of internal rotation of the left hip. Muscle strength is 5/5 except for the hip abductors which are 3 +/5. There is slightly less development (atrophy) of the left abductor musculature. Mobility testing of the hip is normal. No tenderness is noted on soft-tissue palpation. Flexibility testing is inconclusive secondary to pain.

Presumptive Diagnosis: Incomplete stress fracture of the left femoral neck.

Physical Examination Clues:

1. Painful limp, indicating a protective mechanism in response to an injury.
2. Painful limited internal rotation of the hip, indicating probable hip joint pathology because the "Y" capsular ligament tightens in internal rotation creating a capsular pattern.
3. Weak or atrophic abductor musculature: The abductor muscles, when contracting during unilateral stance phase of gait, not only assist in the maintenance of balance but also protects the superior aspect of femoral neck from experiencing excessive varus bending stress with each step. This action is termed a "tension band effect," and is present in many areas of the body as a means by which soft tissues reduce or eliminate what would otherwise be catastrophic tensile forces from acting on bony elements of the body. Failure of this muscle action due to relative weakness resulted in a femoral neck stress fracture.

PARADIGM FOR OSTEOARTHRITIS OF THE HIP DUE TO CONGENITAL HIP DYSPLASIA (CDH)

A 40-year-old female patient presents with a complaint of left groin pain. She gives no history of injury now or in the past. She was the product of a breech birth and achieved normal developmental milestones. About 1 year ago she began to notice episodic discomfort in her left groin which radiated to the inner aspect of her thigh. Pain was in proportion to her level of weight-bearing activity. She was beginning to notice a slight limp on walking more than 15 minutes or standing for more than 30 minutes. She is having difficulty entering and exiting her new sports car and has difficulty in cutting her toenails. She reports no pain at rest, but does report stiffness on arising in the morning and after prolonged periods of sitting. She does not perceive any noises with movement, and does not report symptoms of "pins and needles" or tingling in the lower extremity. There are no other family members affected similarly, and she has no other significant medical history.

Physical examination demonstrates a well-developed, well-nourished woman who walks with a slight abductor limp. Her stride lengths are equal as are her leg lengths. She uses no assistive devices. She has a positive Trendelenburg sign, with no significant weakness in either lower extremity. She mounts and dismounts from the examining table easily and independently. Her musculoskeletal exam is otherwise unremarkable except for a significant lack of internal and external rotation of the left hip.

X-rays confirm a markedly shallow acetabulum with narrowing of the articular "space" and periarticular osteophyte formation. This is a paradigm for secondary osteoarthritis of the hip because of:

The patient's young age
Her being female
The involvement of the left hip
The history of breech birth
No history of trauma or excessive loading to the hip

CHAPTER 12

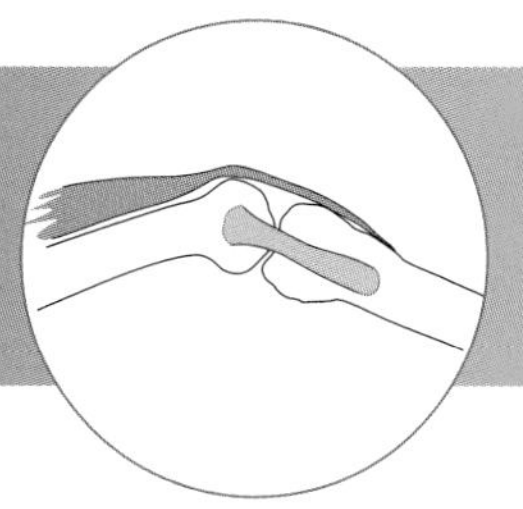

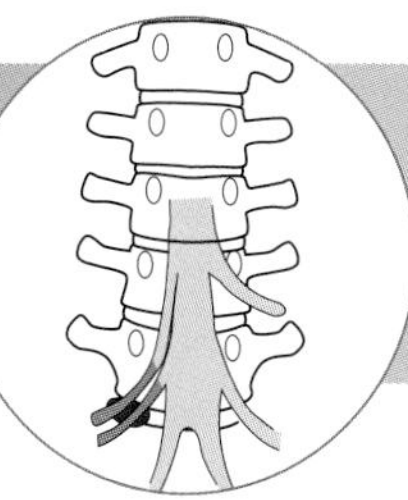

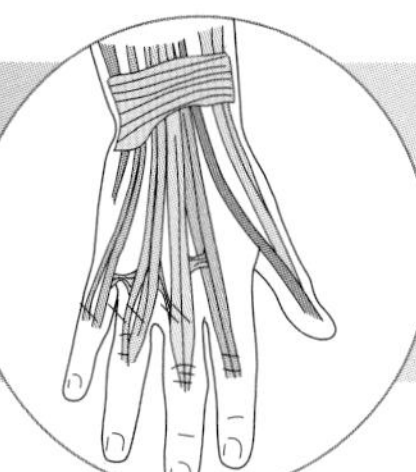

The Knee

FURTHER INFORMATION

Please refer to Chapter 2 for an overview of the sequence of a physical examination. For purposes of length and to avoid having to repeat anatomy more than once, the palpation section appears directly after the section on subjective examination and before any section on testing, rather than at the end of each chapter. The order in which the examination is performed should be based on your experience and personal preference as well as the presentation of the patient.

Functional Anatomy

The knee is the largest synovial joint of the body. It is also one of the most complex. The knee is composed of three bones (femur, tibia, and patella) and two articulations (tibiofemoral and patellofemoral). It lies midway along the lower extremity and permits flexion to occur within the lower extremity. This ability to bend the lower extremity has obvious implications for daily functions, as well as assisting in the mechanical efficiency of the body during locomotion.

The tibiofemoral joint is formed by two large, bulbous femoral condyles resting on a relatively flat tibial plateau. As a result, it is inherently unstable. The tibiofemoral articulation can potentially move without limit in four directions: flexion–extension, varus–valgus, external–internal rotation, and anterior–posterior translation (or glide). The amount of movement that can, in fact, occur differs from individual to individual. This movement is stabilized and limited by muscles (dynamically) and ligaments (statically). Accessory soft tissues such as the menisci, by virtue of their concave shape, increase stability of the knee joint by increasing the articular congruity the tibial plateau presents to the femoral condyles (Figure 12.1).

The geometry of the articular surfaces also contributes to the knee joint's stability (i.e., the concave femoral trochlea and convex patellar articular surface of the patellofemoral articulation) (Figure 12.2).

There are two pairs of major ligaments (medial and lateral collateral ligaments, anterior and posterior cruciate ligaments) and many minor or capsular ligaments stabilizing the knee joint. Although it is not possible to truly injure one ligament alone, an isolated ligament sprain is defined as an injury in which there is clinically significant injury to only one of the four major knee ligaments.

The medial collateral ligament and lateral collateral ligament lie parallel to the longitudinal axis of the knee. As such, they, respectively, prevent excessive valgus or varus displacement of the tibia relative to the femur (Figure 12.3).

The anterior cruciate ligament (ACL) and posterior cruciate ligament lie intra-articularly and extrasynovially in the midline of the knee (Figure 12.4).

Musculoskeletal Examination, Fourth Edition. Jeffrey M. Gross, Joseph Fetto and Elaine Rosen.

Companion website: www.wiley.com/go/musculoskeletalexam

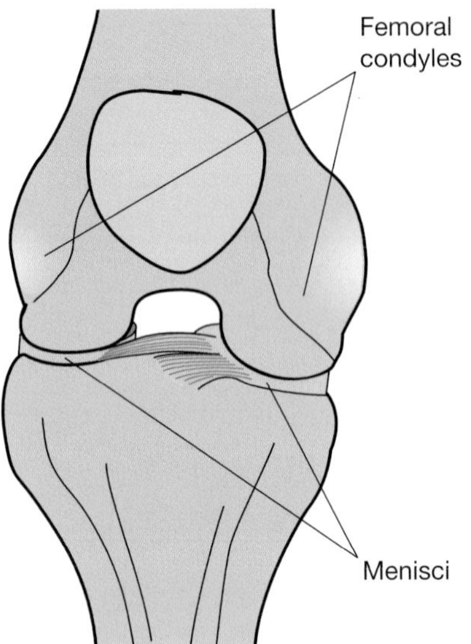

Figure 12.1 The concave surface of the menisci increases the stability of the knee joint by increasing the congruity of the surface presented to the femoral condyles.

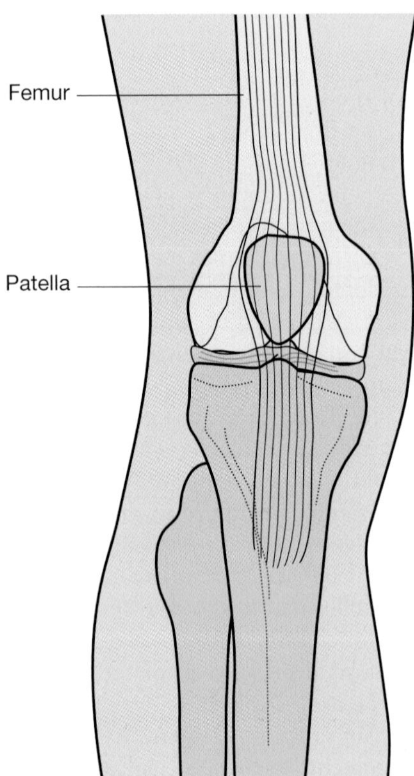

Figure 12.2 The patellofemoral articulation is composed of the convex patella lying within the trochlear groove of the femur.

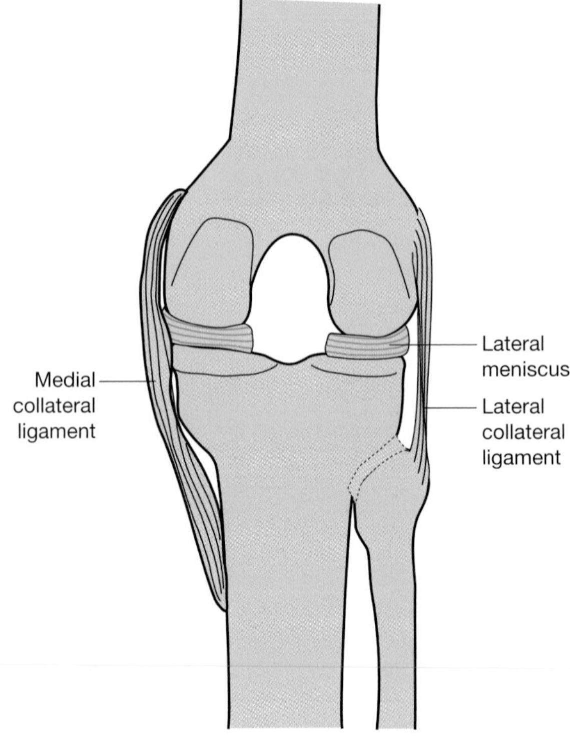

Figure 12.3 The medial collateral ligament and lateral collateral ligament lie parallel to the longitudinal axis of the knee. They provide stability against side-to-side (varus–valgus) deforming forces.

The posterior cruciate ligament is about 50% larger in diameter than the ACL. It has two functions. It acts as a linkage between the posterior cortex of the femur and the posterior cortex of the tibia about which tibial motion may occur, much like a gate hinge (Figure 12.5). It prevents posterior displacement of the tibia on the femur.

The function of the ACL can be deduced from its location within the knee. It is directed anterior to posterior and medial to lateral from near the anterior tibial spine to the posteromedial intercondylar aspect of the lateral femoral condyle. It prevents anterior displacement of the tibia on the femur. It "wraps around" the posterior cruciate ligament, becoming tighter with internal rotation of the tibia on the femur (Figure 12.6). As such, it also prevents excessive internal rotational movement of the tibia on the femur.

Injuries therefore that occur with excessive anterior displacement or internal rotation of the tibia jeopardize the integrity of the ACL.

Once a ligament (or ligaments) is compromised, there will be excessive movement and displacement

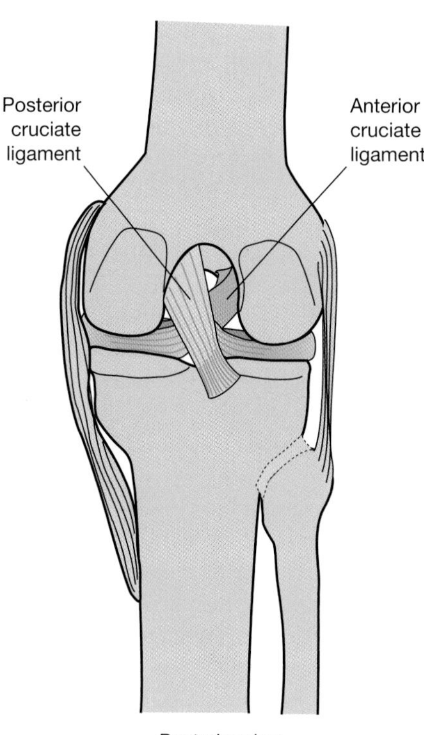

Figure 12.4 The anterior cruciate ligament and posterior cruciate ligament lie within the knee joint (intra-articular), but they are extrasynovial structures.

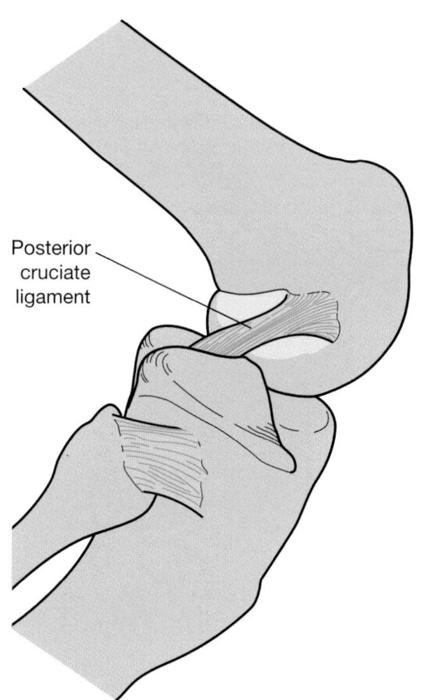

Figure 12.5 The posterior cruciate ligament is the flexible linkage between the posterior cortices of the femur and tibia. It acts as a pivot point much like a gatepost about which the knee rotates.

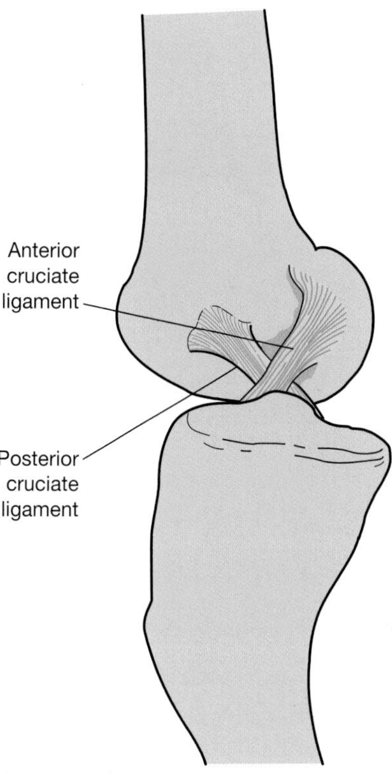

Figure 12.6 The anterior cruciate ligament wraps around the posterior cruciate ligament as it courses anterior to posterior, medial to lateral, from the intraspinous region of the tibia to the posteromedial surface of the lateral femoral condyle.

of the knee in one or more planes of knee movement. This increased laxity creates excessive sheer stress on the articular structure. This will result in accelerated erosion of the articular and meniscal surfaces and increased synovial fluid production due to synovial tissue irritation (synovitis).

The frequency of ACL injury and the severity of its consequences warrant additional comment.

A balance exists within the knee, maintaining stability against anterior displacement of the tibia on the femur (anterior drawer). This balance between the forces destabilizing the knee and those designed to resist anterior displacement of the tibia can be depicted figuratively (Figure 12.7). Anterior stability of the knee relies primarily on the ACL. This is supplemented by the dynamic pull of the hamstrings, the buttressing effect of the posterior horn of the menisci, and improved by the flexion of the knee, which enhances the efficiency of the hamstring pull and presents a more convex surface of the femoral condyles with which the menisci have better purchase.

Acting to destabilize the knee are the anteriorly directed pull of the quadriceps muscles, the forward

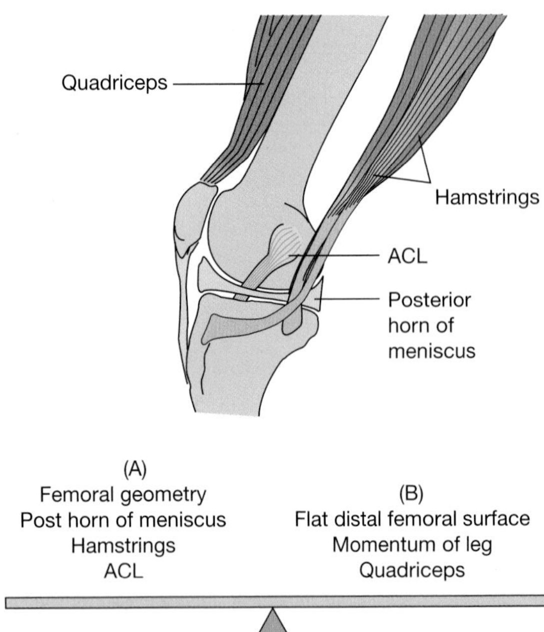

Figure 12.7 A balance exists between the structures that stabilize the knee against anterior displacement of the tibia on the femur and the structures and forces attempting to move the tibia anteriorly on the femur (anterior drawer).

momentum of extending the leg, and the extended position of the knee, which serves to reduce the mechanical advantage of the hamstrings while presenting a relatively flat distal femoral surface, which is less conforming to the meniscal surfaces.

As such, if the ACL is compromised by injury, it is theoretically possible to reduce the effects of its absence by increasing hamstring function and avoiding knee extension, thereby reducing the possibility of the knee experiencing an anterior subluxation event ("giving way" or "buckling"). However, the ability of an individual to accomplish this compensation will be directly dependent on the neuromuscular status and specific activities. For example, extension of the knee during jumping has a high likelihood of resulting in anterior subluxation of the tibia while the individual is in the air. Sudden reduction of this subluxation with ground contact and knee flexion will give the sensation of the bones slipping within the knee as the tibia and posterior horn of the menisci (particularly that of the lateral meniscus) return to a normal relationship to the femur. This sudden reduction usually results in the knee "buckling" or "giving way." This action has been demonstrated to be accurate by laboratory investigation. It is the same mechanism as that produced by the clinical test called the *pivot shift* (Fetto and Marshall, 1979). The ultimate results of such repeated events are sheer fatigue and tearing of the posterior horns of the menisci and premature osteoarthritic degeneration of the articular surfaces of the knee.

The patella has the thickest articular cartilage of any bone in the body. This is a direct result of the significant loads it experiences during activities such as running, jumping, and stair climbing (up to six times body weight). The patella is a sesamoid bone within the quadriceps mechanism. As such, it displaces the quadriceps tendon anteriorly so as to increase the mechanical advantage of the quadriceps by 25% (Figure 12.8).

Because of the tremendous loads experienced by the patella, the nutrients of the synovial fluid are forced deeper into its articular cartilage than that of any other articular surface. This permits the chondrocytes of the patellar articular cartilage to continue multiplying to a greater depth than would otherwise be possible. The hips are wider apart than are the knees. This results in a valgus angle between the femur and

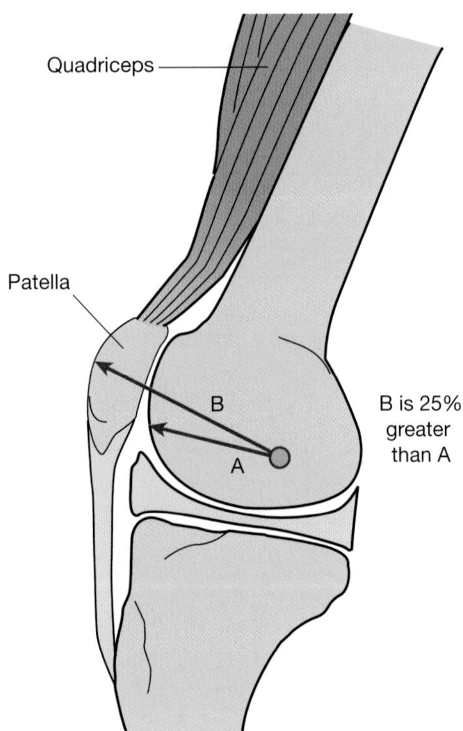

Figure 12.8 The function of the patella as a sesamoid bone with the quadriceps–patellar tendon is to displace the quadriceps anteriorly. This effectively increases the mechanical advantage of the quadriceps' ability to extend the knee by 25%.

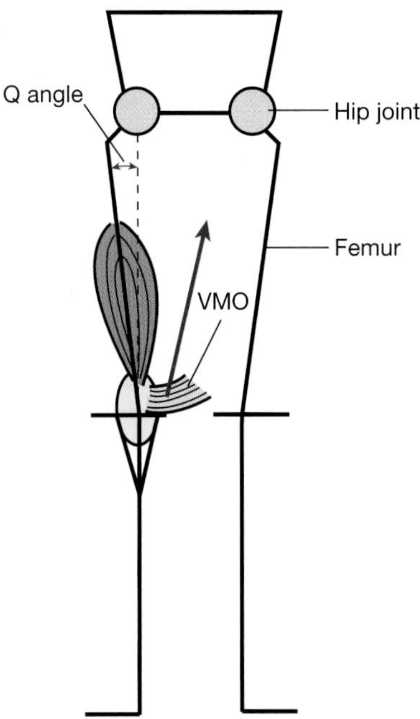

Figure 12.9 The Q angle measures the tendency of the patella to track laterally. It is the angle formed between the mid axis of the femur and the line extending from the midpoint of the patella to the tibial tubercle. Patellofemoral lateral subluxation and related tracking pathologies are associated with Q angles of more than 15 degrees. The normal Q angle for females is generally a few degrees more than that for males.

the tibia of about 7 degrees. Because the quadriceps lies along the axis of the femur, when it contracts, there will be a resultant lateral displacement vector on the patella. This creates a traction load on the medial peripatellar soft tissues, driving the patella toward lateral subluxation out of the femoral trochlea. This displacement or tendency toward lateral tracking is resisted by the oblique fibers of the vastus medialis.

Any imbalance in these forces in favor of lateral displacement of the patella will result in several potential pathological situations: excessive tensile loading of the medial peripatellar soft tissues (capsule, plica), noncontact deterioration of the medial patellar articular facet cartilage, and excessive compression loading of the lateral patellar facet, with secondary articular erosion or soft-tissue impingement. The latter two conditions lead to a prearthritic condition termed *chondromalacia patellae (chondro* means "cartilage," *malacia* means "softening").

The frequency toward these pathologies can be predicted by measuring magnitude of the angulation within the quadriceps–patellar tendon mechanism. This angle has been termed the Q angle (Figure 12.9) (see p. 340, 342, Figure 12.12 for further description).

Observation

The examination should begin in the waiting room before the patient is aware of the examiner's observation. Information regarding the degree of the patient's disability, level of functioning, posture, and gait can be observed. The clinician should pay careful attention to the patient's facial expressions with regard to the degree of discomfort the patient is experiencing. The information gathered in this short period could be very useful in creating a total picture of the patient's condition. Note whether the patient is able to sit with the knees flexed to 90 degrees or whether the involved knee is extended. This will help you to understand the degree of discomfort the patient experiences with movement and the amount of range available.

Observe the patient as he or she goes from sitting to standing. How difficult is it for the patient to change the position of the knee? Can the patient achieve full extension? Can he or she evenly distribute weight between both lower extremities? Look at the alignment of the hip. Femoral anteversion can cause patellofemoral malalignment syndromes.

Pay attention to the alignment of the knee from both the anterior and lateral views. Does the patient appear to have an excessive degree of genu valgum or varum? Genu valgum creates an increase in the Q angle (explained on see p. 338, 340, 342) and is also a cause of patellofemoral malalignment syndromes. Increased Q angles can create a predisposition to patella subluxation. The patient will also have increased stress placed on the medial collateral ligament.

Is genu recurvatum present? Note the position of the patella. Is a tibial torsion present? Observe the alignment of the feet with and without shoes. Move around the patient and check the knee for signs of edema and muscle wasting.

Observe the swing and stance phases of gait, noticing the ability to move quickly and smoothly from flexion to extension. Note any gait deviations and whether the patient is using or requires an assistive device. The details and implications of gait deviations are discussed in Chapter 14.

Subjective Examination

The knee joint is much more mobile than the hip joint. However, under normal conditions it is very stable. It is easily susceptible to trauma and degenerative changes (see pp. 335–39). It is important to note the mechanism of injury if the patient has sustained a trauma. The patient may have noticed tearing, popping, or catching occurring during the incident. Does the patient report any clicking, buckling, or locking? The direction of the force, the activity the patient was participating in at the time of the injury, and the type of shoes he or she was wearing contribute to your understanding of the resulting problem. Note the degree of pain, swelling, and disability reported at the time of the trauma and during the initial 24 hours.

You should determine the patient's functional limitations. Is the patient able to ascend and descend steps without difficulty? Can he or she walk up or downhill? Is the patient able to squat or kneel? Can the patient sit in one position for a prolonged period of time? Is the patient stiff when he or she arises in the morning or after sitting?

The patient's disorder may be related to age, gender, ethnic background, body type, static and dynamic posture, occupation, leisure activities, and general activity level.

Location of the symptoms may give you some insight into the etiology of the complaints. For example, if the pain is located over the anteromedial aspect of the knee, it may be coming from a torn medial meniscus or from an L4 radiculopathy.

(Please refer to Box 2.1, p. 15 for typical questions for the subjective examination.)

Gentle Palpation

It is easiest to begin the palpatory examination with the patient in the supine position since asymmetry is easier to observe with the knee in the extended position. You should examine the knee to see if it is swollen, either locally or generally. Note any areas of ecchymosis, bruising, muscle girth asymmetry, bony incongruities, incisional areas, or open wounds. Generalized edema may be secondary to metabolic or vascular disorders. Hypertrophic bone is a sign of osteoarthritis.

Observe the skin for any dystrophic changes (loss of hair, decrease in temperature, thickening of the nails) which may indicate the presence of complex regional pain syndrome (reflex sympathetic dystrophy). You should not have to use deep pressure to determine areas of tenderness or malalignment. It is important to use a firm but gentle pressure, which will enhance your palpatory skills. If you have a sound basis of cross-sectional anatomy, you will not need to physically penetrate through several layers of tissue to have a good sense of the underlying structures. Remember that if you increase the patient's pain at this point in the examination, the patient will be very reluctant to allow you to continue, or may become more limited in his or her ability to move.

Palpation is most easily performed with the patient in a relaxed position. Although palpation can be performed with the patient standing, non-weight-bearing positions are preferred. The sitting position with the patient's leg hanging over the edge of the examining table allows for optimal palpation of the knee region. It provides easy access to all aspects of the joint and exposes the joint lines secondary to the traction force that is offered by gravity. The examiner should sit on a rolling stool and face the patient.

Anterior Aspect

Bony Structures

Patella

The patella is very superficial and easily located on the anterior surface of the knee. This large sesamoid bone can be situated in a superior, inferior, medial, or lateral direction, instead of the normal resting position, while the knee is positioned in extension. The patella tracks within the trochlear groove. Its resting position should be at the midpoint on a line drawn between the femoral condyles. The patella and its tendon should be of equal length with the knee in extension, without any muscle contraction.

The patella may be superiorly displaced (patella alta), inferiorly displaced (patella baja), medially displaced (squinting patella), and laterally displaced (bullfrog's, fish, grasshopper eyes) (Figure 12.10). Squinting patella can be caused by medial femoral or lateral tibial torsion.

The patella should lie flat when viewed from the lateral and superior aspects. Medial and lateral tilts can produce abnormal wear on the posterior aspect of the patella and its cartilage, causing patellofemoral compression syndrome. With the patient sitting, the inferior pole of the patella should be at the same level as the tibiofemoral joint line.

Tenderness to palpation can be secondary to a contusion or fracture of the patella following a direct insult. Pain, swelling, and tenderness at the inferior pole of the patella in an adolescent may indicate Larsen–Johansson disease (osteochondritis of the inferior pole). Pain with patellar compression may be indicative of chondromalacia patellae.

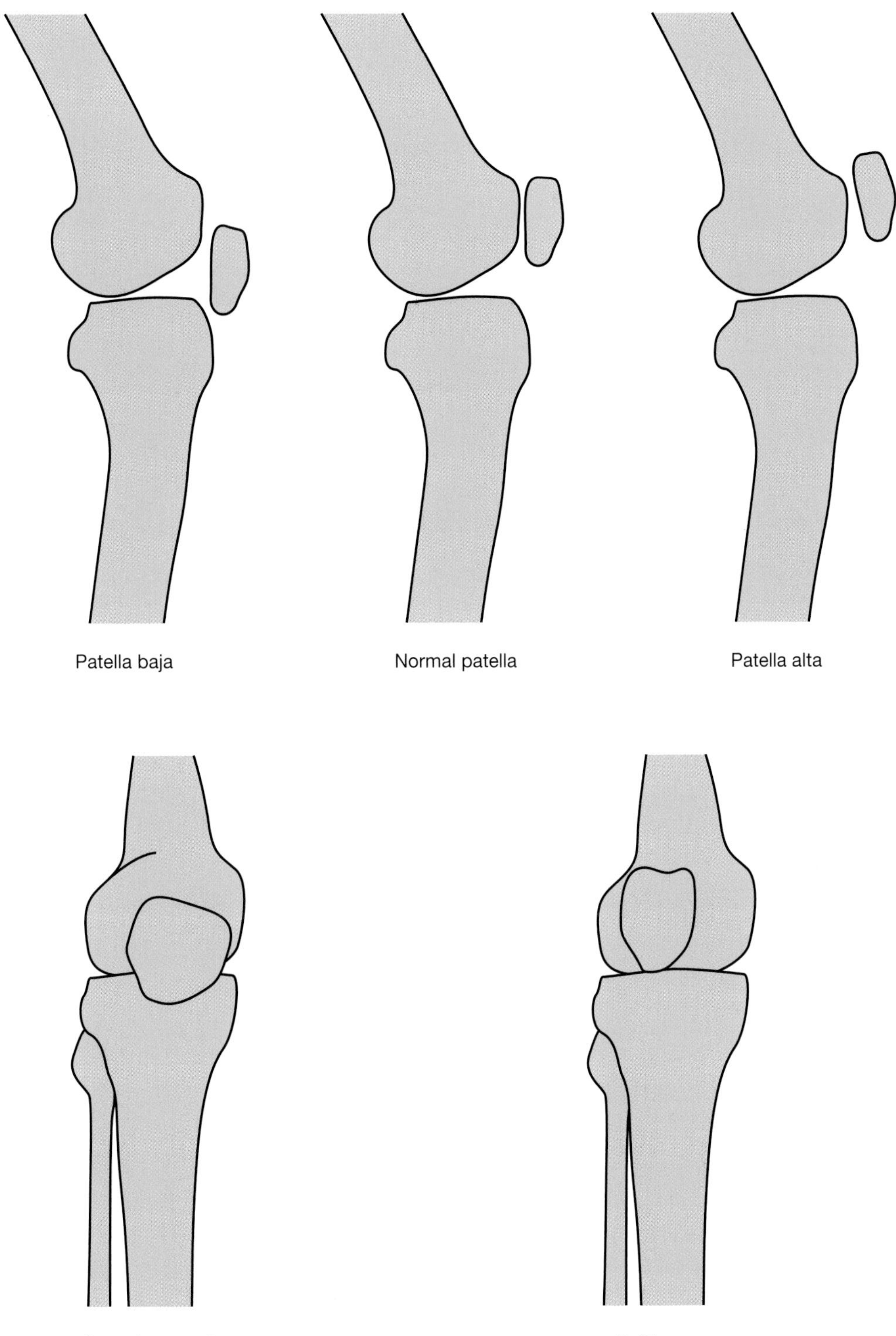

Figure 12.10 Patella alta, baja, squinting, and bullfrog eyes.

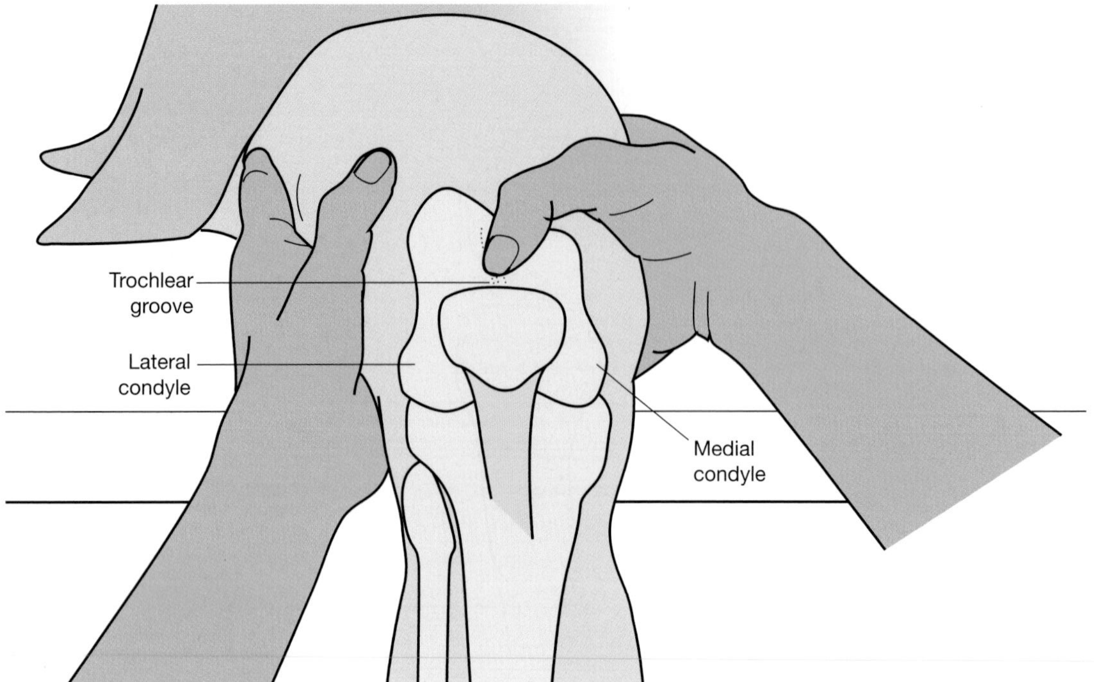

Figure 12.11 Palpation of the trochlear groove.

The trochlear groove is the channel in which the patella glides. It is partially palpable with the knee in flexion. This causes the patella to be inferiorly displaced. Place your thumbs superior to the most cranial portion of the patella between the medial and lateral femoral condyles and you will palpate an indentation, which is the trochlear groove (Figure 12.11). The patella is stabilized within the trochlea by virtue of the surface geometry and the patellofemoral ligaments and the patellar tendon.

This is an appropriate time to measure the Q (quadriceps) angle. Draw a line between the anterior superior iliac spine and the center of the patella. Draw a second line between the center of the patella and the tibial tubercle. Measure the angle formed by the intersection of the two lines (Figure 12.12). Normal findings should be between 10 and 15 degrees in males and 10 to 19 degrees in females. The tibial tubercle should line up with the midline or the lateral half of the patella in the sitting position. Therefore, the Q angle should be 0 degree when the patient is in the sitting position.

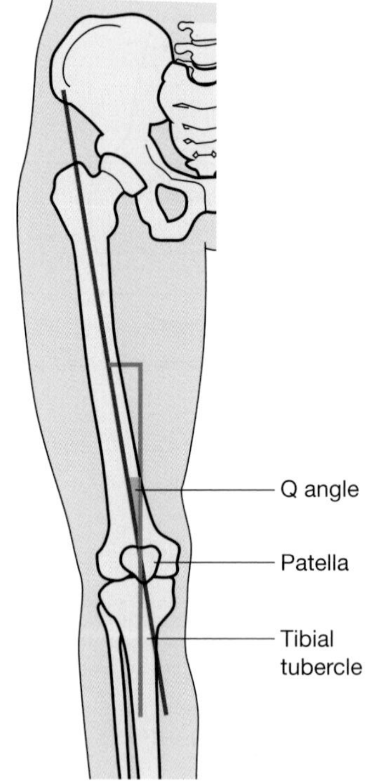

Figure 12.12 Measurement of the Q angle.

Tibial Tuberosity

Place your fingers on the midpoint of the inferior pole of the patella. Approximately 2 in. caudad to that point is a superficial prominence, which is the tibial

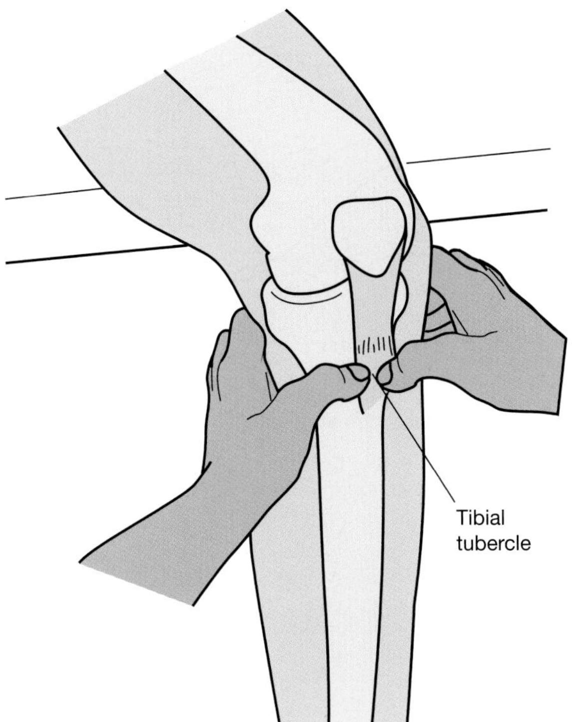

Figure 12.13 Palpation of the tibial tubercle.

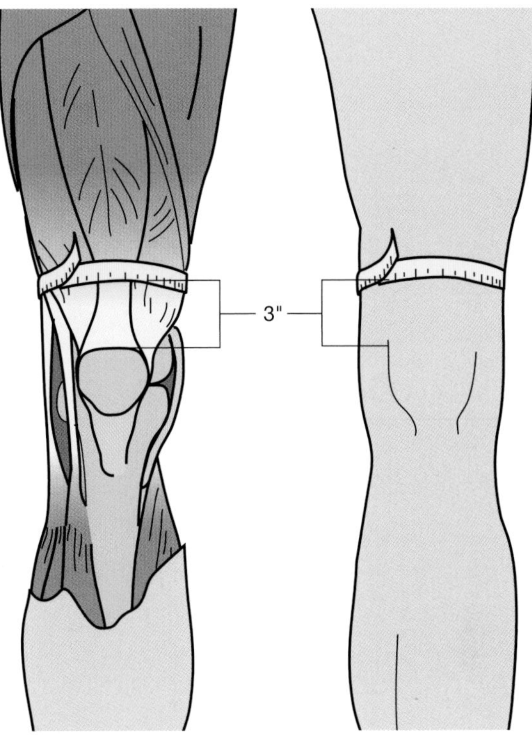

Figure 12.14 Measurement of thigh girth.

tuberosity. This serves as the attachment for the infrapatellar ligament (Figure 12.13). If the tibial tubercle is excessively prominent, the patient may have had osteochondrosis of the tibial apophysis (Osgood–Schlatter disease).

Soft-Tissue Structures

Quadriceps Muscle

Place your fingers over the anterior aspect of the thigh and palpate the large expanse of the quadriceps muscle. This four-muscle group attaches to the superior aspect of the patella. The muscle bulk is most obvious with isometric contraction of the knee in extension. The vastus medialis and lateralis are the most prominent of the muscles, with the medialis extending slightly more inferiorly. Vastus medialis obliquus (VMO) atrophy is very common following knee trauma, immobilization, or surgery. It is helpful to observe and then palpate both knees simultaneously for comparison. Both muscles should be symmetrical and without any visible defect. You can compare the girth measurements using a tape measure. Thigh girth may be increased secondary to edema or decreased due to atrophy. Measurements should be taken at regular intervals bilaterally starting approximately 3 in. proximally to the superior pole of the patella (Figure 12.14). A focal point of tenderness or a lump in the muscle can be caused by a strain, hematoma, or tumor.

Patellar (Infrapatellar) Ligament (Tendon)

Place your hands on the medial inferior aspect of the patella and palpate the bandlike structure running inferiorly to the tibial tubercle. The infrapatellar fat pad is situated immediately posterior to the ligament and may be tender to palpation. Inflammation of the fat pad creates a generalized effusion and is readily visible (Figure 12.15). Tenderness of the tendon may be secondary to patellar tendinitis (jumper's knee), which is related to overuse.

Bursae

Bursae are not commonly palpable unless they are inflamed and enlarged. However, since bursitis is a common occurrence in the knee, you should familiarize yourself with their anatomical locations. Inflammation of any of these bursae will create localized effusions, which are easily palpable.

The prepatellar bursa is located just anterior to the patella. This bursa creates greater freedom of

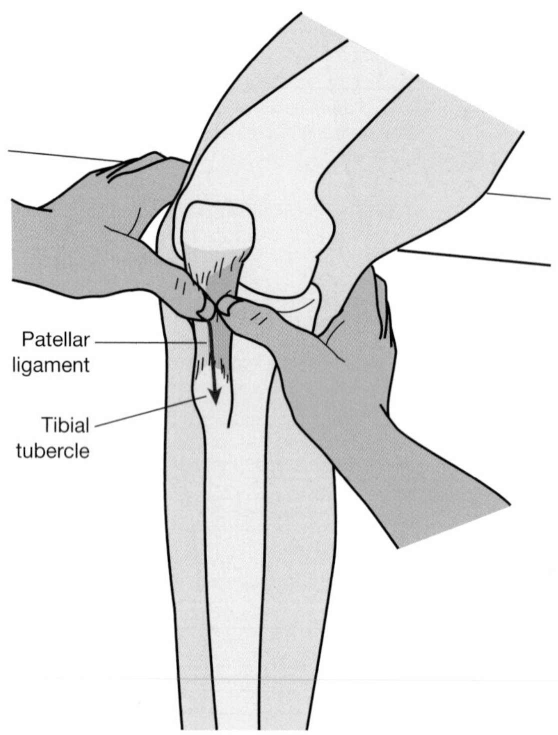

Figure 12.15 Palpation of the patellar ligament.

movement of the skin covering the anterior aspect of the patella. Inflammation of the prepatellar bursa can be caused by excessive kneeling and is referred to as *housemaid's/carpenter's knee.*

The superficial infrapatellar bursa is located just anterior to the patella ligament. Inflammation can occur secondary to prolonged kneeling and is referred to as *Parson's knee.*

The deep infrapatellar bursa is located directly behind the patellar ligament (Figure 12.16).

Medial Aspect

Bony Structures

Medial Femoral Condyle

Place your thumbs on either side of the infrapatellar ligament and allow them to drop into the indentation. This places you at the joint line. Allow your fingers to move medially and superiorly first over the sharp eminence and then allow your fingers to travel over the smooth rounded surface of the medial femoral condyle. The medial femoral condyle is wider and protrudes more than the lateral femoral condyle (Figure 12.17). Localized tenderness may be secondary to osteochondritis dissecans.

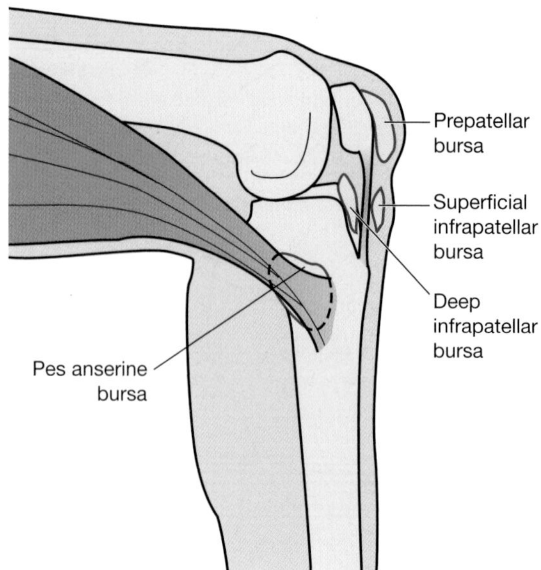

Figure 12.16 Location of the bursae of the knee.

Adductor Tubercle

Allow your fingers to move further cranially from the midline of the medial femoral condyle, and at the very top of the dome you will be on the adductor tubercle. You will know that you are in the correct

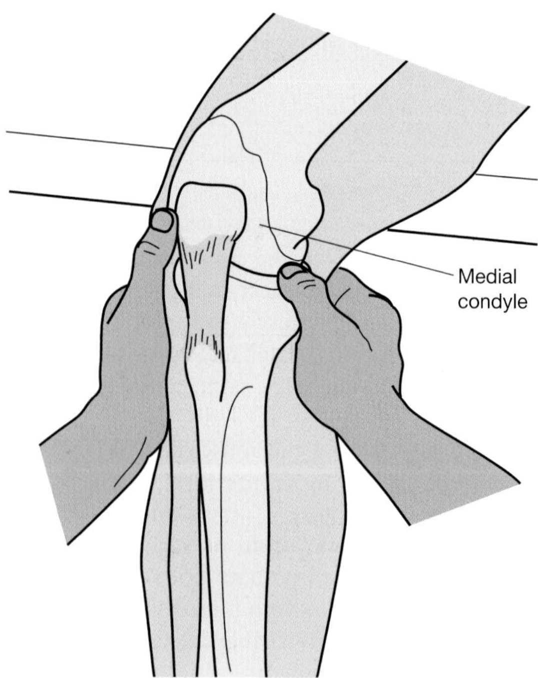

Figure 12.17 Palpation of the medial femoral condyle.

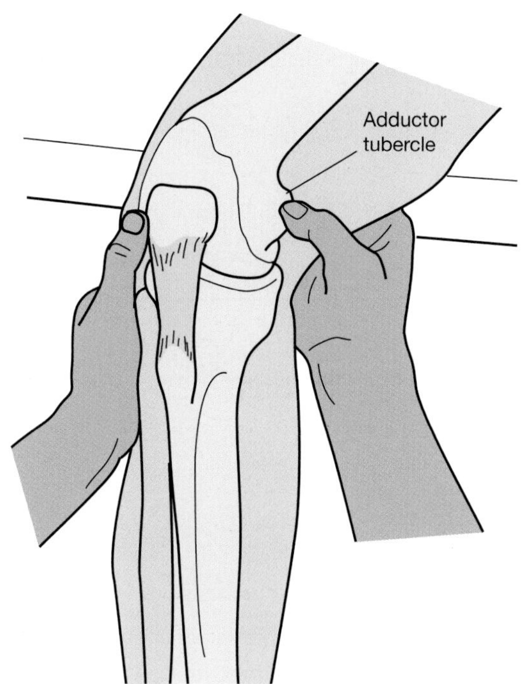

Figure 12.18 Palpation of the adductor tubercle.

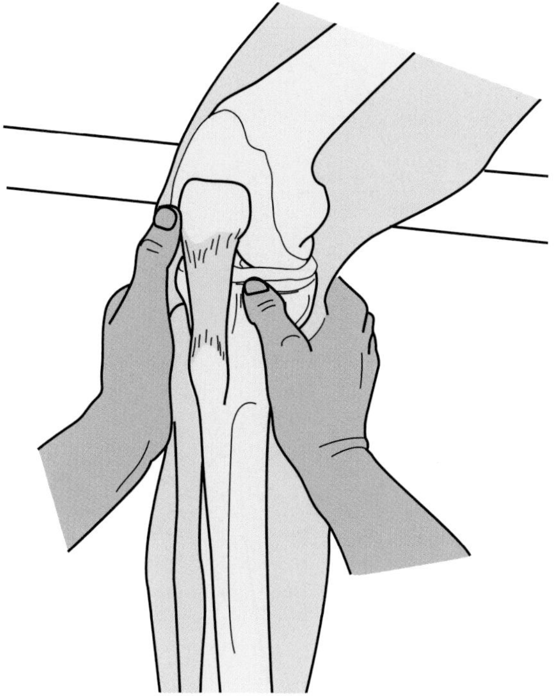

Figure 12.19 Palpation of the medial tibial plateau.

place if the adductors are isometrically contracted and you can palpate their attachment at the tubercle (Figure 12.18). Tenderness can be secondary to an adductor magnus strain.

Medial Tibial Plateau

Allow your fingers to rest in the indentation medial to the infrapatellar ligament and press in a posterior and inferior direction. You will feel the eminence along the edge of the medial tibial plateau as your fingers move medially along the joint line (Figure 12.19). The coronary ligaments are located along the anteromedial joint line. They are more easily palpated with the tibia passively internally rotated, which allows the medial border of the tibia to move posteriorly.

Soft-Tissue Structures

Medial Meniscus

The medial meniscus is located between the medial femoral condyle and the medial tibial plateau. It is anchored by the coronary ligaments and attached to the medial collateral ligament. The meniscus is pulled anteriorly by the medial femoral condyle as the tibia is internally rotated, making it slightly more accessible to palpation (Figure 12.20). If an injury causes

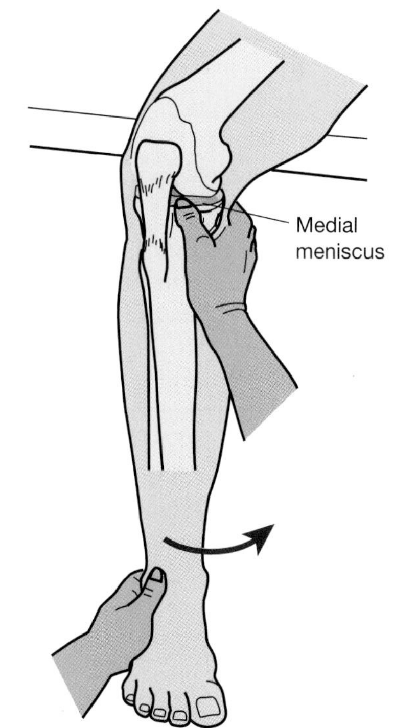

Figure 12.20 Palpation of the medial meniscus.

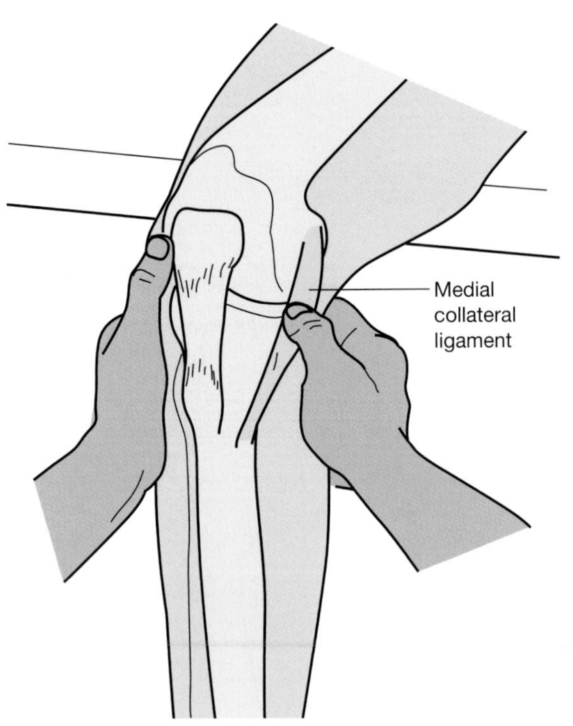

Figure 12.21 Palpation of the medial collateral ligament.

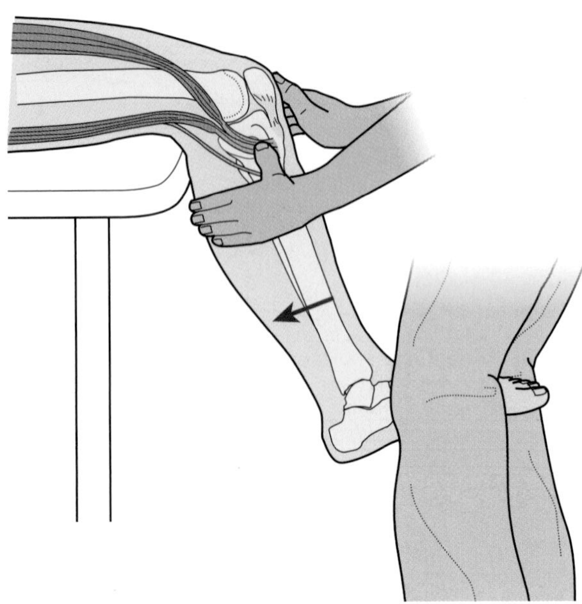

Figure 12.22 Palpation of the pes anserinus.

a tearing of the medial meniscus, tenderness to palpation will be noted along the joint line. Tears in the medial meniscus are very common. They may be coupled with injury to the medial collateral and ACLs. This is referred to as the unhappy triad of O'Donoghue.

Medial Collateral Ligament

The medial collateral ligament is attached from the medial epicondyle of the femur to the medial condyle and shaft of the tibia. The ligament is not easily palpable since it is very flat. You can approximate its general location by following the joint line with your fingers moving in an anterior and then posterior direction. The ligament will obliterate the midjoint line (Figure 12.21). The medial collateral ligament is responsible for the valgus stability of the knee joint. It can be easily injured by a force directed at the lateral aspect of the knee (valgus strain). A lesion of the upper border of the ligament with subsequent periosteal damage is known as Pellegrini–Stieda disease.

Sartorius, Gracilis, and Semitendinosus Muscles (Pes Anserinus)

The pes anserinus is located on the posteromedial aspect of the knee, attaching to the inferior portion of the medial tibial plateau approximately 5–7 cm below the joint line. This common aponeurosis of the tendons of gracilis, semitendinosus, and sartorius muscles adds additional support to the medial aspect of the knee joint and protects the knee during valgus stress. Place your hand medial and slightly posterior to the tibial tubercle. You will feel a bandlike structure that becomes evident. Stabilize the patient's leg by holding it between your knees. Resist knee flexion by using your legs as the resistance to make the tendons more evident (Figure 12.22). The semitendinosus tendon is palpated as a cordlike structure, located at the medial posterior aspect of the knee.

Pes Anserine Bursa

The pes anserine bursa is located between the tibia and the insertion of the pes anserine aponeurosis. Like the other bursae in the knee, it is not readily palpable unless it is inflamed, in which case it will feel swollen and boggy. (Figure 12.16).

Lateral Aspect

Bony Structures

Lateral Femoral Condyle

Place your fingers on either side of the infrapatellar ligament and allow them to drop into the indentation. This places you at the joint line. Allow your fingers to move in a lateral and superior direction until

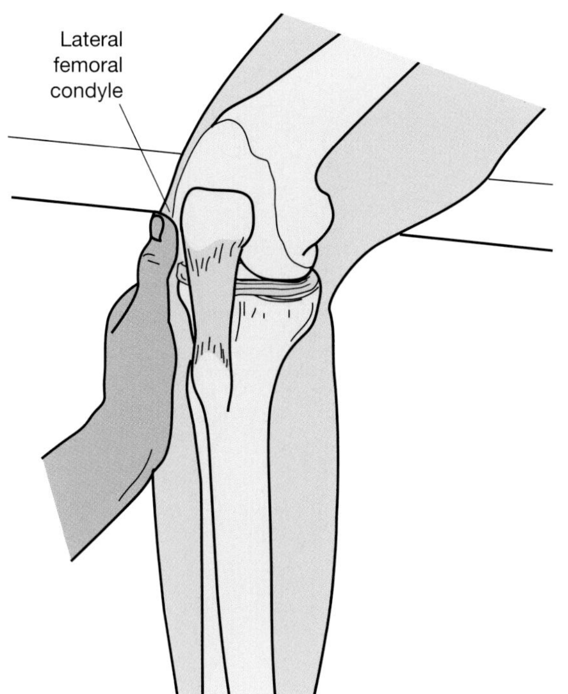

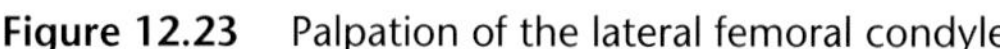

Figure 12.23 Palpation of the lateral femoral condyle.

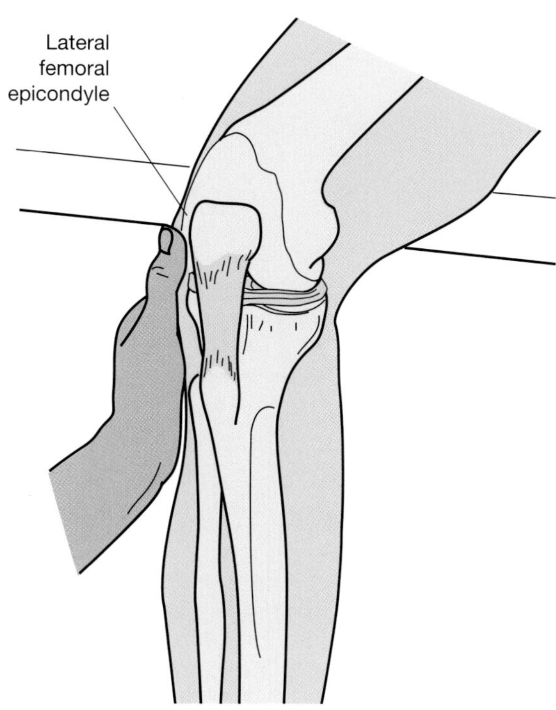

Figure 12.24 Palpation of the lateral femoral epicondyle.

you reach the eminence of the lateral femoral condyle. If you continue to move laterally along the joint line with the tibia, you will feel the popliteus tendon and attachment, and then a groove. You will then palpate a flat, almost concave surface of the condyle (Figure 12.23).

Lateral Femoral Epicondyle

As you continue to move laterally past the concavity of the lateral femoral condyle, you will feel the prominence of the lateral femoral epicondyle (Figure 12.24).

Lateral Tibial Plateau

Allow your fingers to rest on the lateral aspect of the infrapatellar ligament and press in a posterior and inferior direction. You will feel the eminence along the edge of the lateral tibial plateau as your fingers move laterally along the joint line (Figure 12.25).

Lateral Tubercle (Gerdy's Tubercle)

Place your fingers on the lateral tibial plateau and move inferiorly. You will locate a prominence just lateral to the tibial tubercle. This is the lateral tubercle (Figure 12.26). This can be tender at the insertion of the iliotibial band.

Fibular Head

Place your middle finger over the lateral femoral epicondyle. Allow your finger to move in an inferior direction crossing the joint line and you will locate the fibular head and move your fingers in a superior direction and you will feel a bandlike structure (lateral collateral ligament) standing away from the joint (Figure 12.27). The popliteus muscle is located underneath the lateral collateral ligament and separates the ligament from the lateral meniscus (Figure 12.28). The popliteus can be palpated, after a groove, slightly posterior to the lateral collateral ligament along the joint line. The lateral collateral ligament is responsible for the varus stability of the knee joint. It can be injured when the individual sustains a medial force to the knee. If a sprain has occurred, the ligament will be tender to palpation (Figure 12.29).

Iliotibial Tract

The iliotibial tract is a strong band of fascia that is attached superiorly to the iliac crest. It ensheathes the tensor fasciae lata and a large part of the gluteus maximus inserts into it. Inferiorly, it attaches to the lateral condyle of the tibia (Gerdy's tubercle) where it blends

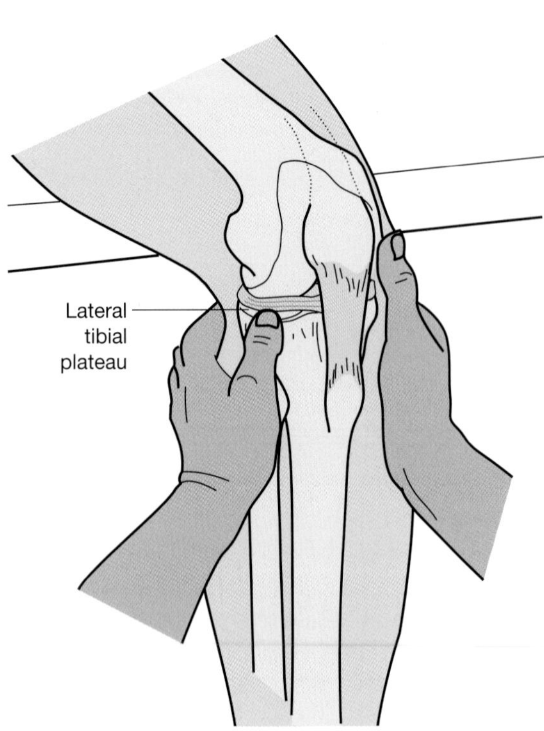

Figure 12.25 Palpation of the lateral tibial plateau.

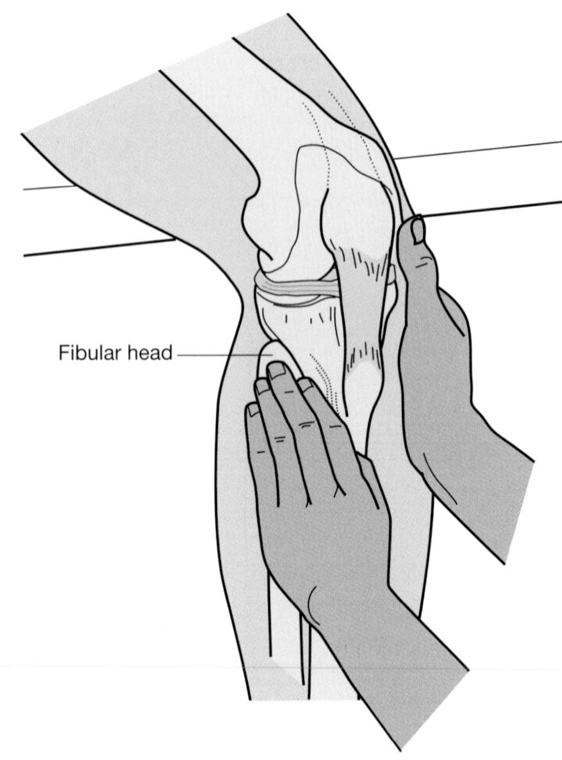

Figure 12.27 Palpation of the fibular head.

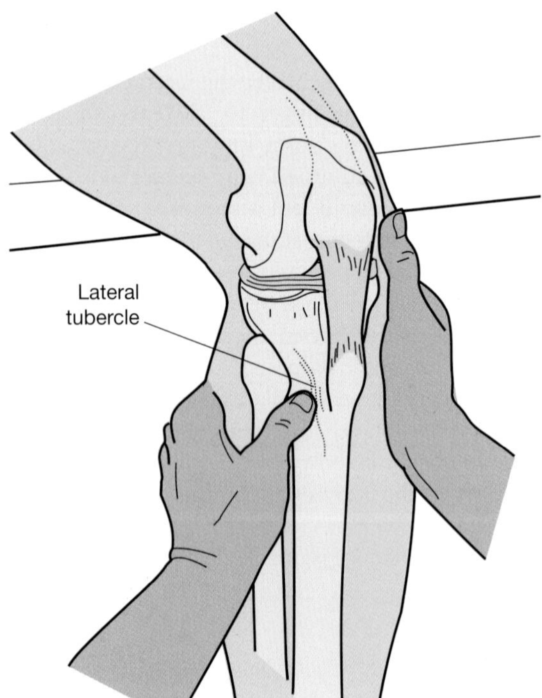

Figure 12.26 Palpation of the lateral tibial tubercle (Gerdy's tubercle).

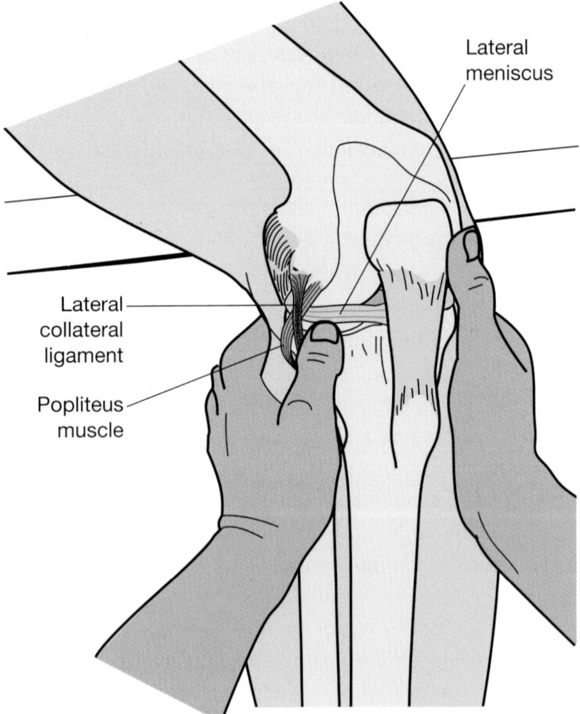

Figure 12.28 Palpation of the lateral meniscus.

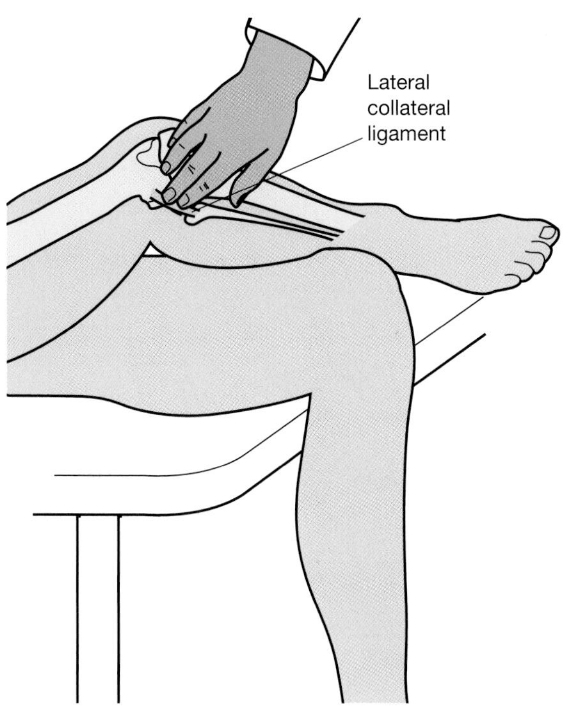

Figure 12.29 Palpation of the lateral collateral ligament.

with an aponeurosis from the vastus lateralis. You can locate it by placing your hand on the band, which is visible on the anterolateral aspect of the knee when the knee is extended (Figure 12.30). It is tightest when the knee is flexed between 15 and 30 degrees.

Common Peroneal (Fibular) Nerve

Place your fingers along the posterior aspect of the fibular head. Allow your fingers to travel behind the head, just below the insertion of the biceps femoris. The common peroneal (fibular) nerve is very superficial and you can roll it under your fingers. Remember not to apply too much pressure because you can induce a neurapraxia. The nerve can normally be tender to palpation. Enlargement of the nerve is commonly noted in Charcot–Marie–Tooth disease. Damage to the common peroneal nerve will cause a foot drop, creating difficulty during the heel strike and swing phases of gait (Figure 12.31).

Posterior Aspect

Bony Structure

There are no bony structures that are best palpated on the posterior aspect.

Soft-Tissue Structures

Biceps Femoris

Have the patient lie in the prone position with the knee flexed. The biceps femoris will become a prominent cordlike structure that is easily palpable proximal to its attachment to the fibular head. You can increase its prominence by providing resistance to knee flexion (Figure 12.32).

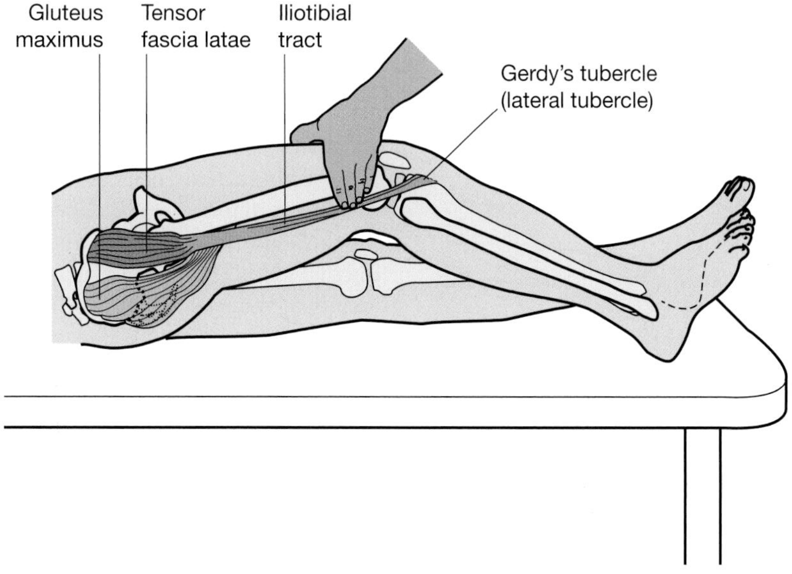

Figure 12.30 Palpation of the iliotibial band.

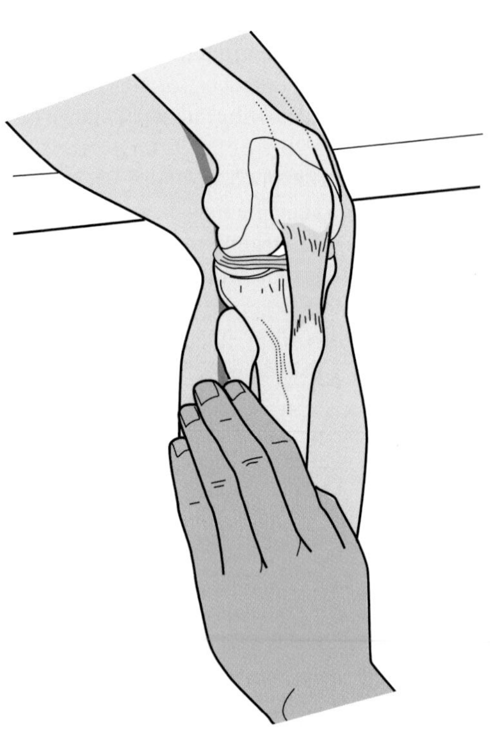

Figure 12.31 Location of the common (fibular) peroneal nerve.

Gastrocnemius

The gastrocnemius muscle is palpable on the posterior surface of the medial and lateral femoral condyles with the patient in the prone position and the knee extended. The muscle can be made more distinct by resisting either knee flexion or ankle plantar flexion. The muscle belly is located further distally over the mid portion of the posterior aspect of the tibia. Tenderness can be indicative of a strain of the muscle. Localized tenderness and effusion can be indicative of a deep venous thrombosis (Figure 12.33).

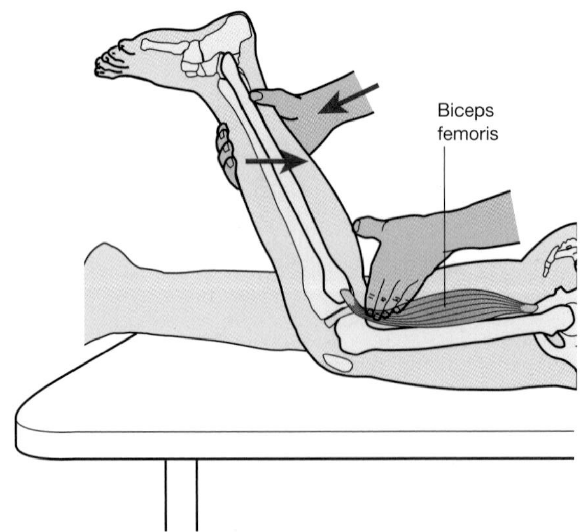

Figure 12.32 Palpation of the biceps femoris.

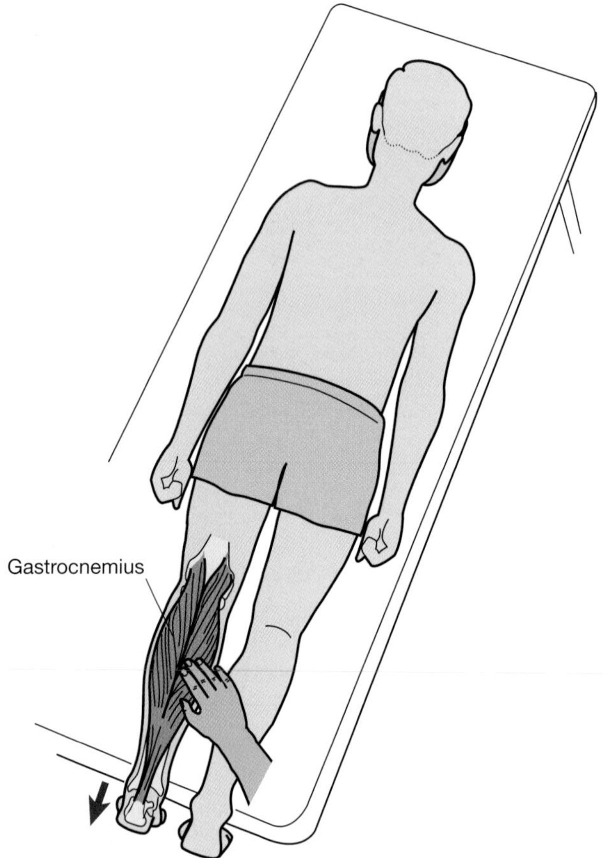

Figure 12.33 Palpation of the gastrocnemius.

Popliteal Fossa

The popliteal fossa is formed on the superior aspect by the biceps femoris on the lateral side, and the tendons of the semimembranosus and semitendinosus on the medial side. The inferior aspect is defined by the two heads of the gastrocnemius (Figure 12.34).

Popliteal Vein, Artery, and Nerve

The popliteal nerve is the most superficial structure passing within the popliteal fossa. This structure is not normally palpable. Deep to the nerve, the popliteal vein is located and is also not normally palpable. The popliteal artery is the deepest of the structures and can be palpated with deep, firm pressure through the superficial fascia. The popliteal pulse is much

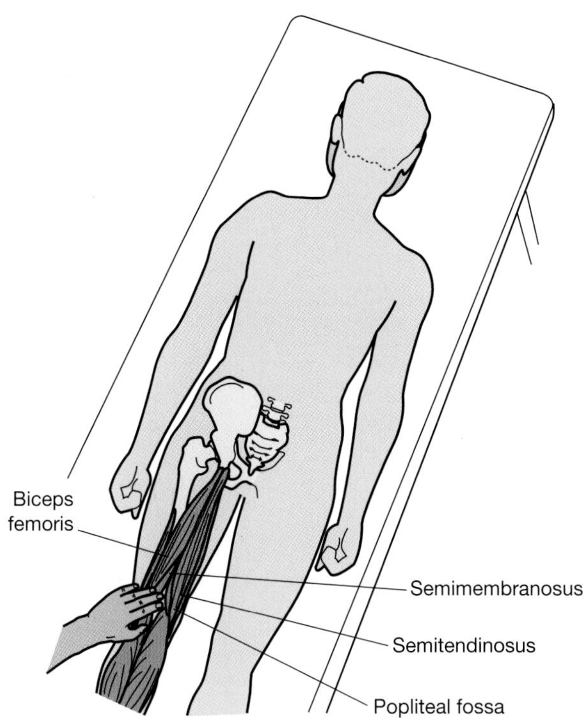

Figure 12.34 The popliteal fossa.

easier to palpate when the knee is flexed between 60 and 90 degrees, relaxing the muscle and connective tissue.

A comparison should be made between the dorsalis pedis and tibialis posterior pulses to rule out vascular compression. If you palpate an irregular lump on the artery, it may be an aneurysm.

Semimembranosus Muscle

The major insertion of the semimembranosus tendon is at the posteromedial aspect of the tibia, 1 cm distal to the joint line of the knee. The tendon is about 6 mm in diameter and is surrounded by a large synovial sleeve. Because of its proximity to the medial joint line, inflammation of the tendon and/or its sheath can be misinterpreted as medial joint line pain. Semimembranosus inflammation may be the result of repetitive or excessive stretching of the muscle.

Gastrocnemius-Semimembranosus Bursa

The gastrocnemius-semimembranosus bursa is located in the popliteal fossa. It is not normally palpable unless it becomes inflamed. It is then known as a Baker's cyst. It is more easily visible and palpable if the patient's knee is in extension. The cyst is easily moveable and is normally painless (Figure 12.35).

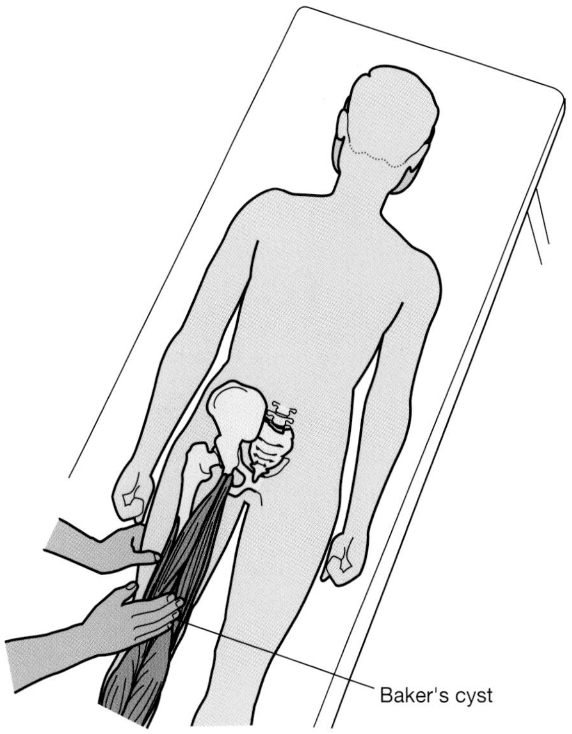

Figure 12.35 Baker's cyst.

Any type of knee effusion can cause a Baker's cyst to develop.

Trigger Points

Trigger points of the quadriceps and hamstring muscles can refer pain distally to the knee. Common trigger point locations for these muscles are illustrated in Figures 12.36 and 12.37.

Active Movement Testing

The two major movements of the knee joint are flexion and extension on the transverse axis. Internal and external rotation on the vertical axis can also be performed with the knee in 90 degrees of flexion. To accomplish the full range of flexion and extension, the tibia must be able to rotate. These are designed to be quick, functional tests designed to clear the joint. If the motion is pain free at the end of the range, you can add an additional overpressure to "clear" the joint. If the patient experiences pain during any of these movements, you should continue to explore whether the etiology of the pain is secondary to contractile or

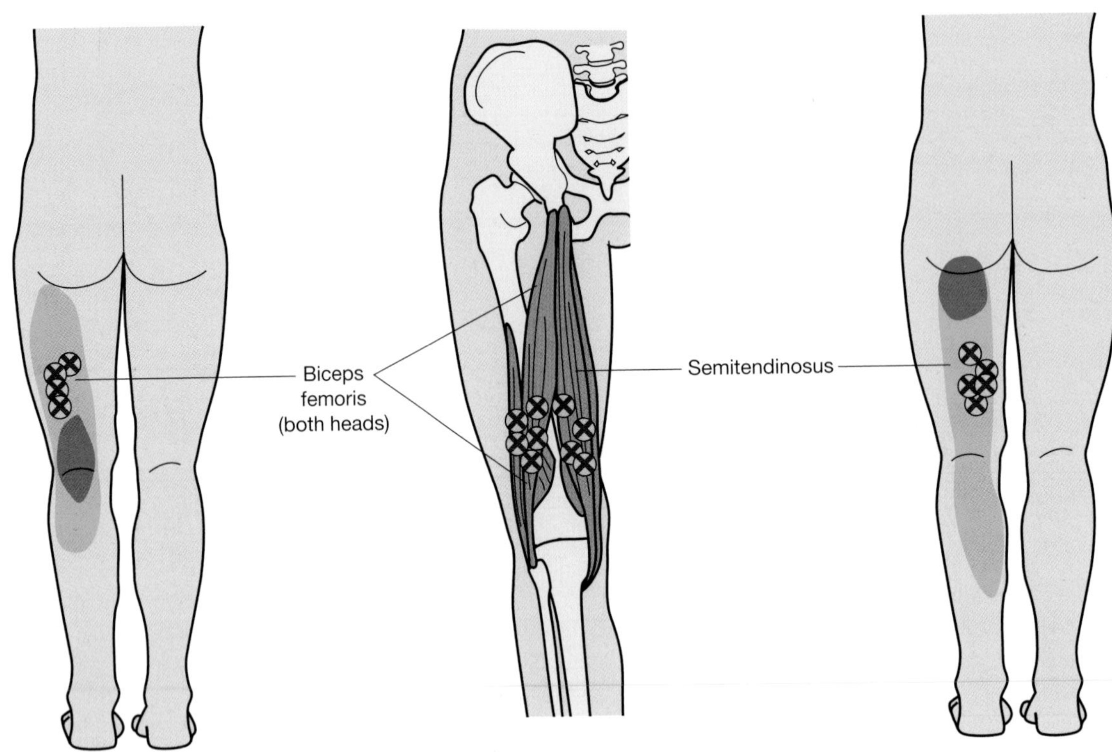

Figure 12.36 Trigger points in the right hamstring muscle are represented by the X's. Referred pain pattern distributions are represented by the stippled regions. (Adapted with permission from Travell and Rinzler, 1952.)

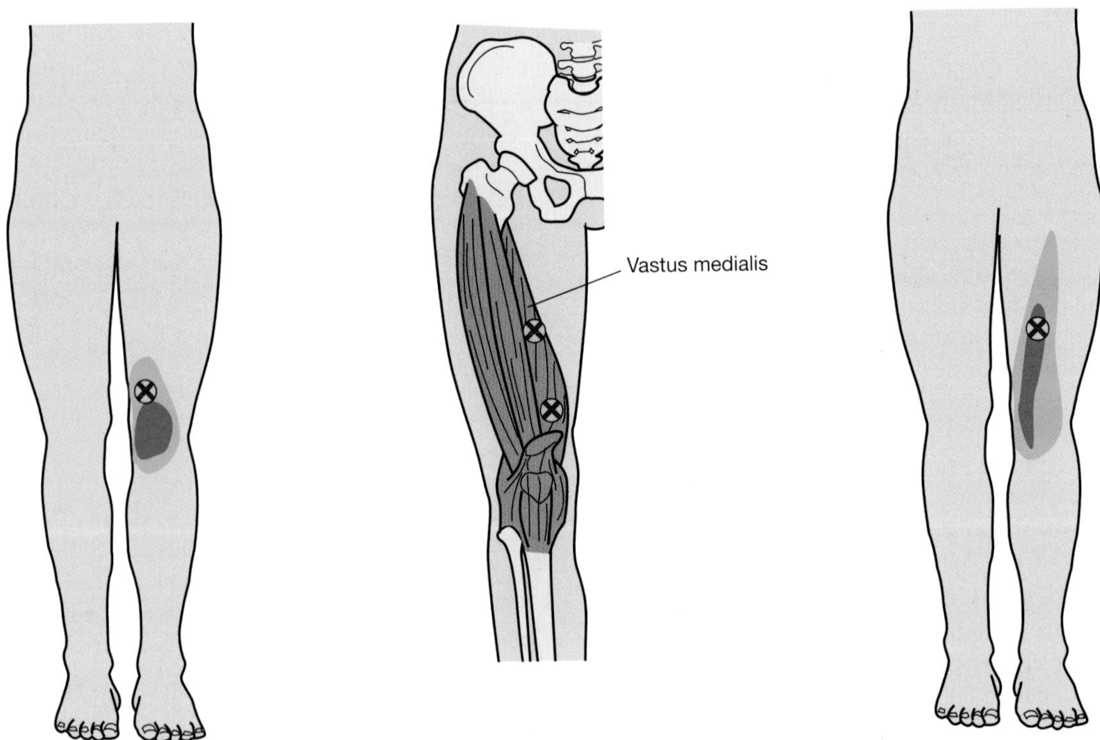

Figure 12.37 Trigger points in the quadriceps muscle are depicted above. The stippled regions are areas of referred pain from the trigger points, noted by the X's. (Adapted with permission from Travell and Rinzler, 1952.)

noncontractile structures by using passive and resistive testing.

A quick screening examination of the movements can be accomplished by asking the patient to perform a full, flat-footed squat and then to return to full extension. Flexion of the knee can also be accomplished in the prone position, during which the patient is asked to bend the knee toward the buttock and then return the leg to the table. Internal and external rotation can be observed by asking the patient to turn the tibia medially and then laterally while he or she is in the sitting position with the legs dangling off the edge of the table.

Passive Movement Testing

Passive movement testing can be divided into two categories: physiological movements (cardinal plane), which are the same as the active movements, and mobility testing of the accessory movements (joint play, component). You can determine whether the noncontractile (inert) elements are the cause of the patient's problem by using these tests. These structures (ligaments, joint capsule, fascia, bursa, dura mater, and nerve root) (Cyriax, 1982) are stretched or stressed when the joint is taken to the end of the available range. At the end of each passive physiological movement, you should sense the end feel and determine whether it is normal or pathological. Assess the limitation of movement and see if it fits into a capsular pattern. The capsular pattern of the knee is a greater restriction of flexion than extension so that with 90 degrees of limited flexion there is only 5 degrees of limited extension. Limitation of rotation is only noted when there is significant limitation of flexion and extension (Kaltenborn, 2011).

Physiological Movements

You will be assessing the amount of motion available in all directions. Each motion is measured from the anatomical starting position, which is the knee extended with the longitudinal axes of both the femur and tibia in the frontal plane. They normally meet at an angle of 170 degrees (Kaltenborn, 2011).

Flexion

The best position for measuring flexion is the prone position with the patient's foot over the edge of the table. If the rectus femoris appears to be very shortened, you should place the patient in the supine position. Place your hand over the distal anterior aspect of the tibia and bend the leg toward the buttock. The normal end feel for this movement is soft tissue from the contact between the gastrocnemius and the hamstrings. If the rectus femoris is the limiting factor, the end feel is abrupt and firm (ligamentous) (Magee, 2008; Kaltenborn, 2011). Normal range of motion is 0–135 degrees (American Academy of Orthopedic Surgeons, 1965) (Figure 12.38).

Extension

Full extension is achieved when the patient is placed in either the prone or the supine position. When testing in supine, place one hand over the anterior distal surface of the femur to stabilize and the other under the posterior surface of the tibia and move the leg into extension. The normal end feel is abrupt and firm (ligamentous) because of tension in the posterior capsule and ligaments (Magee, 2008; Kaltenborn, 2011). The normal range of motion is zero degree (Figure 12.39) (American Academy of Orthopedic Surgeons, 1965).

Medial and Lateral Rotation

You can measure medial and lateral rotation with the patient either in the sitting position with the leg dangling off the end of the table or in the prone position with the knee flexed. Place your hand over the distal part of the leg, proximal to the ankle joint, and rotate the tibia first in a medial direction to the end of the available range, back to the midline, and then in a lateral direction to the end of the available range. The normal end feel is abrupt and firm (ligamentous) (Magee, 2008; Kaltenborn, 2011). Normal range of motion is 20–30 degrees of medial rotation of the tibia and 30–40 degrees of lateral rotation of the tibia (Magee, 2008) (Figure 12.40).

Mobility Testing of Accessory Movements

Mobility testing of accessory movements will give you information about the degree of laxity present in the joint. The patient must be totally relaxed and comfortable to allow you to move the joint and obtain the most accurate information. The joint should be placed in the maximal loose-packed (resting) position to allow for the greatest degree of joint movement.

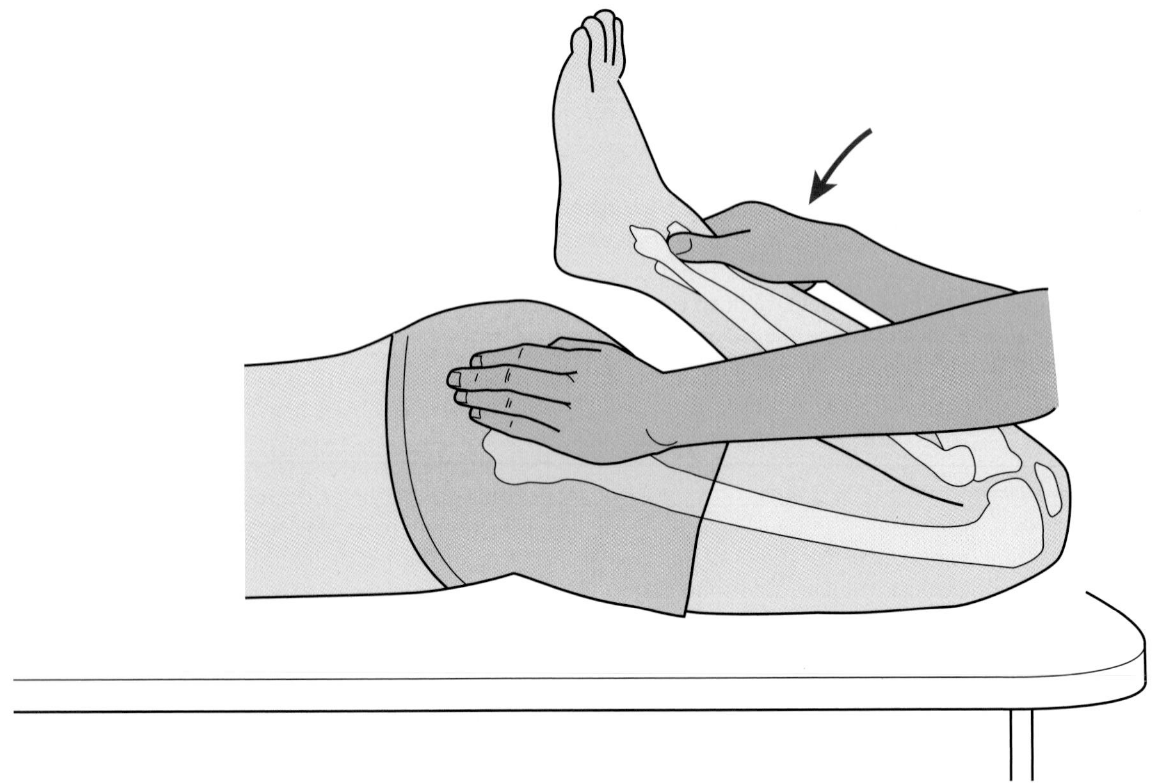

Figure 12.38 Passive flexion of the knee.

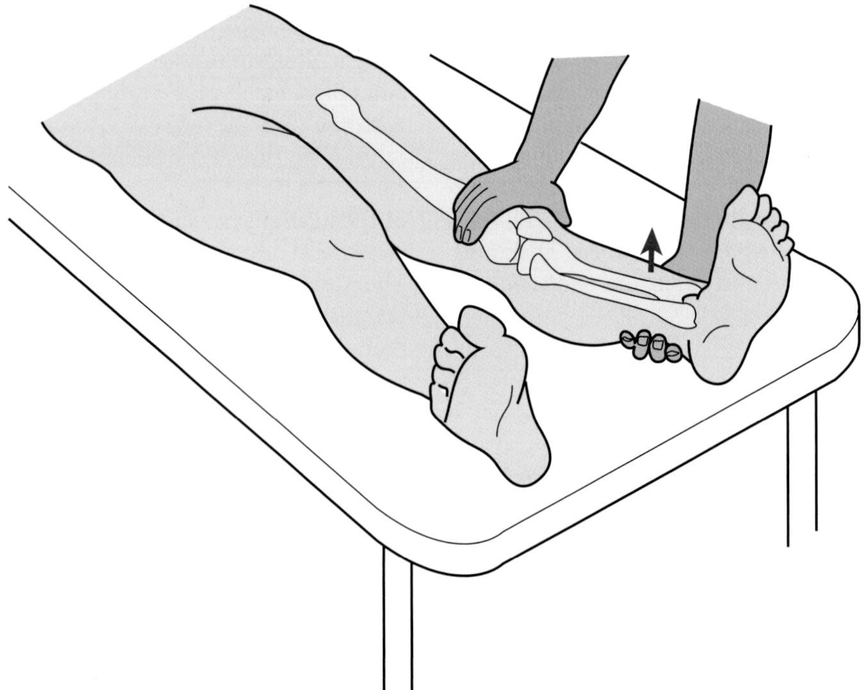

Figure 12.39 Passive extension of the knee.

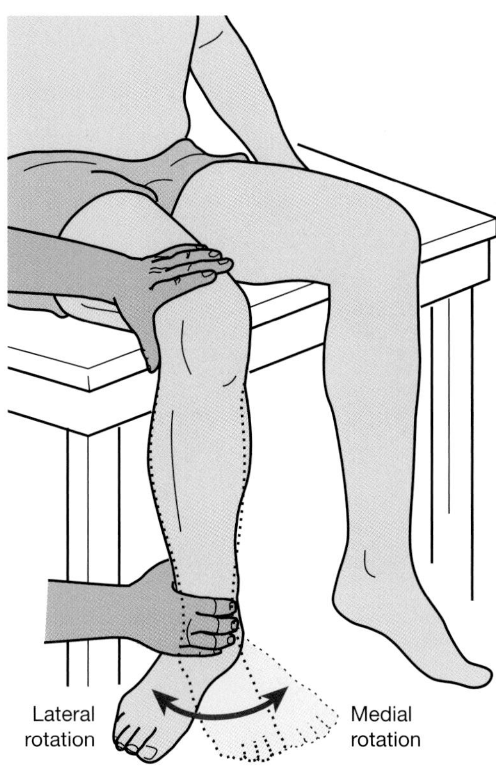

Figure 12.40 Passive lateral and medial rotation of the tibia.

The resting position of the knee is 25 degrees of flexion (Kaltenborn, 2011).

Traction

Place the patient in the supine position with the hip flexed to approximately 60 degrees and the knee flexed approximately 25 degrees. Stand to the side of the patient, facing the lateral aspect of the leg to be tested. Stabilize the femur by grasping the distal medial aspect of the femur with your index finger at the joint line, to enable you to palpate. Stabilize the leg against your trunk. Hold the distal end of the tibia, proximal to the malleoli from the medial aspect. Pull the tibia in a longitudinal direction producing traction in the tibiofemoral joint (Figure 12.41).

Ventral Glide of the Tibia

Place the patient in the supine position with the knee flexed to approximately 90 degrees. Stand on the side of the patient, with your body facing the patient. You can rest your buttock on the patient's foot to stabilize it. Place your hands around the tibia, allowing your

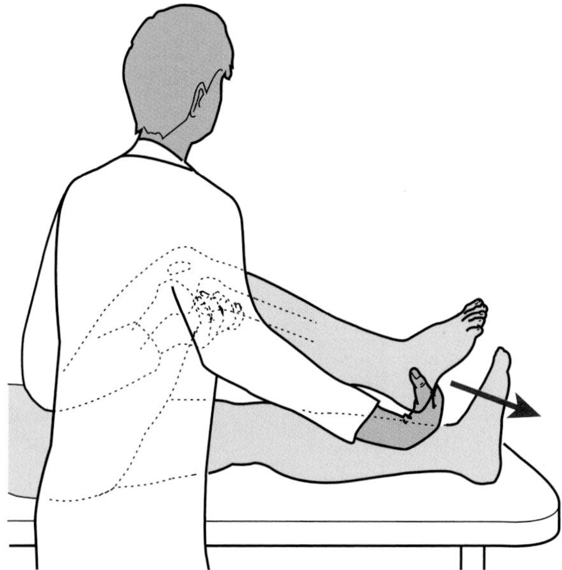

Figure 12.41 Traction of the tibiofemoral joint—mobility testing.

thumbs to rest on the medial and lateral joint lines, to enable you to palpate the joint line. Pull the tibia in an anterior direction until all the slack has been taken up. This not only tests for anterior mobility of the femoral tibial joint, but also tests for the integrity of the ACL. The test for the ACL is referred to as the *anterior drawer test* (Figure 12.42).

Medial and lateral rotation of the tibia can be added to the anterior drawer test to check for rotational instability. Medial rotation increases the tension in the intact posterolateral structures and decreases the degree of anterior displacement. Lateral rotation increases the tension in the intact posteromedial structures and decreases anterior displacement of the tibia even when the ACL is compromised (Figure 12.43) (see pp. 367–368, Figure 12.70). This is referred to as the Slocum test.

Posterior Glide of the Tibia

Place the patient in the supine position with the knee flexed to approximately 90 degrees. Stand on the side of the patient, with your body facing the patient. You can rest your buttock on the patient's foot to stabilize it. Place your hands around the tibia so that the heels of your hands are resting on the medial and lateral tibial plateaus and your fingers are wrapped around the medial and lateral joint spaces. Push the tibia in a posterior direction until all the slack has been taken up. This not only tests for posterior mobility of the

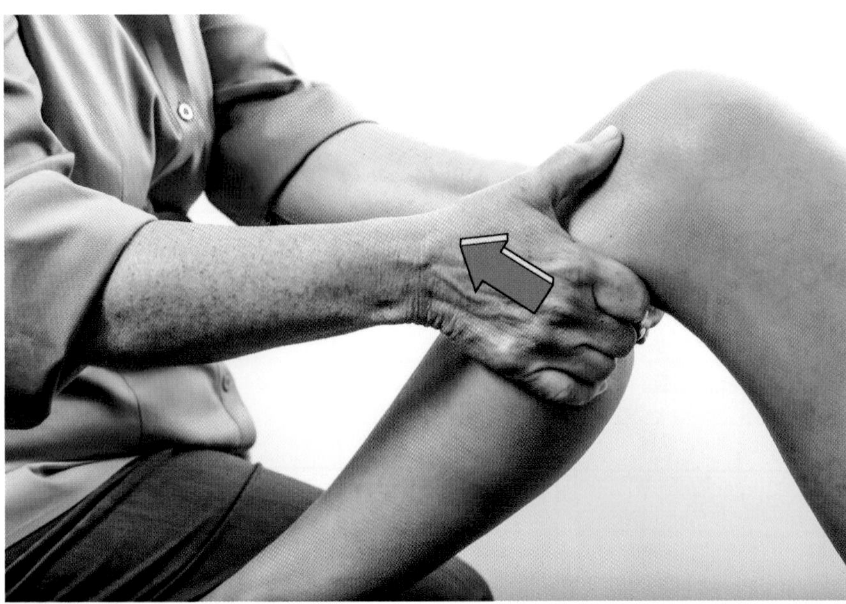

Figure 12.42 Anterior glide of the tibia which is also known as the anterior drawer test when testing for ligamentous stability.

femoral tibial joint, but also tests for the integrity of the posterior cruciate ligament. The test for the posterior cruciate ligament is referred to as the *posterior drawer test* or the *gravity test* (Figure 12.44). Medial and lateral tibial rotation can be added to check for posterior medial and lateral stability and is known as Hughston's draw sign (Magee, 2008).

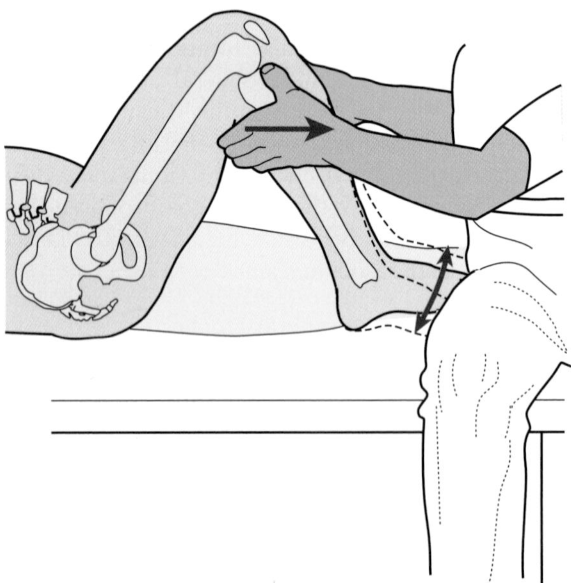

Figure 12.43 Anterior drawer test with medial and lateral rotation, also known as the Slocum test when testing for ligamentous stability.

Medial and Lateral Gapping (Varus–Valgus Stress)

Place the patient in the supine position, and stand on the side of the table and face the patient. Hold the patient's ankle between your elbow and trunk to secure the leg. Extend your arm proximally to the joint space on the medial aspect of the knee, allowing you to palpate. Place your other hand on the distal lateral aspect of the patient's femur, as the stabilizing force. Allow the patient's knee to flex approximately 30 degrees. Apply a valgus force to the knee by pulling the distal aspect of the tibia in a lateral direction while maintaining your stabilization on the lateral part of the femur. This will create a gapping on the medial side of the knee joint. You should expect to feel a normal abrupt and firm (ligamentous) end feel (Magee, 2008; Kaltenborn, 2011). If there is increased gapping, a different end feel, or a "clunk" as you release, you should suspect a loss of integrity of the medial collateral ligament. This procedure should be repeated with the patient's knee in extension. If you have a positive finding in both the flexed and the extended position, involvement of the posterior cruciate ligament in addition to the medial collateral ligament should be suspected (Figure 12.45).

To test the integrity of the lateral collateral ligament, the same test should be repeated by reversing your hand placements. This will allow you to create a varus force, creating gapping on the lateral aspect of the knee joint (Figures 12.46a and 12.46b).

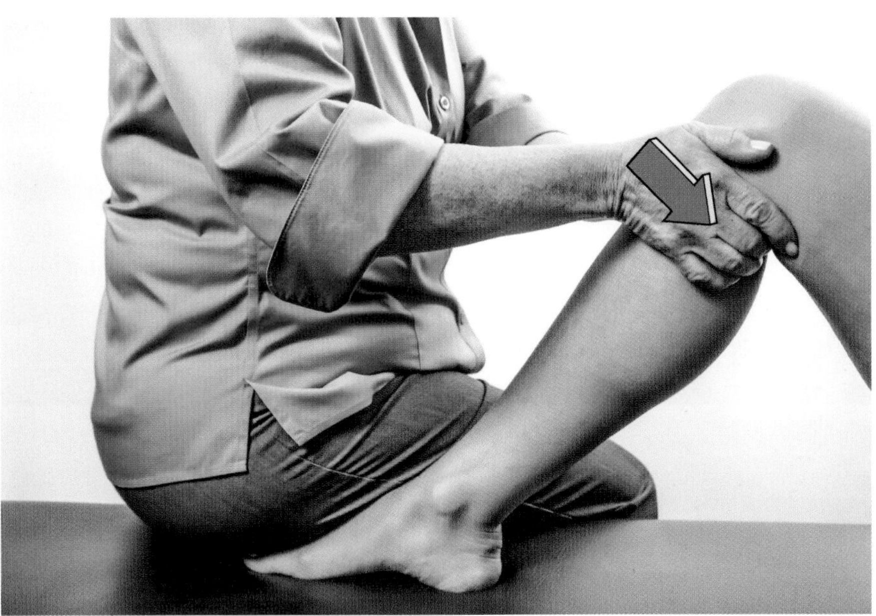

Figure 12.44 Posterior glide of the tibia. Also known as the posterior drawer test when testing for ligamentous stability.

Medial and Lateral Glide of the Tibia

Place the patient in the supine position so that the knee is at the end of the table. Face the patient and secure the ankle between your legs. Place your stabilizing hand on the distal medial aspect of the femur just proximal to the joint line. Your mobilizing hand should be on the proximal lateral part of the tibia just distal to the joint line. Use your mobilizing hand to push in a medial direction until all the slack has been taken up. You should feel an abrupt and firm (ligamentous) end feel (Magee, 2008; Kaltenborn, 2011). This tests for normal mobility of medial glide of the tibia (Figure 12.47).

Testing for normal mobility of lateral glide can be assessed in the same manner by reversing your hand placements (Figure 12.48).

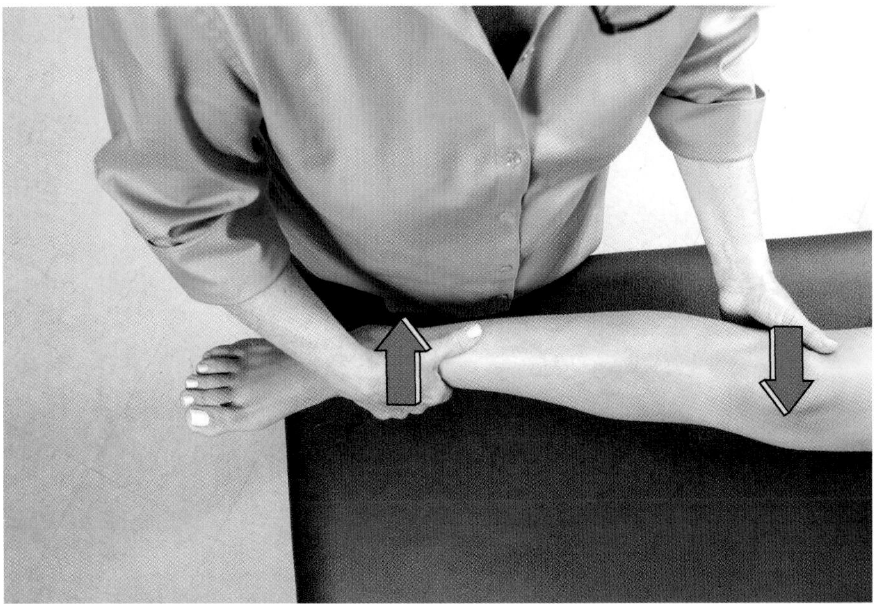

Figure 12.45 Valgus strain (medial gapping).

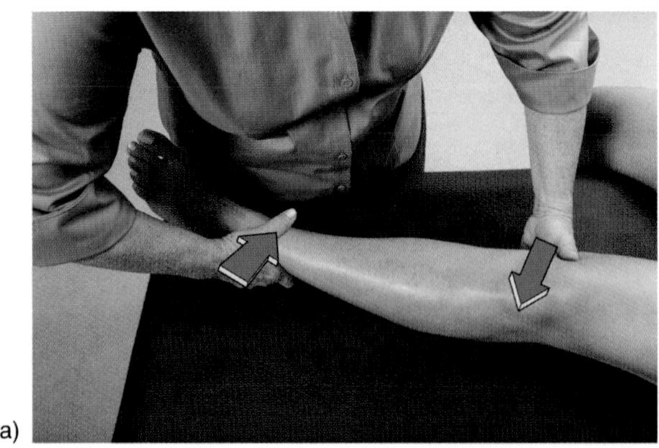
(a)

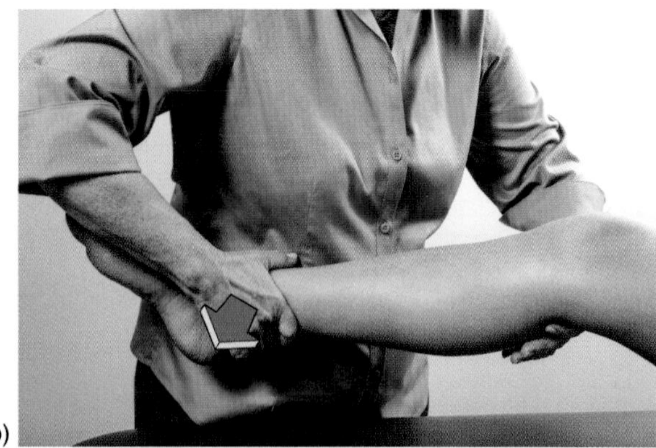
(b)

Figure 12.46 (a) Varus strain (lateral gapping). (b) Varus strain with flexion of the knee.

Patellar Mobility

Place the patient in the supine position, with a small towel placed underneath the knee to avoid full extension. Stand on the stand of the table, facing the patient. With both hands, grasp the patella between your thumb and index and middle fingers. Distract the patella by lifting it away from the femur (Figure 12.49).

Stand so that you are facing the lateral aspect of the patient's lower extremity. Place your extended thumbs on the lateral aspect of the patella. Push your thumbs simultaneously in a medial direction. This will create medial glide of the patella (Figure 12.50). Lateral glide can be accomplished by placing your hands on the medial aspect of the patella. The patella should move approximately one-half its width in both medial

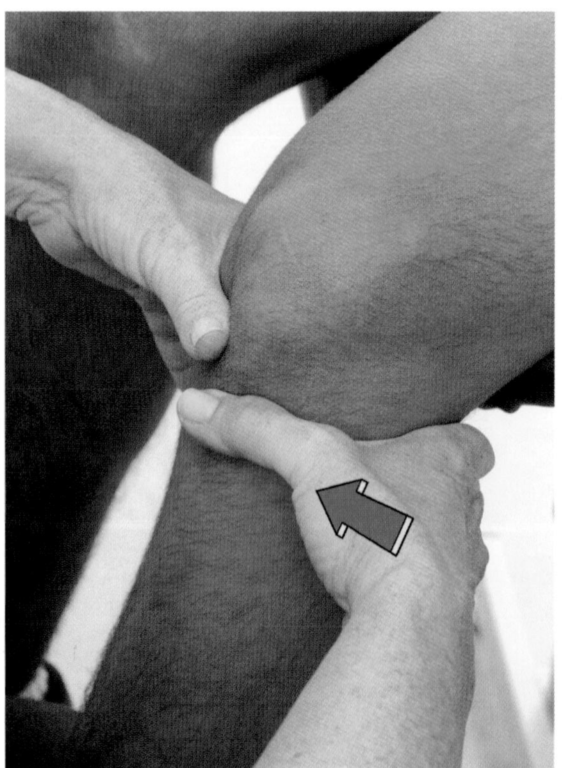

Figure 12.47 Medial glide of the tibia—mobility testing.

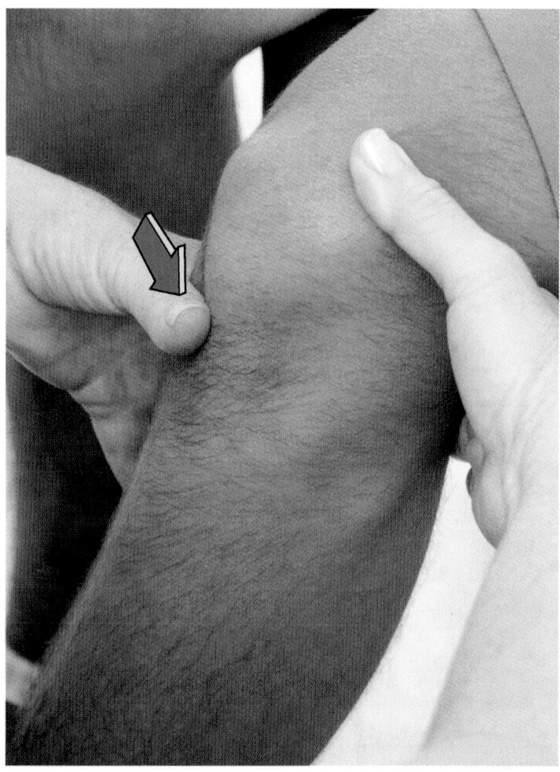

Figure 12.48 Lateral glide of the tibia—mobility testing.

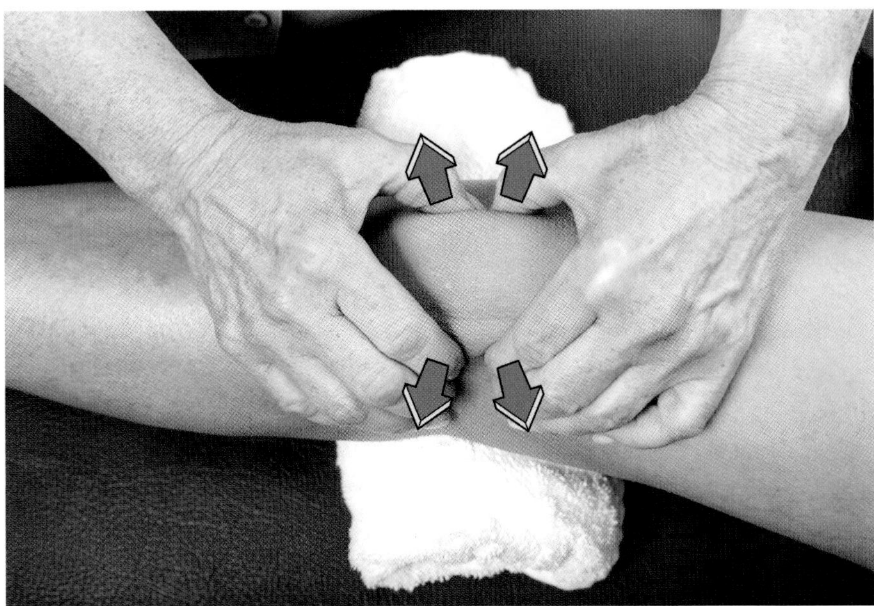

Figure 12.49 Distraction of the patella—mobility testing.

and lateral glides in extension. The lateral glide is easier to perform and has a greater excursion than the medial glide (Figure 12.51). Inferior glide can be accomplished by turning so that you face the patient's foot. Place the heel of one hand over the superior pole of the patella, allowing your arm to rest on the patient's thigh. Place your other hand on top of the first hand and push in an inferior (caudad) direction (Figure 12.52). This will test inferior mobility of the patella. It is important to remember not to create any compressive forces on the patella during the glide.

Resistive Testing

The primary movements of the knee to be examined are flexion and extension. Resisted internal and external rotation of the tibia can also be tested. The ability

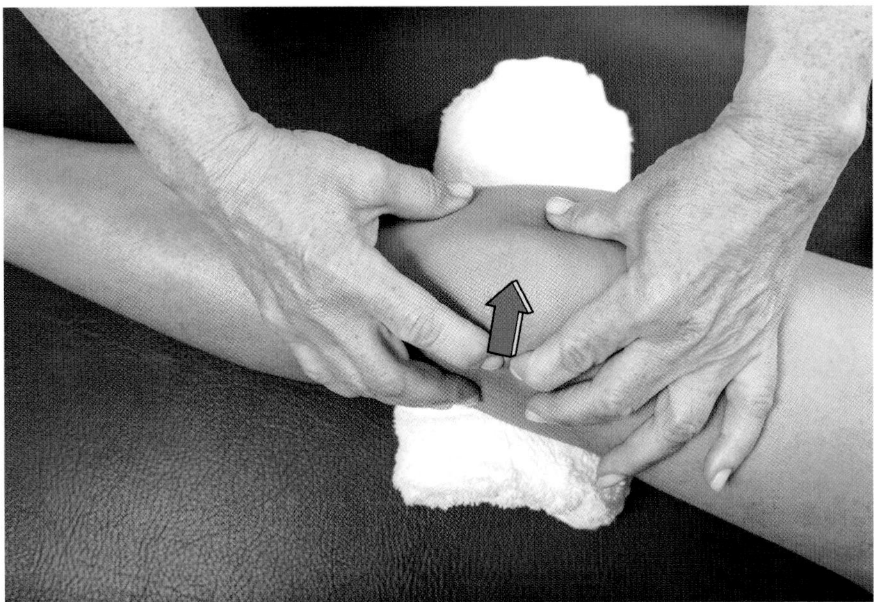

Figure 12.50 Medial glide of the patella—mobility testing.

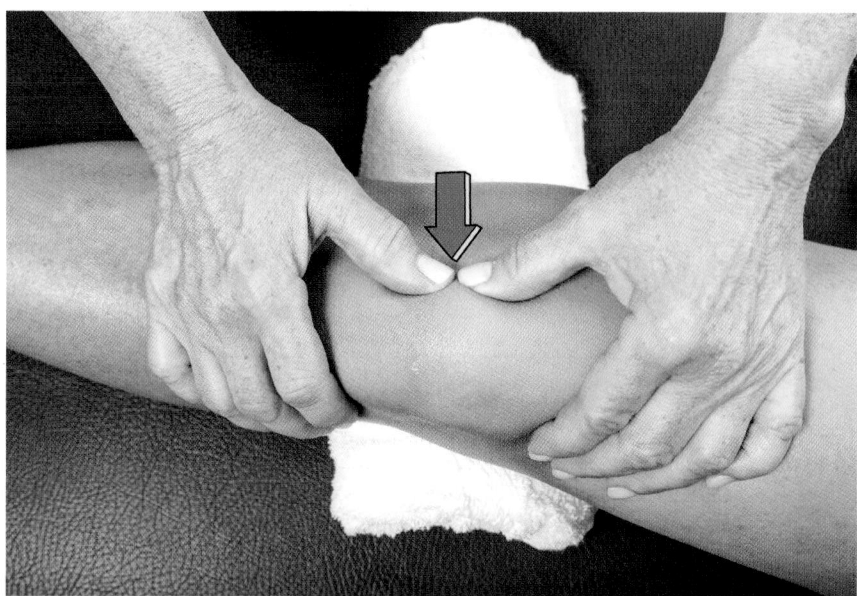

Figure 12.51 Lateral glide of the patella—mobility testing.

to resist rotational forces is especially important when damage has occurred to the ligamentous stabilizers of the knee.

Flexion

The flexors of the knee are the hamstrings—semitendinosus, biceps femoris, and semimembranosus (Figure 12.53). The hamstrings are assisted by the sartorius, gracilis, and popliteus muscles. Except for the popliteus muscle, all the knee flexors cross the hip as well. As the hip is flexed, the strength of the hamstrings as knee flexors increases.

- Position of patient: Prone with the hip in neutral (Figure 12.54).
- Resisted test: Ask the patient to bend the knee so as to bring the heel toward the buttock. Resist the movement by placing one hand posteriorly above

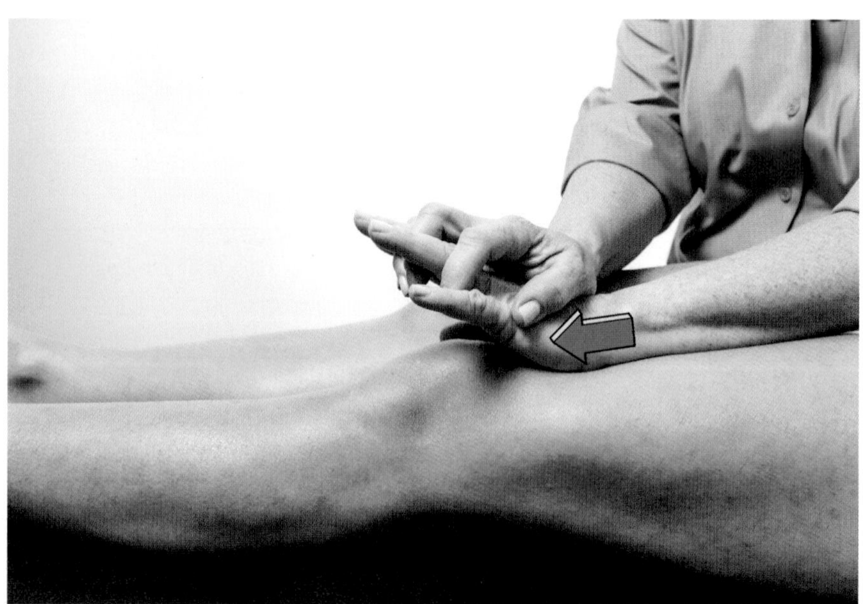

Figure 12.52 Inferior glide of the patella—mobility testing. Remember not to compress the patella.

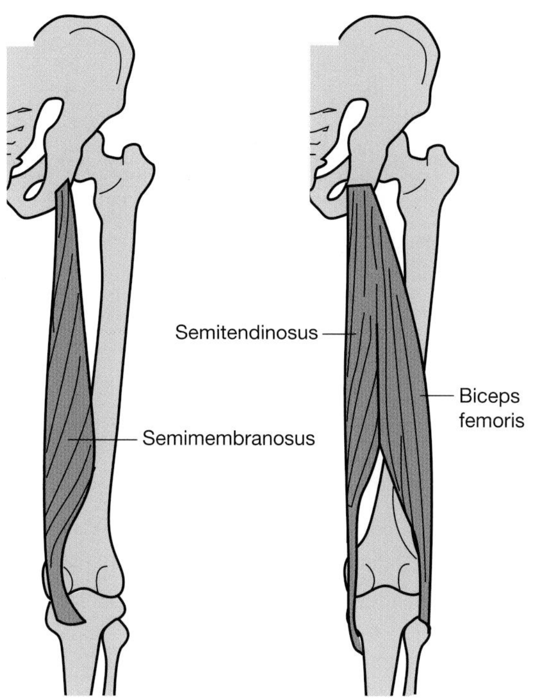

Figure 12.53 The primary knee flexors. Note that the long head of the biceps is innervated by the tibial portion of the sciatic nerve and the short head of the biceps femoris is innervated by the peroneal portion of the sciatic nerve.

the ankle. Stabilize the patient's thigh downward with the other hand. Note: Medial and lateral hamstrings may be relatively isolated by rotating the thigh and leg medially to test the medial hamstrings and laterally to test the lateral hamstrings.

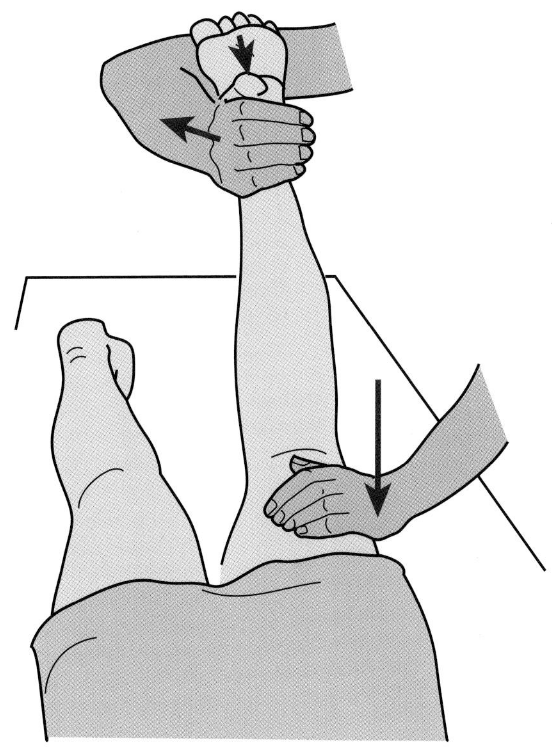

Figure 12.54 Testing knee flexion.

Testing knee flexion with gravity eliminated is performed in the same manner, except that the patient is in the side-lying position (Figure 12.55).

Painful resisted knee flexion may be due to tendinitis of the hamstring muscles or the muscles of the pes anserinus. A popliteal (Baker's) cyst may also cause pain during knee flexion.

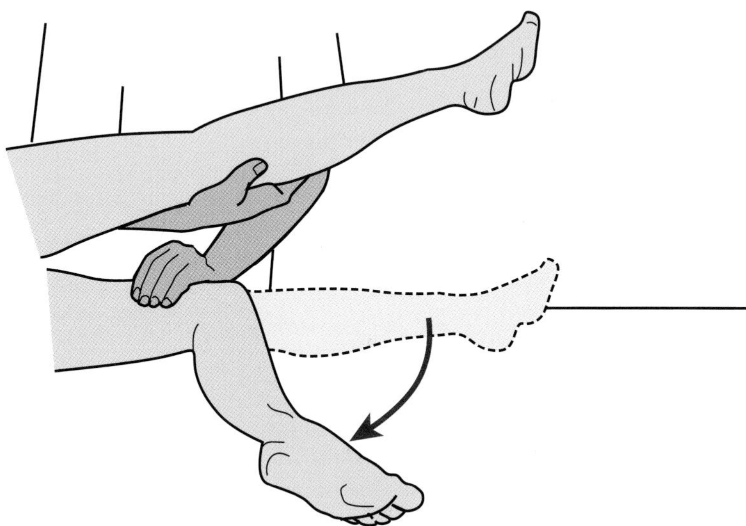

Figure 12.55 Testing knee flexion with gravity eliminated.

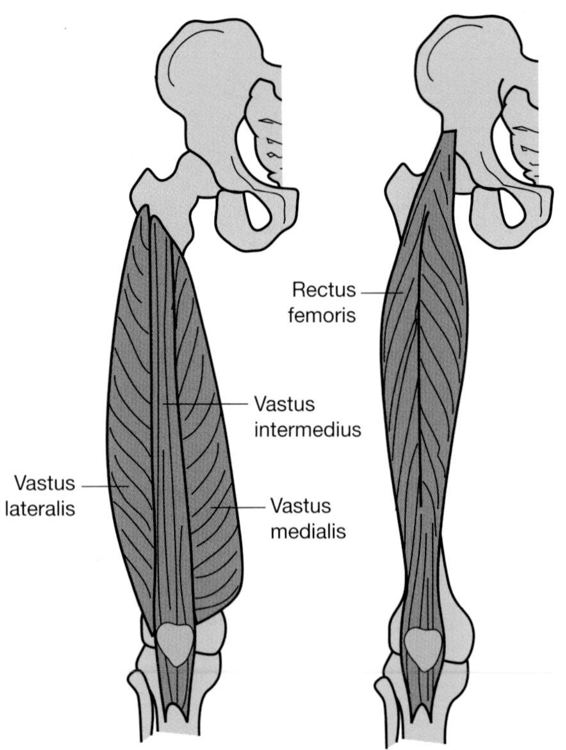

Figure 12.56 The primary extensors of the knee. Note that the rectus femoris muscle also crosses the hip joint and acts as a hip flexor as well as a knee extensor.

Weakness of knee flexion results in an abnormal gait. A hyperextension deformity of the knee may result from lack of dynamic stability. Isolated weakness of the medial or lateral hamstrings will result in knee instability on the same side of the joint as the weakness. For example, weakness of the lateral hamstrings causes a tendency toward varus deformity of the knee on weight bearing.

Extension

The primary extensor of the knee is the quadriceps femoris muscle (Figure 12.56). The rectus femoris also crosses the hip as well and assists in hip flexion.

- Position of patient: Sitting with the legs hanging over the edge of the table. Place a rolled towel or small pillow under the patient's knee and distal part of the thigh to act as a cushion (Figure 12.57).
- Resisted test: Ask the patient to extend the knee while applying downward pressure with your hand above the ankle.

Testing knee extension with gravity eliminated is performed with the patient lying on the side and the knee initially bent. The patient attempts to extend the knee while the leg is resting on the table (Figure 12.58).

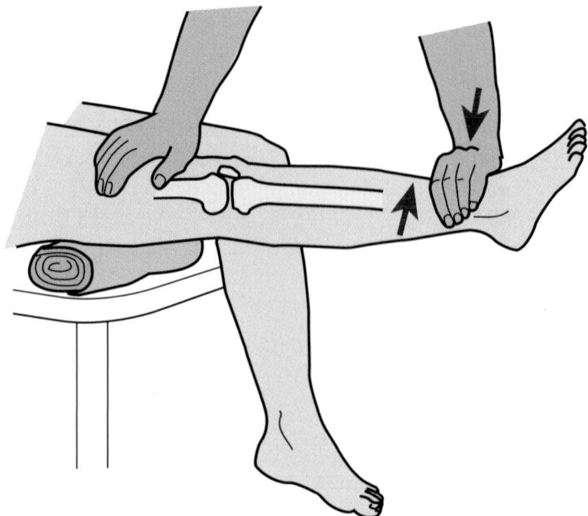

Figure 12.57 Testing knee extension.

Painful resisted knee extension may be due to patellar tendinitis, also known as *jumper's knee*. Disorders of the patellofemoral joint may also be painful if knee extension is tested in a position of extreme knee flexion. This position increases the force within the patellofemoral joint.

Weakness of knee extension causes difficulty in getting out of a chair, climbing stairs, and walking up an incline. An abnormal gait also results.

Rotation

The medial hamstrings, sartorius, gracilis, and popliteus muscles are medial rotators of the tibia (Figure 12.59). This rotation occurs as the knee is unlocked from its extended position during initiation of knee flexion.

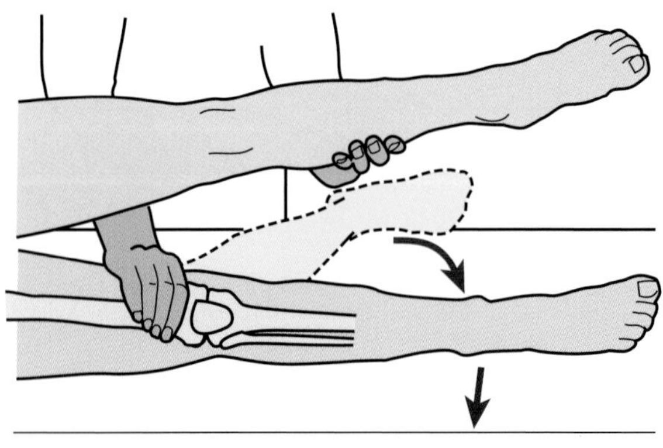

Figure 12.58 Testing knee extension with gravity eliminated.

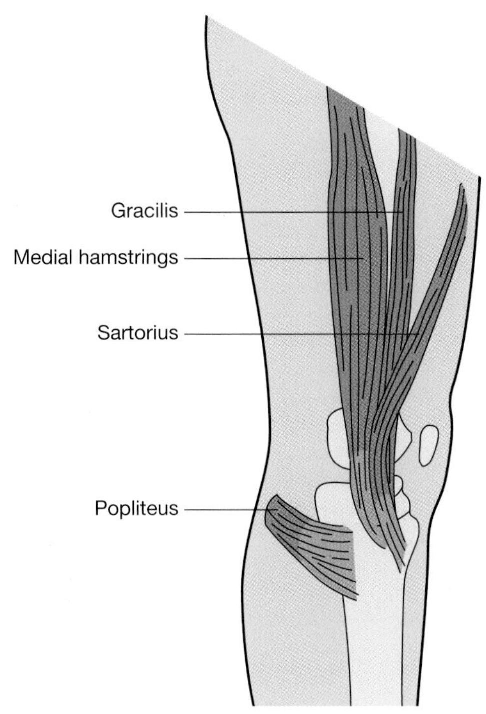

Figure 12.59 The medial rotators of the knee.

The lateral rotators of the tibia are the biceps femoris and tensor fasciae latae muscles (see Figure 12.59). All the rotators of the knee act as dynamic stabilizers in conjunction with the ligaments.

- Position of patient: Sitting upright with the knees bent over the edge of the table (Figure 12.60).
- Resisted test: Take the tibia with both hands and ask the patient to attempt to rotate it. Have the patient twist the tibia medially and then laterally as you resist this movement.

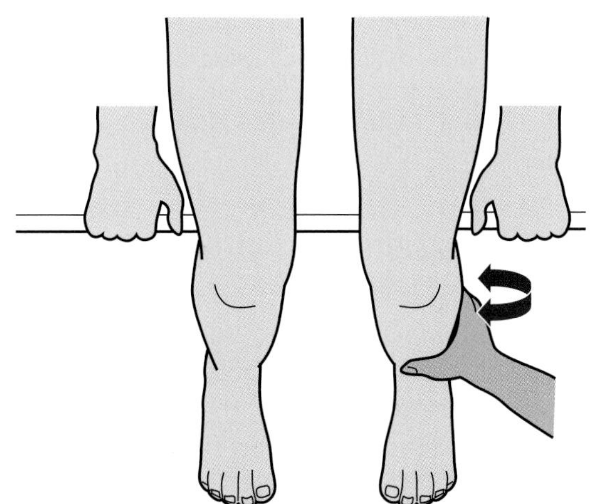

Figure 12.60 Testing medial and lateral rotation of the knee.

Neurological Examination

Motor

The innervation and spinal levels of the muscles that function across the knee joint are listed in Table 12.1.

Reflexes

Knee Jerk

The knee jerk is performed to test the L3 and L4 nerve roots (Figure 12.61). To test the knee jerk, place the patient in the supine position. Elevate the leg behind the knee with one hand so that it is flexed approximately 20–30 degrees. Take the reflex hammer and tap the patellar tendon below the patella to observe the response. Look for contraction of the quadriceps muscle with or without elevation of the foot from the table. Perform the test bilaterally for comparison. Loss of this reflex may be due to a radiculopathy of the L3 or L4 nerve roots, or damage to the femoral nerve or quadriceps muscle.

Hamstring Jerk

The medial and lateral hamstring reflexes are performed to test the L5–S1 (medial hamstring) and S1 and S2 (lateral hamstring) root levels (Figure 12.62). The patient is prone with the knee flexed and the leg supported. Place your thumb over the medial or lateral hamstring tendon and tap your thumb with the reflex hammer. Look for contraction of the hamstring muscle exhibited by knee flexion. Compare both sides.

Sensation

Light touch and pinprick sensation should be examined after the motor examination. The dermatomes for the anterior aspect of the knee are L2 and L3. Please refer to Figure 12.63 for the exact locations of the key sensory areas of these dermatomes. We have included dermatome drawings from more than one anatomy text to emphasize the variability that exists among patients and anatomists. The peripheral nerves providing sensation in the knee region are shown in Figure 12.64.

Infrapatellar Nerve Injury

The infrapatellar branch of the saphenous nerve may be cut during surgery of the knee. Tinel's sign may be

Table 12.1 Movements of the Knee: The Muscles and Their Nerve Supply, as well as Their Nerve Root Derivations Are Shown

Movement	Muscles	Innervation	Root Levels
Flexion of knee	Biceps femoris	Sciatic	L5, S1, S2
	Semitendinosus	Sciatic	L5, S1, S2
	Semimembranosus	Sciatic	L5, S1
	Gracilis	Obturator	L2, L3
	Sartorius	Femoral	L2, L3
	Popliteus	Tibial	L4, L5, S1
	Gastrocnemius	Tibial	S1, S2
Extension of knee	Rectus femoris	Femoral	L2, L3, L4
	Vastus medialis	Femoral	L2, L3, L4
	Vastus intermedius	Femoral	L2, L3, L4
	Vastus lateralis	Femoral	L2, L3, L4
Medial rotation of flexed leg	Popliteus	Tibial	L4, L5, S1
	Semimembranosus	Sciatic	L5, S1
	Sartorius	Femoral	L2, L3
	Gracilis	Obturator	L2, L3
	Semitendinosus	Sciatic	L5, S1, S2
Lateral rotation of flexed leg	Biceps femoris	Sciatic	L5, S1, S2

obtained by tapping on the medial aspect of the tibial tubercle (Figure 12.65). A positive response would be tingling or tenderness.

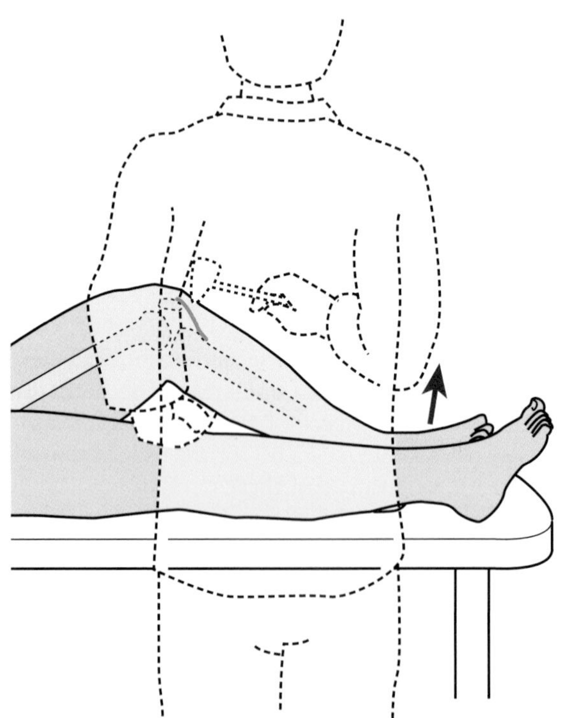

Figure 12.61 The patient is positioned for the patellar reflex. The reflex can also be obtained with the patient seated, by tapping on the patellar tendon with the knee flexed.

Referred Pain Patterns

Pain in the region of the knee may be referred from the ankle and hip. Pain in the knee that is referred from the hip is usually felt medially. An L3, L4, or L5 radiculopathy can also be perceived as pain in the knee (Figure 12.66).

Special Tests

Flexibility Tests

An estimation of quadriceps flexibility can be performed by asking the patient to take the lower leg with one hand and bend the knee and foot behind him or her so as to bring the heel toward the buttocks (Figure 12.67). The patient may compensate for a tight rectus femoris by rotating the pelvis anteriorly and flexing the hip. Hamstring flexibility is described in Chapter 11.

Tests for Stability and Structural Integrity

There is an abundance of testing procedures with associated eponyms that have been developed in an effort to test the stability of the anterior and posterior cruciate ligaments in various planes. Some of the more commonly used tests are described in this section. A clear understanding of the functional anatomy of the cruciate ligaments is necessary in order to appreciate

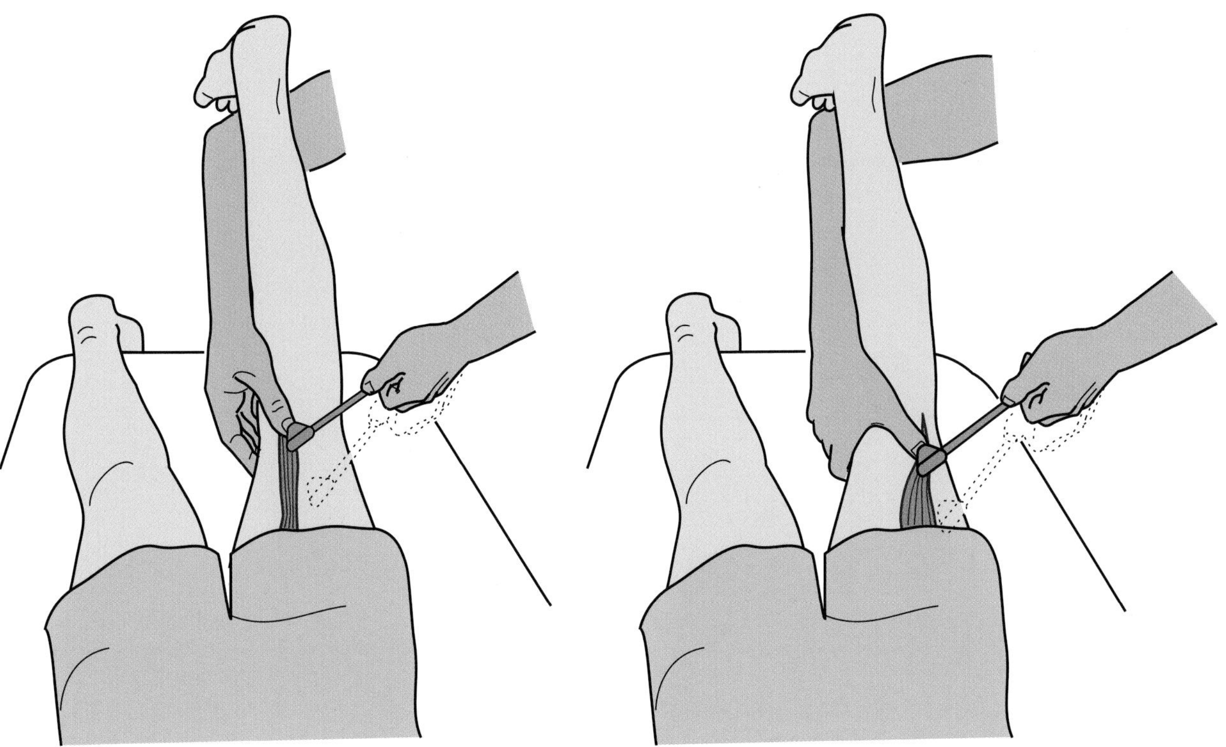

Figure 12.62 Testing the medial and lateral hamstring reflexes is performed with the patient in this position.

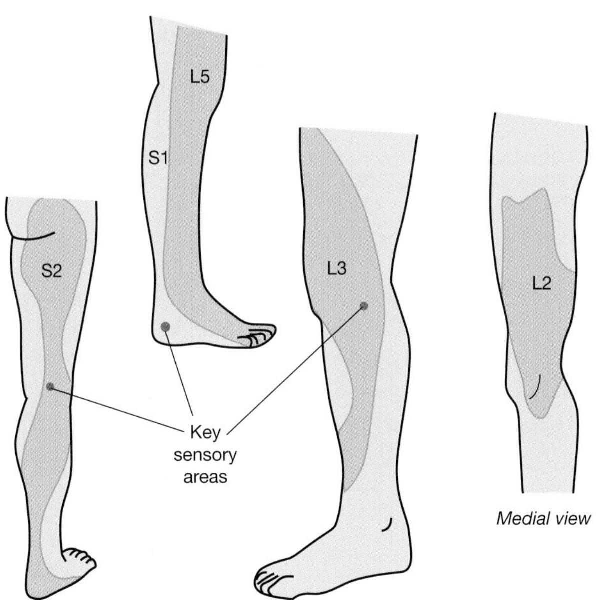

Figure 12.63 The dermatomes in the region of the knee. Note that the key sensory area for L3 is medial to the patella. The key sensory area for S2 is depicted in the popliteal fossa. The key sensory area for S1 is located distal to the lateral malleolus and calcaneus.

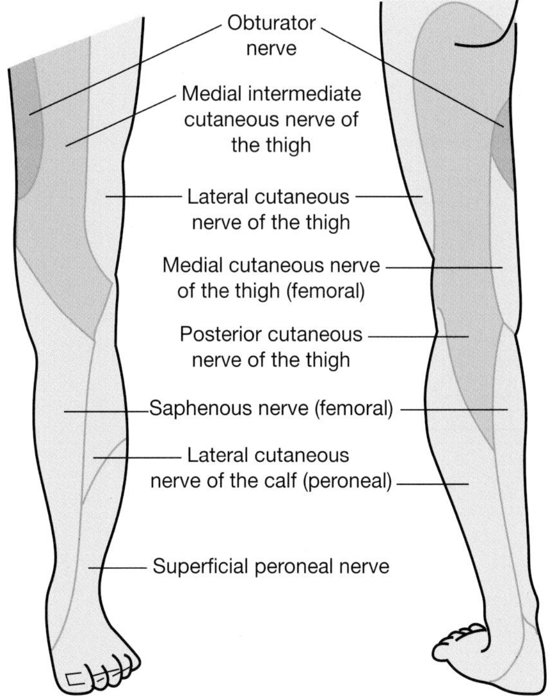

Figure 12.64 The nerve distributions to the skin of the anterior and posterior aspects of the thigh and leg.

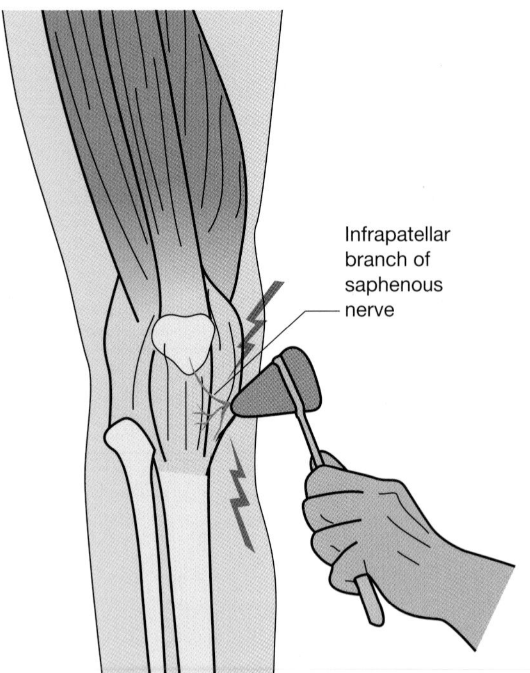

Figure 12.65 The infrapatellar branch of the saphenous nerve can be injured during surgery. This will cause numbness or tingling in the distribution of this nerve medial to the patella. Tapping the region of the nerve with a reflex hammer will cause a tingling sensation, known as Tinel's sign.

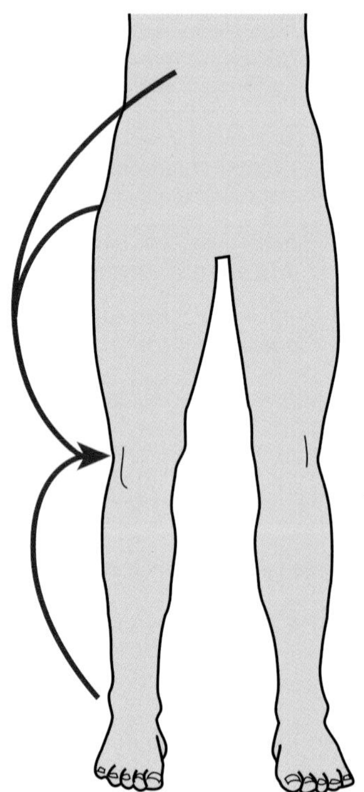

Figure 12.66 Pain may be referred to and from the knee.

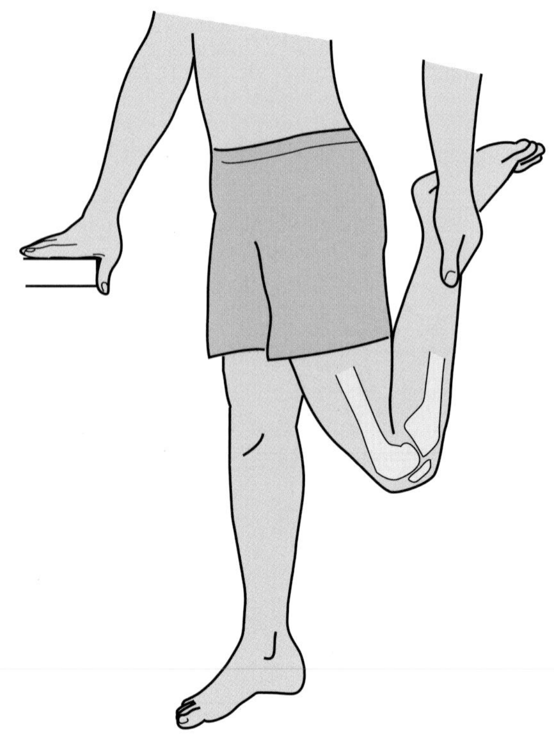

Figure 12.67 The patient is shown stretching the quadriceps muscle and displaying normal flexibility of the muscle.

the purpose of the various tests. Many of the tests reveal subtle responses and require a great deal of experience to interpret (Figure 12.68).

Anterior Stability Tests

In testing the anterior and posterior cruciate ligaments, you should first examine the patient for anterior and posterior instability of the tibia. This can be accomplished with the anterior drawer and posterior drawer tests, which are performed with the knee in 90 degrees of flexion. These tests were described earlier in this chapter (see pp. 355–356, Figure 12.43) (http://www.youtube.com/watch?v=vEQw-G1Vr18).

Lachman Test

This test is used to elicit excessive anterior movement of the tibia that results from damage to the ACL. The test is performed with the patient in the supine position and the knee flexed to about 30 degrees. Use one hand to stabilize the thigh while trying to displace the tibia anteriorly. A positive test result implies damage to the ACL (Figure 12.69). As with all tests of stability, you must examine the opposite side for comparison (http://www.youtube.com/watch?v=vEQw-G1Vr18).

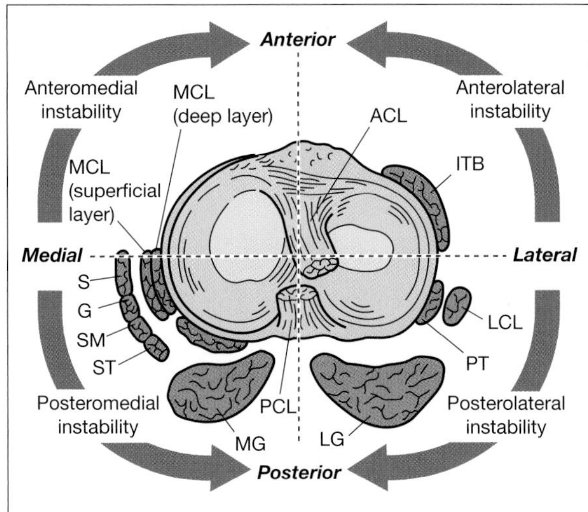

Figure 12.68 Knee instability. ACL, anterior cruciate ligament; PCL, posterior cruciate ligament; MCL, medial collateral ligament; LCL, lateral collateral ligament; G, gracilis; PT, popliteus tendon; ITB, iliotibial band; SM, semimembranosus; ST, semitendinosus; MC, medial head of gastrocnemius; LC, lateral head of gastrocnemius; S, sartorius. This figure was originally published in Magee DJ. *Orthopedic Physical Assessment*, 4th edn. Philadelphia: WB Saunders, 2002 Copyright Elsevier.

Anterior Medial and Lateral Instability Tests

In testing anteromedial and anterolateral instability, the goal is to reproduce the "giving way" phenomenon that the patient recognizes after injury to the ACL. The test may be performed beginning with the patient's knee extended or beginning with the patient's knee flexed. A sudden jerk, which is the giving way phenomenon, is noted by the patient and the examiner as the knee is moved from the extended to a flexed position, or from the flexed to an extended position.

Slocum Test

This test can be used to define damage in the anterior cruciate and medial collateral ligaments (Figures 12.70a and 12.70b) (http://www.youtube.com/watch?v=Z8zre1EfShA).

The patient is in the supine position and the hip is flexed to 45 degrees. The knee is flexed to 80–90 degrees. Place the leg and foot in 15 degrees of lateral rotation and sit on the foot to stabilize it in this position. Take the lower leg with both of your hands and attempt to pull the tibia anteriorly. The test result will be positive when anterior movement occurs primarily on the medial side of the knee. This test can also be performed with the leg and foot in 30 degrees of medial rotation. When excessive movement of the lateral part of the tibia is noted, the test result is positive and indicates ACL and posterolateral capsular damage.

Additional tests for anteromedial and anterolateral instability include the Losee test, the crossover test, the Noyes test, and the Nakajima test.

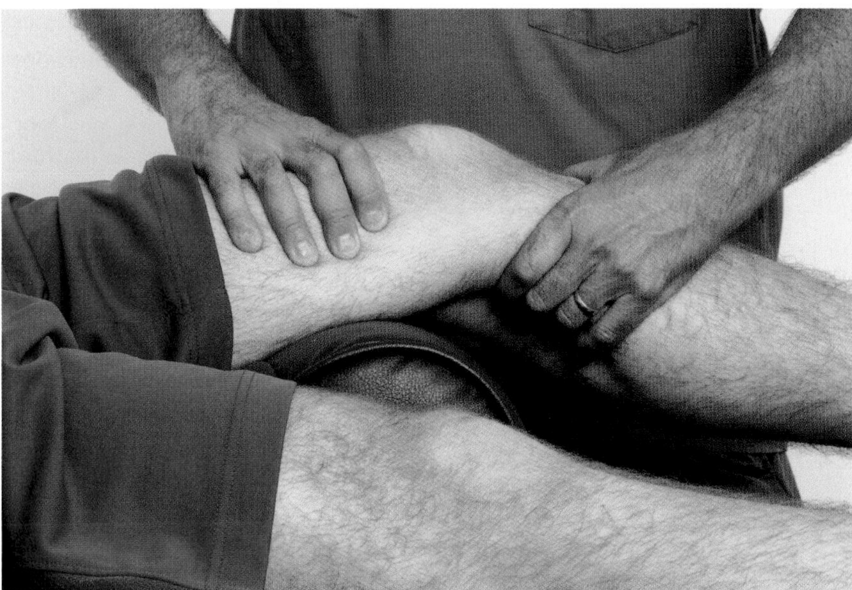

Figure 12.69 The position of the examiner and patient for the Lachman test. It is very important that the patient be relaxed for this test.

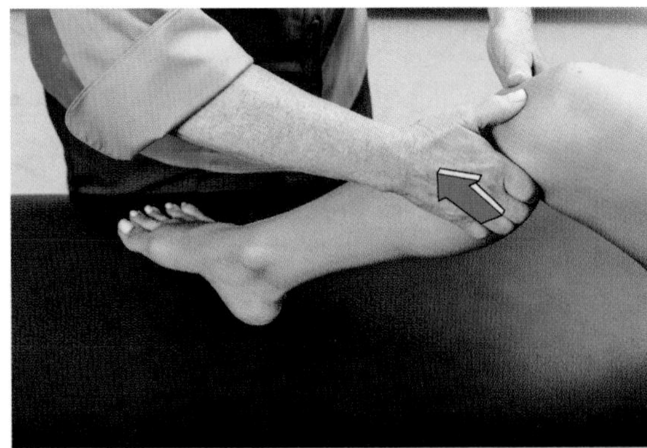
(a)

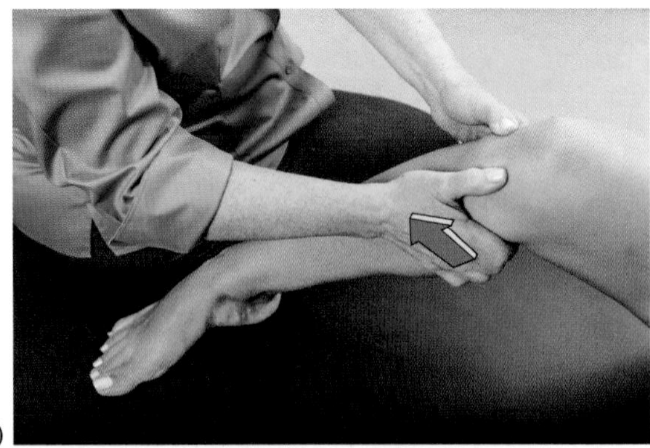
(b)

Figure 12.70 (a) The Slocum test. Note that the leg is in lateral rotation. The test result is positive when anterior drawer fails to tighten in 15 degrees of lateral rotation of the leg. This occurs with damage to the anterior cruciate and medial collateral ligaments. (b) This is the same test performed with the foot in medial rotation. The test result is positive when anterior drawer does not decrease with medial rotation. This results from damage to the anterior cruciate ligament and posterolateral secondary restraints.

Pivot Shift Test (Macintosh)

The patient is placed in the supine position with the hip extended. Take the affected foot in one hand and medially rotate the tibia on the femur. The other hand is placed behind the patient's knee so that a valgus stress and flexion maneuver can be performed simultaneously. At about 25–30 degrees of flexion, there is a sudden jerk and you will feel and see the lateral femoral condyle jump anteriorly on the lateral tibial plateau. This is a positive test result and signifies a rupture of the ACL. As the knee is flexed further, the tibia suddenly reduces (Figure 12.71) (http://www.youtube.com/watch?v=vEQw-G1Vr18).

Posterior Stability Tests

"Reverse" Lachman Test

This test is used to elicit excessive posterior movement of the tibia that results from damage to the posterior cruciate ligament. The test is performed with the patient in the prone position with the knee flexed to about 60 degrees. Use one hand to stabilize the thigh while trying to displace the tibia posteriorly with the other hand (Figure 12.72) (http://www.youtube.com/watch?v=Z8zre1EfShA).

Hughston (Jerk) Test

This test is performed similarly to the pivot shift test. However, the starting position is with the patient's knee flexed to 90 degrees. Again, take one hand and rotate the tibia medially while using the other hand behind the knee to apply a valgus and extension stress. Here, the lateral femoral condyle starts out in a forward subluxed position relative to the tibia. As the knee is extended and at about 20 degrees, a subluxation of the tibia occurs. This subluxation reduces in full extension. This is a positive test result and indicates a rupture of the ACL (Figure 12.73) (http://www.youtube.com/watch?v=xCndb5pLY_Y).

Posterior Medial and Lateral Stability

Hughston Posteromedial and Posterolateral Drawer Test

This test is performed similarly to the posterior drawer test. This test can be used to define damage in the posterior cruciate and medial and lateral collateral ligaments (Figure 12.74) (http://www.youtube.com/watch?v=tWajO9K8Os0).

The patient is in the supine position and the hip is flexed to 45 degrees. The knee is flexed to 80–90 degrees. Place the leg and foot in 15 degrees of lateral rotation and sit on the foot to stabilize it in this position. Take the lower leg with both of your hands and attempt to push the tibia posteriorly. When excessive movement of the lateral part of the tibia is noted, the test result is positive and indicates posterior cruciate ligament, lateral collateral ligament, and posterolateral capsular damage.

This test can also be performed with the leg and foot in 30 degrees of medial rotation. When excessive movement of the medial part of the tibia is noted, the test result is positive and indicates posterior cruciate ligament, medial collateral ligament, and posteromedial capsular damage.

Medial and Lateral Stability Tests

In testing for the stability of the medial and lateral collateral ligaments, you should first examine the patient

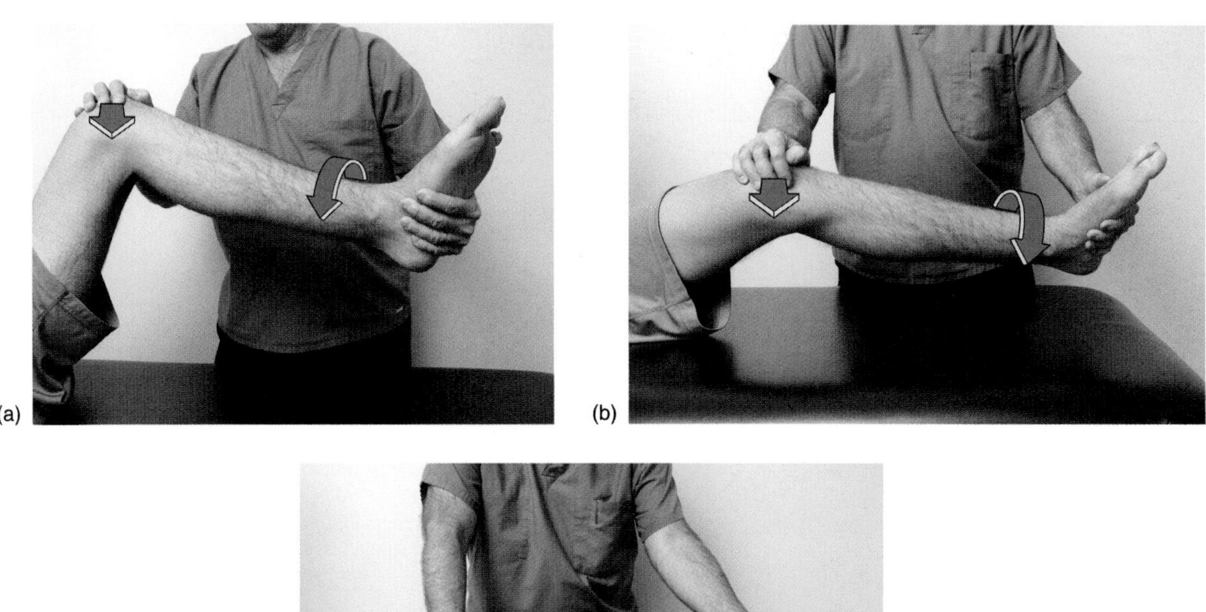

Figure 12.71 Position for the lateral pivot shift test. (a) Note that the patient's knee is fully extended. Internally rotate the leg and apply a valgus stress. (b) At 20 degrees, a subluxation occurs, and reduces in full extension.

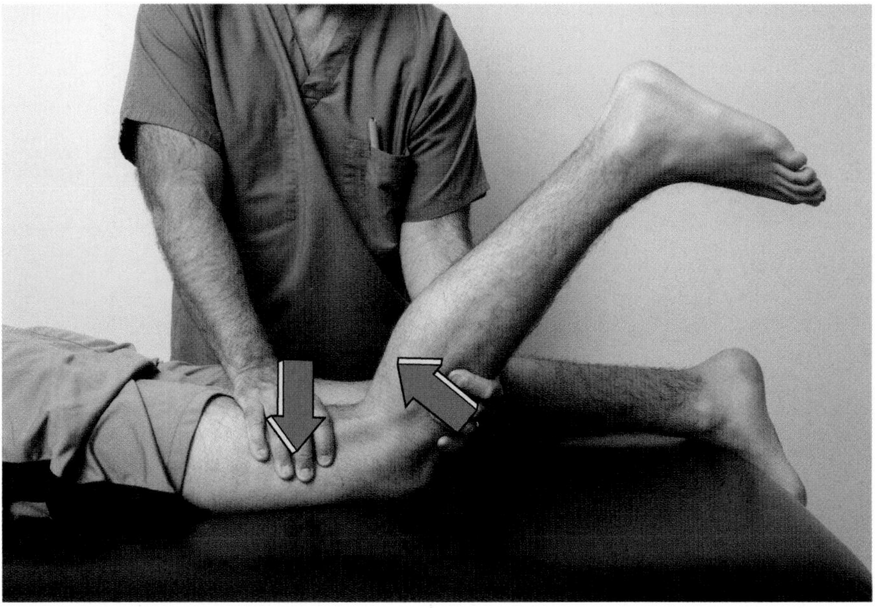

Figure 12.72 The position for performing the reverse Lachman test. The test result is positive when the tibia is able to be subluxed posteriorly on the femur. The patient should be fully relaxed while performing this test.

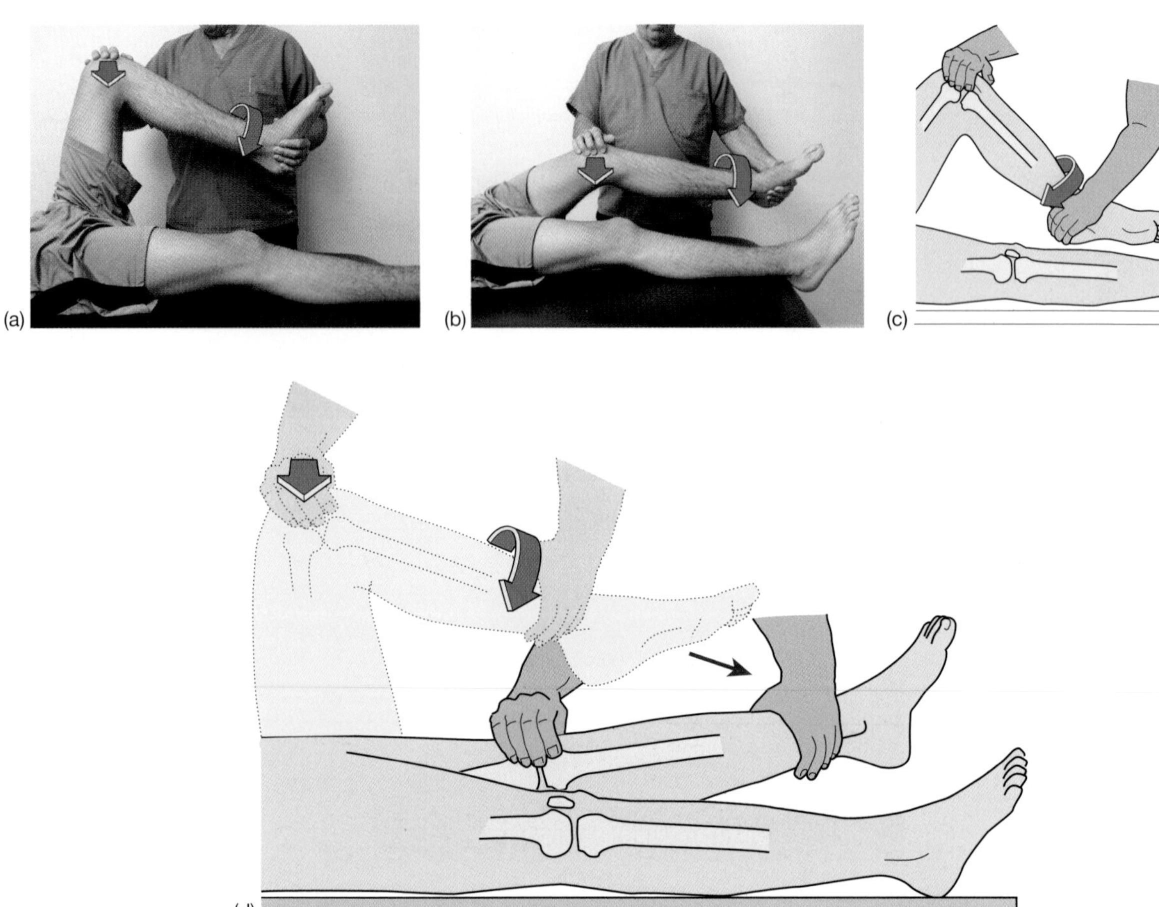

Figure 12.73 The Hughston jerk test. (a) Note the initial starting position with the knee in 90 degrees of flexion and the leg internally rotated as a valgus stress is applied. (b) and (c) Note that the patient's knee is extended while maintaining internal rotation of the leg and valgus stress at the knee. (d) At 20 degrees, a subluxation of the tibia occurs, and reduces in full extension.

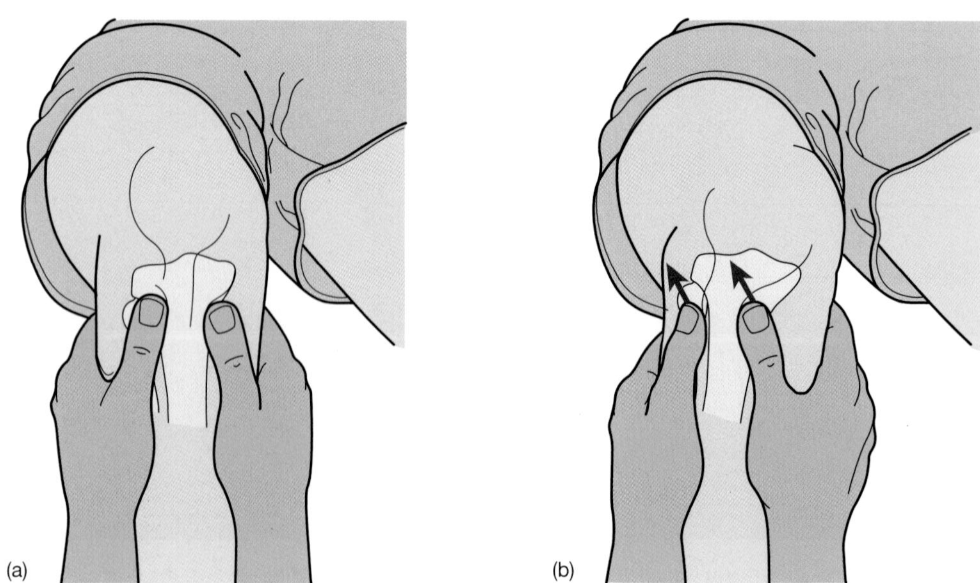

Figure 12.74 Hughston posterolateral drawer test. (a) Starting position, (b) the test is positive as shown.

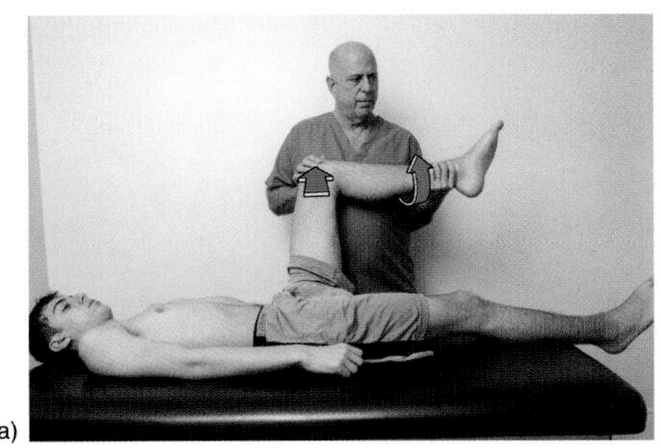

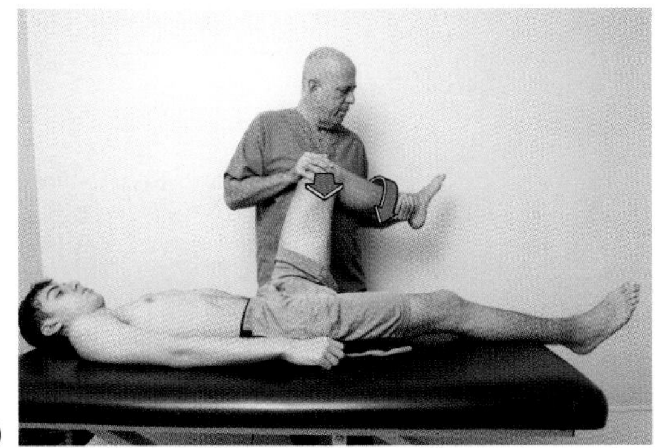

Figure 12.75 (a) McMurray's test is performed with the leg externally rotated, and applying a varus stress to test the medial meniscus. (b) McMurray's test is performed with the leg internally rotated, and applying a valgus stress to test for the lateral meniscus.

for medial and lateral instability of the tibia. This can be accomplished with the varus (adduction) and valgus (abduction) stress tests. These tests were described earlier in this chapter.

Tests for Meniscal Damage

The goal of these tests is to assess the presence of meniscal injury. The tests are performed by applying a stress to the knee that reproduces pain or a click as the torn meniscus is impinged by the tibia and femur.

McMurray's Test

This test can be performed to examine the lateral and medial menisci. The patient is placed in a supine position with the test knee completely flexed, so that the heel approaches the buttock. Put your hand on the knee so that the thumb and index fingers are along the joint line of the knee. Take the other hand and rotate the tibia externally (laterally), while applying a varus stress. A painful click on rotation is significant for damage to the lateral meniscus (Figure 12.75a).

If the tibia is rotated internally (medially) while applying a valgus stress, the medial meniscus can be examined (Figure 12.75b).

The test can be performed in a position of less than full flexion. With more extension, the further anterior portions of the meniscus can be examined. The result of McMurray's test can also be positive in the presence of osteochondritis dissecans of the medial femoral condyle (http://www.youtube.com/watch?v=fkt1TOn1UfI).

Bounce Home Test

The purpose of this test is to examine for a blockage to extension that may result from a torn meniscus. The patient is placed in a supine position. Take the heel of the patient's foot and cup it in your hand and then flex the patient's knee fully. Allow the patient's knee to extend passively. If the patient's leg does not extend fully, or if the end feel is rubbery, there is a blockage to extension and the test result is positive (Figure 12.76) (http://www.youtube.com/watch?v=52reQsXQAZk).

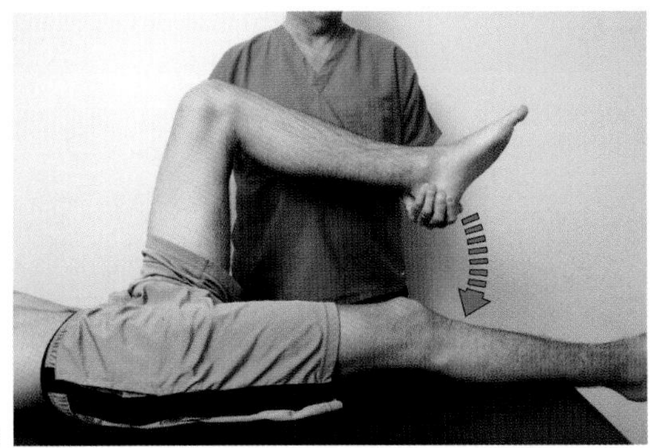

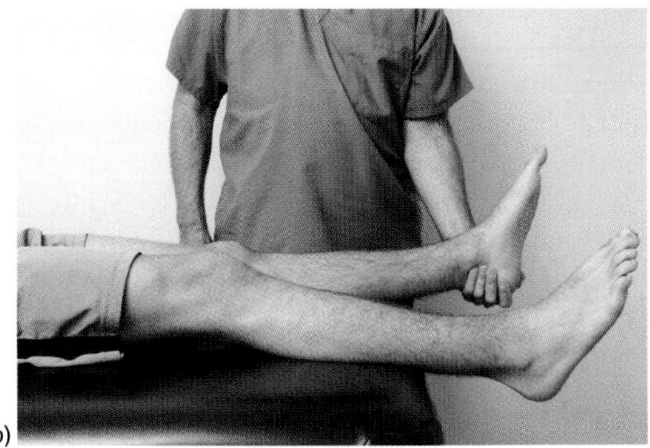

Figure 12.76 The bounce home test looks for damage to the torn menisci. The patient's foot is cupped in the hand and the knee is allowed to lower into extension. If the knee does not reach full extension, or if spongy end feel is noted, the test result is positive. (a) Mid position. (b) End position.

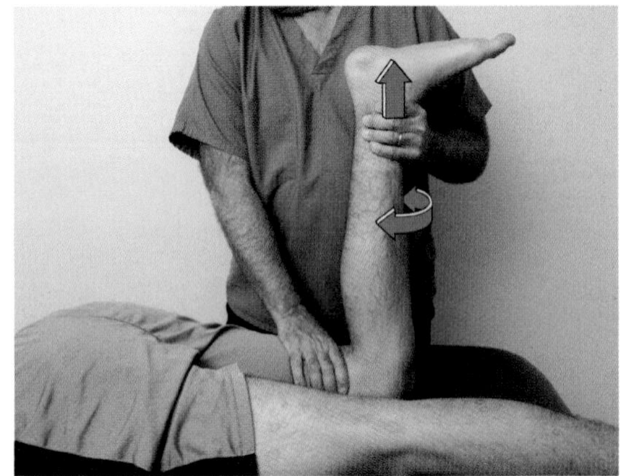
(a)

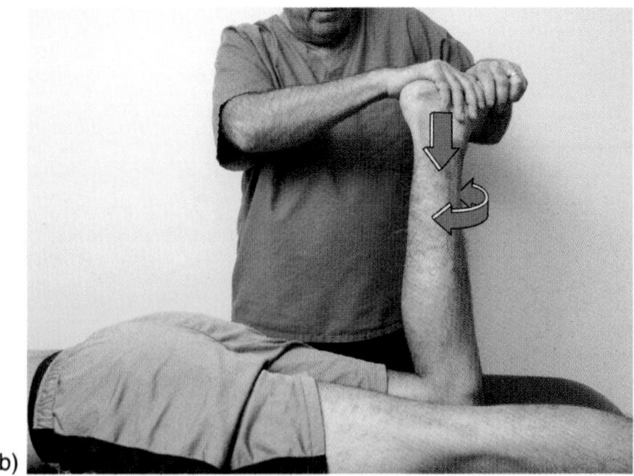
(b)

Figure 12.77 The grinding/distraction test of Apley. The tibia is rotated first with a distraction force on the leg and then with a compression force. Distraction with rotation tests the collateral ligaments (a), while compression with rotation tests the menisci (b).

Apley (Grinding, Distraction) Test

This test is performed to assess whether medial or lateral joint line pain is due to meniscus or collateral ligament damage. The test is performed with the patient in the prone position. The knee is flexed to 90 degrees, and the patient's thigh is stabilized by the weight of your knee. Hold the patient's ankle with your hand and rotate the tibia internally and externally while applying a downward force on the foot. Pain during compression with rotation is significant for meniscal damage. Perform the same rotation medially and laterally, but this time pulling upward on the foot and ankle so as to distract the tibia from the femur. If rotation with distraction is painful, the patient is more likely to have a ligamentous injury (Figures 12.77a and 12.77b) (http://www.youtube.com/watch?v=w57I1cYXlCA).

Patellofemoral Joint Tests

Apprehension (Fairbanks) Test

This test is used to diagnose prior dislocation of the patella. The patient is placed in a supine position with the quadriceps muscles as relaxed as possible. The knee is flexed to approximately 30 degrees while you carefully and gently push the patella laterally. The test result is positive if the patient feels like the patella is going to dislocate and abruptly contract the quadriceps (Figure 12.78) (http://www.youtube.com/watch?v=O701WBDDmzY).

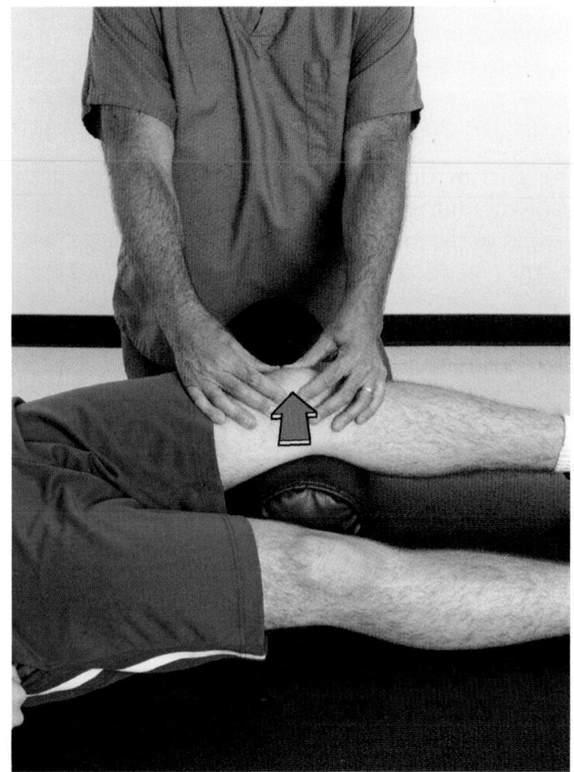

Figure 12.78 The apprehension test for patellar subluxation and dislocation.

Clarke's Sign (Patella Grind Test)

This test is used to diagnose patellofemoral dysfunction. The patient is in supine with the knee in extension. Using your hand as shown in Figure 12.79, hold the superior border of the patella. Ask the patient to contract their quadriceps muscle while you continue to push downwards. If the patient is able to complete the muscle contraction without pain, the test is considered to be negative (Figure 12.79) (http://www.youtube.com/watch?v=0VfKRLFz4xo).

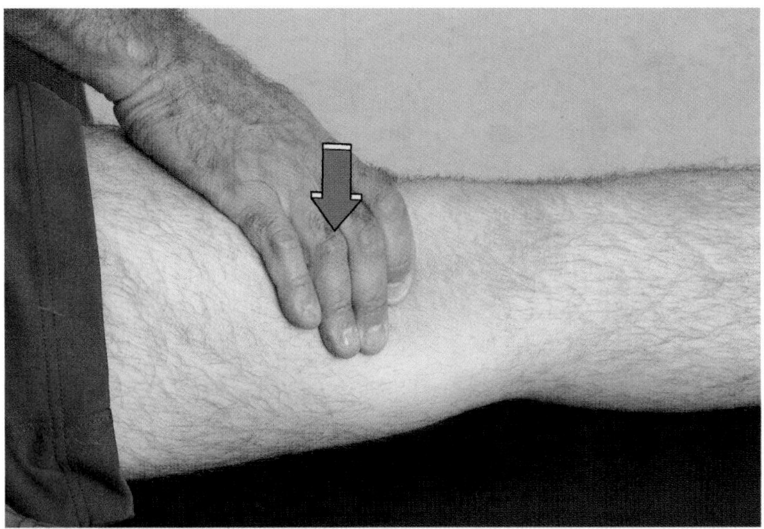

Figure 12.79 Clarke's sign. Apply downward pressure on the proximal patella as the patient actively contracts the quadriceps.

Patellofemoral Arthritis (Waldron) Test

This test is used to detect the presence of patellofemoral arthritis. The patient is asked to perform several deep knee bends slowly. Place your hand over the patella so that you can palpate the patella as the patient bends and straightens. Tell the patient to inform you if there is pain during the bending or straightening. The presence of crepitus during a complaint of pain is positive for patellofemoral joint disease.

Test for Plica

Medial and lateral plicae are synovial thickenings that connect from the femur to the patella. In some individuals, these synovial thickenings are overdeveloped and may be pinched in the patellofemoral joint or may be painful. The plicae can be examined by having the patient lie in the supine position with the thigh relaxed. Test for the medial plica by pushing the patella medially with one hand. Then attempt to pluck the plica like a guitar string on the medial aspect of the patella. Check for lateral patellar plica by pushing the patella laterally with one hand and attempting to pluck the plica on the lateral aspect of the patella.

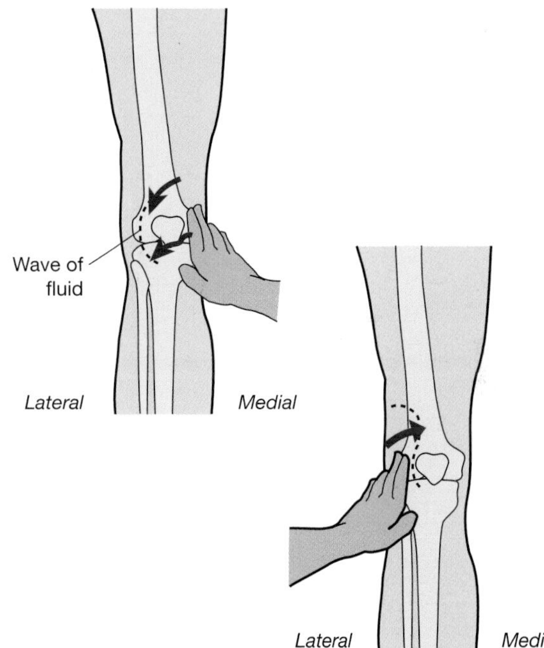

Figure 12.80 The wipe test for swelling in the knee. Attempt to move the fluid from medial to lateral first. Then attempt to wipe the fluid from lateral to medial over the patella. If a bulge of fluid is noted inferior and medial to the patella, the test result is positive for a small joint effusion.

Tests for Joint Effusion

Wipe Test

This test is sensitive to detecting small amounts of joint fluid. The patient lies in the supine position with the knee extended, if possible. Fluid is first massaged across the suprapatellar pouch from medial to lateral. Next, try to move the fluid from lateral to medial, using a wiping action over the patella. If you see a bulge of fluid inferomedially to the patella, a joint effusion is present (Figure 12.80) (http://www.youtube.com/watch?v=Uhw7_zRKOwE).

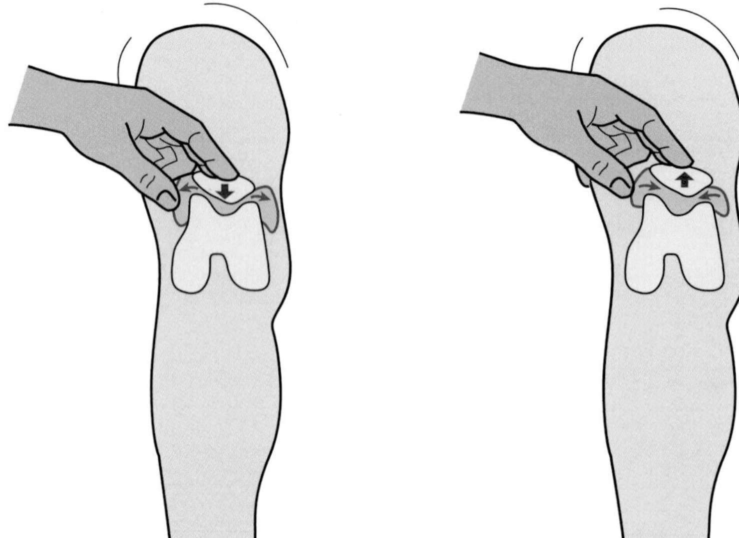

Figure 12.81 Test for large knee effusion showing a ballotable patella with fluid exiting on either side of the patella with downward compression.

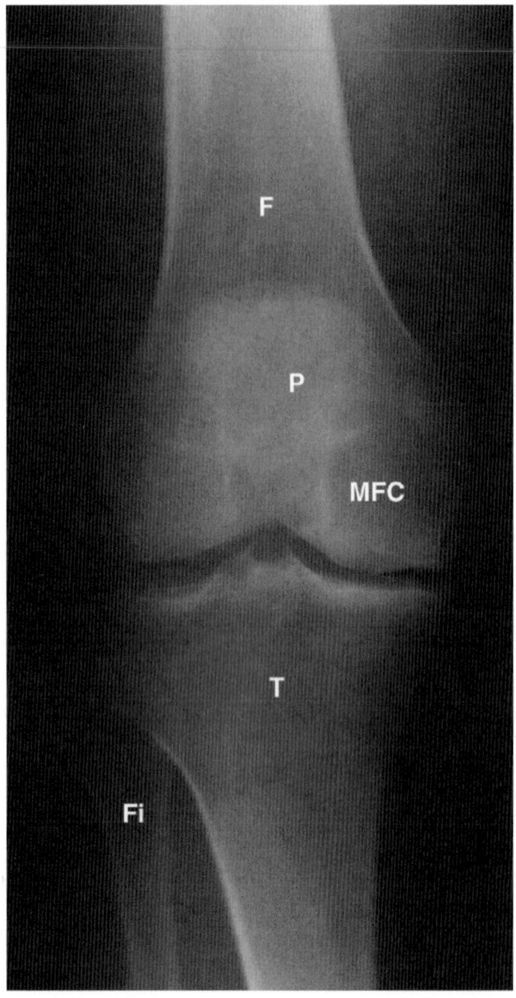

Figure 12.82 Anteroposterior view of the knee.

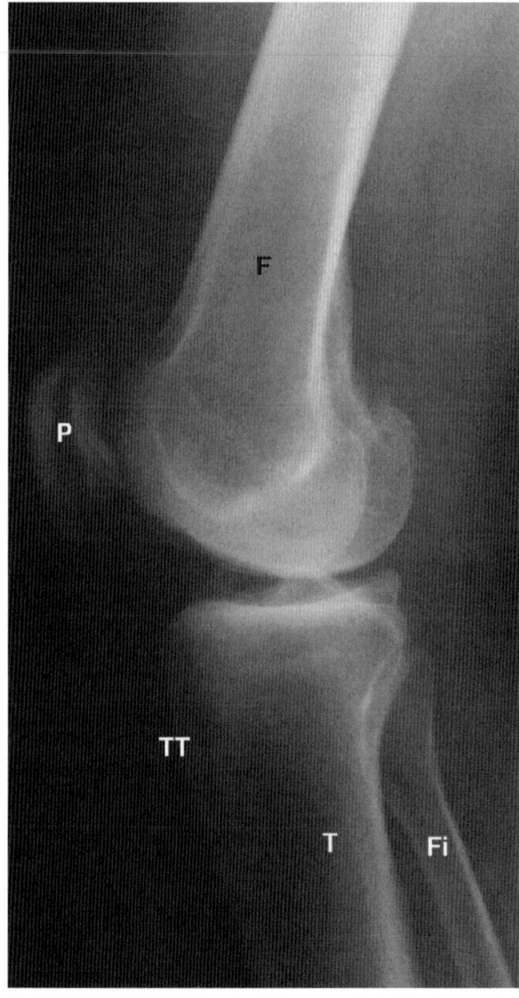

Figure 12.83 Lateral view of the knee.

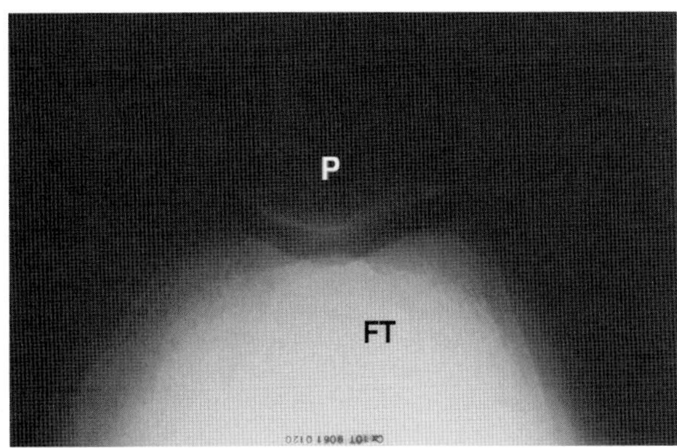

Figure 12.84 "Skyline" view of the patella.

Ballotable Patella

If a large effusion is suspected, you can test for it by having the patient lie in the supine position with the knee extended as much as possible. Push down on the patella. The fluid will flow to either side and then return underneath the patella when the pressure on the patella is released, causing the patella to rebound upward (Figure 12.81) (http://www.youtube.com/watch?v=ULBAyfwkaE).

Radiological Views

Radiological views are shown in Figures 12.82, 12.83, 12.84, 12.85, and 12.86.

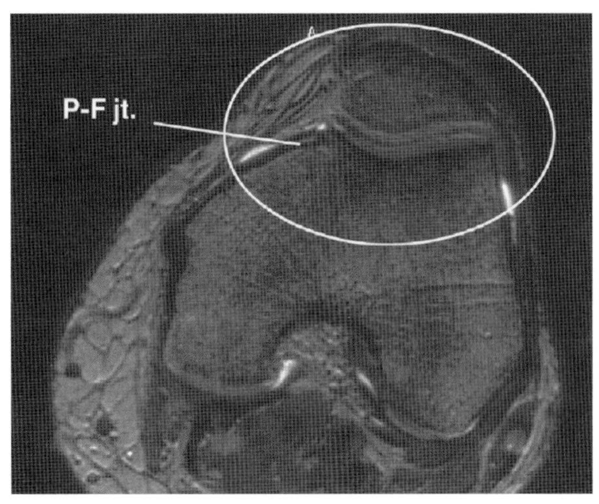

Figure 12.85 MRI of the patellofemoral joint.

F = Femur
T = Tibia
P = Patella
P-F jt. = Patellofemoral joint
Fi = Fibula
MFC = Medial femoral condyle
TT = Tibial tubercle
FT = Femoral trochlear groove
A = Anterior cruciate ligament
B = Posterior cruciate ligament

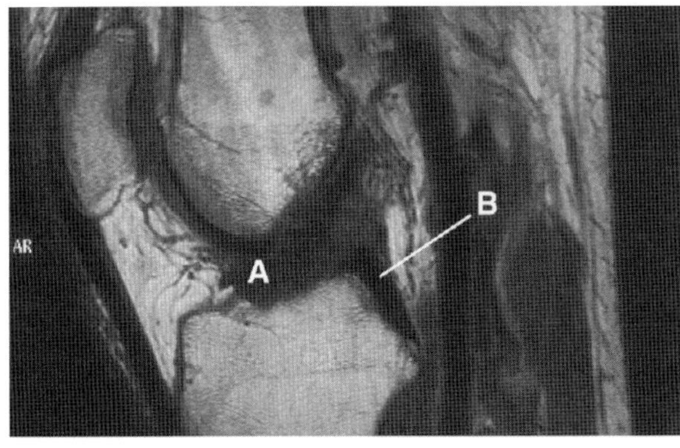

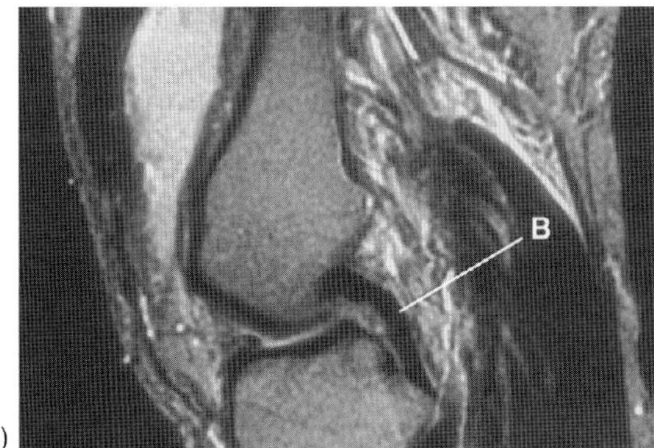

Figure 12.86 Sagittal view of the knee.

SAMPLE EXAMINATION

History: 25-year-old snow skier presents with painful swelling and decreased range of motion of the left knee and limited weight-bearing tolerance, 2 days after a fall. He is an intermediate skier who, while attempting to turn to the right, "caught an edge." His ski tips crossed and he fell forward over the skis. He perceived acute pain in the left knee. He had difficulty trying to stand up. He was uncertain as to whether he heard or felt a "pop." He was able to complete the run down the hill, although slowly and with some difficulty. He had swelling of the knee overnight. He had no prior history of injury to the extremity.

Physical Examination: Moderate swelling and effusion of the left knee. Limited range of motion of 20–70 degrees of flexion. Muscle testing was inconclusive secondary to pain. There was pain at the posterolateral knee. He had inconclusive anterior drawer, Lachman test, Slocum test and pivot shift signs due to pain and limited range of motion of the left knee. Negative sag sign, posterior drawer test, reverse Lachman test, Hughston's test, varus and valgus stress, Fairbanks and Clarke sign, McMurray test. Neurovascular examination was normal.

Presumptive Diagnosis: Acute ACL sprain.

Physical Examination Clues: (1) History clearly describes the mechanism of injury: indicating potential injury was sustained by the ACL, because the ACL in the static stabilizer (ligament) of the knee which resists internal rotation. (2) Posterolateral knee pain, indicating that there was a combined extension, internal rotational stress applied to the knee to cause pain in this area of the joint. This further raises suspicion of an ACL injury because of the ACL's function in a static stabilizer of the knee against excessive internal rotational movement. When the ligament fails under excessive loading, this stress is then translated further to the posterolateral aspect of the knee joint. (3) Delayed onset of swelling and effusion classic for an acute ACL sprain; indicating an accumulating hemarthrosis which can be exquisitely painful and restrictive to movement. (4) The absence of special testing for the medial collateral ligament, lateral collateral ligament, posterior cruciate ligament, meniscus, and patella and the absence of medial joint line or medial peripatellar discomfort, indicating no apparent or significant injury to the medial collateral ligament, medial meniscus, patella, or patellar retinaculum.

PARADIGM OF A KNEE LIGAMENT INJURY

Medial Collateral Ligament Insufficiency

A young athlete presents with a complaint of "knee instability" and "giving way" when pivoting or changing direction. This symptom is followed, not preceded, by medial knee pain and swelling. The patient gives a history of prior injury to the knee. The traumatic event described by the patient implies the mechanism of injury to have been one of excessive valgus stress. At the time of the original injury the patient recalls feeling a "tearing" sensation emanating from the medial knee joint. Pain was localized to the medial aspect of the knee and proximal tibia. Swelling, although not evident at the time of injury, was apparent and significant over the next 12 hours. The patient's symptoms seem to resolve completely with 6 weeks of rest and protection of the knee. However, on returning to sports and vigorous activities, the patient found the knee to be somewhat unstable and painful.

His symptoms became more frequent, even to occur with daily activities. There have been no episodes of "locking" or limitation in range of knee motion. On physical examination, the patient had no limp and a full range of knee motion. Patellofemoral and tibiofemoral alignment were unremarkable. There was pain on palpation of the medial collateral ligament. Valgus stress on the knee revealed a discernable gap and was mildly painful. Minimal soft-tissue swelling was present. There was no increased anterior excursion of the tibia on the femur during an anterior drawer test. There was a negative pivot shift sign. Meniscal signs were negative; and x-rays were read as normal.

This is a paradigm of ligament injury because of:

A history of injury
A characteristic mechanism of injury
Instability not precipitated by pain
Normal bony alignment
Unremarkable x-rays

CHAPTER 13

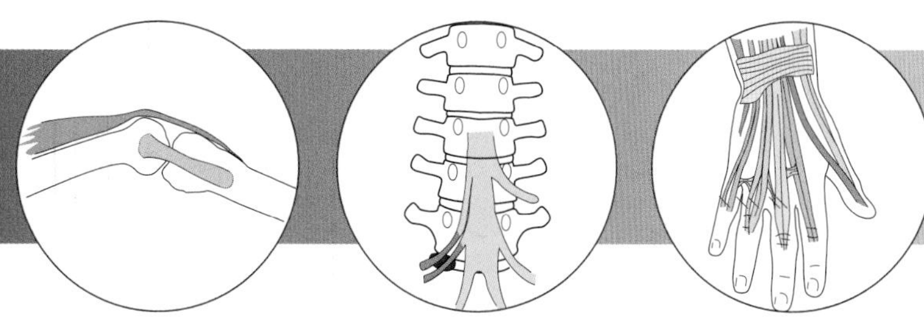

The Ankle and Foot

FURTHER INFORMATION

Please refer to Chapter 2 for an overview of the sequence of a physical examination. For purposes of length and to avoid having to repeat anatomy more than once, the palpation section appears directly after the section on subjective examination and before any section on testing, rather than at the end of each chapter. The order in which the examination is performed should be based on your experience and personal preference as well as the presentation of the patient.

Functional Anatomy

The Ankle

The ankle is a synovial articulation composed of three bones: the tibia, the fibula, and the talus. Although intimately interrelated with the foot, the ankle and foot have separate and distinct functions. The ankle is the simpler of the two structures. It is an extraordinarily stable linkage between the body and its base of support, the foot. Generally, the ankle lies lateral to the body's center of gravity. Therefore, the ankle joint is subjected to varus as well as compressive loading (Figure 13.1). The structure of the ankle is that of a bony mortise. It is bounded medially by the malleolar process at the distal end of the tibia, superiorly by the flat surface of the distal end of the tibia (the tibial plafond), and laterally by the malleolar process of the distal end of the fibula. The smaller fibular malleolus extends distally and posteriorly relative to the medial malleolus. As a result, the transmalleolar axis is externally rotated approximately 15 degrees to the coronal axis of the leg (Figure 13.2). Anteriorly, the mortise is deepened by the anterior tibiofibular ligament. Posteriorly, it is buttressed by the bony distal projection of the tibia (posterior malleolus) and the posterior tibiofibular ligament. Within this mortise is set the body of the talus. The talus articulates with the tibial plafond by its large superior convexity (the dome). It also presents an articular surface to each of the malleoli. The dome of the talus is wider anteriorly than it is posteriorly. As such, the talus becomes firmly wedged within the ankle mortise on dorsiflexion. This creates medial–lateral tension across the distal tibiofibular syndesmosis and ligament. The intact ankle mortise primarily allows the talus a single plane of motion (flexion–extension), with only a modest amount of anterior–posterior glide. Therefore, this increased stability of the ankle during dorsiflexion affords the means to isolate and assess medial–lateral ankle ligament integrity and subtalar inversion–eversion mobility.

The ankle is solely responsible for transmission of all weight-bearing forces between the body and the foot. The ankle is remarkably immune to the otherwise universally observed degenerative changes of

Musculoskeletal Examination, Fourth Edition. Jeffrey M. Gross, Joseph Fetto and Elaine Rosen.

Companion website: www.wiley.com/go/musculoskeletalexam

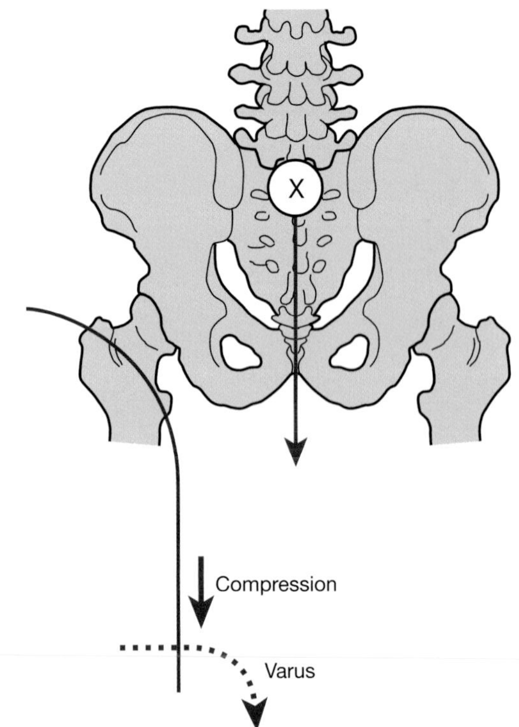

Figure 13.1 The ankle is lateral to the center of gravity and therefore is subject to a varus stress as well as compression.

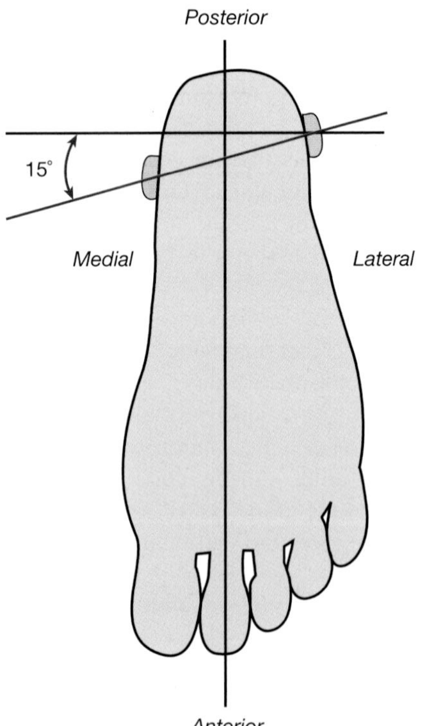

Figure 13.2 The transmalleolar axis is externally rotated 15 degrees.

senescence, seen in other large synovial articulations. This unusual and unique sparing of the ankle joint is probably a consequence of a combination of factors, including the ankle's requirement of limited degrees of freedom and its extreme degree of stability. However, to accommodate the severe stresses of daily activities and changes in ground contours, the ankle is complemented by a complex of accessory articulations that comprise the foot. The most significant of these is the subtalar (talocalcaneal) articulation.

The Foot

The primary functions of the foot are to provide a stable platform of support to attenuate impact loading of the extremity during locomotion, and to assist in the efficient forward propulsion of the body. To accomplish these tasks, the foot is made up of three sections. These sections—the hindfoot, the midfoot, and the forefoot—are in turn composed of multiple mobile and semirigid articulations that afford foot conformity to varying surface topographies. The bony elements of the foot are arranged to form a longitudinal and a transverse arch. These arches are spanned across the plantar aspect by soft-tissue tension bands that act as shock absorbers during impact (Figure 13.3a).

The foot has 26 bones distributed among the hindfoot, midfoot, and forefoot (Figure 13.3b). The hindfoot represents one-third of the total length of the foot. It contains the two largest bones of the foot, the calcaneus and the talus. The larger is the calcaneus (heel bone). The calcaneus lies beneath and supports the body of the second bone, the talus. The talus (ankle bone) is the only bony link between the leg and the foot. The tibia articulates with the talus in the middle of the hindfoot.

The midfoot contains the small, angular navicular, cuneiforms (medial, middle, and lateral), and cuboid bone. The midfoot makes up slightly more than one-sixth of the overall length of the foot. Little movement occurs within the midfoot articulations.

The forefoot represents the remaining one-half of the overall length of the foot. It is composed of miniature long bones, 5 metatarsals and 14 phalanges.

Structural integrity of the foot is dependent on the combination of articular geometry and soft-tissue support. All articulations of the foot are synovial. The soft-tissue support is provided by static (ligamentous) and dynamic (musculotendinous) stabilizers. The failure of either articular or soft-tissue structural integrity will result in ankle dysfunction, foot

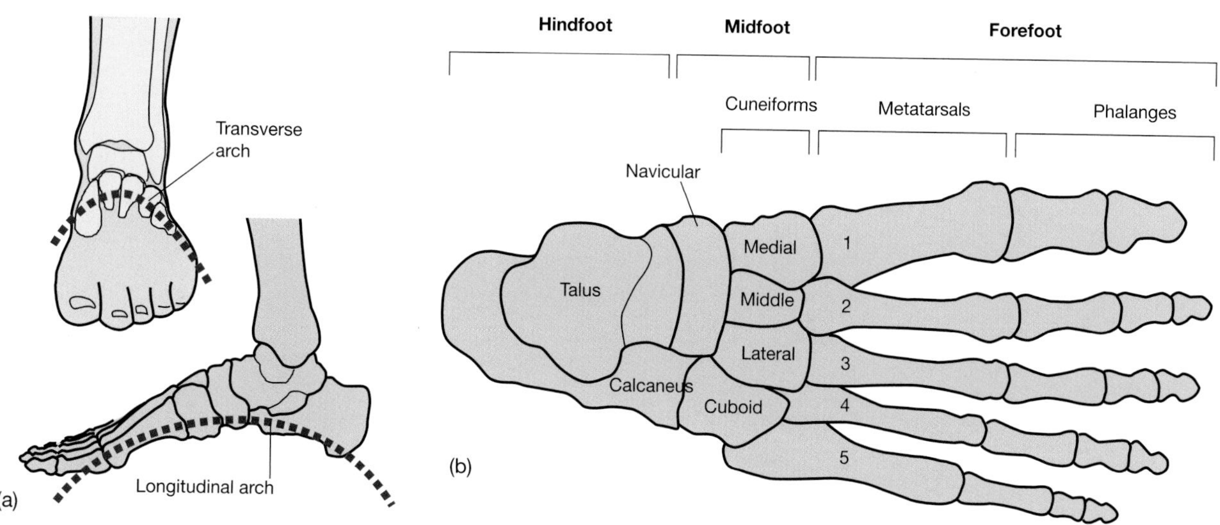

Figure 13.3 (a) Longitudinal and transverse arches are formed by the bones of the foot. The soft tissues that span these arches act to dampen the forces of impact during ambulation. (b) The 26 bones of the foot are divided into three sections.

dysfunction, reduced efficiency, arthritis, and bony failure (fatigue fractures).

The support of the talus is afforded posteriorly by the anterior calcaneal facet and distally by the navicular bone. There is a void of bony support at the plantar aspect between the calcaneus and navicular, beneath the talar head. Support of the talar head across this void is totally dependent on soft tissues that span this gap (Figure 13.4a). Statically, this support is provided by the fibrocartilaginous plantar calcaneonavicular (spring) ligament. Dynamically, the talocalcaneonavicular articulation is supported by the tibialis posterior tendon and its broad plantar insertion onto the plantar medial aspect of the midfoot. Because the head of the talus is only supported by soft tissue, in the presence of soft-tissue or ligamentous laxity and muscular weakness, the head of the talus can sag in a plantar direction. This will force the calcaneus and foot laterally, with medial rotation of the foot about its long axis. This rotation of the foot beneath the talus has been termed *pronation.* The primary locus of pronation is therefore at the subtalar joint. Rotation of the subtalar joint causes the talus to twist within the ankle mortise. There is little possibility for movement of the talus within the ankle mortise due to the rigid anatomy of that joint. Therefore, this torsional load is transmitted through the talus to the leg and lower extremity, with a resultant internal rotational torque on the leg and a supination torque on the midfoot (talonavicular, calcaneocuboid, and naviculocuneiform articulations) (Figure 13.4b).

Pronation serves two critical functions. First, it dampens impact loading of the medial arch of the foot during locomotion, which would otherwise exceed the tolerance of the medial arch. Second, pronation of the talus creates a relative internal rotational torque of the leg, external rotation valgus of the calcaneus, and abduction–supination of the midfoot. This configuration passively stretches the triceps surae (gastrocsoleus) at its attachment to the supramedial aspect of the calcaneus. It also stretches the tibialis posterior, flexor digitorum longus, and flexor hallucis longus and toe flexors as it begins to lift the heel from the foot in midstance. This passive stretching of these muscles serves to increase their mechanical efficiency.

The forefoot is composed of five digits. Each digit has a long bone (metatarsal) and two or more phalanges. These articulations of the forefoot are basically hinge joints. Their stability is primarily due to medial and lateral ligaments. Volarly, the interphalangeal joints are stabilized against excessive dorsiflexion by firm volar ligaments called *plates.*

The digits of the foot can be divided into three columns (Figure 13.4c). The medial digit is the largest. It is more than twice the dimension of any of the other digits. This reflects its greater importance in weight-bearing and push-off activity. The second ray, together with the first, forms the medial column of the forefoot. The third ray represents the "stable" or minimally mobile central column of the foot. The lateral two rays are progressively more capable of movement. They combine to form the lateral column of the forefoot, the fifth metatarsal being the most mobile of

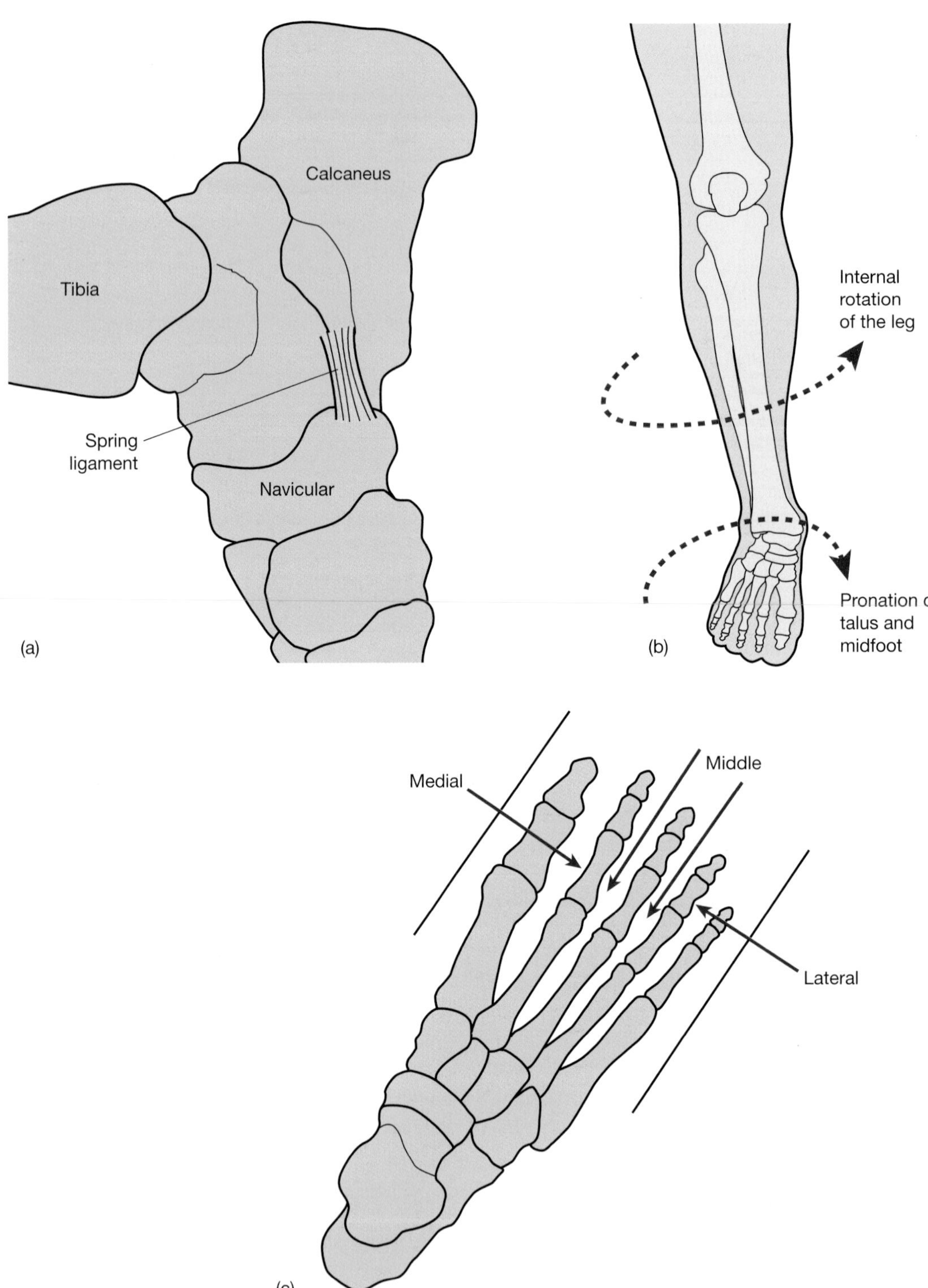

Figure 13.4 (a) A void exists between the navicular anteriorly and the calcaneus posteriorly. It is occupied by the spring ligament. (b) Pronation of the talus results in internal rotation of the leg and a supination torque at the midfoot. (c) The bones of the foot are aligned in three columns—medial (digits 1, 2), middle (digit 3), and lateral (digits 4, 5).

all the digits. Because of the insertion of the peroneus brevis tendon onto the base of the fifth metatarsal, it is the site of excessive traction load when the foot is supinated during an injury such as a typical ankle sprain. The resultant excessive traction of the peroneal tendon on the base of the fifth metatarsal leads to the commonly seen fifth metatarsal fracture and more complex Jones fracture of the metatarsal shaft.

Observation

The examination should begin in the waiting room before the patient is aware of the examiner's observation. Information regarding the degree of the patient's disability, level of functioning, posture, and gait can be observed. The clinician should pay careful attention to the patient's facial expressions with regard to the degree of discomfort the patient is experiencing. The information gathered in this short period can be very useful in creating a total picture of the patient's condition.

Note whether the patient is allowing the foot to rest in a weight-bearing position. Assess the patient's willingness and capability to use the foot. How does the patient get from sitting to standing? Is the patient able to ambulate? Observe the heel-strike and push-off phases of the gait pattern. Note any gait deviations and whether the patient is using or requires the use of an assistive device. Details of any gait deviations are described in Chapter 14.

The patient can be observed in both the weight-bearing and non-weight-bearing positions. Observe the patient's shoes. Notice the wear pattern. Ask the patient to remove his or her shoes and observe the bony and soft-tissue contour and the bony alignment of the foot. Common bony deformities that you might see include: pes cavus, pes planus, Morton's foot, splaying of the forefoot, mallet toe, hammer toes, claw toes, hallux valgus, hallux rigidus, tibial torsion, and bony bumps (i.e., pump bump). Soft-tissue problems include: calluses, corns, plantar warts, scars, sinuses, and edema. You should also observe the patient's toenails. Look for muscular atrophy, especially in the gastrocnemius. Observe for signs of vascular insufficiency including shiny skin, decreased hair growth, decreased temperature, and thickening of the toenails. Pay attention to the integrity of the medial arch during weight-bearing compared to non-weight-bearing. Check the alignment of the calcaneus and notice if there is increased inversion or eversion during weight-bearing.

Subjective Examination

The ankle and foot are subjected to large forces during the stance phase of the gait cycle. Although the foot is very agile and adapts well to changing terrain, it is vulnerable to many injuries. In addition, the foot often presents with static deformities because of the constant weight-bearing stresses placed on it. The foot can also be involved in systemic diseases such as diabetes and rheumatoid arthritis. Does the patient present with a previous history of any systemic diseases?

You want to determine the patient's functional limitations. Has he or she noticed a gradual change in the shape or structure of the foot? Has the patient noticed generalized or localized swelling? Did the swelling come on suddenly or over a long period? Has the patient been participating regularly in a vigorous activity like running? What are the patient's usual activities? What is the patient's occupation? Are abnormal stresses placed on the feet because of his or her job? Is the patient able to stand on toes or heels without difficulty? Is the patient stiff when he or she arises in the morning or after sitting? Is the patient able to ascend and descend steps? Can he or she adapt to ambulating on various terrains? Does one particular terrain offer too much of a challenge?

Does any portion of the foot feel numb or have altered sensation? Paresthesias in the ankle and foot may be secondary to radiculopathy from L4, L5, S1, or S2. Cramping in the calf or foot after walking may be secondary to claudication.

If the patient reports a history of trauma, it is important to note the mechanism of injury. The direction of the force, the activity in which the patient was participating in at the time of the injury, and the type of shoes he or she was wearing contribute to your understanding of the resulting problem. The degree of pain, swelling, and disability noted at the time of the trauma and during the first 24 hours should be noted. Does the patient have a previous history of the same or similar injury?

It is also important to note the type of shoes the patient is using and whether he or she changes to appropriate shoes for different activities. Does the patient use an orthotic in the shoe that is well constructed and properly fit to the foot? The patient's disorders may be related to age, gender, ethnic background, body type, static and dynamic posture, occupation, leisure activities, hobbies, and general activity level. (Please refer to Box 2.1, see p. 15 for typical questions for the subjective examination.)

Gentle Palpation

Begin the palpatory examination with the patient in the supine position. You should examine the ankle and foot to see if it is swollen, either locally or generally. Note any areas of bruising, muscle girth asymmetry, abnormal bony contours, incisional areas, or open wounds. Generalized edema may be secondary to metabolic or vascular disorders. Observe the skin for dystrophic changes and consider the presence of reflex sympathetic dystrophy if there are any positive findings.

You should not have to use deep pressure to determine areas of tenderness or malalignment. It is important to use firm but gentle pressure, which will enhance your palpatory skills. By having a sound basis of cross-sectional anatomy, you will not need to physically penetrate through several layers of tissue to have a good sense of the underlying structures. Remember that if you increase the patient's pain at this point in the examination, the patient will be very reluctant to allow you to continue, or may become more limited in his or her ability to move.

Palpation is most easily performed with the patient in a relaxed position. Although palpation may be performed with the patient standing, non-weight-bearing positions are preferred. The sitting position with the patient's leg hanging over the edge of the examining table allows for optimal palpation of most of the structures in the ankle joint and foot, and provides easy access to all aspects. The examiner should sit on a rolling stool and face the patient.

Medial Aspect

Bony Structures

Medial Malleolus

Place your fingers along the anterior shaft of the tibia and follow it inferiorly. You will feel the prominence of the medial malleolus at the distal medial aspect of the tibia. The medial malleolus is larger and normally anterior compared to the lateral malleolus. It articulates with the medial aspect of the talus and lends medial stability to the ankle joint (Figure 13.5). See p. 372, Figure 13.4 for more information.

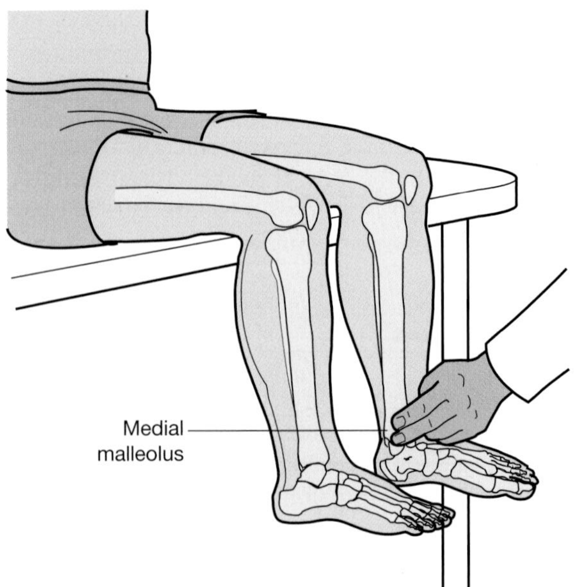

Figure 13.5 Palpation of the medial malleolus.

Sustentaculum Tali

Allow your fingers to move just distal to the medial malleolus and you will find the small protrusion of the sustentaculum tali. It is easier to locate this if the foot is everted. Although the sustentaculum tali is a very small structure, it provides inferior support for the talus. The spring ligament attaches here (Figure 13.6).

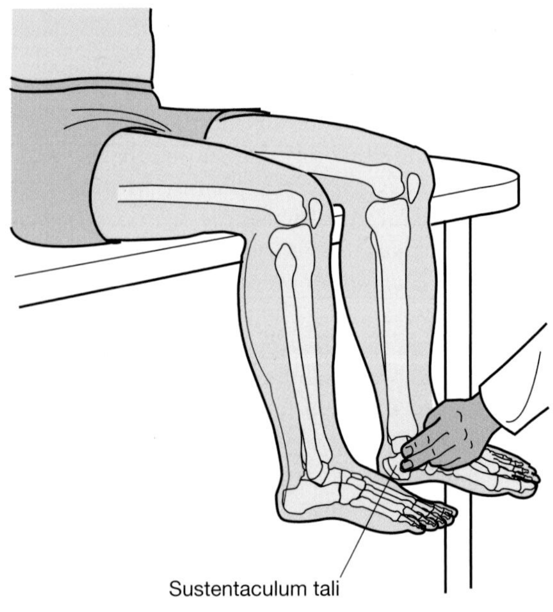

Figure 13.6 Palpation of the sustentaculum tali.

Navicular Tubercle

If you continue distally along the medial border of the foot, the next large protuberance is the navicular tubercle (Figure 13.7). The tibionavicular portion of the deltoid ligament attaches here. A very prominent

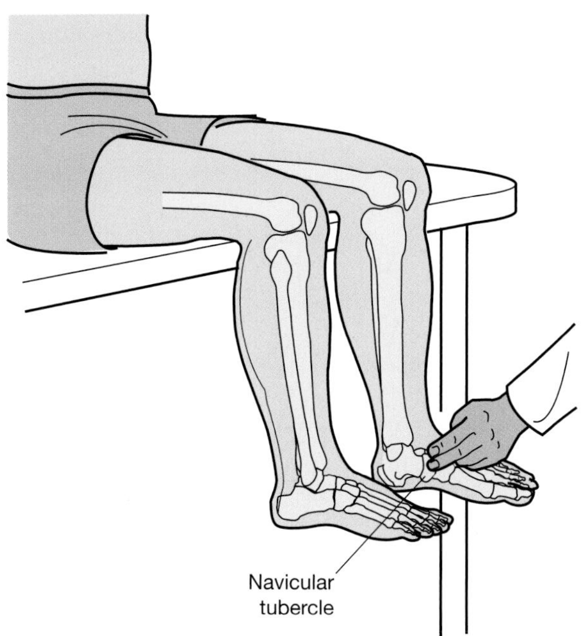

Figure 13.7 Palpation of the navicular tubercle.

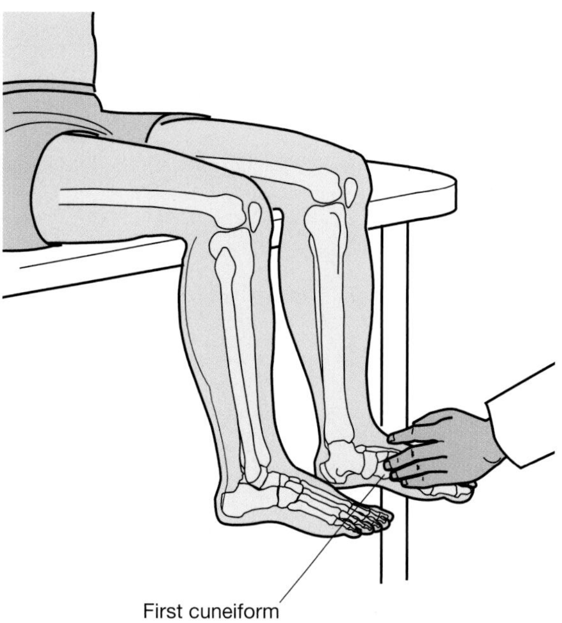

Figure 13.8 Palpation of the cuneiform bones.

navicular tubercle may become callused and irritated by the medial aspect of the shoe.

Cuneiform Bones

Allow your finger to continue distally from the navicular tubercle. In the space between the navicular and the base of the first metacarpal lies the first cuneiform bone. There are three cuneiform bones and they articulate with the first three metatarsals. They are extremely difficult to distinguish individually (Figure 13.8).

First Metatarsal and Metatarsophalangeal Joint

The base of the first metatarsal flares out and is palpable at the joint line with the first cuneiform. Continue to palpate the shaft of the bone until you feel the articulation with the proximal phalanx of the great toe (Figure 13.9). The first metatarsophalangeal joint is commonly involved in hallux valgus (Figure 13.10) and can be very painful and disfiguring. This joint is also a common site of acute gout.

Soft-Tissue Structures

Deltoid Ligament (Medial Collateral Ligament)

The deltoid ligament is a strong, triangular band that runs from the medial malleolus to the navicular tubercle, the sustentaculum tali, and the talus. This ligament is stronger and larger than the lateral ligaments but not as distinct to palpation. Place your fingers inferior to the medial malleolus and evert the foot. You will feel the tightness of the deltoid ligament under your fingers (Figure 13.11). Injury with

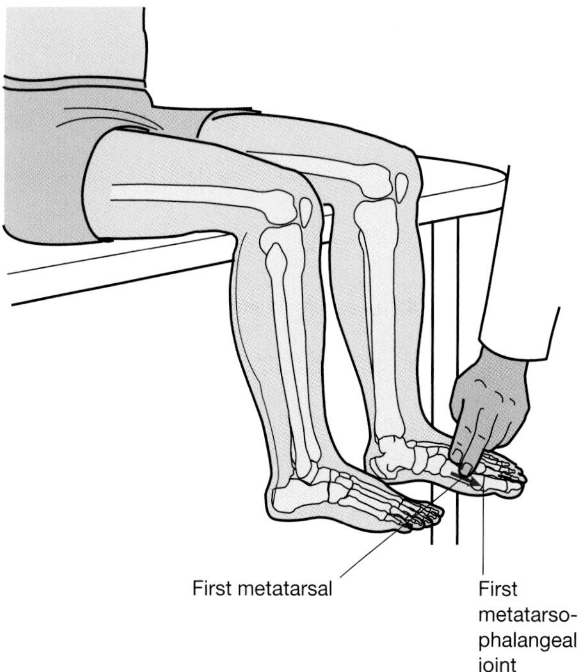

Figure 13.9 Palpation of the first metatarsal and the metatarsophalangeal joint.

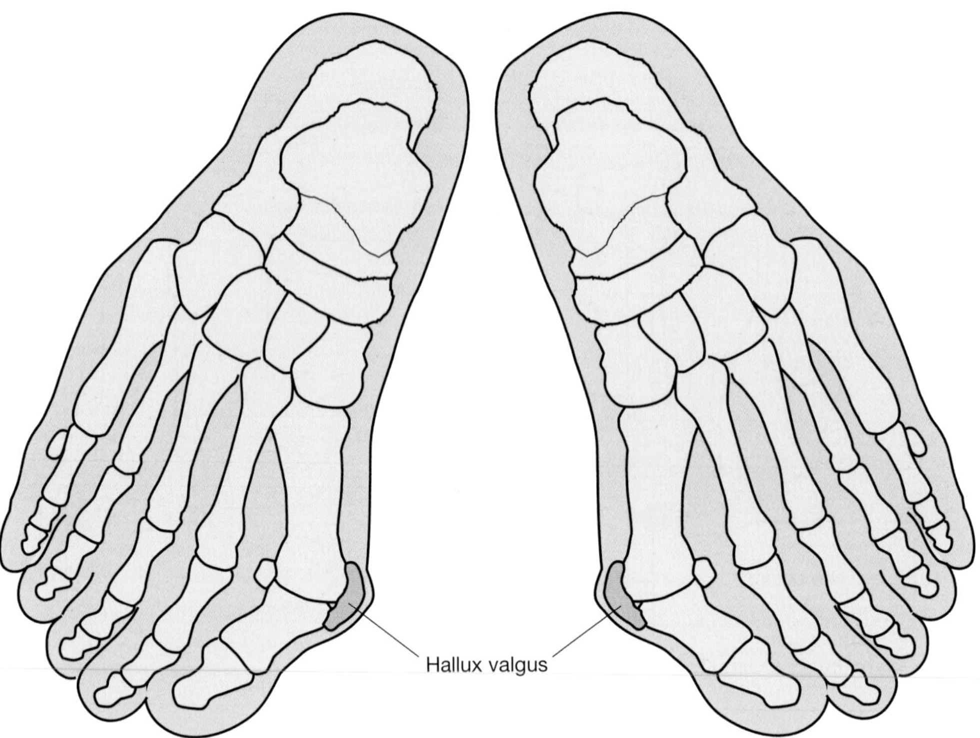

Figure 13.10 Hallux valgus.

eversion of the ankle often results in an avulsion fracture of the tibia, rather than a sprain of the ligament.

Tibialis Posterior

Place your fingers between the inferior aspect of the medial malleolus and the navicular and you will find the band of the tibialis posterior tendon. The tendon becomes more distinct when you ask the patient to invert and plantarflex the foot (Figure 13.12).

Flexor Digitorum Longus

After locating the tibialis posterior, move proximally so that you are posterior to the medial malleolus.

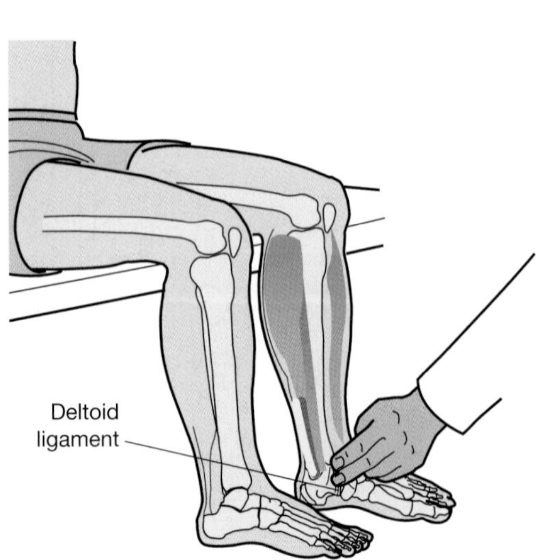

Figure 13.11 Palpation of the deltoid ligament.

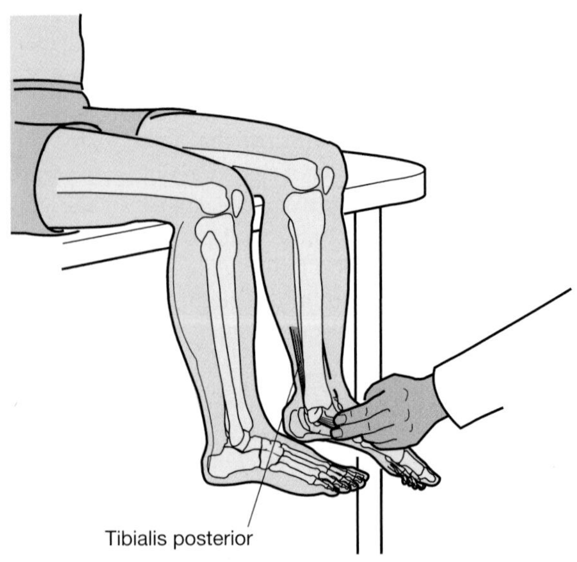

Figure 13.12 Palpation of the tibialis posterior.

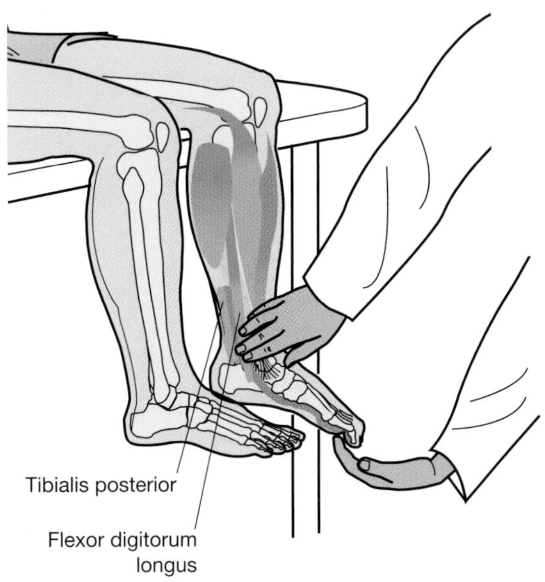

Figure 13.13 Palpation of the flexor digitorum longus.

The next tendon posterior to it is the flexor digitorum longus. This tendon is not as distinct as the tibialis posterior. However, you can sense it becoming tense under your finger as you resist toe flexion (Figure 13.13).

Posterior Tibial Artery

Place your fingers posterior to the medial malleolus. Make sure that the patient's foot is in a neutral position and that all the muscles are relaxed. The posterior tibial artery is located between the tendons of the flexor digitorum longus and the flexor hallucis longus (Figure 13.14). Gently palpate the pulse. Do not press too firmly or you will obliterate the pulse. It is helpful to compare the intensity from one ankle to the other. This is a reliable and clinically significant pulse to palpate since it is a major blood supply to the foot. It may be difficult to locate if the patient is either edematous or obese. Absence of the posterior tibial pulse may be indicative of occlusive arterial disease.

Posterior Tibial Nerve

The posterior tibial nerve follows along with the posterior tibial artery. It is slightly posterior and deep to the artery (Figure 13.15). The nerve itself is not palpable, but it is of great clinical significance in that it is the major nerve supply to the sole of the foot.

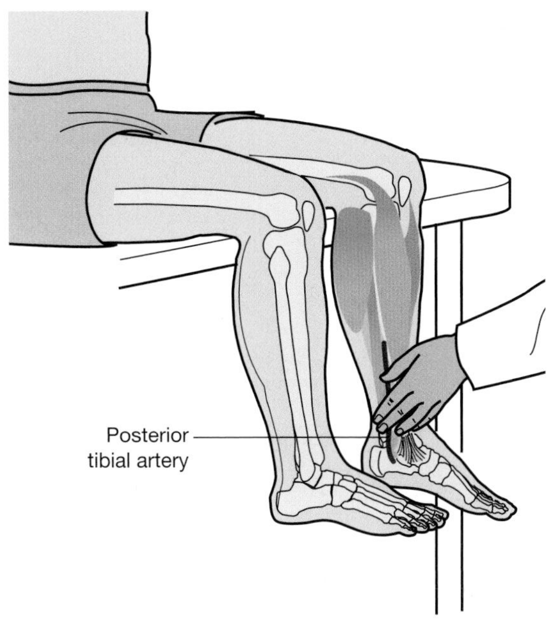

Figure 13.14 Palpation of the posterior tibial artery.

Flexor Hallucis Longus

The tendon of the flexor hallucis longus grooves around the distal posterior aspect of tibia, talus, and the inferior aspect of the sustentaculum tali. It is the most posterior of the tendons on the medial aspect of the ankle. It is not palpable because it is so deep. All three tendons (tibialis posterior, flexor digitorum

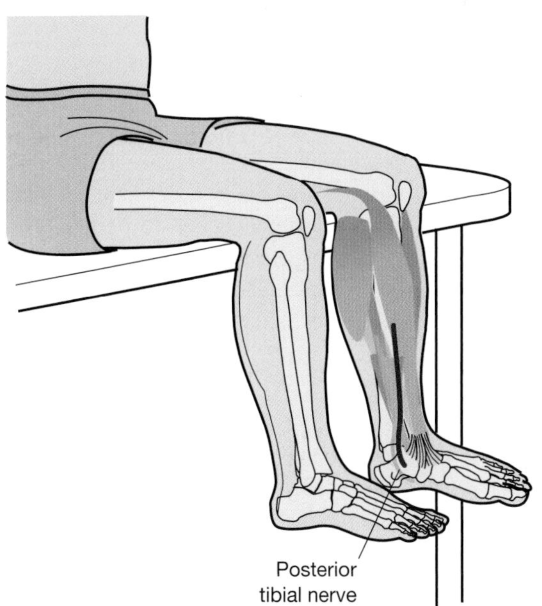

Figure 13.15 Location of the posterior tibial nerve.

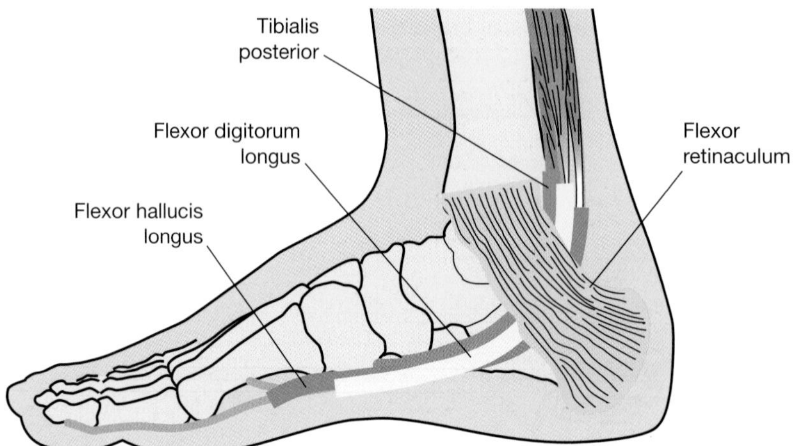

Figure 13.16 Location of the flexor retinaculum and tibialis posterior, flexor digitorum longus, tibial artery, tibial nerve, and flexor hallucis longus.

longus, and flexor hallucis longus) and the neurovascular bundle lie under the flexor retinaculum, which creates the tarsal tunnel (Figure 13.16, 13.89). Compression causes tarsal tunnel syndrome with resulting neuropathy of the posterior tibial nerve.

The order of these structures as they pass through the space between the medial malleolus and Achilles tendon can be remembered by the mnemonic "Tom, Dick, an' Harry" representing tibialis posterior, flexor digitorum longus, artery, nerve, and flexor hallucis longus.

Long Saphenous Vein

Place your finger on the medial malleolus and move anteriorly approximately 2.5–3.0 cm and you will palpate the long saphenous vein (Figure 13.17). This vein is very superficial and easily accessible for placement of intravenous catheters when upper-extremity sites are inaccessible. Inspect the length of the vein for varicosities and pay attention to any indications of thrombophlebitis.

Dorsal Aspect

Bony Structures

Inferior Tibiofibular Joint

Allow your fingers to move inferiorly along the anterior aspect of the tibia until you reach the depression of the talus. Move laterally and you will detect a slight indentation before you reach the inferior aspect of the fibula (Figure 13.18). You cannot palpate a distinct joint line because the inferior tibiofibular ligament overlies the anterior aspect of the joint. Mobility can be detected when the fibula is glided in an anterior/posterior direction.

Body of the Talus

Place your thumb and index finger at the distal aspect of the tibia at a level that is at the inferior portion of

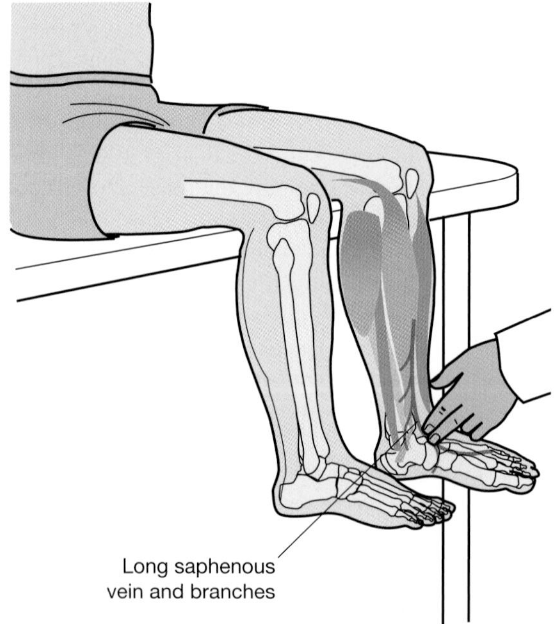

Figure 13.17 Palpation of the long saphenous vein.

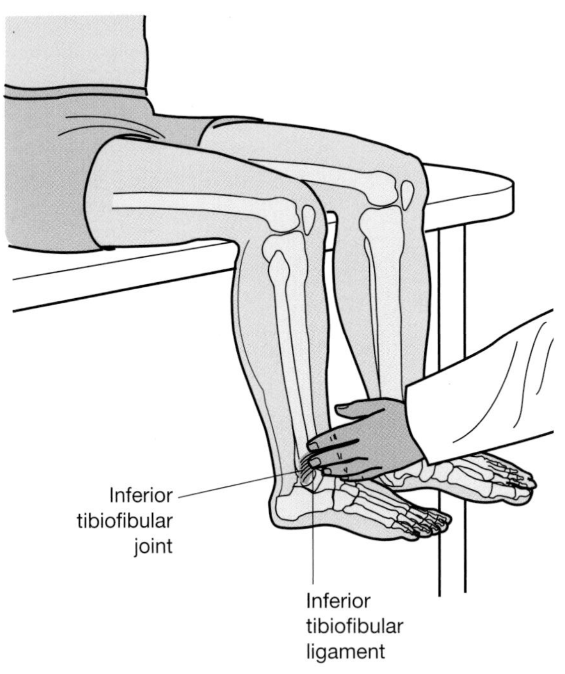

Figure 13.18 Palpation of the inferior tibiofibular joint.

the medial malleolus. You will feel a depression when the ankle is at zero degrees. Bring the foot into plantar flexion and you will feel the dome of the talus come under your palpating fingers. Move the forefoot into inversion and eversion and you will be able to feel movement of the body of the talus and find its neutral position (Figure 13.19).

Sinus Tarsi

Place your finger medial to the inferior aspect of the lateral malleolus, into an indentation (Figure 13.20). You will be able to palpate the small bulge of the extensor digitorum brevis. Deep to the soft tissue you can feel the lateral aspect of the neck of the talus, which becomes more prominent in inversion.

Soft-Tissue Structures

Tibialis Anterior Tendon

Place your fingers anterior to the medial malleolus. The first and most prominent tendon that you will locate is the tibialis anterior. This tendon becomes more distinct as you ask the patient to dorsiflex and invert the foot (Figure 13.21). The tibialis anterior is the strongest of the dorsiflexors and weakness of the muscle will result in a drop foot.

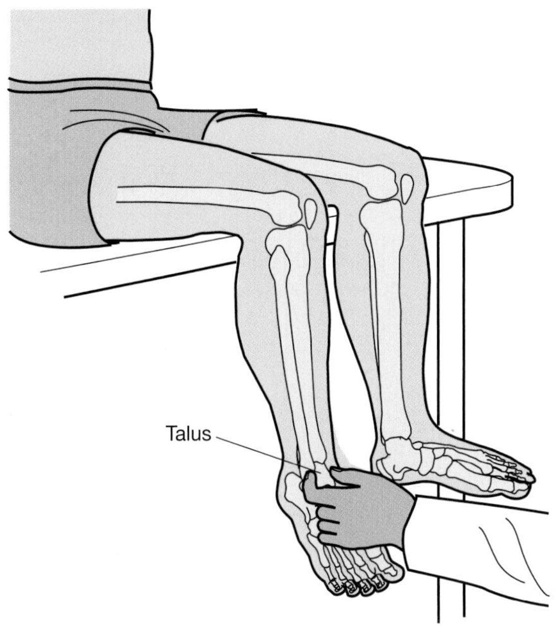

Figure 13.19 Palpation of the talus.

Extensor Hallucis Longus

Allow your fingers to continue laterally from the tibialis anterior and you will come to the tendon of the extensor hallucis longus. The tendon becomes more distinct as you ask the patient to extend the great toe. You can visually trace the tendon as it travels distally to its attachment on the base of the distal phalanx of the hallux (Figure 13.22).

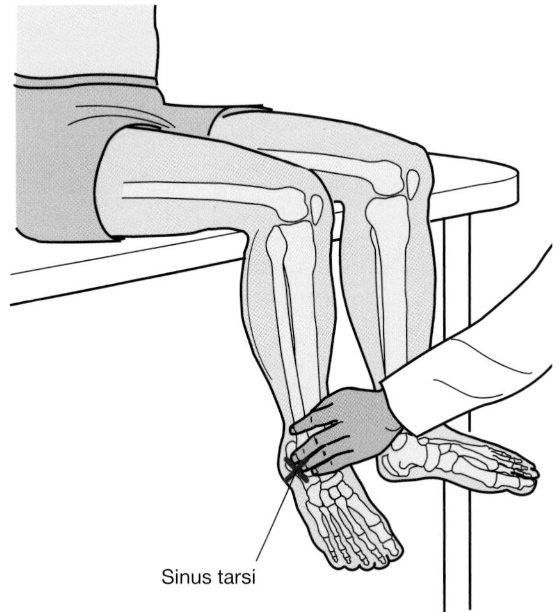

Figure 13.20 Palpation of the sinus tarsi.

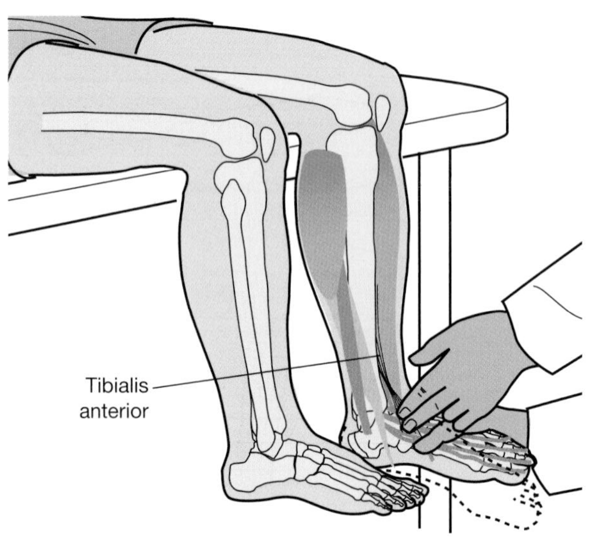

Figure 13.21 Palpation of the tibialis anterior.

Extensor Digitorum Longus Tendon

Allow your fingers to continue laterally from the extensor hallucis longus and you will come to the extensor digitorum longus. The tendon becomes more distinct as you ask the patient to extend the toes. You can visualize this tendon as it splits into four components and attaches into the middle and distal phalanges of toes two through five (Figure 13.23).

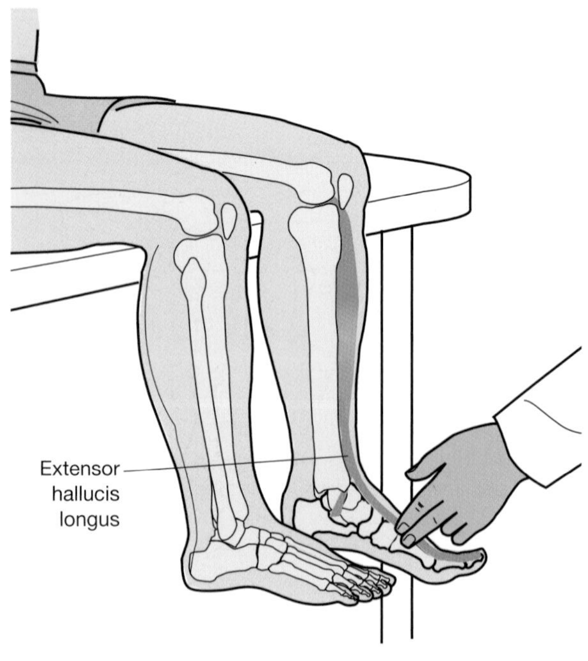

Figure 13.22 Palpation of the extensor hallucis longus.

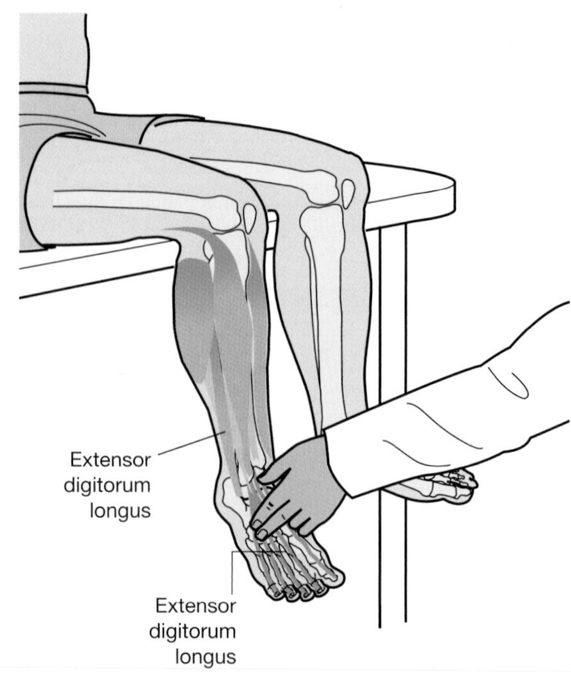

Figure 13.23 Palpation of the extensor digitorum longus.

Dorsal Artery of the Foot (Dorsalis Pedis Pulse)

Place your fingers on the dorsal surface of the foot over the anterior aspect of the talus. The dorsalis pedis pulse can be located lateral to the extensor hallucis longus and medial to the first tendon of the extensor digitorum longus (Figure 13.24). The pulse is easily palpable as it is very superficial. However, this pulse can be congenitally absent.

Extensor Digitorum Brevis

Place your fingers over the lateral dorsal aspect of the foot just anterior to the lateral malleolus in the sinus tarsi. You will feel a soft bulge which is likened to a puff ball. It is sometimes blue in appearance. This is the extensor digitorum brevis (Figure 13.25). The muscle belly becomes more distinct as the patient extends the lateral four toes.

Lateral Aspect

Bony Structures

Lateral Malleolus

Place your fingers along the lateral aspect of the leg along the fibular shaft and follow it inferiorly. You will come to the prominence of the lateral malleolus (Figure 13.26). It projects more inferiorly than its medial counterpart. You can compare the relative

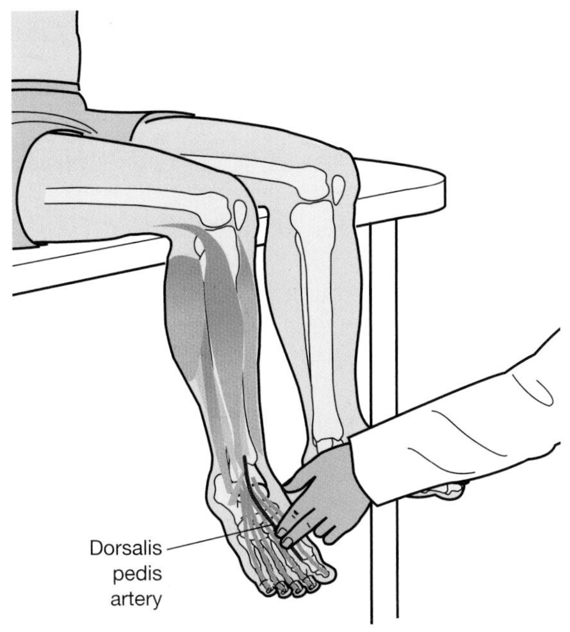

Figure 13.24 Palpation of the dorsal artery (dorsalis pedis) of the foot.

positions by placing your index finger and thumb over both the medial and lateral malleoli from the anterior aspect and compare their locations. The lateral malleolus adds additional stability to the lateral aspect of the mortise and helps to resist eversion sprains.

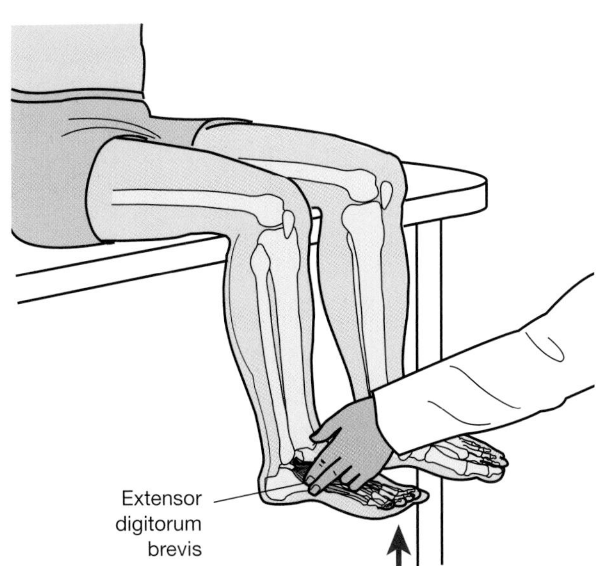

Figure 13.25 Palpation of the extensor digitorum brevis.

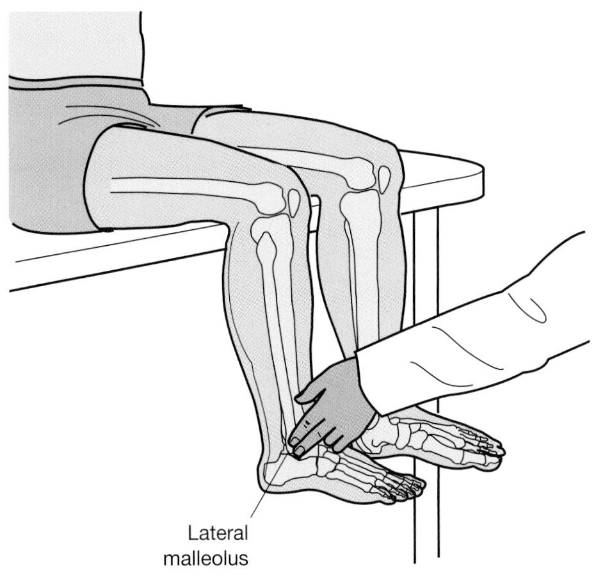

Figure 13.26 Palpation of the lateral malleolus.

Peroneus Tubercle

Place your fingers on the lateral malleolus and move slightly inferiorly and continue distally. You will be palpating the peroneus tubercle, which was created as the separation between the peroneus brevis and longus tendons as they travel along the lateral calcaneus (Figure 13.27).

Cuboid

Place your fingers inferior to the lateral malleolus and find the lateral aspect of the calcaneus. Allow your

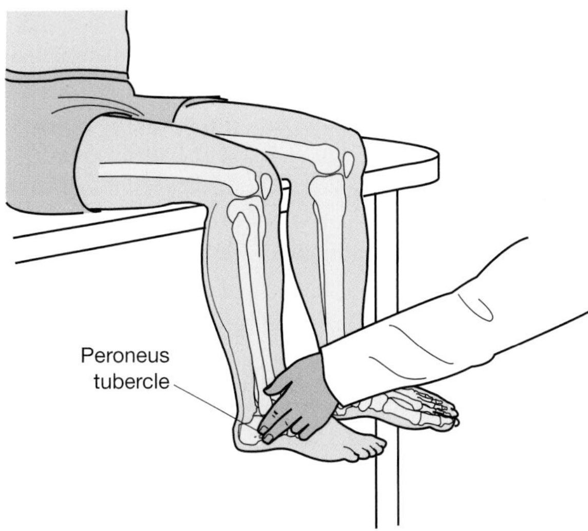

Figure 13.27 Palpation of the peroneus tubercle.

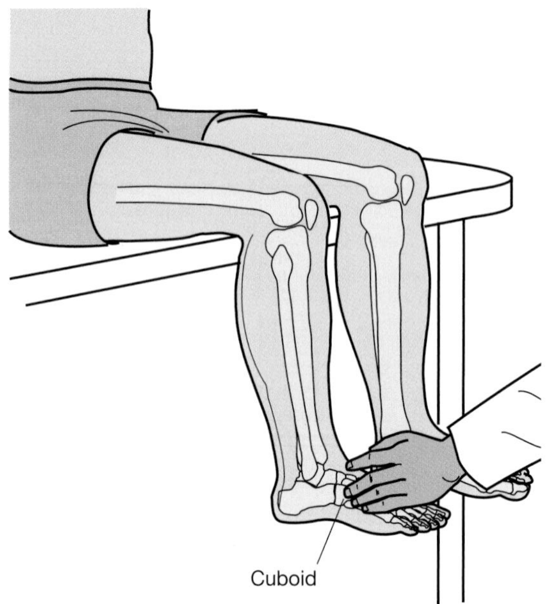

Figure 13.28 Palpation of the cuboid.

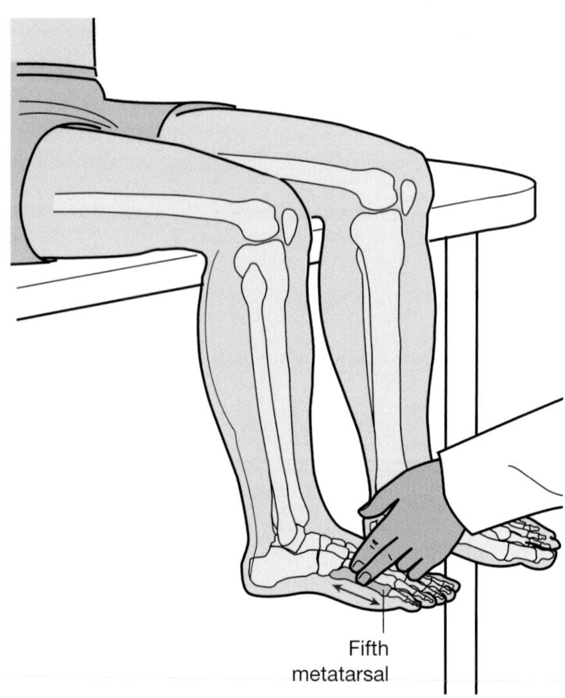

Figure 13.29 Palpation of the fifth metatarsal.

fingers to travel anteriorly along the lateral aspect of the foot until you feel an indentation. You will be along the cuboid. To check your location, follow a little more distally and you will palpate the articulation with the fifth metatarsal (Figure 13.28). The groove that you have palpated is for the tendon of the peroneus longus as it passes to its attachment on the plantar aspect of the foot. The cuboid may be tender to palpation, especially when it has dropped secondary to trauma.

Fifth Metatarsal

Continue distally from the cuboid and you will palpate the flare of the fifth metatarsal base, its styloid process. You can continue along the lateral aspect of the foot and palpate the shaft of the fifth metatarsal until you come to the fifth metatarsophalangeal joint (Figure 13.29). The peroneus brevis attaches to the base of the fifth metatarsal. A fracture here is known as a Jones fracture.

Soft-Tissue Structures

Anterior Talofibular Ligament

Place your fingers over the sinus tarsi and you will locate the anterior talofibular ligament as it passes from the lateral malleolus to the talar neck (Figure 13.30).

The ligament is not distinctly palpable. However, increased tension can be noted under your finger when the patient inverts and plantarflexes the foot. This ligament becomes vertically oriented in plantar flexion and is therefore the most commonly ruptured

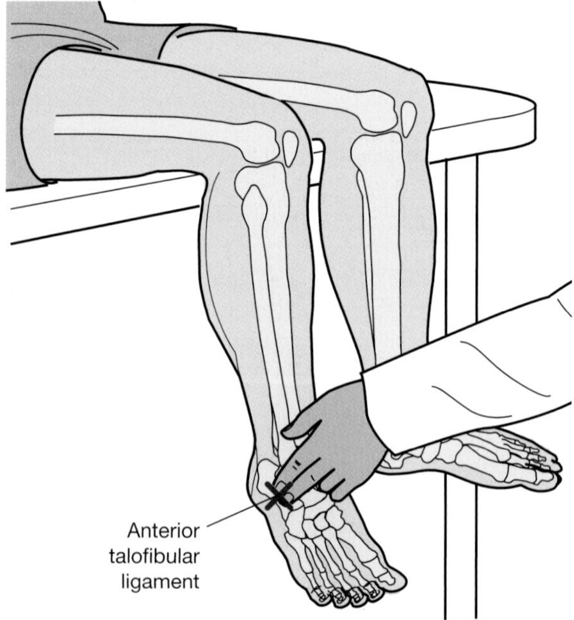

Figure 13.30 Palpation of the anterior talofibular ligament.

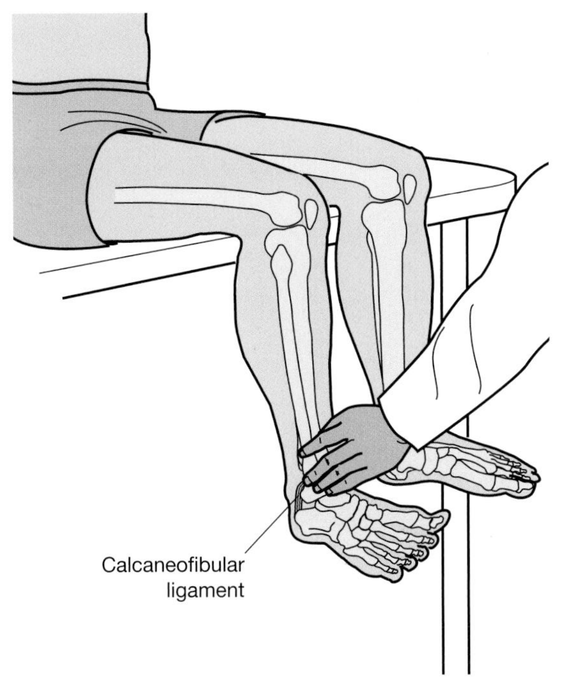

Figure 13.31 Palpation of the calcaneofibular ligament.

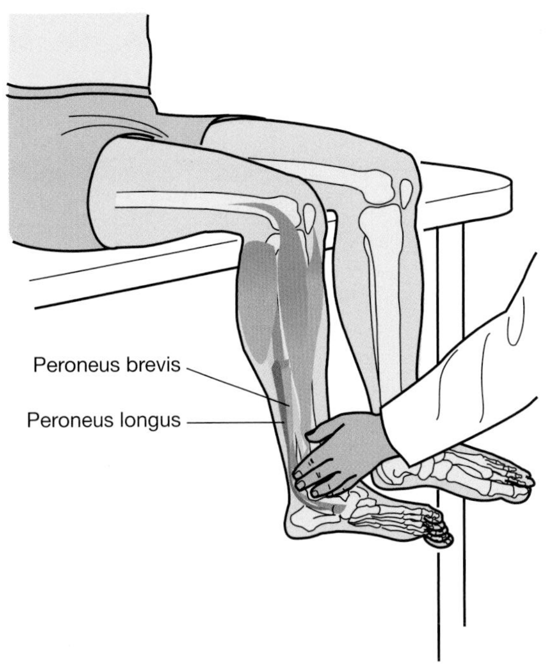

Figure 13.32 Palpation of the peroneus longus and brevis.

in ankle injuries. Edema and tenderness will be found over the sinus tarsi following a sprain of this ligament.

Calcaneofibular Ligament

Place your fingers between the lateral malleolus and the lateral aspect of the calcaneus and you will find the tubular cord of the calcaneofibular ligament (Figure 13.31). The ligament becomes more distinct as you ask the patient to invert the ankle. This ligament can also be torn during inversion injuries of the ankle and, coupled with injury to the anterior talofibular ligament, creates lateral instability of the ankle.

Posterior Talofibular Ligament

The posterior talofibular ligament runs from the lateral malleolus to the posterior tubercle of the talus. The ligament is very strong and deep. It is not palpable.

Peroneus Longus and Brevis Tendons

Place your fingers posterior and slightly inferior to the lateral malleolus. You will find the tendons of the peroneus longus and brevis. The brevis is closer to the malleolus and the longus is just posterior to the malleolus. The tendon is made more distinct by asking the patient to evert the foot (Figure 13.32). You can visualize the tendon of the peroneus brevis distally to its attachment on the base of the fifth metatarsal. A tender thickening that is palpable inferior to the lateral malleolus may be indicative of stenosing tenosynovitis of the common peroneal tendon sheath. Painful snapping of the tendons can occur if they sublux anteriorly to the lateral malleolus.

Posterior Aspect

Bony Structures

Calcaneus

The large dome of the calcaneus is easily palpable at the posterior aspect of the foot. You will notice that the calcaneus becomes wider as you approach the base (Figure 13.33). Excessive prominence of the superior tuberosity of the calcaneus often occurs in women who wear high heels and has been called a pump bump.

Soft-Tissue Structures

Tendocalcaneus (Achilles Tendon)

Place your fingers at the posterior aspect of the calcaneus and move them proximally to the lower one-third of the calf. Palpate the thick common tendon of the gastrocnemius and soleus, referred to as the Achilles tendon (Figure 13.34). Tenderness may be noted if the patient has overused the muscle and has

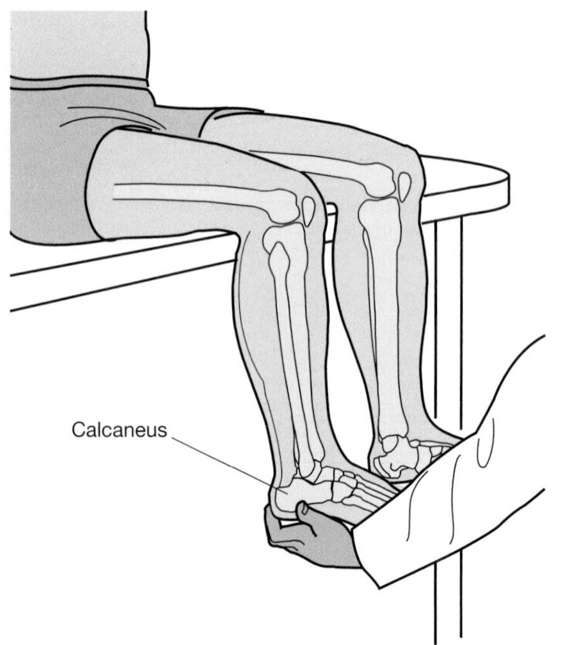

Figure 13.33 Palpation of the calcaneus.

developed a tenosynovitis. Swelling may be noted and crepitus can be perceived with movement. The tendon can be ruptured secondary to trauma. Discontinuity of the tendon can be tested clinically and yields a positive Thompson sign (see pp. 408, 411, Figure 13.92).

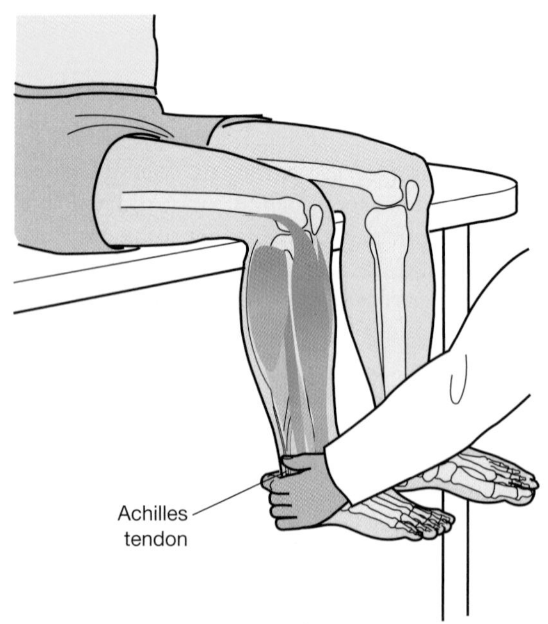

Figure 13.34 Palpation of the tendocalcaneus (Achilles tendon).

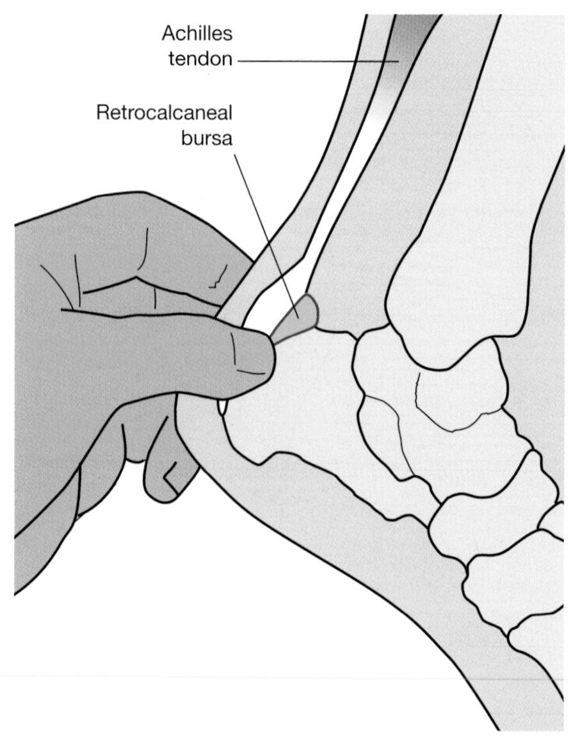

Figure 13.35 Location of the retrocalcaneal bursa.

Palpation of the disruption of the tendon may be difficult because of the secondary swelling. The patient will be unable to actively plantarflex the ankle.

Retrocalcaneal Bursa

The retrocalcaneal bursa separates the posterior aspect of the calcaneus and the overlying Achilles tendon. It is not normally palpable unless it is inflamed from increased friction (Figure 13.35).

Calcaneal Bursa

The calcaneal bursa separates the distal attachment of the tendocalcaneus and the overlying skin. This bursa is not normally palpable (Figure 13.36).

If thickness, tenderness, or edema is noted in the posterior calcaneal area, the patient may have bursitis. The calcaneal bursa is often irritated by wearing improperly fitting shoes that rub against the posterior aspect of the foot.

Plantar Surface

Bony Structures

Medial Tubercle of the Calcaneus

Place your fingers on the plantar surface of the calcaneus and move them anteriorly to the dome. You will

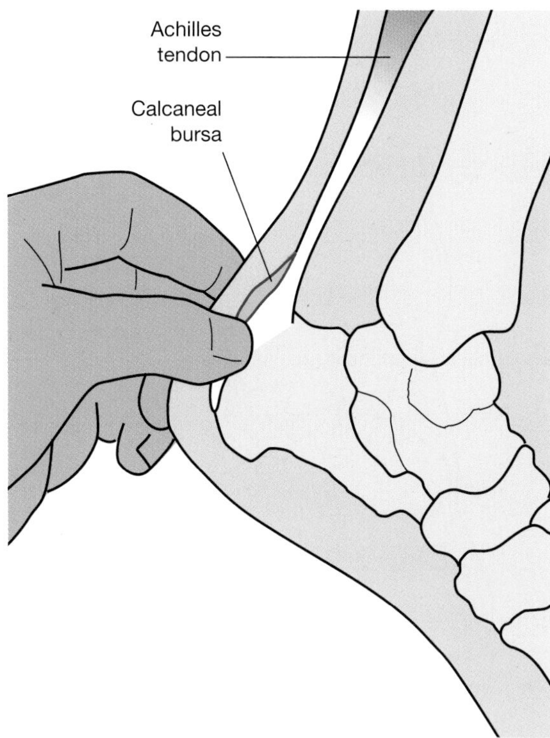

Figure 13.36 Location of the calcaneal bursa.

feel a flattened area that is not very distinct. You can confirm your location by abducting the great toe and palpating the attachment of the abductor hallucis. If you move medially, you will feel the attachments of the flexor digitorum brevis and the plantar aponeurosis (Figure 13.37). The medial tubercle bears weight and is the site of the development of heel spurs. If a spur is present, the tubercle will be very tender to palpation. The most common cause of a spur is chronic plantar fasciitis.

Sesamoid Bones

Find the lateral aspect of the first metatarsophalangeal joint and allow your fingers to travel to the inferior aspect. You will feel two small sesamoid bones when you press superiorly on the ball of the foot. These sesamoid bones are located in the tendon of the flexor hallucis brevis and help to more evenly distribute weight-bearing forces (Figure 13.38). The sesamoid bones will also facilitate the function of the flexor hallucis brevis, especially during toe off.

Metatarsal Heads

Allow your fingers to travel slightly proximally from the inferior portion of the first metatarsophalangeal joint until you feel the first metatarsal head. Move

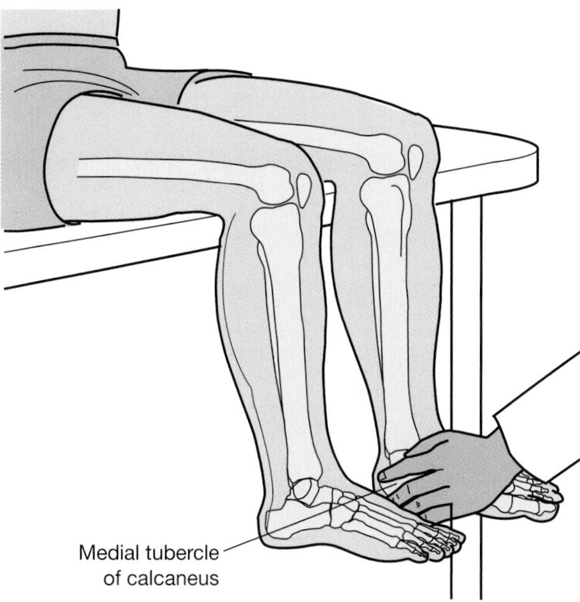

Figure 13.37 Palpation of the medial tubercle of the calcaneus.

laterally and palpate the heads of metatarsals two through five (Figure 13.39). You should feel that the first and fifth metatarsal heads are the most prominent because of the shape of the transverse arch of the foot (Figure 13.40). Sometimes you will notice a drop of the second metatarsal head, which will increase the weight-bearing surface. You will also palpate increased callus formation in this area. Tenderness and swelling between the metatarsals may be

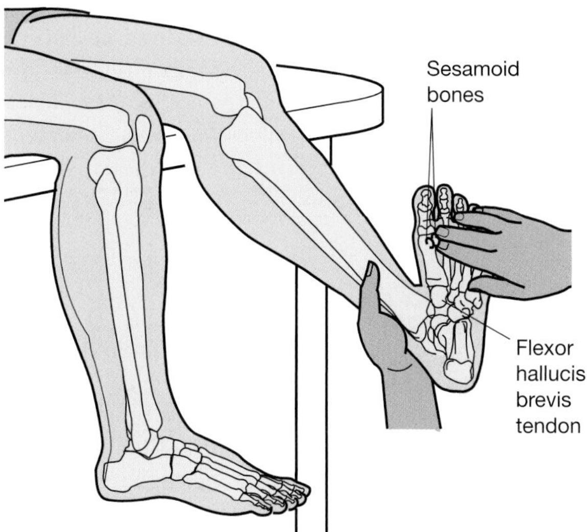

Figure 13.38 Palpation of the sesamoid bones.

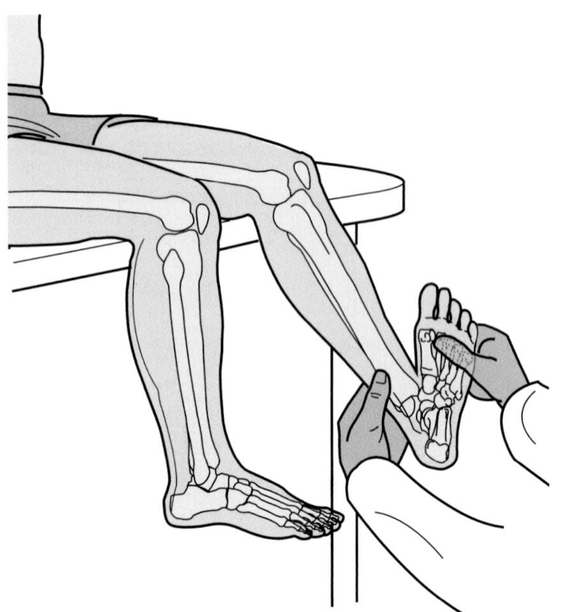

Figure 13.39 Palpation of the metatarsal heads.

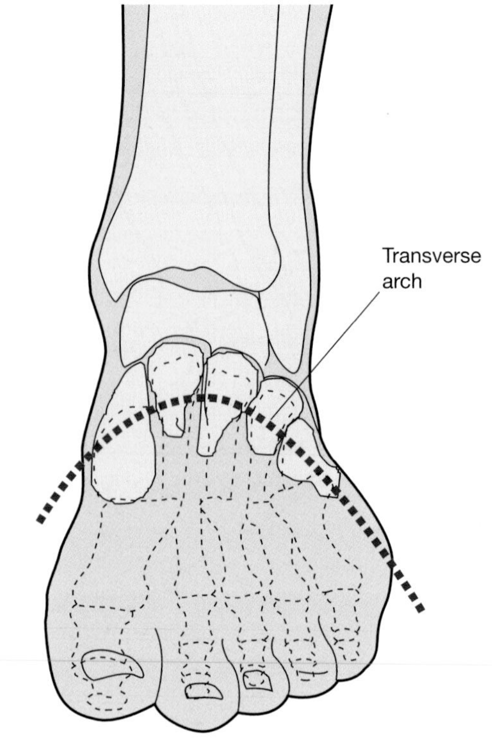

Figure 13.40 Transverse arch of the foot.

indicative of a neuroma. Morton's neuroma is the most common neuroma and is usually found between the third and fourth metatarsals.

Soft-Tissue Structures

Plantar Aponeurosis (Plantar Fascia)

The plantar aponeurosis consists of strong longitudinal fibers that run from the calcaneus and divide into five processes before attaching onto the metatarsal heads. The plantar aponeurosis plays an integral part in the support of the medial longitudinal arch (Figure 13.41). Focal tenderness and nodules on the plantar surface may be indicative of plantar fasciitis. Under normal circumstances, the plantar surface should be smooth and without any nodules. It should not be tender to palpation.

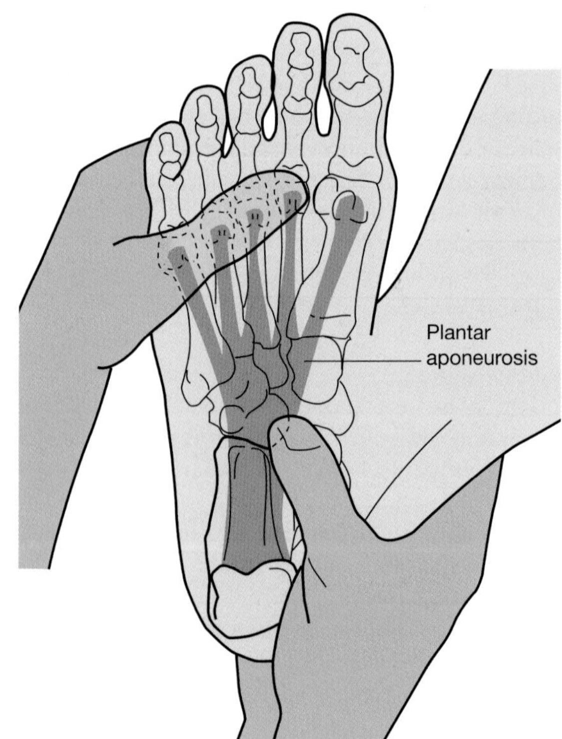

Figure 13.41 Palpation of the plantar aponeurosis (plantar fascia).

Toes

Under normal circumstances, the toes should be flat and straight. The great toe should be longer than the second. If the second toe is longer, it is referred to as a *Morton's toe* (Figure 13.42) and is due to a short first metatarsal. Observe the toes for alignment, callus or corn formation, color, and temperature. Calluses and corns can be found on top of the joint surfaces, beneath the toes, and between them.

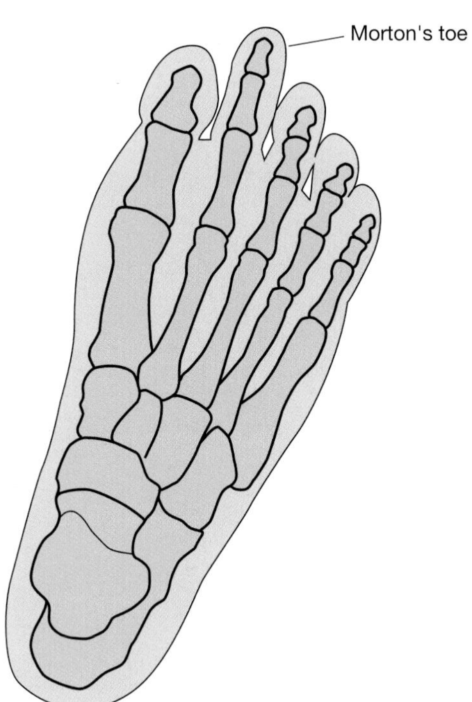

Figure 13.42 Morton's toe.

Claw Toes

The patient will present with hyperextension of the metatarsophalangeal joints and flexion of the proximal and distal interphalangeal joints (Figure 13.43). The patient will often have callus formation over the dorsal aspect of the toes. This is caused by rubbing from the patient's shoes due to decreased space that results from the deformity. Calluses will also be noted at the tip of the toes because of the increased amount of distal weight-bearing. Patients with pes cavus often develop claw toes.

Hammer Toes

The patient will present with hyperextension of the metatarsophalangeal joint, flexion of the proximal interphalangeal joint, and hyperextension of the distal interphalangeal joint (Figure 13.44). The patient will often have callus formation over the dorsal aspect of the proximal interphalangeal joint secondary to increased pressure from the top of the shoe.

Active Movement Testing

Active movement tests should be quick, functional tests designed to clear the joint. They are designed to

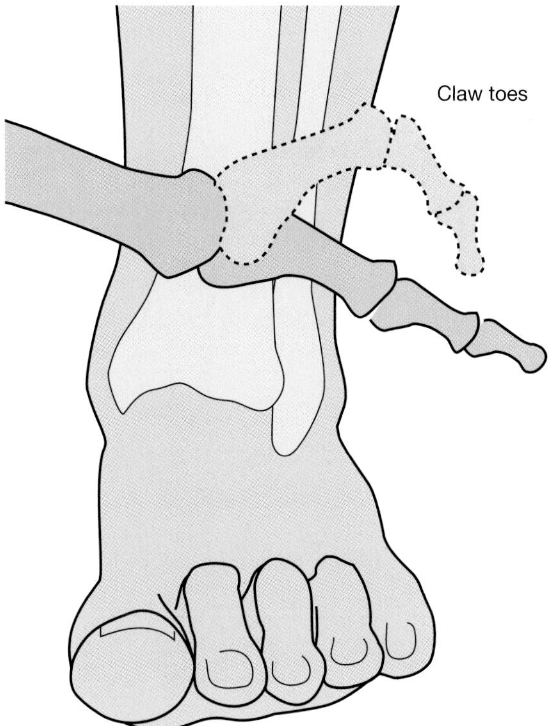

Figure 13.43 Claw toes.

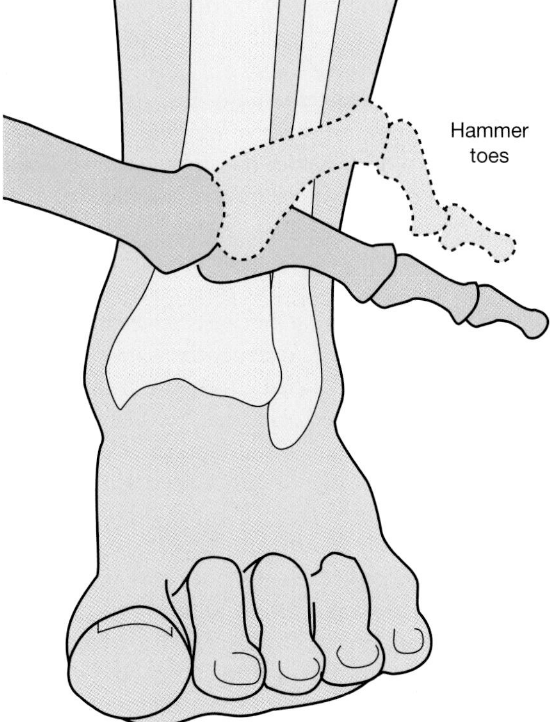

Figure 13.44 Hammer toes.

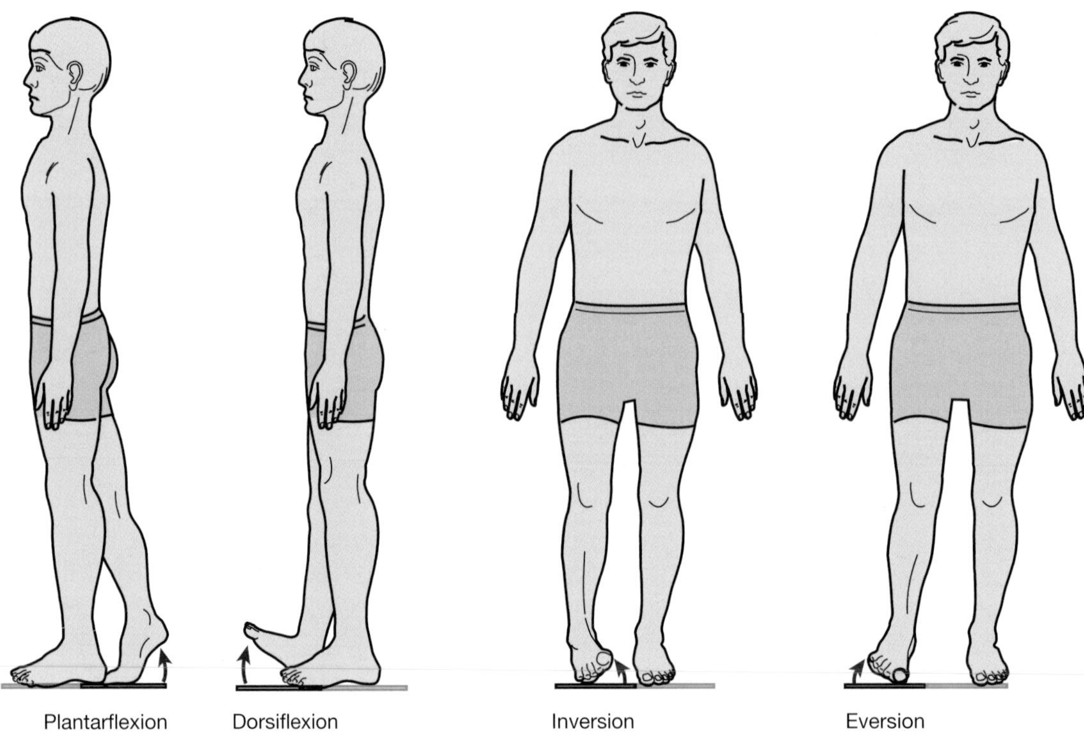

Figure 13.45 Active movement testing for inversion and eversion.

help you see if the patient has a gross restriction. You should always remember to compare the movement from one side to the other. If the motion is pain free at the end of the range, you can add an additional overpressure to "clear" the joint. If the patient experiences pain in any of these movements, you should continue to explore whether the etiology of the pain is secondary to contractile or noncontractile structures by using passive and resistive testing.

Active movements of the ankle and foot should be performed in both weight-bearing and non-weight-bearing (supine or long sitting) positions. In the weight-bearing position, instruct the patient to stand and walk on the toes to check for plantar flexion and toe flexion, and to stand and walk on the heels to test for dorsiflexion and toe extension. Then instruct the patient to stand on the lateral border of the foot to test for inversion, and then the medial border of the foot to test for eversion (Figure 13.45).

In the non-weight-bearing position, instruct the patient to pull the ankle up as far as possible, push it down, and turn it in and then out. This will check for dorsiflexion, plantar flexion, inversion, and eversion. Then have the patient bring up the toes, curl them, and spread them apart. This will check for toe extension, flexion, abduction, and adduction (Figure 13.46).

Passive Movement Testing

Passive movement testing can be divided into two areas: physiological movements (cardinal plane), which are the same as the active movements, and mobility testing of the accessory movements (joint play, component). You can determine whether the noncontractile (inert) elements are causative of the patient's problem by using these tests. These structures (ligaments, joint capsule, fascia, bursa, dura mater, and nerve root) (Cyriax, 1982) are stretched or stressed when the joint is taken to the end of the available range. At the end of each passive physiological movement, you should sense the end feel and determine whether it is normal or pathological. Assess the limitation of movement and see if it fits into a capsular pattern. The capsular patterns of the foot and ankle are as follows: talocrural joint—greater restriction of plantar flexion than dorsiflexion; subtalar joint—greater restriction of varus than valgus; midtarsal joint—most restriction in dorsiflexion, followed by plantar flexion, adduction, and medial rotation; first metatarsophalangeal joint—greater restriction of extension than flexion; interphalangeal joints—greater restriction of extension than flexion (Magee, 2008; Kaltenborn, 2011).

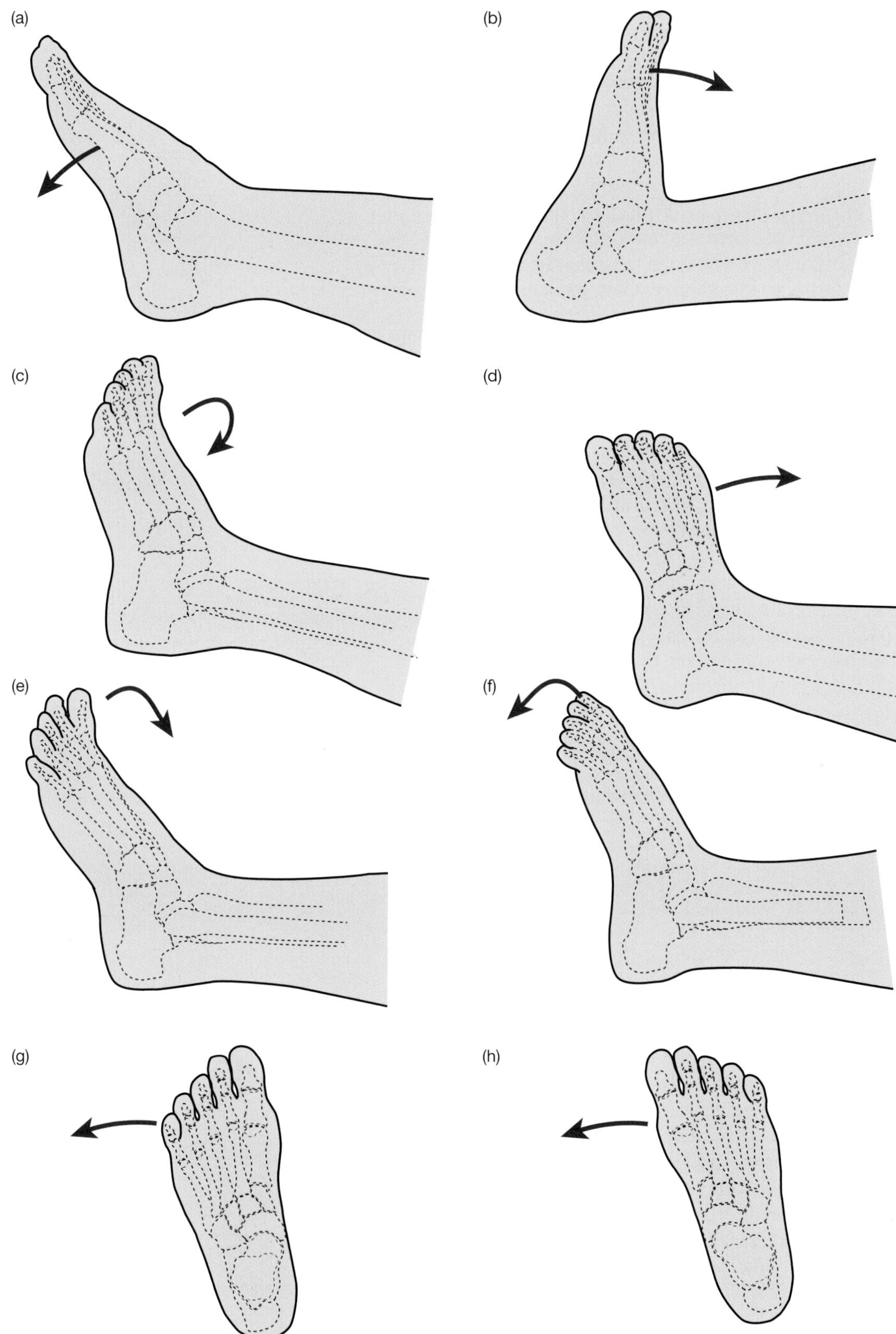

Figure 13.46 Active movement testing in non-weight-bearing of: (a) plantar flexion, (b) dorsiflexion, (c) inversion, (d) eversion, (e) toe extension, (f) flexion, (g) abduction, and (h) adduction.

Physiological Movements

You will be assessing the amount of motion available in all directions. Each motion is measured from the anatomical starting position. In the talocrural joint this is when the lateral aspect of the foot creates a right angle with the longitudinal axis of the leg. In addition, a line passing through the anterior superior iliac spine and through the patella must be aligned with the second toe. The starting position for the toes is when the longitudinal axes through the metatarsals form a straight line with the corresponding phalanx.

Dorsiflexion

You can measure dorsiflexion with the patient either in the sitting position with the leg dangling over the side of the treatment table or in the supine position. This motion takes place in the talocrural joint. Place the patient so that the knee is flexed at 90 degrees and the foot is at 0 degrees of inversion and eversion. Place one hand over the distal posterior aspect of the leg to stabilize the tibia and fibula and prevent movement at the knee and hip. Place your other hand with the palm flattened under the plantar surface of the foot directing your fingers toward the toes. Bend the ankle in a cranial direction. The normal end feel is abrupt and firm (ligamentous) because of the tension from the tendocalcaneus and the posterior ligaments (Magee, 2008; Kaltenborn, 2011). The normal range of motion is 0–20 degrees (Figure 13.47) (American Academy of Orthopedic Surgeons, 1965).

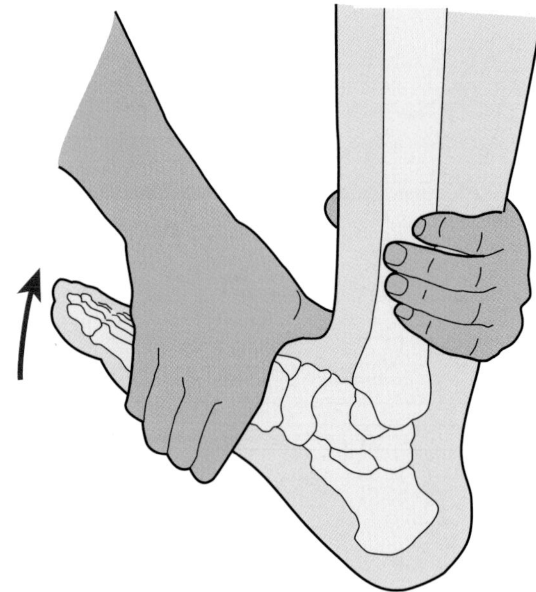

Figure 13.47 Passive movement testing of dorsiflexion.

Plantar Flexion

You can measure plantar flexion with the patient either in the sitting position with the leg dangling over the side of the treatment table or in the supine position. This motion takes place in the talocrural joint. Place the patient so that the knee is flexed at 90 degrees and the foot is at 0 degrees of inversion and eversion. Place one hand over the distal posterior aspect of the leg to stabilize the tibia and fibula and prevent movement at the knee and hip. Place your other hand with the palm flattened over the dorsal surface of the foot directing your fingers laterally. Push the foot in a caudal direction avoiding any inversion or eversion. The normal end feel is abrupt and firm (ligamentous) because of the tension in the anterior capsule and the anterior ligaments (Magee, 2008; Kaltenborn, 2011). A hard end feel may result from contact between the posterior talar tubercle and the posterior aspect of the tibia. The normal range of motion is 0–50 degrees (Figure 13.48) (American Academy of Orthopedic Surgeons, 1965).

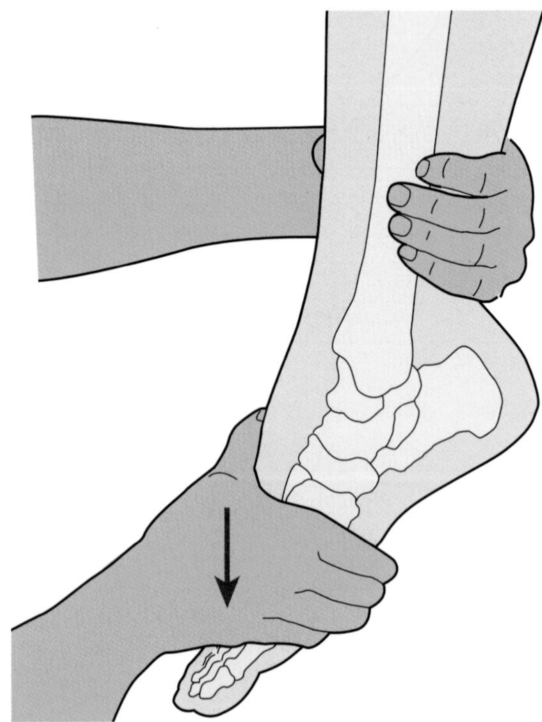

Figure 13.48 Passive movement testing of plantar flexion.

Inversion

Place the patient in the sitting position with the leg dangling over the side of the treatment table and the knee flexed to 90 degrees or in the supine position with the foot over the end of the treatment table. Make sure that the hip is at zero degrees of rotation, and adduction and abduction. Inversion, which is a combination of supination, adduction, and plantar flexion, takes place at the subtalar, transverse tarsal, cuboideonavicular, cuneonavicular, intercuneiform, cuneocuboid, tarsometatarsal, and intermetatarsal joints. Place one hand over the distal medial and posterior aspect of the leg to stabilize the tibia and fibula and prevent movement at the knee and hip. Place your hand over the distal lateral aspect of the foot with your thumb on the dorsal surface and the other four fingers under the metatarsal heads. Turn the foot in a medial and superior direction. The normal end feel is abrupt and firm (ligamentous) because of the tension in the joint capsules and the lateral ligaments (Magee, 2008; Kaltenborn, 2011). The normal range of motion is 0–35 degrees (Figure 13.49) (American Academy of Orthopedic Surgeons, 1965).

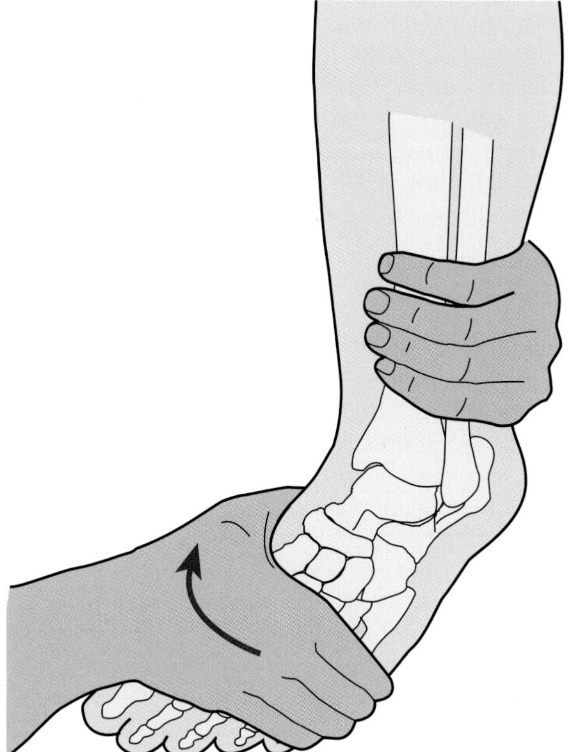

Figure 13.49 Passive movement testing of inversion.

Eversion

Place the patient in the sitting position with the leg dangling over the side of the treatment table and the knee flexed to 90 degrees or in the supine position with the foot over the end of the treatment table. Make sure that the hip is at zero degrees of rotation, and adduction and abduction. Eversion, which is a combination of pronation, abduction, and dorsiflexion, takes place at the subtalar, transverse tarsal, cuboideonavicular, cuneonavicular, intercuneiform, cuneocuboid, tarsometatarsal, and intermetatarsal joints. Place one hand over the distal lateral and posterior aspect of the leg to stabilize the tibia and fibula and prevent movement at the knee and hip. Place your hand under the distal plantar aspect of the foot with your thumb on the first metatarsal and the other four fingers around the fifth metatarsal. Turn the foot in a lateral and superior direction. The normal end feel is abrupt and firm (ligamentous) (Magee, 2008; Kaltenborn, 2011) because of the tension in the joint capsules and the medial ligaments. The normal range of motion is 0–15 degrees (Figure 13.50) (American Academy of Orthopedic Surgeons, 1965).

Subtalar (Hindfoot) Inversion

Place the patient in the prone position with the foot over the end of the treatment table. Make sure that the

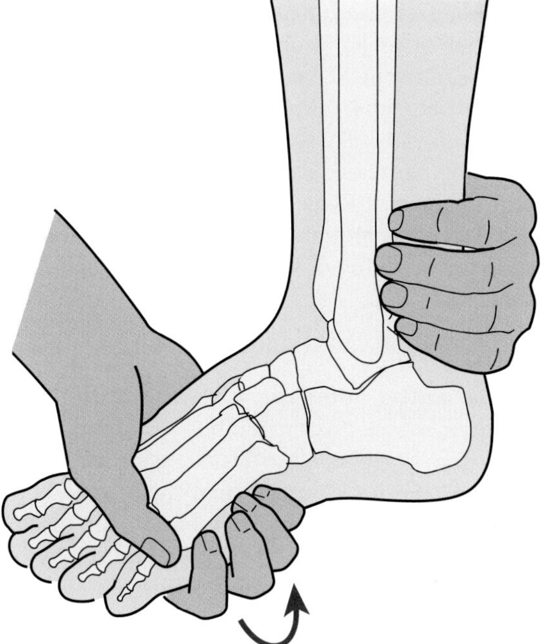

Figure 13.50 Passive movement testing of eversion.

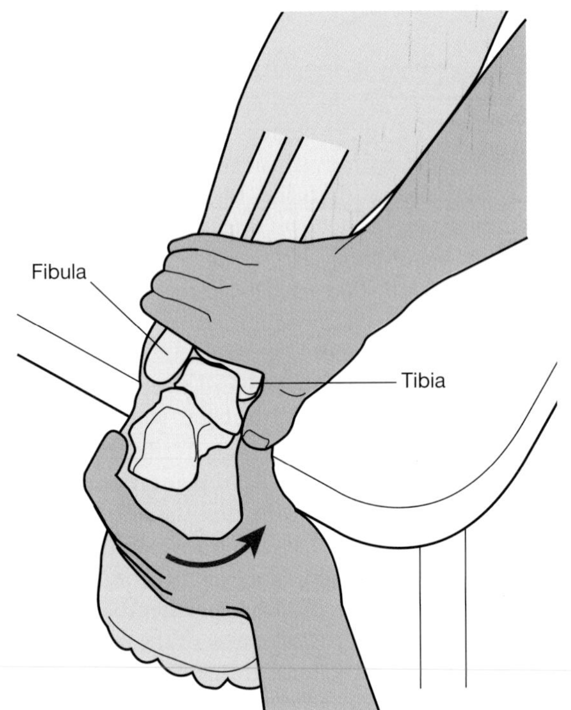

Figure 13.51 Passive movement testing of subtalar (hindfoot) inversion.

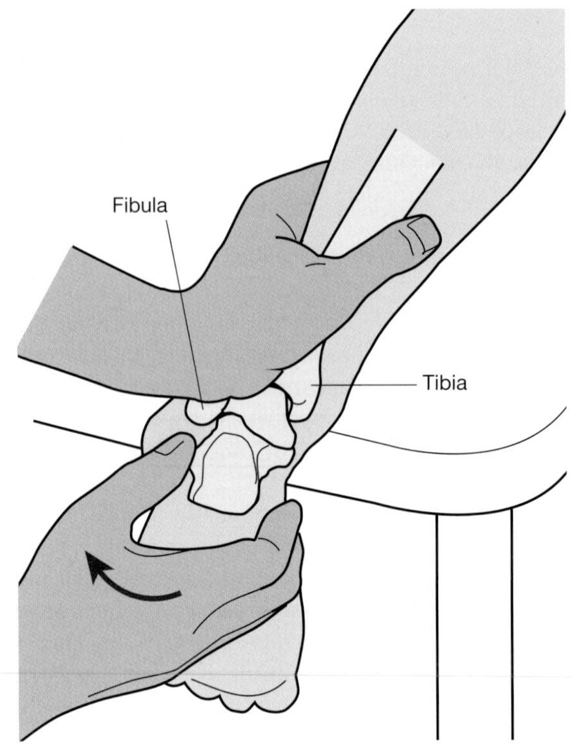

Figure 13.52 Passive movement testing of subtalar (hindfoot) eversion.

hip is at zero degrees of flexion–extension, abduction–adduction, and rotation, and that the knee is at zero degrees of extension. Place one hand over the middle posterior aspect of the leg to stabilize the tibia and fibula and prevent motion in the hip and knee. Place your other hand on the plantar surface of the calcaneus, grasping it between your index finger and thumb. Rotate the calcaneus in a medial direction. The normal end feel is abrupt and firm (ligamentous) because of the tension in the joint capsule and the lateral ligaments (Magee, 2008; Kaltenborn, 2011). Normal range of motion is 0–5 degrees (Figure 13.51) (American Academy of Orthopedic Surgeons, 1965).

Subtalar (Hindfoot) Eversion

Place the patient in the prone position with the foot over the end of the treatment table. Make sure that the hip is at zero degrees of flexion–extension, abduction–adduction, and rotation, and that the knee is at zero degrees of extension. Place one hand over the middle posterior aspect of the leg to stabilize the tibia and fibula and prevent motion in the hip and knee. Place your other hand on the plantar surface of the calcaneus, grasping it between your index finger and thumb. Rotate the calcaneus in a lateral direction. The normal end feel is abrupt and firm (ligamentous) because of the tension in the joint capsule and the medial ligaments (Magee, 2008; Kaltenborn, 2011). If the end feel is hard, it may be due to contact between the calcaneus and the sinus tarsi. Normal range of motion is 0–5 degrees (Figure 13.52) (American Academy of Orthopedic Surgeons, 1965).

Forefoot Inversion

Place the patient in the sitting position with the leg dangling over the side of the treatment table and the knee flexed to 90 degrees or in the supine position with the foot over the end of the treatment table. Make sure that the hip is at zero degrees of rotation, and adduction and abduction. Place one hand under the calcaneus to stabilize the calcaneus and talus and prevent dorsiflexion at the talocrural joint and inversion of the subtalar joint. Place your other hand over the lateral aspect of the foot over the metatarsals with your thumb on the dorsal aspect facing medially and the other four fingers on the plantar surface. Move the foot medially. The normal end feel is abrupt and firm (ligamentous) because of the tension in the joint capsule and the lateral ligaments (Magee, 2008;

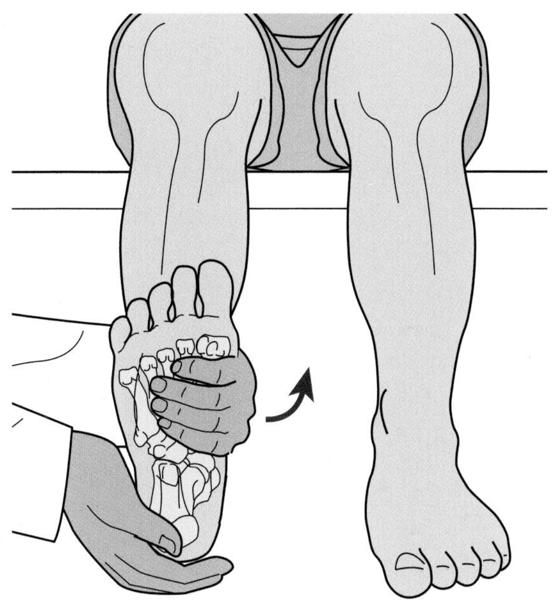

Figure 13.53 Passive movement testing of forefoot inversion.

Kaltenborn, 2011). Normal range of motion is 0–35 degrees (Figure 13.53) (American Academy of Orthopedic Surgeons, 1965).

Forefoot Eversion

Place the patient in the sitting position with the leg dangling over the side of the treatment table and the knee flexed to 90 degrees or in the supine position with the foot over the end of the treatment table. Make sure that the hip is at zero degrees of rotation, and adduction and abduction. Place one hand under the calcaneus to stabilize the calcaneus and talus and prevent dorsiflexion at the talocrural joint and inversion of the subtalar joint. Place your other hand under the distal plantar aspect of the foot with your thumb on the medial aspect of the first metatarsophalangeal joint and the other four fingers around the fifth metatarsal. Move the foot laterally. The normal end feel is abrupt and firm (ligamentous) because of the tension in the joint capsule and the medial ligaments (Magee, 2008; Kaltenborn, 2011). Normal range of motion is 0–15 degrees (Figure 13.54) (American Academy of Orthopedic Surgeons, 1965).

Flexion of the Metatarsophalangeal Joint

Place the patient in the sitting position with the leg dangling over the side of the treatment table and the knee flexed to 90 degrees or in the supine position with the foot over the end of the treatment table. Make sure that the metatarsophalangeal joint is at zero degrees of abduction–adduction. The interphalangeal joints should be maintained at zero degrees of flexion–extension. If the ankle is allowed to plantarflex or the interphalangeal joints of the toe being tested are allowed to flex, the range of motion will be limited by increased tension in the extensor digitorum longus and extensor hallucis longus. Place one hand around the distal metatarsals with your thumb on the plantar surface and the fingers across the dorsum to stabilize the foot and prevent plantar flexion. The other hand holds the hallux between the thumb and index finger and flexes the metatarsophalangeal joint. The normal end feel is abrupt and firm (ligamentous) because of the tension in the capsule and the collateral ligaments (Magee, 2008; Kaltenborn, 2011). Normal range of motion is 0–45 degrees for the hallux (Figure 13.55) (American Academy of Orthopedic Surgeons, 1965).

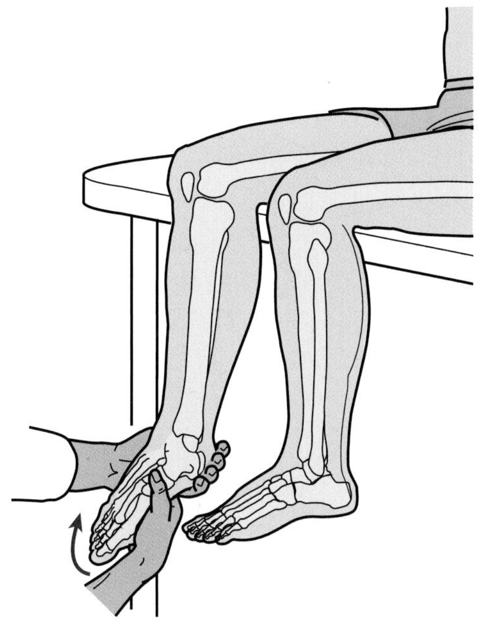

Figure 13.54 Passive movement testing of forefoot eversion.

Extension of the Metatarsophalangeal Joint

Place the patient in the sitting position with the leg dangling over the side of the treatment table and the knee flexed to 90 degrees or in the supine position with the foot over the end of the treatment table. Make sure that the metatarsophalangeal joint is at

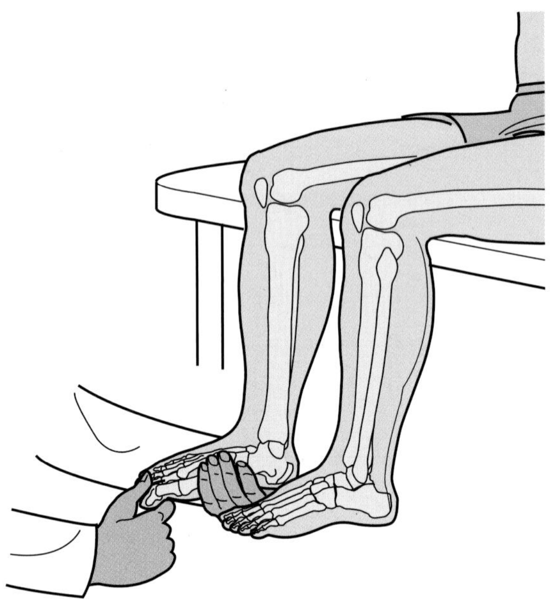

Figure 13.55 Passive movement testing of flexion of the metatarsophalangeal joint.

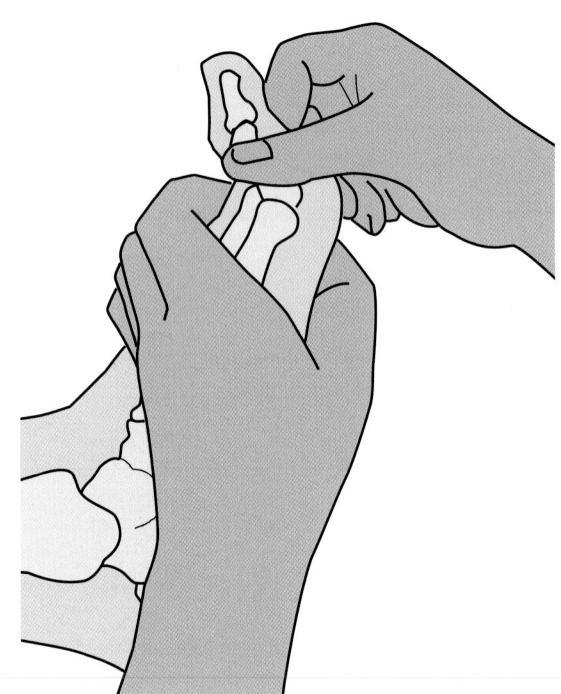

Figure 13.56 Passive movement testing of extension of the metatarsophalangeal joint.

zero degrees of abduction–adduction. The interphalangeal joints should be maintained at zero degrees of flexion–extension. If the ankle is allowed to dorsiflex or the interphalangeal joints of the toe being tested are allowed to extend, the range of motion will be limited by increased tension in the flexor digitorum longus and flexor hallucis longus. Place one hand around the distal metatarsals with your thumb on the plantar surface and the fingers across the dorsum to stabilize the foot and prevent dorsiflexion. The other hand holds the hallux between the thumb and index finger and extends the metatarsophalangeal joint. The normal end feel is abrupt and firm (ligamentous) because of the tension in the plantar capsule, the plantar fibrocartilaginous plate, the flexor hallucis longus, flexor digitorum brevis, and the flexor digiti minimi muscles (Magee, 2008; Kaltenborn, 2011). Normal range of motion is 0–70 degrees for the hallux (Figure 13.56) (American Academy of Orthopedic Surgeons, 1965).

Mobility Testing of the Accessory Movements

Mobility testing of accessory movements will give you information about the degree of laxity present in the joint. The patient must be totally relaxed and comfortable to allow you to move the joint and obtain the most accurate information. The joint should be placed in the maximal loose packed (resting) position to allow for the greatest degree of joint movement. The resting position of the ankle and foot are as follows: talocrural joint, 10 degrees of plantar flexion and midway between maximal inversion and eversion; distal and proximal interphalangeal joints, slight flexion; metatarsophalangeal joints, approximately 10 degrees of extension (Kaltenborn, 2011).

Dorsal and Ventral Glide of the Fibula at the Superior Tibiofibular Joint

Place the patient in the supine position with the knee flexed to approximately 90 degrees. Sit on the side of the treatment table and on the patient's foot to prevent it from sliding. Stabilize the tibia by placing your hand on the proximal ventral aspect. Hold the fibular head by placing your thumb anteriorly and your index finger posteriorly. Pull the fibular head in both a ventral-lateral and then a dorsal-medial direction (Figure 13.57).

Ventral Glide of the Fibula at the Inferior Tibiofibular Joint

Place the patient in the prone position with the foot over the end of the treatment table. Place a rolled

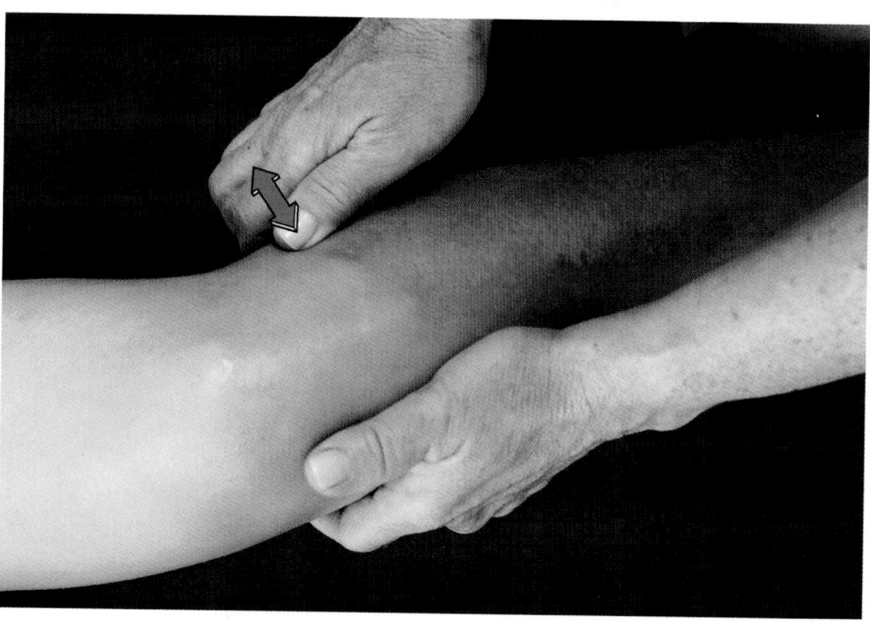

Figure 13.57 Mobility testing of dorsal and ventral glide of the fibula at the superior tibiofibular joint.

towel or a wedge under the distal anterior aspect of the tibia, just proximal to the mortise. Stand at the end of the table facing the medial plantar aspect of the patient's foot. Stabilize the tibia by placing your hand on the medial distal aspect. Using your hand on the posterior aspect of the lateral malleolus, push the fibula in an anterior direction (Figure 13.58).

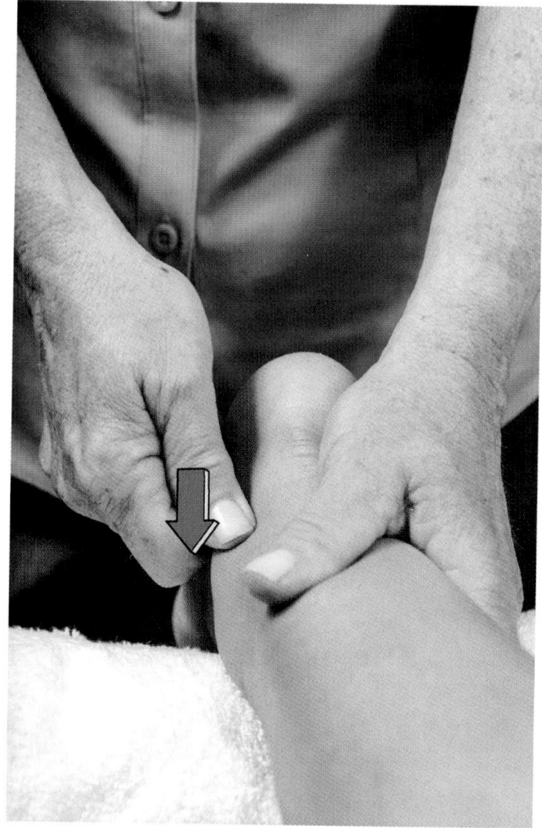

Figure 13.58 Mobility testing of ventral glide of the fibula at the inferior tibiofibular joint.

Traction of the Talocrural Joint

Place the patient in the supine position so that the calcaneus is just past the end of the treatment table. Stand at the end of the table facing the plantar aspect of the foot. Stabilize the tibia by placing your hand on the distal anterior aspect, just proximal to the mortise. Hold the foot so that your fifth finger is over the talus with your other four fingers resting over the dorsum of the foot. Allow your thumb to hold the plantar surface of the foot facing the first metatarsophalangeal joint. Pull the talus in a longitudinal direction, until all the slack is taken up. This produces distraction in the talocrural joint (Figure 13.59).

Traction of the Subtalar Joint

Place the patient in the supine position with the foot at zero degrees of dorsiflexion so that the calcaneus is just past the end of the treatment table. Stand at

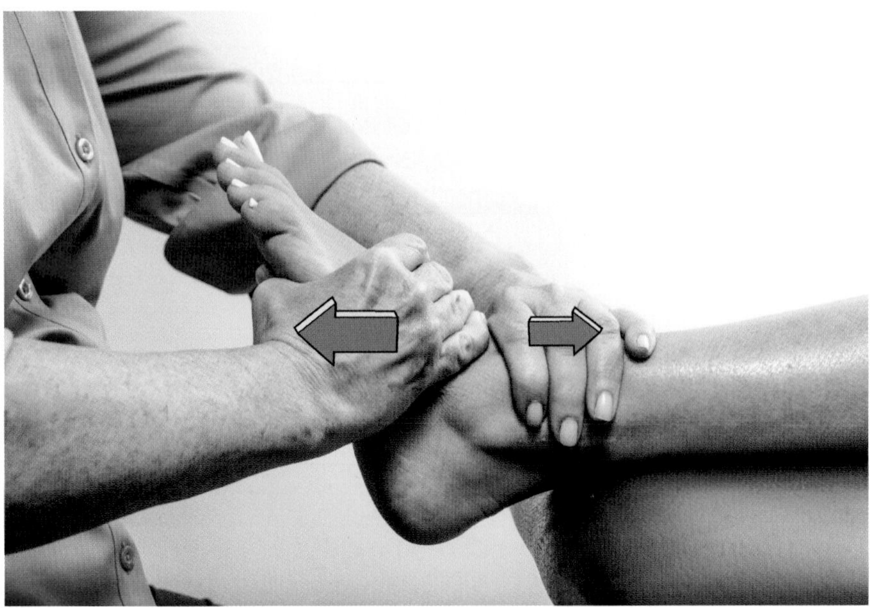

Figure 13.59 Mobility testing of traction of the talocrural joint.

the end of the table facing the plantar aspect of the foot. Maintain the dorsiflexion angle by resting the patient's foot on your thigh. Stabilize the tibia and the talus by placing your hand over the anterior aspect of the talus and the distal anterior aspect of the tibia, just distal to the mortise. Hold the posterior aspect of the calcaneus and pull in a longitudinal direction, until all the slack is taken up, producing distraction in the subtalar joint (Figure 13.60).

Dorsal and Plantar Glide of the Cuboid–Metatarsal Joint

Place the patient in the supine position with the knee flexed to approximately 90 degrees. Stand at the side of the treatment table facing the medial side of the foot. Stabilize the cuboid on the lateral side with your second and third fingers on the dorsal aspect and your thumb on the plantar aspect. Hold the base of the

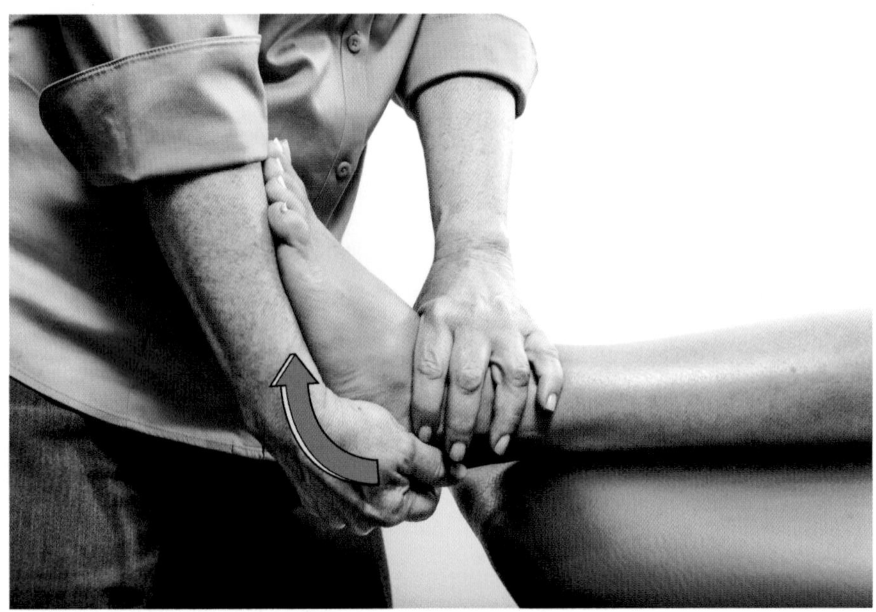

Figure 13.60 Mobility testing of traction of the subtalar joint.

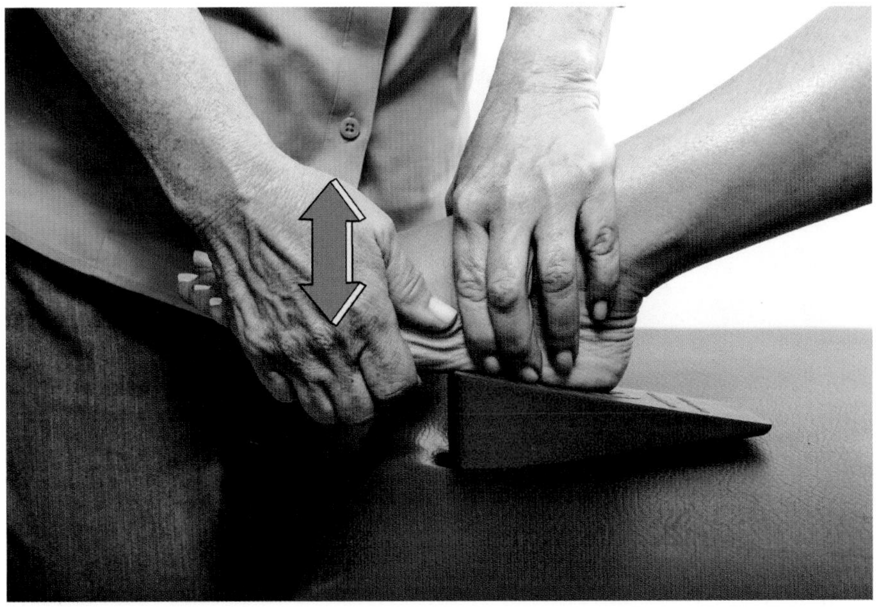

Figure 13.61 Mobility testing of dorsal and plantar glide of the cuboid–metatarsal joint.

fourth and fifth metatarsals with your second and third fingers on the plantar aspect and your thumb on the dorsal aspect. Glide the metatarsals first in a dorsal direction taking up all the slack, and then in a plantar direction (Figure 13.61).

Dorsal and Plantar Glide of the Talonavicular Joint

Place the patient in the prone position and the foot in the resting position on a wedge placed under the anterior talus. Stand at the side of the treatment table facing the lateral side of the foot. Stabilize the talus on the medial side with your second and third fingers, and on the lateral side with your thumb. Use your thumb, second and third fingers to glide the navicular in a dorsal direction to check for restriction in dorsiflexion. (Figure 13.62).

Dorsal and Plantar Glide of the Metatarsals

Place the patient in the supine position with the knee flexed to 90 degrees and the foot flat on the treatment table. Stand on the side of the table facing the dorsal aspect of the patient's foot. Stabilize the second metatarsal from the medial aspect of the foot using your thumb on the dorsal aspect and wrapping your fingers around the first metatarsal toward the plantar aspect. Hold the third metatarsal with your thumb on the dorsal aspect and your fingers on the plantar aspect. Move the third metatarsal in a dorsal direction until all the slack is taken up, allow it to come back to the neutral position, and then move it in a plantar direction. This test can be repeated by stabilizing the second metatarsal and mobilizing the first metatarsal, by stabilizing the third metatarsal and mobilizing the fourth metatarsal, and by stabilizing the fourth metatarsal and mobilizing the fifth metatarsal (Figure 13.63).

Traction of the First Metatarsophalangeal Joint

Place the patient in the supine position with the knee extended. Sit on the side of the treatment table on the lateral aspect of the foot. Stabilize the first metatarsal with your thumb on the dorsal aspect and your fingers wrapped around the plantar surface just proximal to the joint line. Hold the foot against your body for additional stabilization. Hold the first proximal phalanx with your thumb and index fingers. Pull the phalanx in a longitudinal direction until all the slack is taken up, creating traction in the first metatarsophalangeal joint (Figure 13.64).

Resistive Testing

Muscle strength of the ankle is tested in plantar flexion and dorsiflexion. Inversion and eversion of the foot occur at the subtalar joint and are also tested. The toes are examined for flexion and extension strength.

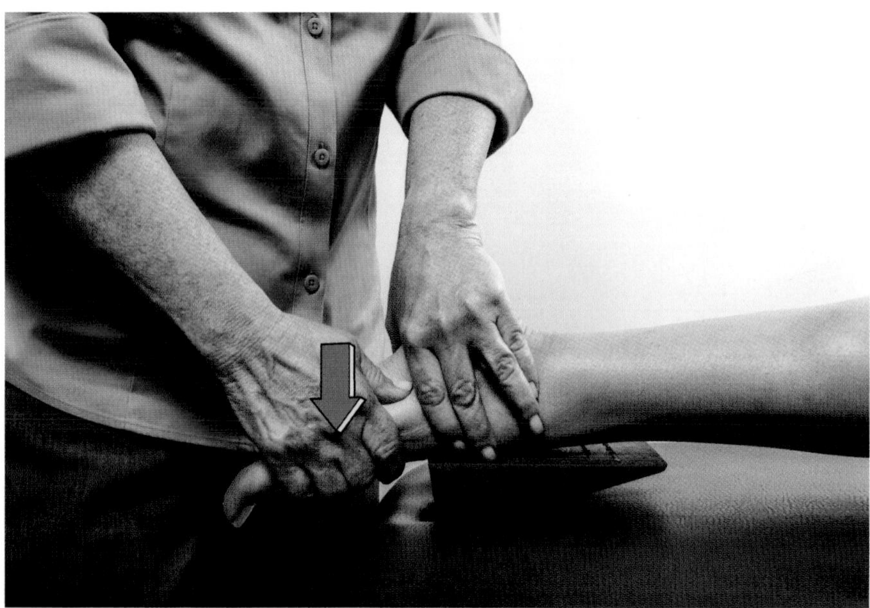

Figure 13.62 Mobility testing of dorsal glide of the talonavicular joint.

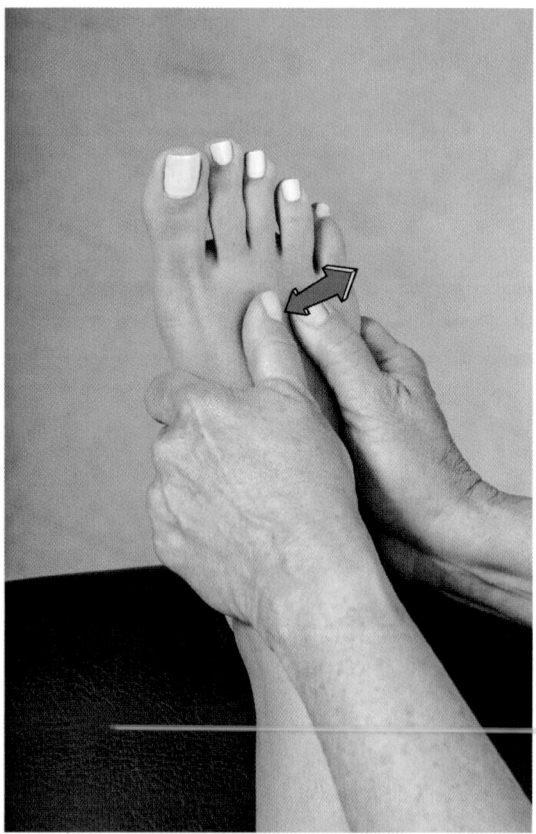

Figure 13.63 Mobility testing of dorsal and plantar glide of the metatarsals.

In testing muscle strength of the foot and ankle, it is important to watch for evidence of muscle substitution. Observe the forefoot for excessive inversion, eversion, plantar flexion, or dorsiflexion. The toes should be observed for movement while testing the ankle. If the ankle muscles are weak, the patient will recruit the flexors or extensors of the toes in an effort to compensate.

Ankle Plantar Flexion

The primary plantar flexors of the ankle are the gastrocnemius and soleus muscles (Figure 13.65). Additional muscles that assist are the tibialis posterior, peroneus longus and brevis, flexor hallucis longus, flexor digitorum longus, and plantaris muscles. All the ankle plantar flexors pass posterior to the ankle joint. It is imperative to observe for downward rotation of the calcaneus. Excessive toe flexion in an attempt to plantarflex the ankle is a result of substitution by the long toe flexors. Excessive inversion during attempts to plantar flex is due to substitution by the tibialis posterior muscle. Excessive eversion is due to substitution by the peroneus longus muscle. The foregoing information is important when the patient is unable to perform normal plantar flexion in a standing position due to weakness of the gastrocsoleus muscle group.

- Position of patient: Standing upright on the foot to be tested (Figure 13.66).

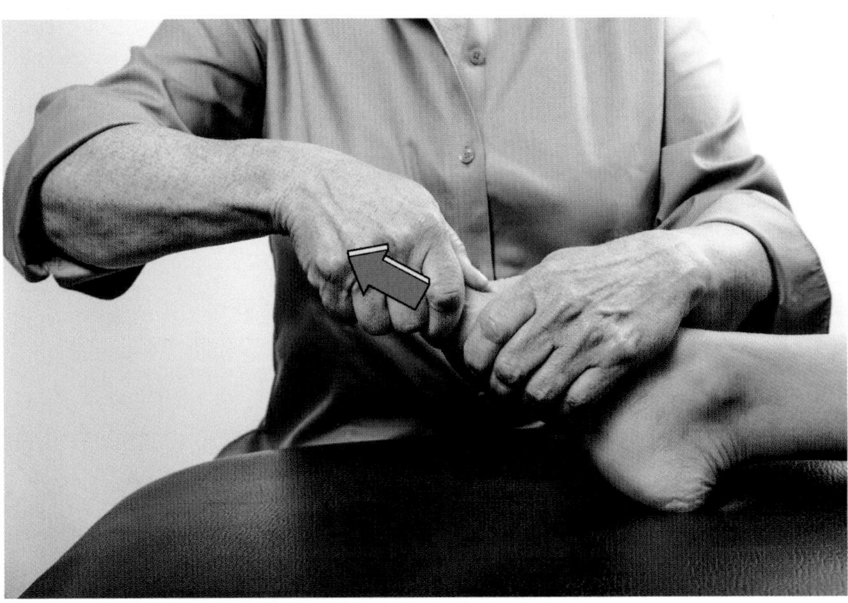

Figure 13.64 Mobility testing of traction of the first metatarsophalangeal joint.

- Resisted test: Ask the patient to stand up on the toes. Resistance is supplied by the body weight of the patient.

Testing plantar flexion of the ankle with gravity eliminated is performed with the patient in a side-lying position and the ankle in neutral position. The patient attempts to plantarflex the foot downward. Observe the patient for substitution by the subtalar invertors/evertors and toe flexors (Figure 13.67).

Painful resisted plantar flexion can be due to Achilles tendinitis or strain of the gastrocnemius or

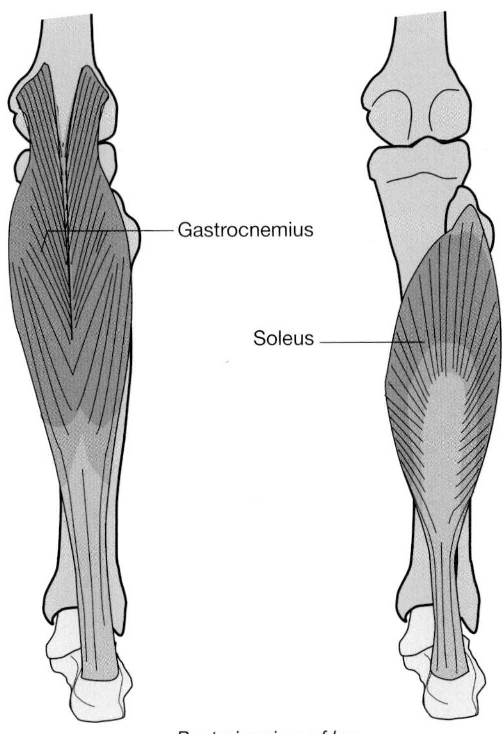

Figure 13.65 Plantar flexors of the ankle.

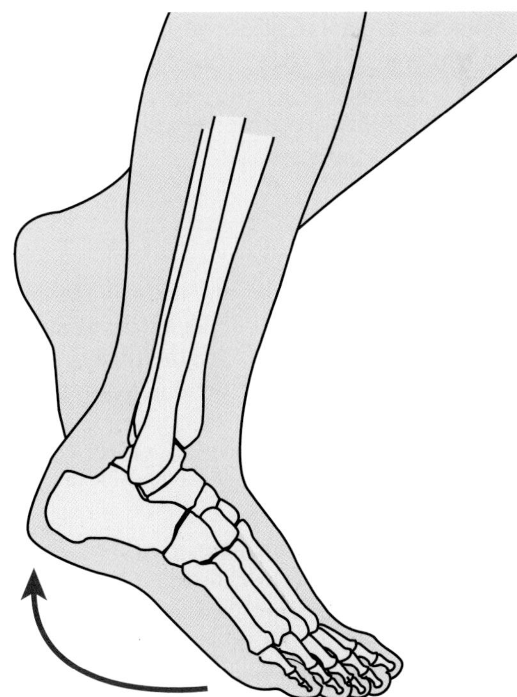

Figure 13.66 Testing ankle plantar flexion.

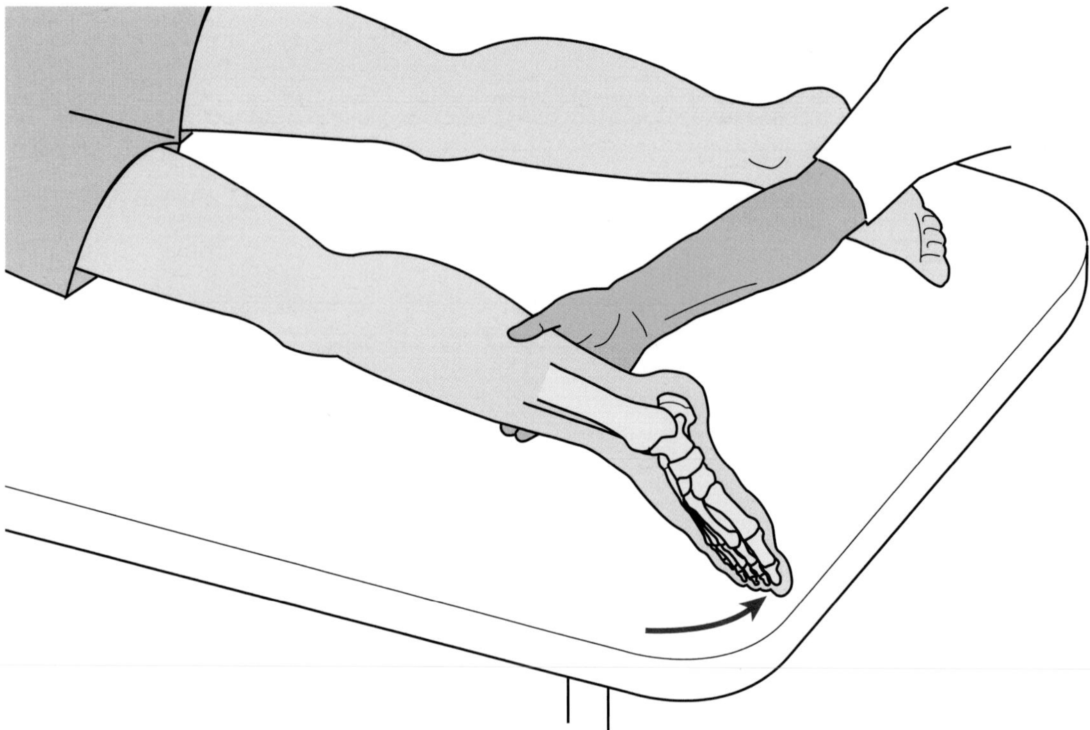

Figure 13.67 Testing plantar flexion with gravity eliminated.

soleus muscle. Pain behind the heel during resisted plantar flexion can be due to retrocalcaneal bursitis.

Weakness of plantar flexion results in an abnormal gait, as well as difficulty with climbing stairs and jumping. Hyperextension deformity of the knee and a calcaneus deformity of the foot may be noted in cases of paralysis (i.e., spina bifida).

Ankle Dorsiflexion

The primary dorsiflexor of the ankle is the tibialis anterior muscle (Figure 13.68). Due to its attachment medial to the subtalar joint axis, the tibialis anterior also inverts the foot. This muscle is assisted by the long toe extensors.

- Position of patient: Sitting with the legs over the edge of the table and the knees flexed to 90 degrees (Figure 13.69).
- Resisted test: Support the patient's lower leg with one hand and apply a downward and everting force to the foot in its midsection as the patient attempts to dorsiflex the ankle and invert the foot. Dorsiflexion can also be tested by asking the patient to walk on his heels with his toes in the air.

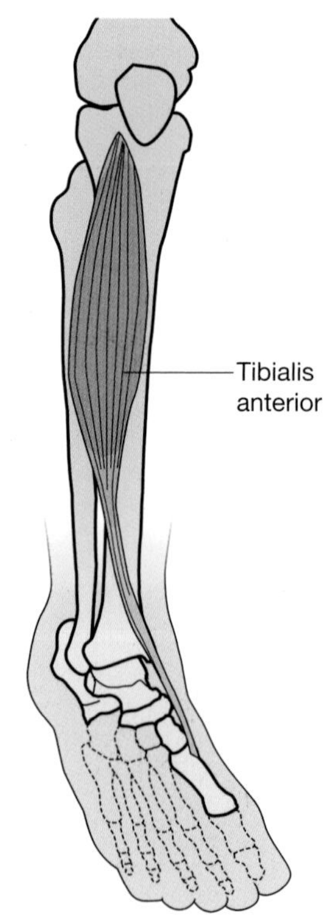

Figure 13.68 The dorsiflexor of the ankle.

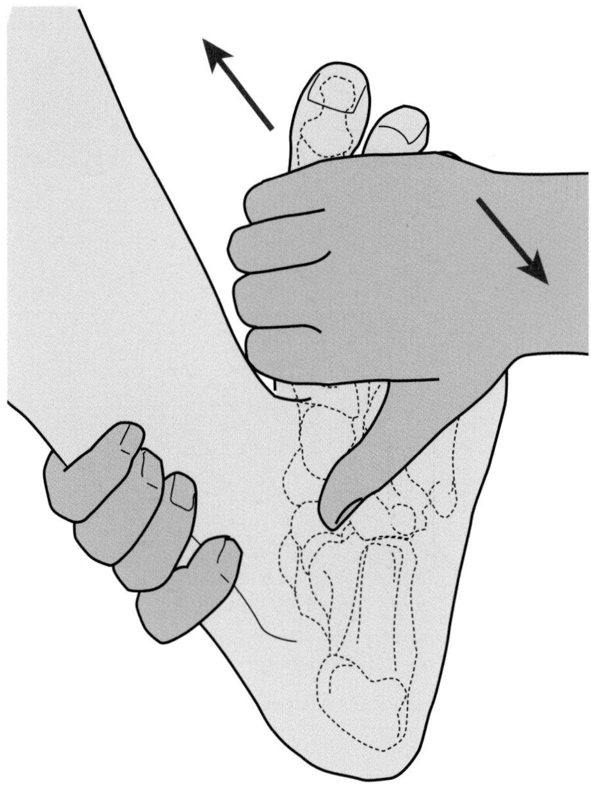

Figure 13.69 Testing dorsiflexion.

Testing dorsiflexion with gravity eliminated is performed by placing the patient in a side-lying position and asking him or her to dorsiflex the ankle. Observe the patient for substitution by the long extensors of the toes. You will see dorsiflexion of the toes if substitution is taking place (Figure 13.70).

Painful resisted dorsiflexion in the anterior tibial region can be due to shin splints at the attachment of the tibialis anterior muscle to the tibia, or an anterior compartment syndrome.

Weakness of dorsiflexion results in foot drop and a steppage gait. An equinus deformity of the foot may result (i.e., as in peroneal palsy).

Subtalar Inversion

Inversion of the foot is brought about primarily by the tibialis posterior muscle (Figure 13.71). Accessory muscles include the flexor digitorum longus and flexor hallucis longus.

- Position of patient: Lying on the side, with the ankle in slight degree of plantar flexion (Figure 13.72).
- Resisted test: Stabilize the lower leg with one hand. The other hand is placed over the medial border of the forefoot. Apply downward pressure on the forefoot as the patient attempts to invert the foot.

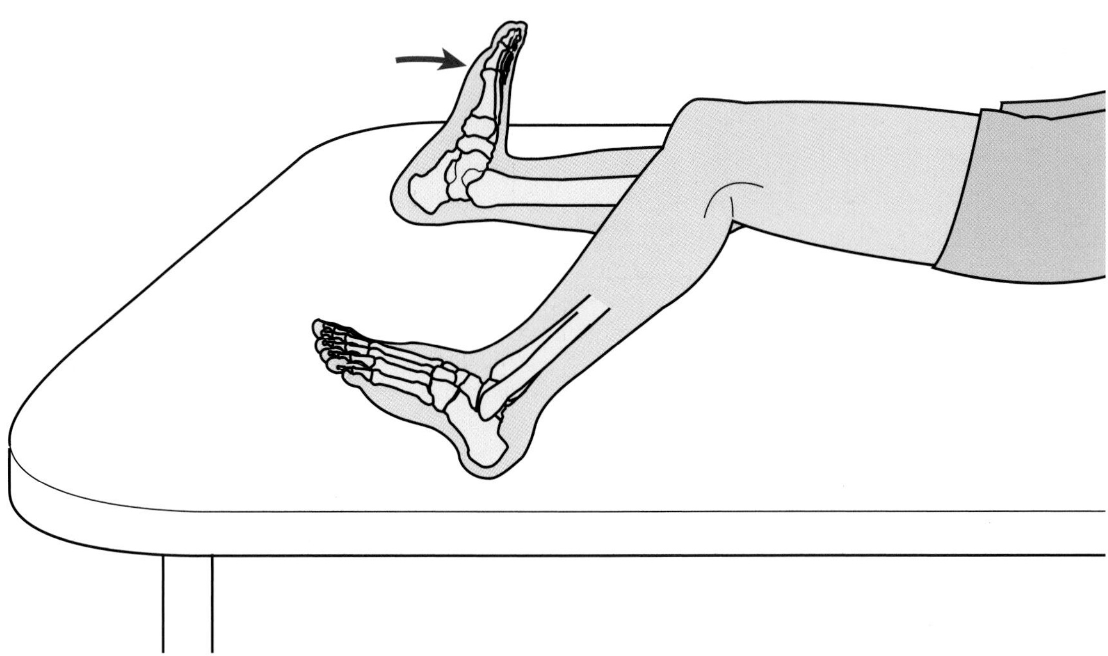

Figure 13.70 Testing dorsiflexion with gravity eliminated.

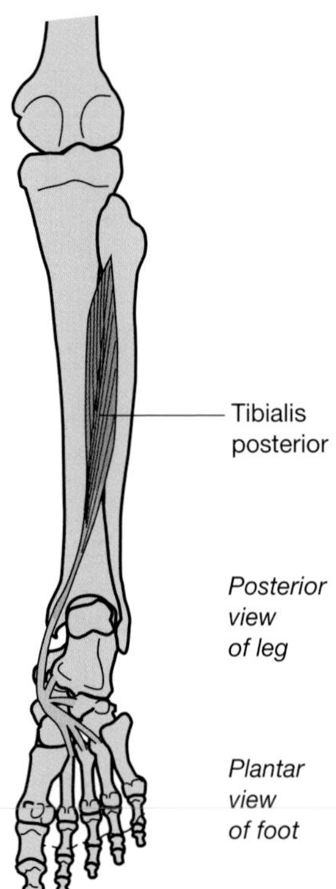

Figure 13.71 The inverters of the foot.

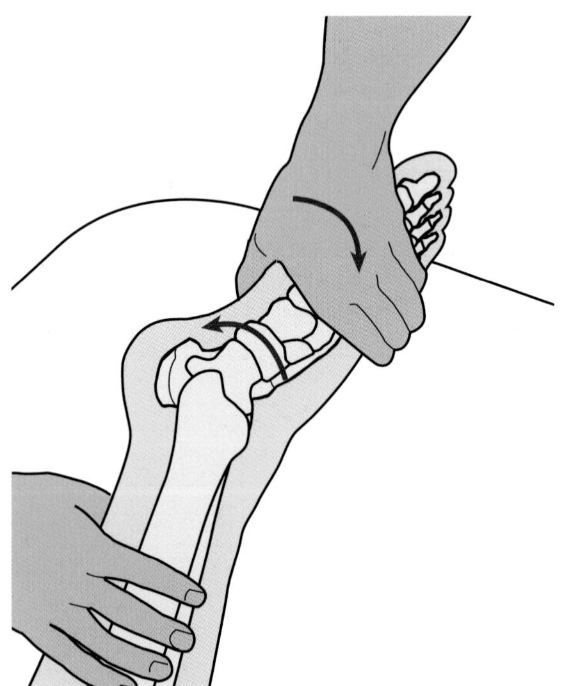

Figure 13.72 Testing subtalar inversion.

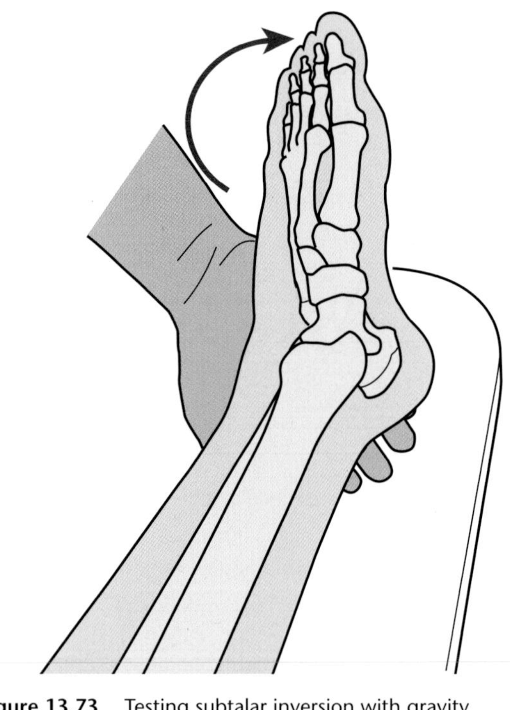

Figure 13.73 Testing subtalar inversion with gravity eliminated.

Testing inversion of the foot with gravity eliminated is performed by having the patient lie in the supine position and attempting to invert the foot through the normal range of motion. Watch for substitution of the flexor hallucis longus and flexor digitorum longus during this procedure, as the toes may flex in an attempt to overcome a weak tibialis posterior (Figure 13.73).

Weakness of foot inversion results in pronation or valgus deformity of the foot and reduced support of the plantar longitudinal arch.

Painful resisted foot inversion can be due to a tendinitis of the tibialis posterior muscle at its attachment to the medial tibia, known as shin splints. Pain can also indicate tendinitis of the tibialis posterior or flexor hallucis longus posterior to the medial malleolus.

Subtalar Eversion

The evertors of the foot are the peroneus longus and peroneus brevis muscles (Figure 13.74). They are assisted by the extensor digitorum longus and peroneus tertius muscles.

- Position of patient: Lying on the non-tested side with the ankle in neutral position (Figure 13.75).

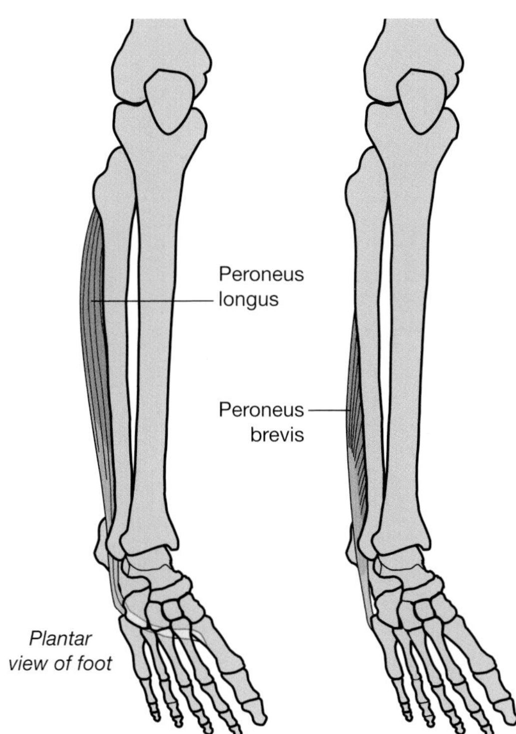

Figure 13.74 The evertors of the foot.

- Resisted test: Stabilize the lower leg of the patient with one hand. The other hand is used to apply a downward pressure on the lateral border of the foot. Ask the patient to raise the lateral border of the foot. This maneuver is more specific for the peroneus brevis.

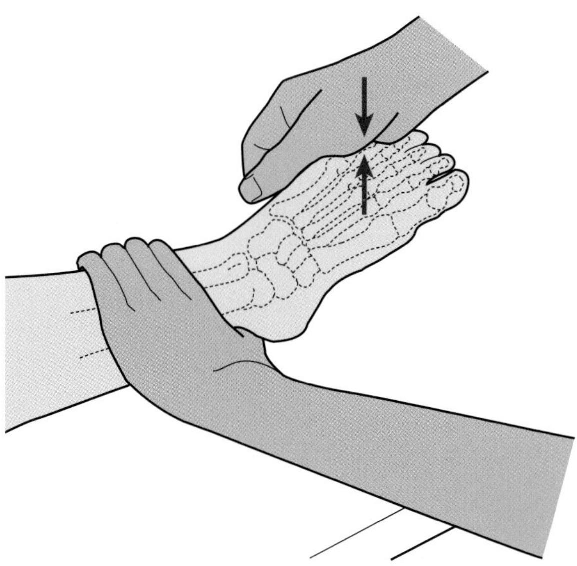

Figure 13.75 Testing subtalar eversion.

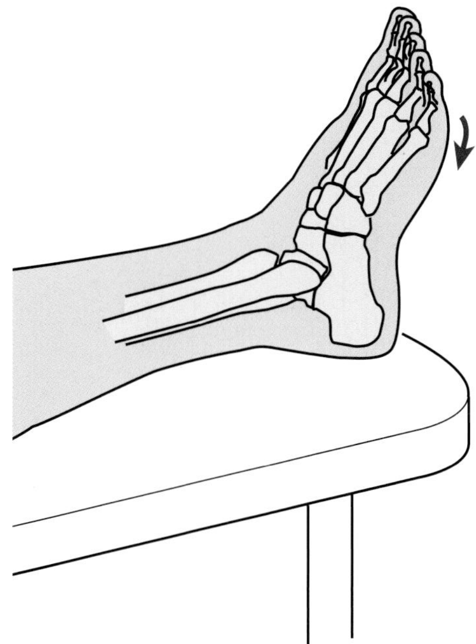

Figure 13.76 Testing subtalar eversion with gravity eliminated.

Testing foot eversion with gravity eliminated is performed by having the patient lie in the supine position and attempting to evert the foot through a normal range of motion. Observe for extension of the toes, as this signifies substitution (Figure 13.76).

Painful resisted foot eversion can be due to tendinitis of the peroneal tendons posterior to the ankle or at the attachment site of the muscles to the fibula. An inversion sprain of the ankle can result in stretching or tearing of the peroneal tendons and painful resisted foot eversion. A snapping sound may be heard as the tendons pass anteriorly over the lateral malleolus.

Weakness of foot eversion may result in a varus position of the foot and cause reduced stability of the lateral aspect of the ankle.

Toe Flexion

The flexors of the toes are the flexor hallucis brevis and longus and the flexor digitorum brevis and longus (Figure 13.77).

- Position of patient: Supine (Figure 13.78).
- Resisted test: Apply an upward pressure to the bottoms of the patient's toes as he or she attempts to flex them. The flexors of the great toe may be examined separately.

Inability to flex the distal phalanx of the toes results from dysfunction of the long flexors.

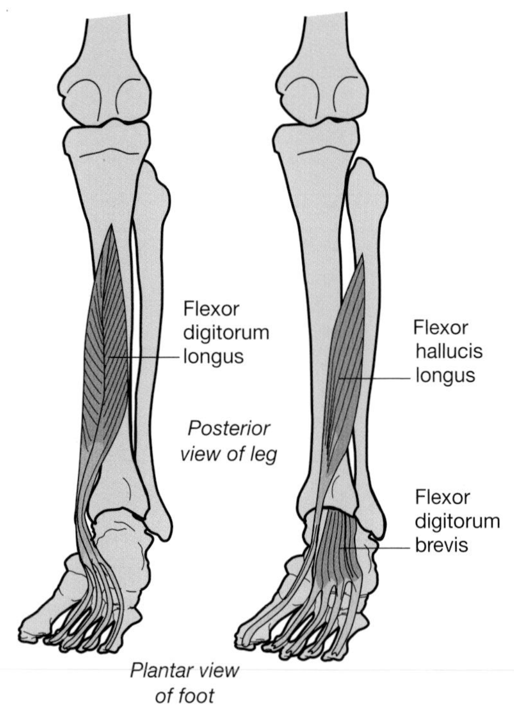

Figure 13.77 The flexors of the toes.

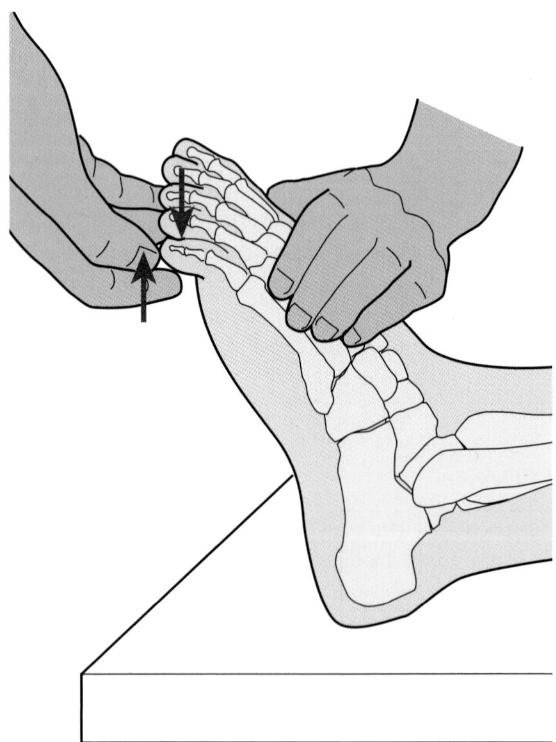

Figure 13.78 Testing toe flexion.

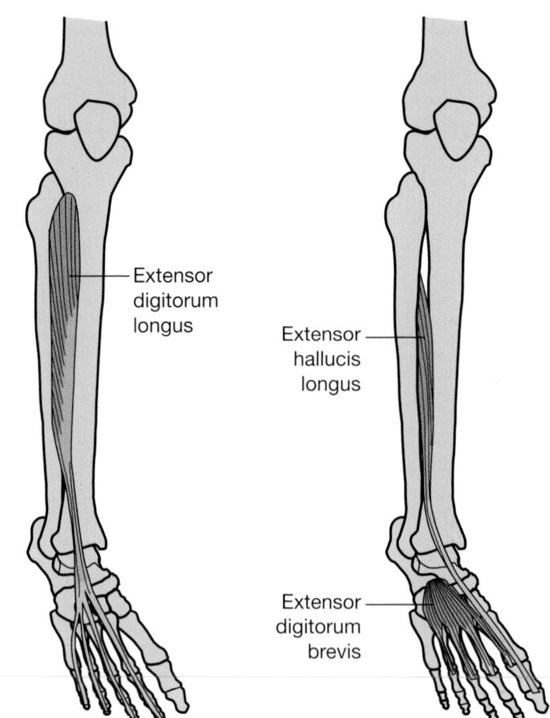

Figure 13.79 The extensors of the toes.

Painful resisted toe flexion may be due to tendinitis of the long flexors.

Toe Extension

The extensors of the toes are the extensor hallucis brevis and longus and the extensor digitorum brevis and longus (Figure 13.79).

- Position of patient: Supine (Figures13.80 and 13.81).
- Resisted test: Apply a downward pressure on the distal phalanx of the great toe, as the patient attempts to extend the toe, to test the extensor hallucis longus. Resistance can be applied to the middle phalanges of the other toes together to test the extensor digitorum longus and brevis.

Weakness of toe extension may result in decreased ability to dorsiflex the ankle and evert the foot. Walking barefoot may be unsafe, due to increased risk of falling as the toes bend under the foot.

Neurological Examination

Motor

The innervation and spinal levels of the muscles that function in the ankle and foot are listed in Table 13.1.

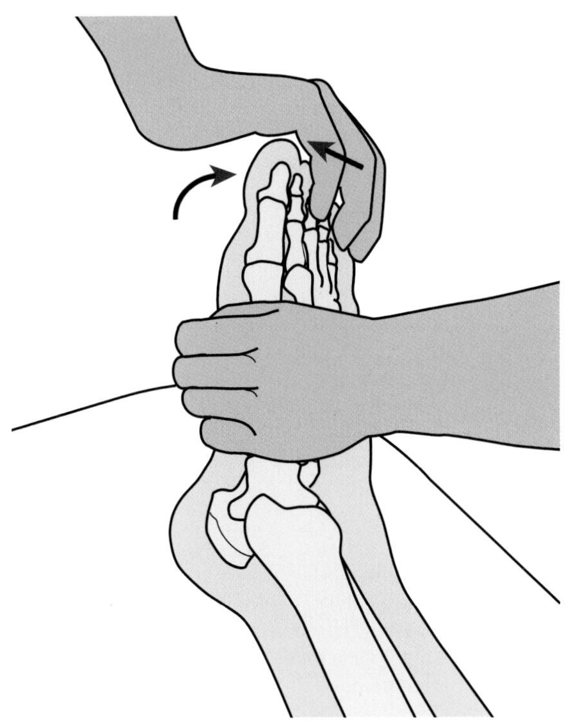

Figure 13.80 Testing toe extension.

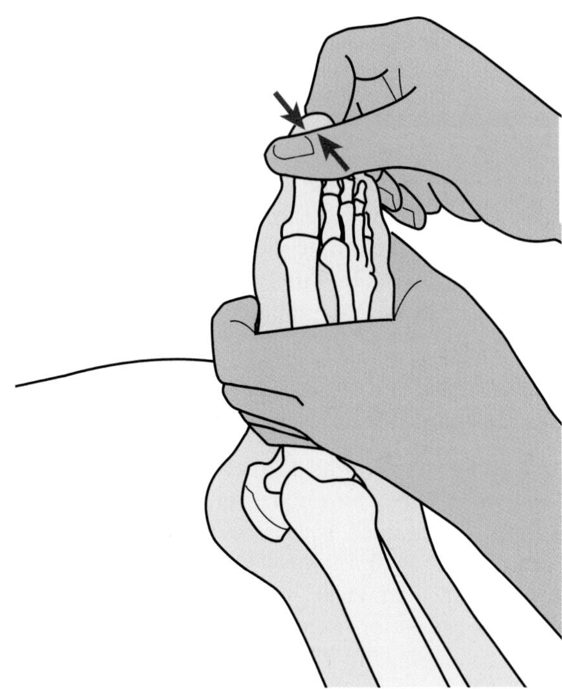

Figure 13.81 Testing great toe extension by the extensor hallucis longus.

Reflexes

The ankle jerk primarily tests the S1 nerve root. It will be diminished or lost in patients with S1 radiculopathy or sciatic or tibial nerve damage. Loss of continuity of the Achilles tendon will also result in loss of an ankle jerk.

The ankle jerk is easily elicited when the patient is relaxed (Figure 13.82). Have the patient sit on the edge of the table with the knees flexed to 90 degrees. Support the ball of the patient's foot gently upward with one hand while asking him or her to relax and try not to assist in dorsiflexion of the foot. Take the reflex hammer and gently tap the Achilles tendon to elicit a plantar flexion response at the ankle. The test can also be performed with the patient prone with the feet off the edge of the table. In this position, the Achilles tendon is tapped with the reflex hammer. Always compare findings bilaterally.

Sensation

Light touch and pinprick sensation should be examined following the motor examination. The dermatomes of the lower leg are L3, L4, L5, S1, and S2 (Figure 13.83). Note the location of the key sensory areas for the L4, L5, and S1 dermatomes. The peripheral nerves providing the sensation to the leg and foot are shown in Figures13.84, 13.85, and 13.86.

Referred Pain Patterns

Pain in the leg and foot may be referred from the lumbar spine, sacrum, hip, or knee (Figure 13.87).

Special Tests

Special Neurological Tests

Tests for Nerve Compression

Peroneal (Fibular) Nerve Compression

The common peroneal (fibular) nerve can be injured where it wraps around the head of the fibula and is close to the skin (Figure 13.88). Tinel's sign may be elicited inferior and lateral to the fibular head by tapping with a reflex hammer. The patient will note a tingling sensation down the lateral aspect of the leg and onto the dorsum of the foot. The patient will have a foot drop.

Table 13.1 Movements of the Ankle and Foot: The Muscles and their Nerve Supply, as well as their Nerve Root Derivations, are Shown

Movement	Muscles	Innervation	Root Levels
Plantar flexion of ankle	Gastrocnemius	Tibial	S1,S2
	Soleus	Tibial	S1,S2
	Flexor digitorum longus	Tibial	L5, S1,S2
	Flexor hallucis longus	Tibial	L5, S1,S2
	Peroneus longus	Superficial peroneal	L5, S1
	Peroneus brevis	Superficial peroneal	L5, S1
	Tibialis posterior	Tibial	L4, L5, S1
Dorsiflexion of ankle	Tibialis anterior	Deep peroneal	L4, L5
	Extensor digitorum longus	Deep peroneal	L4, L5, S1
	Extensor hallucis longus	Deep peroneal	L5, S1
	Peroneus tertius	Deep peroneal	L4, L5, S1
Inversion	Tibialis posterior	Tibial	L4, L5, S1
	Flexor digitorum longus	Tibial	L5, S1,S2
	Flexor hallucis longus	Tibial	L5, S1,S2
	Extensor hallucis longus	Deep peroneal	L5, S1
	Tibialis anterior	Deep peroneal	L4, L5
Eversion	Peroneus longus	Superficial peroneal	L5, S1
	Peroneus brevis	Superficial peroneal	L5, S1
	Extensor digitorum longus	Deep peroneal	L4, L5, S1
	Peroneus tertius	Deep peroneal	L4, L5, S1
Flexion of toes	Flexor digitorum longus	Tibial	L5, S1, S2
	Flexor hallucis longus	Tibial	L5, S1, S2
	Flexor digitorum brevis	Tibial (medial plantar)	L5, S1
	Flexor hallucis brevis	Tibial (medial plantar)	L5, S1
	Flexor digit minimi	Tibial (lateral plantar)	S1, S2
Extension of toes	Extensor digitorum longus	Deep peroneal	L4, L5, S1
	Extensor hallucis longus	Deep peroneal	L5, S1
	Extensor digitorum brevis	Deep peroneal	S1
Abduction of great toe	Abductor hallucis	Tibial (medial plantar)	S1,S2

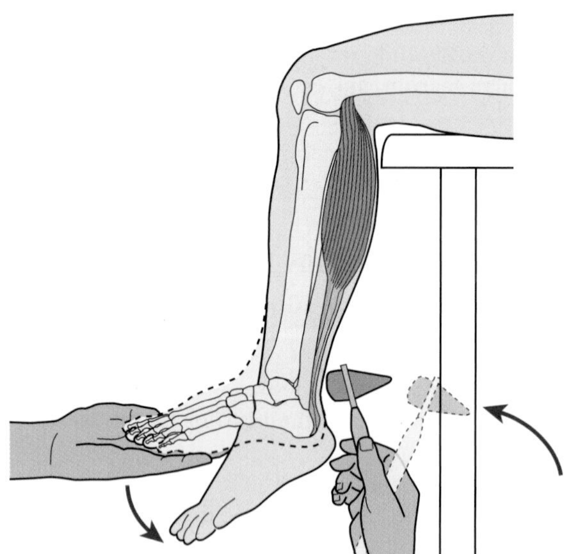

Figure 13.82 Testing the ankle jerk.

Tarsal Tunnel Syndrome

Entrapment of the posterior tibial nerve underneath the flexor retinaculum at the tarsal tunnel may also occur (Figure 13.89). Tinel's sign may be obtained inferior to the medial malleolus by tapping with a reflex hammer.

Tests for Upper Motor Neuron Involvement

Babinski's response and Oppenheim's test are used to diagnose upper motor neuron disease. Babinski's response is obtained by scratching the foot on the plantar aspect from the heel to the upper lateral sole and across the metatarsal heads (Figure 13.90). A positive response is dorsiflexion of the great toe. Flexion of the foot, knee, and hip can occur concomitantly.

Oppenheim's test is performed by running a knuckle or fingernail up the anterior tibial surface. A positive response is the same as for Babinski's response (Figure 13.91).

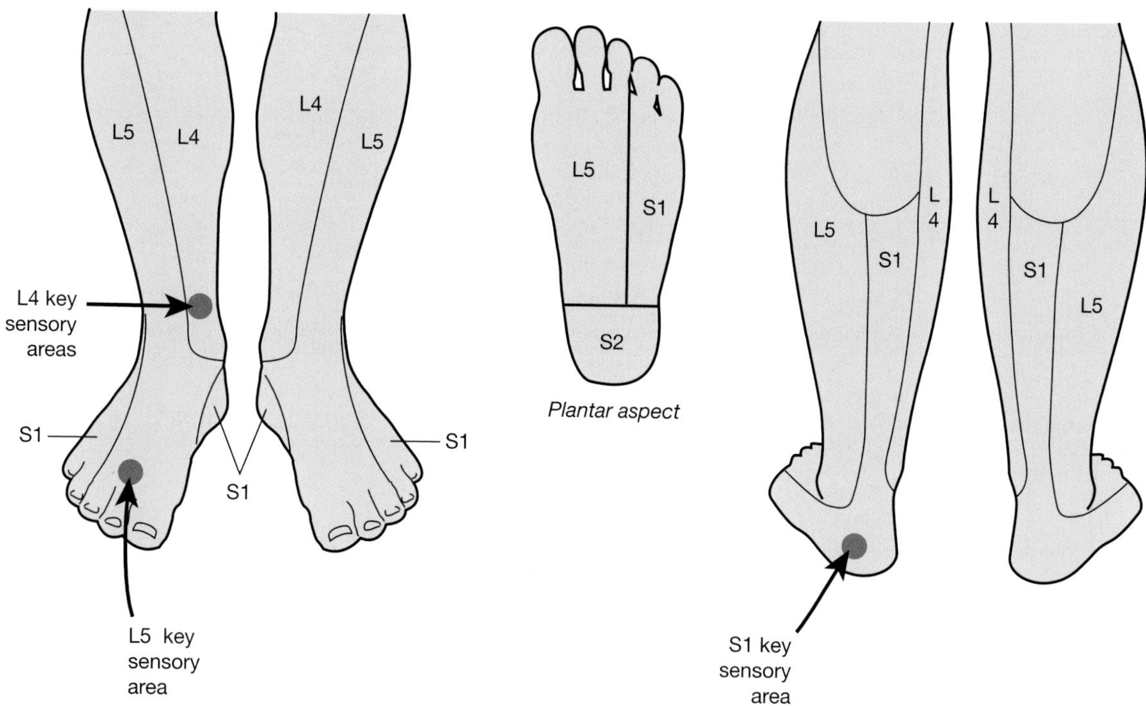

Figure 13.83 The dermatomes of the lower leg, foot, and ankle. Note the key sensory areas for L4, L5, and S1.

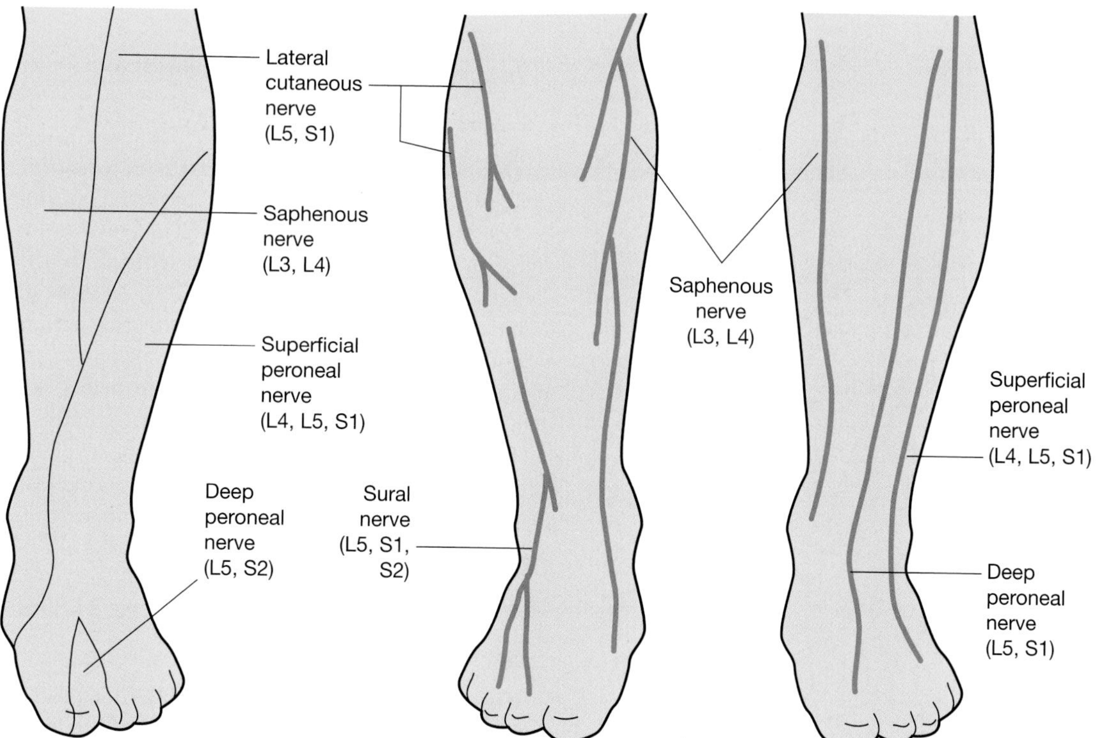

Figure 13.84 Anterior view of the peripheral nerves of the lower leg and foot and their distributions.

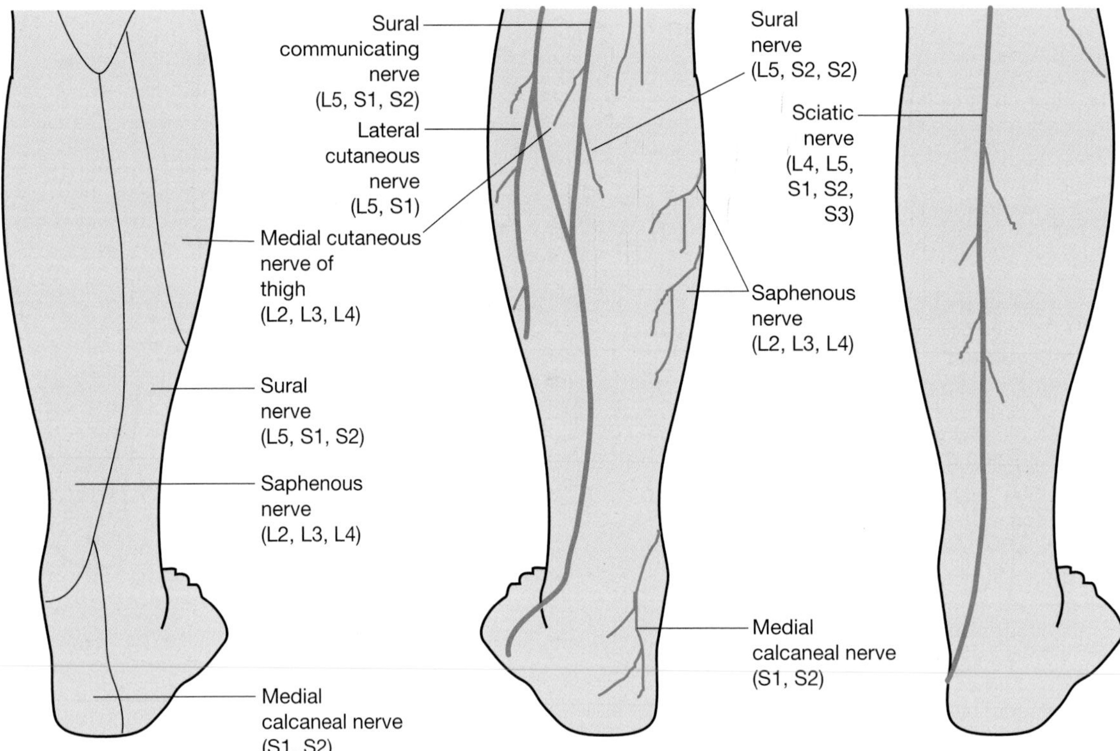

Figure 13.85 Posterior view of the peripheral nerves of the lower leg and foot with their distributions.

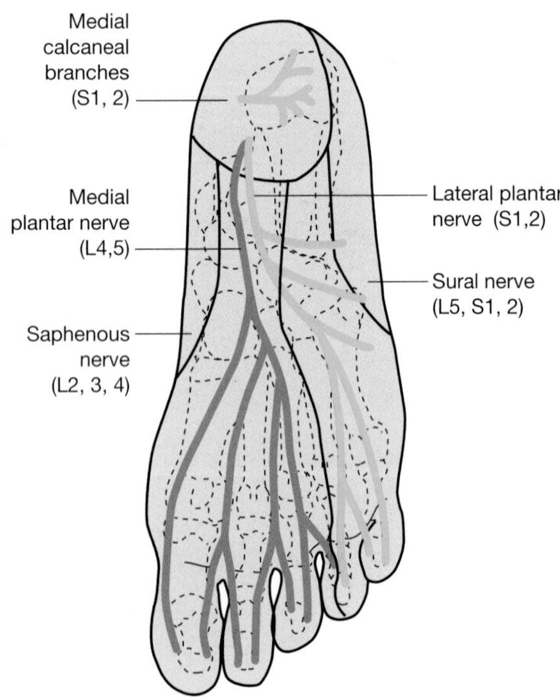

Figure 13.86 The nerves of the plantar surface of the foot.

Tests for Structural Integrity

Ligament and Tendon Integrity

Thompson Test for Achilles Tendon Rupture

This test is performed to confirm rupture of the Achilles tendon (Figure 13.92). The tendon often ruptures at a site 2–6 cm proximal to the calcaneus, which coincides with a critical zone of circulation. The test is performed with the patient prone and the feet dangling over the edge of the table. Squeeze the gastrocnemius muscle firmly with your hand and observe for evidence of plantar flexion. The absence of plantar flexion is a positive test result. Also, observe the patient for excessive passive dorsiflexion and a palpable gap in the tendon (https://www.youtube.com/watch?v=8kxPFjSJj0k).

Anterior Drawer Sign

This test is used to determine whether there is structural integrity of the anterior talofibular ligament, anterior joint capsule, and calcaneofibular band (Figure 13.93). The test is performed with the patient sitting with the knees flexed over the edge of the table,

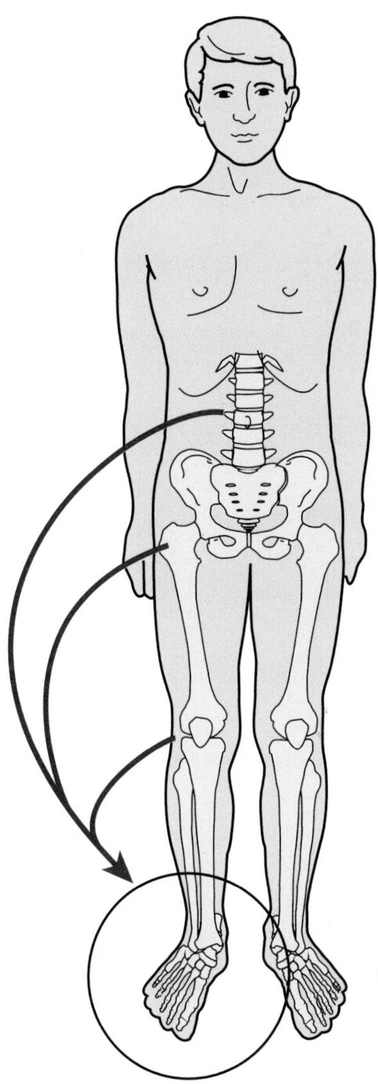

Figure 13.87 Pain in the leg and foot may be due to pathology in the lumbar spine, sacrum, hip, or knee.

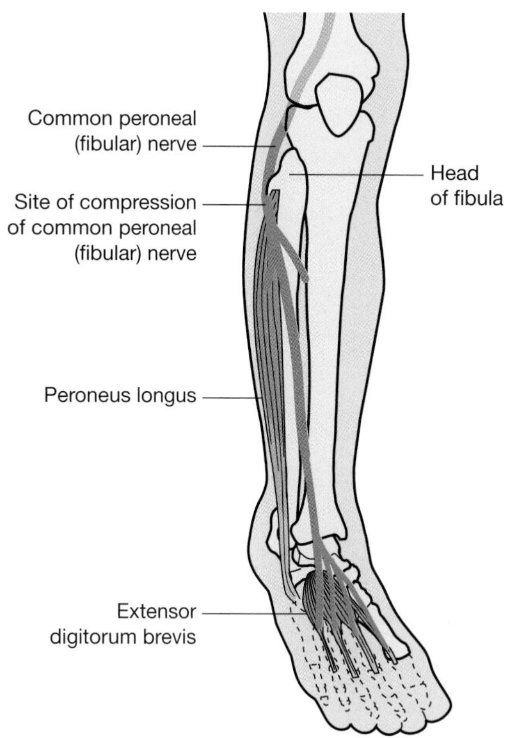

Figure 13.88 The peroneal (fibular) nerve is shown at its most common site of compression, where it wraps around the fibular head.

or in supine. Stabilize the anterior distal tibia with one hand and take the calcaneus in the palm of the opposite hand. Place the ankle in 20 degrees of plantar flexion. This position makes the anterior talofibular ligament perpendicular to the lower leg. Now attempt to bring the calcaneus and talus forward out of the ankle mortise. Excessive anterior movement of the foot, which is often accompanied by a clunk, is a positive anterior drawer sign. This test can also be performed with the patient in the supine position with the hips and knees flexed. The reliability depends in part on the ability of the patient to relax and cooperate (https://www.youtube.com/watch?v=zjauu5gXF2A).

Inversion Stress Test

This test is performed if the anterior drawer test result is positive. This test uncovers damage to the calcaneofibular ligament, which is responsible for preventing excessive inversion. The patient is positioned either seated at the edge of the table or in the supine position (Figure 13.94). Stabilize the anterior distal aspect of the tibia. Cup the patient's heel in your hand and attempt to invert the calcaneus and talus. Excessive inversion movement of the talus within the ankle mortise is a positive test result (https://www.youtube.com/watch?v=v-PcTW5Bj1c).

Bone Integrity

Test for Stress Fractures

Stress fractures are common in the bones of the lower leg and foot. If a stress fracture is suspected, the area of localized tenderness over the bone can be examined with a tuning fork. Placing the tuning fork onto the painful area will cause increased pain in a stress fracture. This test should not be relied on without the benefit of x-rays or MRI testing.

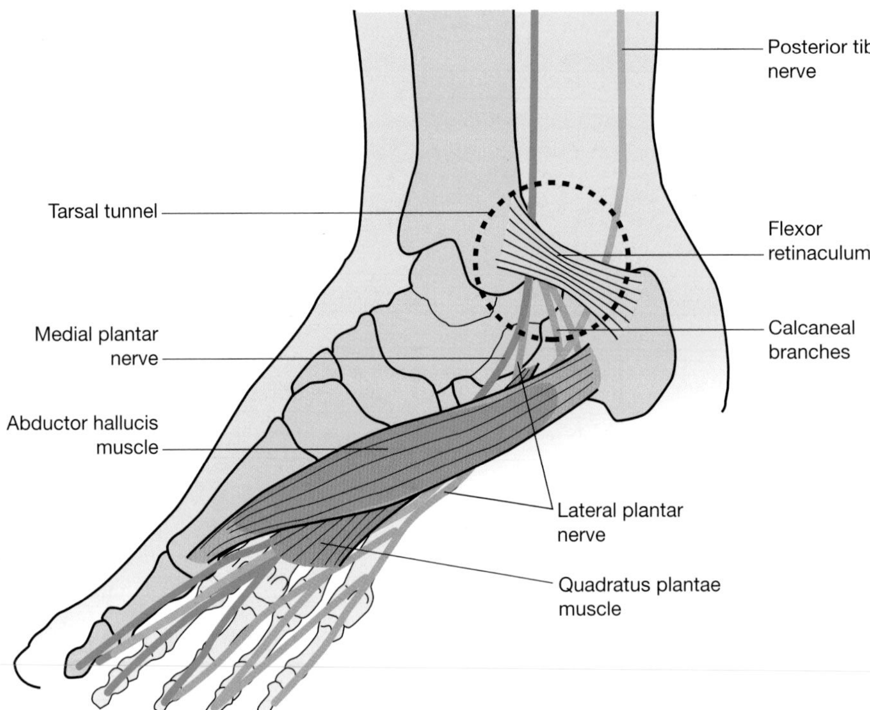

Figure 13.89 The anatomy of the tarsal tunnel. The posterior tibial nerve passes underneath the flexor retinaculum and is subject to compression at this site.

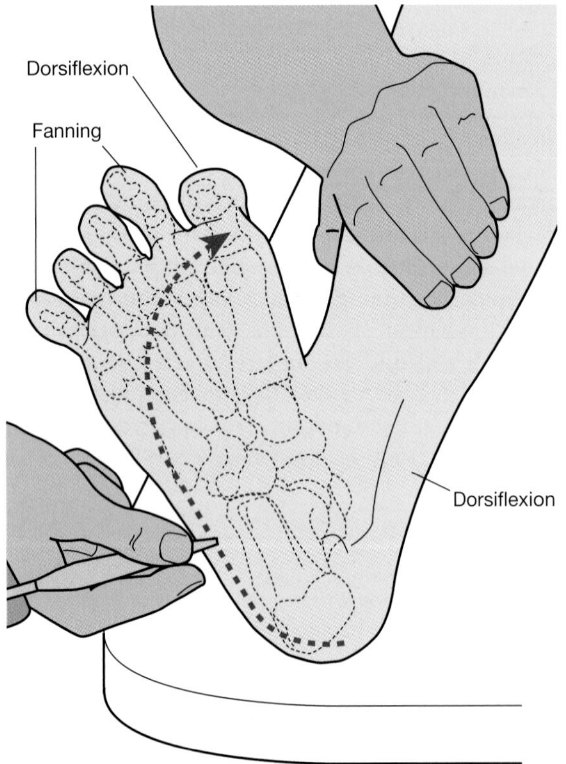

Figure 13.90 Babinski's response is found in patients with upper motor neuron disease.

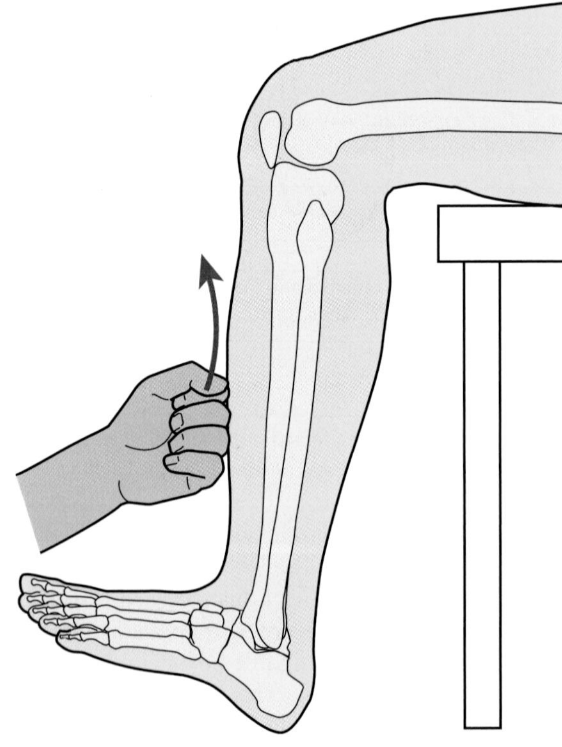

Figure 13.91 Oppenheim's sign is found in patients with upper motor neuron disease.

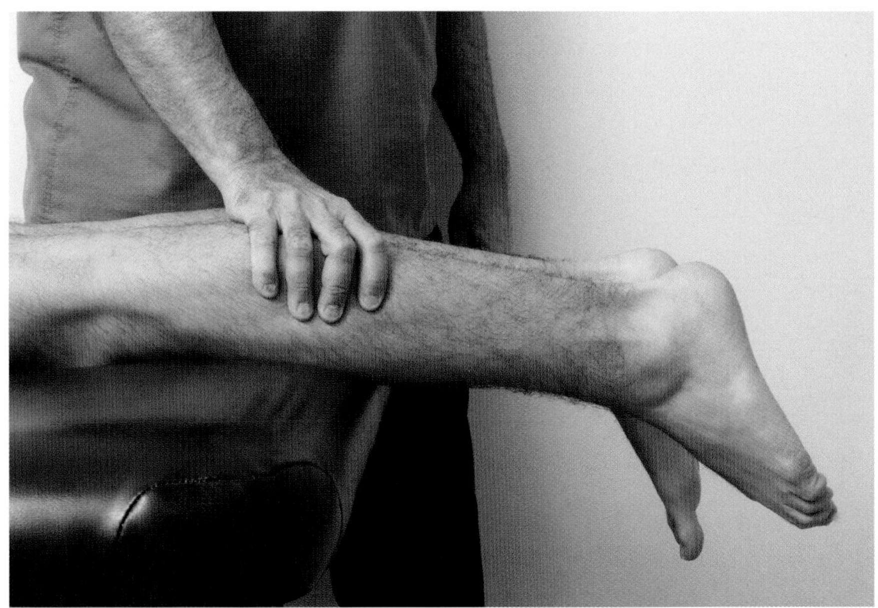

Figure 13.92 The Thompson test for continuity of the Achilles tendon. Absence of plantar flexion on squeezing the calf indicates a ruptured Achilles tendon (or a fused ankle joint).

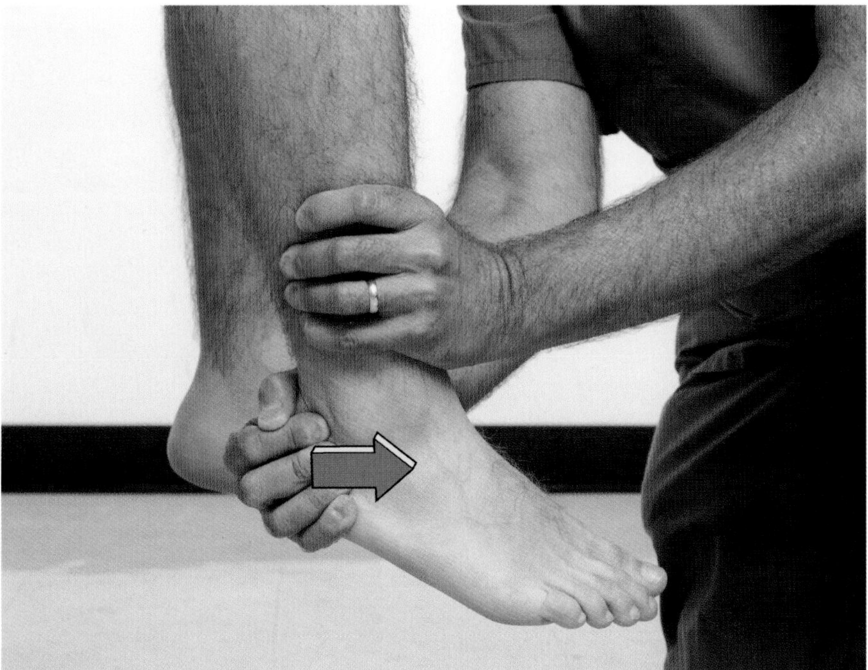

Figure 13.93 Testing anterior drawer of the ankle. Excessive anterior movement of the foot indicates a tear of the anterior talofibular ligament.

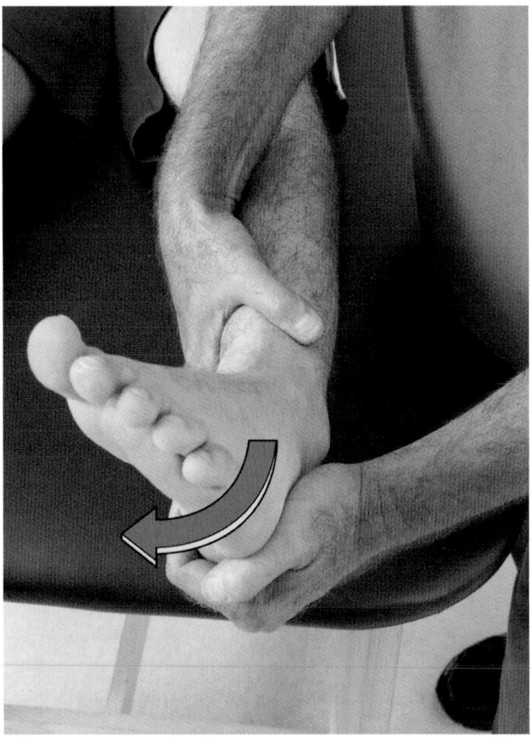

Figure 13.94 Inversion stress test of the ankle. Excessive foot inversion indicates a tear of the calcaneofibular ligament.

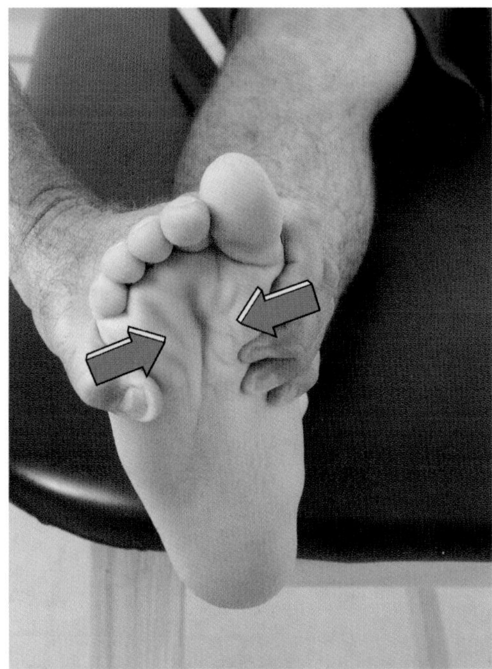

Figure 13.95 Morton's neuromas develop in the second or third web space where the interdigital nerves branch. They may be painful to palpation and metatarsal compression.

Neural Integrity

Test for Morton's Neuroma

A Morton's neuroma develops in the second or third web space where the interdigital nerves branch (Figure 13.95). By holding the foot with your hand and squeezing the metatarsals together, a click may be heard. This occurs in patients with advanced Morton's neuroma and is called a *Moulder's click*.

Vascular Integrity

Homan's Sign

This maneuver is used to aid in the diagnosis of thrombophlebitis of the deep veins of the leg (Figure 13.96). The test is performed by passively dorsiflexing the patient's foot with the knee extended. Pain in the calf is considered a positive Homan's sign. Swelling, tenderness, and warmth of the lower leg are also indicative of deep vein thrombosis.

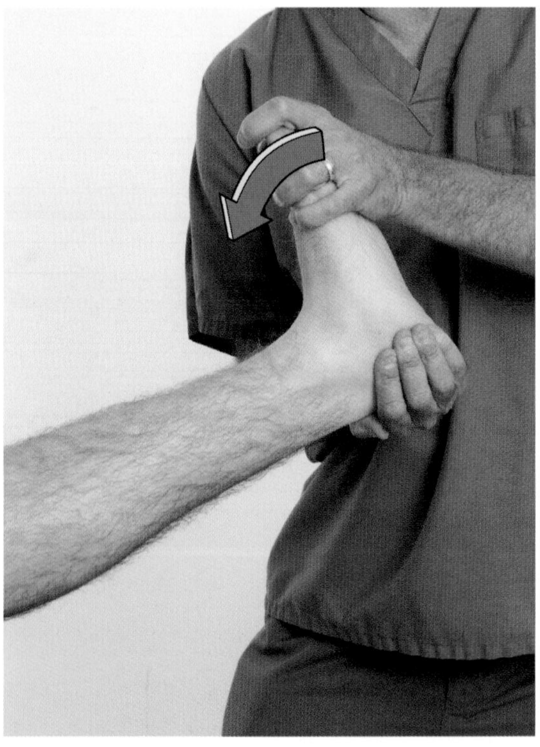

Figure 13.96 Homan's sign is used to test for deep vein thrombophlebitis. This stretching maneuver places the deep veins of the calf on stretch.

Buerger's Test

This test is used to determine if there is arterial insufficiency in the leg. The patient is laid as flat as possible in supine. Support and lift the lower leg to an angle of 30 degrees. Hold the leg in this position for 2 minutes. Observe the color of the leg and foot. If the leg or foot is pale, there is reduced arterial blood flow. Next, have the patient sit up and allow their foot and leg to dangle over the edge of the table. If the toes and then the foot turn bright red (termed *dependent rubor*), there is arterial insufficiency in the leg.

Tests for Alignment

Deviations from normal alignment of the forefoot and hindfoot are common. Abnormal weight-bearing forces due to these deviations cause pain and disorders such as tendinitis, stress fractures, corns, and other pressure problems. Frequently, abnormal alignment patterns, which are initially flexible, become rigid. The most common abnormality is a hindfoot valgus with compensatory forefoot varus, which is known as *pes planus* or a *flat foot*.

Test for Flexible Versus Rigid Flat Foot

A curved medial longitudinal arch should normally be observed when the patient is both sitting and standing. If a medial longitudinal arch is noted in an unloaded position and disappears when the patient stands, this is referred as a *flexible flat foot* (Figure 13.97). If the patient does not have a visible arch in an unloaded position, this is known as a *rigid flat foot* (Figure 13.98).

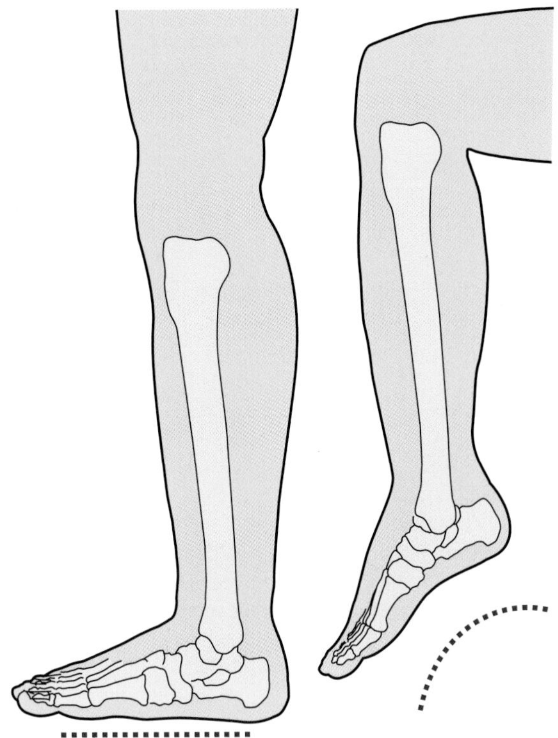

Figure 13.97 Flexible flat feet are only visible in the standing position. The normal plantar arch is noted in an unloaded position.

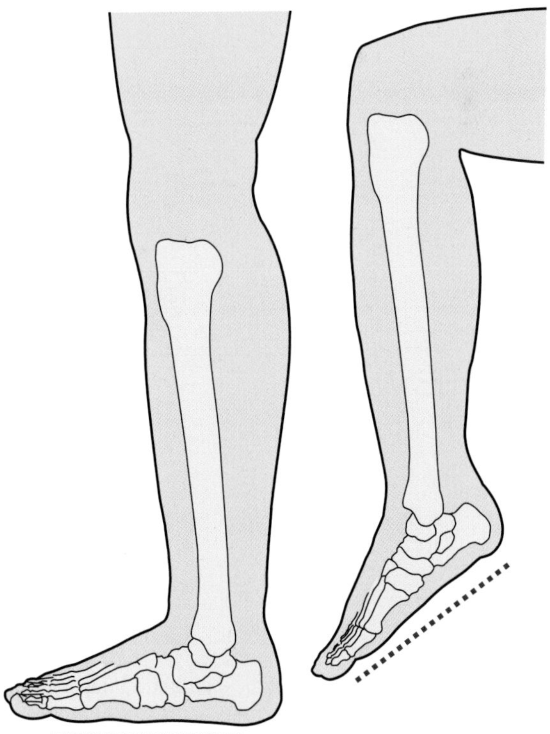

Figure 13.98 Rigid flat feet remain flat in any position.

Test for Medial Longitudinal Arch

Feiss' Line

The patient is in the supine position. Palpate and then mark the medial malleolus and the first metatarsophalangeal joint. Imagine a line between the two structures. Then locate the navicular tubercle and note where it is situated in relation to the line. Have the patient weight-bear and reassess the location of the navicular tubercle. Divide the space between the line and the floor into thirds. The navicular tubercle should normally lie close to the line. If it is lower, the degree of pes planus is determined by its relative location and is graded as first degree pes planus (one-third of the way from the line), second degree if it is two-thirds of the way, and third degree if the navicular tubercle is on the floor (see Figure 2.19).

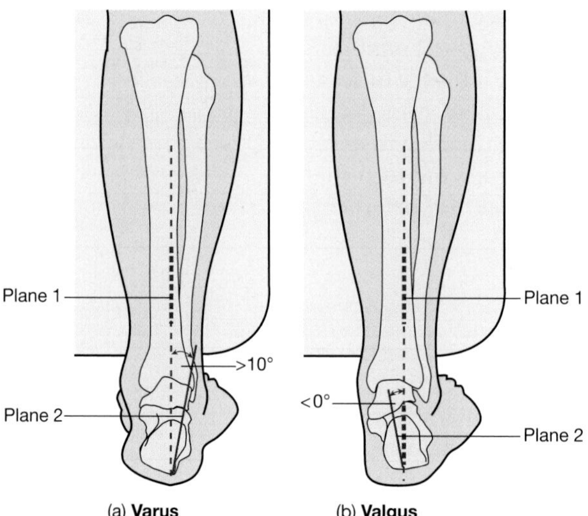

Figure 13.99 Testing for hindfoot varus and valgus. Four lines are drawn on the posterior aspect of the leg, two lines in the distal third of the leg in the midline, and two lines at the attachment of the Achilles tendon to the heel, (a) Here, plane 1 and plane 2 form an angle that is more than 10 degrees and the patient has hindfoot varus. (b) The angle formed in between the two planes is less than zero degrees and hence the patient has hindfoot valgus.

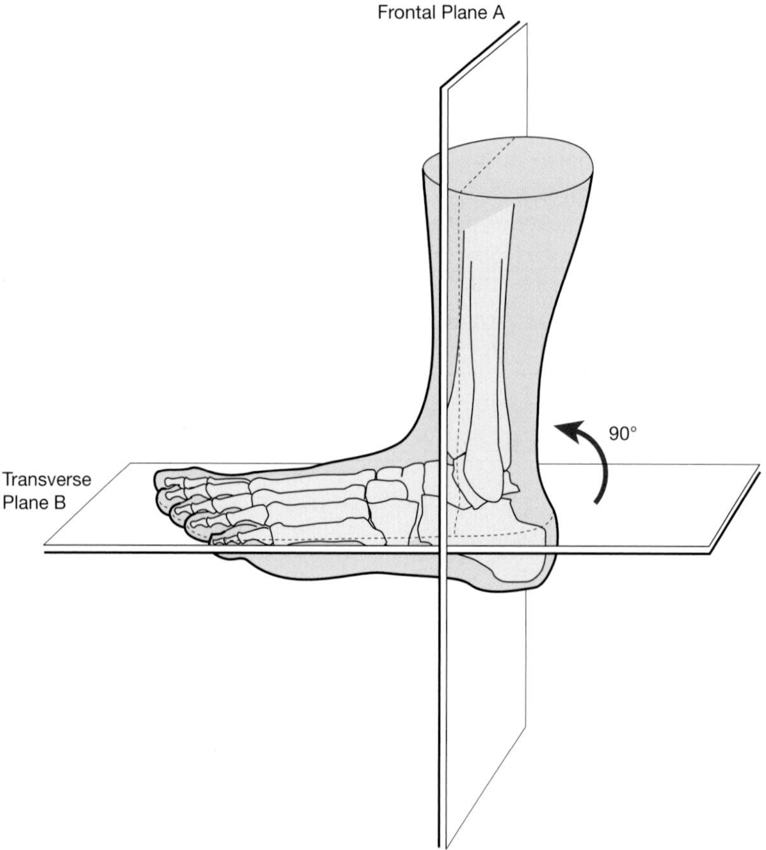

Figure 13.100 Testing for forefoot varus and valgus. With the subtalar joint in neutral position, an imaginary plane B (transverse) passing through the heads of the metatarsals should be perpendicular to the vertical (frontal) A axis. If the medial side of the foot is elevated, there is a forefoot varus deformity. If the lateral side of the foot is elevated, the patient has forefoot valgus deformity.

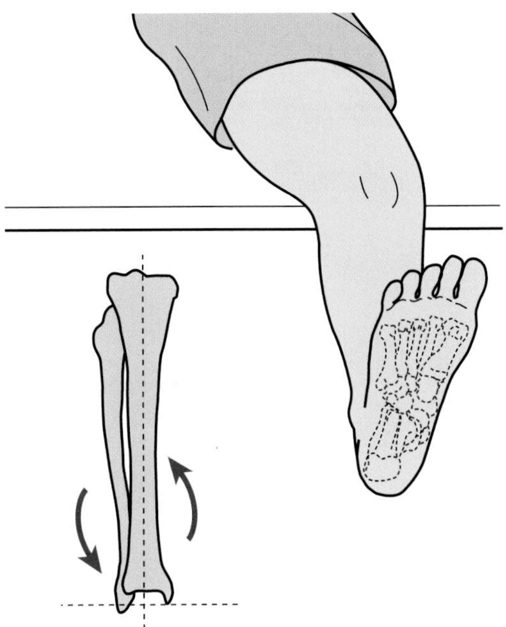

Figure 13.101 Toeing-in may be caused by internal tibial torsion.

Test for Leg–Heel Alignment

This test is used to determine whether a hindfoot valgus or varus condition exists. The patient is placed prone with the test leg extended and the opposite foot crossed over the posterior aspect of the knee on the test leg. A vertical line is drawn along the lower third of the leg in the midline (Figure 13.99). Another vertical line is drawn in the midline of the Achilles insertion into the calcaneus. While the subtalar joint is held in neutral position (described on p. 378),

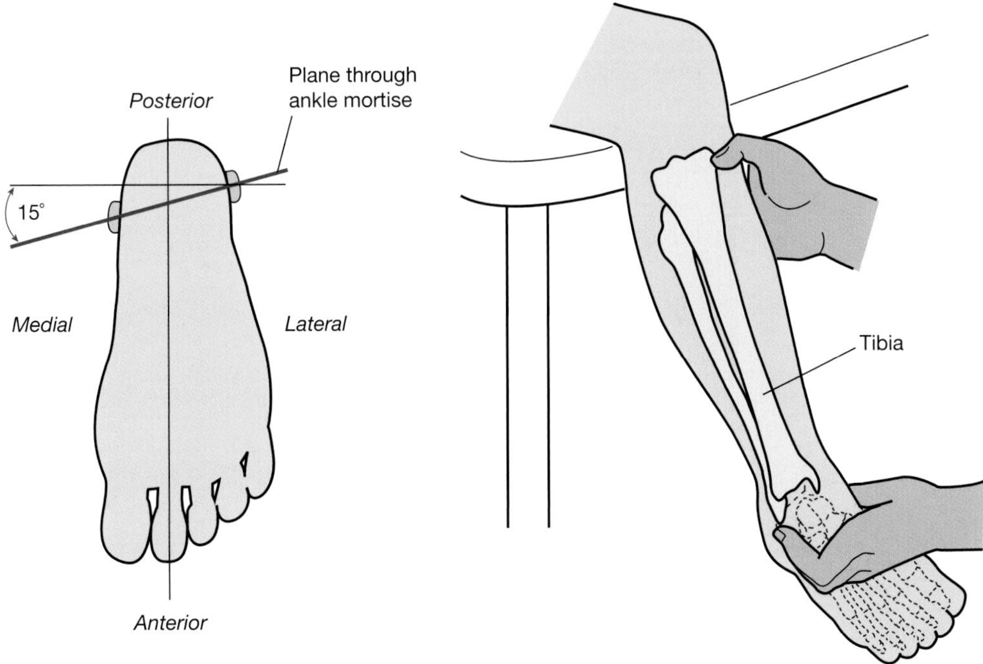

Figure 13.102 A plane extending through the ankle mortise should be externally rotated 15 degrees.

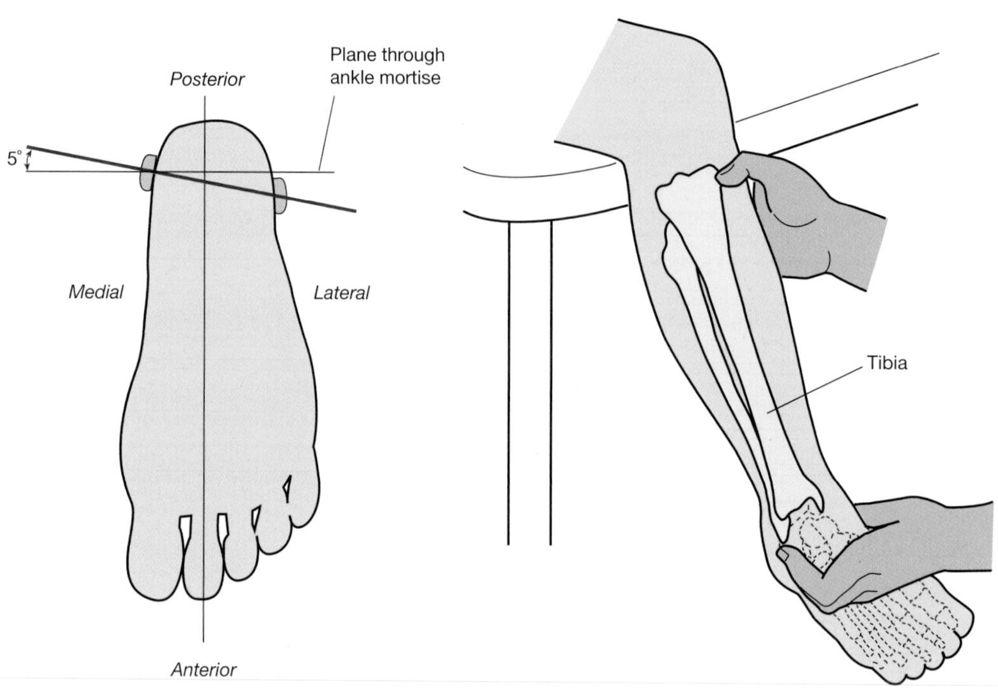

Figure 13.103 An internal tibial torsion, the ankle mortise faces medially less than 13 degrees.

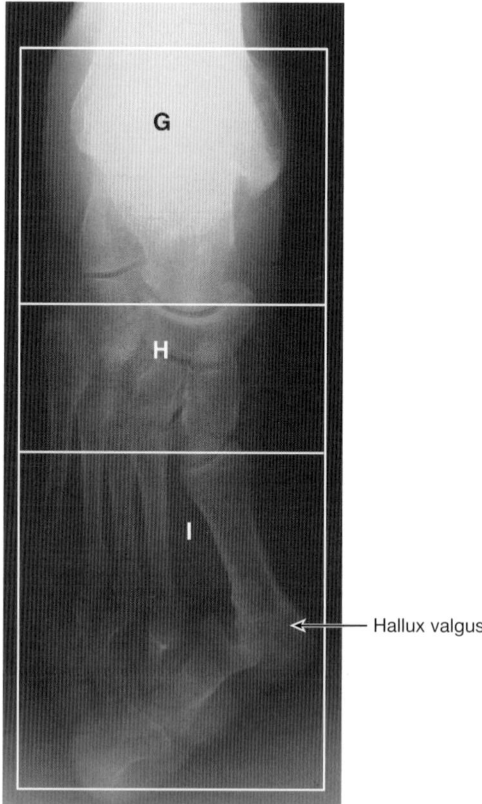

Figure 13.104 Anteroposterior view of the foot.

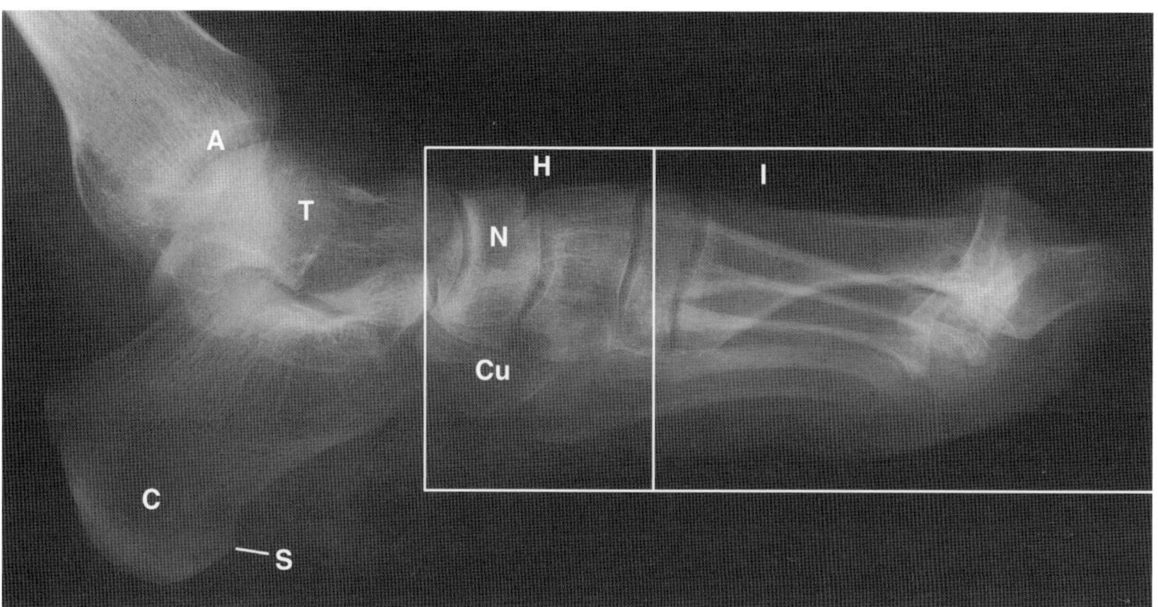

Figure 13.105 Lateral view of the ankle and foot.

the angle formed by the two lines is measured. An angle of approximately 0–10 degrees is normal. If the angle is less than zero degree, the patient has a hindfoot varus.

Test for Forefoot–Heel Alignment

The patient is placed in the supine position with the feet extending off the end of the table. While maintaining the subtalar joint in neutral, take the forefoot with the other hand and maximally pronate the forefoot (Figure 13.100). Now imagine a plane that extends through the heads of the second to the fourth metatarsals. This plane should be perpendicular to the vertical axis of the calcaneus. If the medial side of the foot is elevated, the patient has a forefoot varus. If the lateral side of the foot is elevated, the patient has a forefoot valgus.

Test for Tibial Torsion

At birth, the tibia is internally rotated approximately 30 degrees. By age 3, the tibia is externally rotated 15 degrees. Excessive toeing-in may be caused by internal tibial torsion (Figure 13.101). With the patient sitting on the edge of the table, the examiner imagines a plane that is perpendicular to the tibia and extends through the tibial tubercle. A plane extending through the ankle mortise should be externally rotated 15 degrees (Figure 13.102). If this plane is

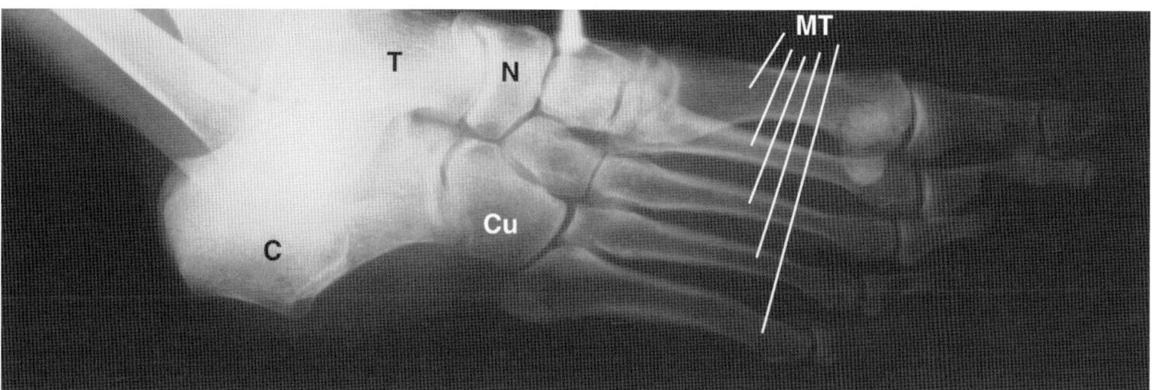

Figure 13.106 Oblique view of the foot.

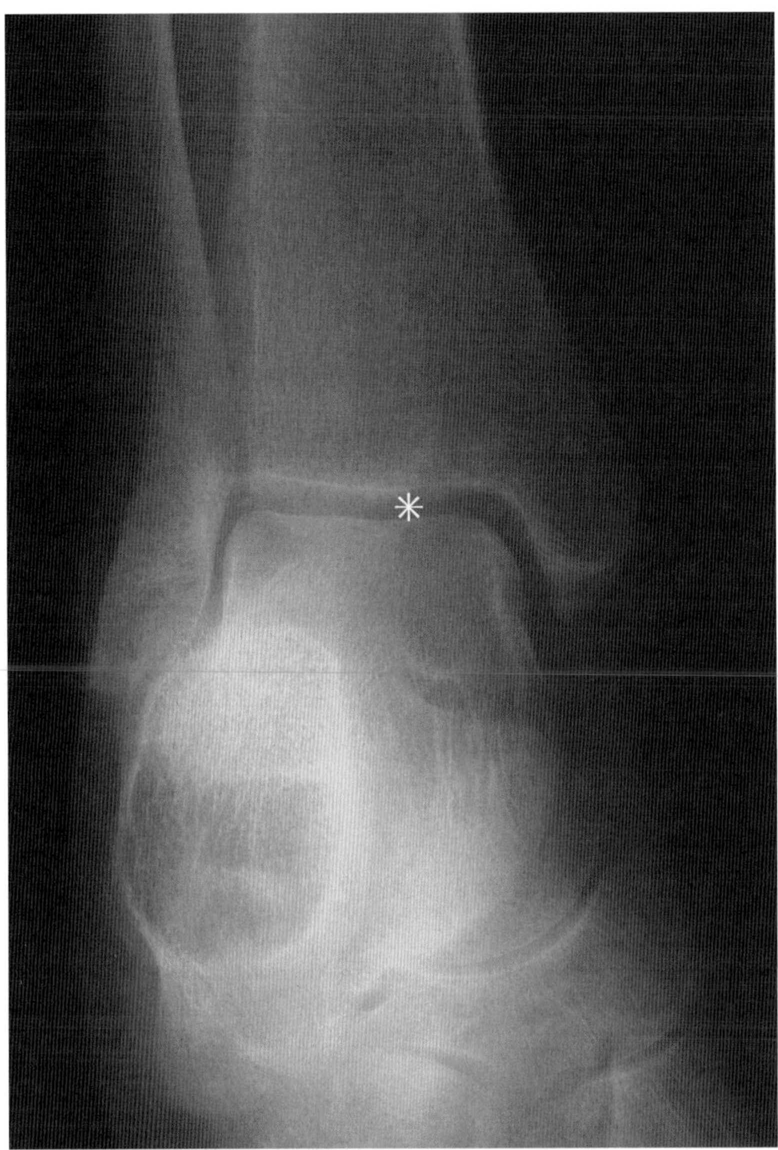

Figure 13.107 View of the ankle mortise (*).

externally rotated less than 13 degrees, the patient has internal tibial torsion (Figure 13.103). If the plane is rotated more than 18 degrees, the patient has external tibial torsion.

Radiological Views

Radiological views are presented in Figures 13.104, 13.105, 13.106, and 13.107.

G = Hindfoot
H = Midfoot
I = Forefoot
A = Ankle
C = Calcaneus
Cu = Cuboid
T = Talus
N = Navicular
S = Spur
MT = Metatarsal

SAMPLE EXAMINATION

History: 20-year-old female training for a marathon for 1 month presents with a 2-week history of right leg pain, aggravated by running. There has been no history of prior trauma. She recently began using lighter weight "racing shoes."

Physical Examination: Well-developed slender female, ambulating comfortably in her usual well-fitting running shoes. There is tenderness on palpation along the anteromedial border of the right tibia. Muscle testing was 5/5; however, patient tended to invert with plantar flexion. Mobility testing of the calcaneus was increased in eversion. Anterior and posterior drawer tests were negative. The patient demonstrates generalized hyperextensibility at the knee and elbow, with flexible pronation of the subtalar joint on weight-bearing. Feiss' line reveals a grade 2 pes planus.

Presumptive Diagnosis: Posterior tibial tendonitis (shin splints).

Physical Examination Clues: (1) Female, indicating possibility of greater musculoskeletal soft-tissue laxity, (2) Excessive musculoskeletal flexibility, indicating potential for greater demand to be placed on dynamic stabilizers (muscles), (3) Posteromedial tibial tenderness, indicating a specific anatomic region and structure at the site of injury. The subtalar joint is stabilized statically by the spring ligament and dynamically by the posterior tibialis muscle and tendon. Increased musculoskeletal laxity results in reduced contribution to joint stability by static stabilizers (ligaments), placing greater demand on the dynamic stabilizers (muscles). In this case, the relative increased laxity in the calcaneonavicular (spring ligament) will expose the posterior tibialis to greater demand and potential overuse failure.

PARADIGM FOR AN OVERUSE SYNDROME OF THE FOOT AND ANKLE

A 22-year-old female jogger presents with a complaint of pain on weight-bearing at the medial aspect of the right heel. She has been "training" for a marathon for the past 2 months and has increased her running from an average of 5 miles per day to 10 miles per day, 6 days per week. There has been no evidence of swelling about the ankle and foot. She describes a pattern of stiffness on arising in the morning which lessens within 15 minutes of walking. The pain, however, returns and increases in proportion to her daily activities.

She gives no history of similar symptoms with her prior training for distance runs. She recently began running in lightweight racing shoes.

On physical examination, the patient has full range of motion in all joints of the lower extremities. She has a well-formed longitudinal arch which decreases in height on weight-bearing. There is a moderate amount of subtalar pronation on unilateral stance and tenderness to palpation along the distal medial aspect of the right calcaneus. Tenderness is also produced with passive dorsiflexion of the foot and toes. Tinel's sign is negative on percussion over the tarsal tunnel. She has multiple subungual hematomas. X-rays are reported to show no abnormalities.

This is a paradigm for chronic overuse syndrome of plantar fascia because:

No history of acute trauma
A significant increase in demand over a relatively short period
Pain on initiation of activities which quickly abates
Return of symptoms in proportion to activities

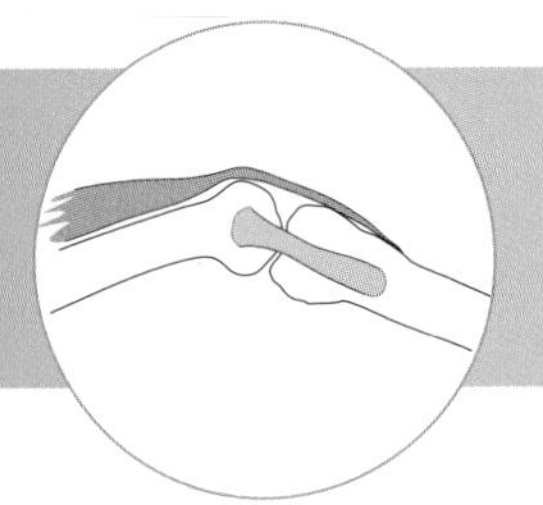
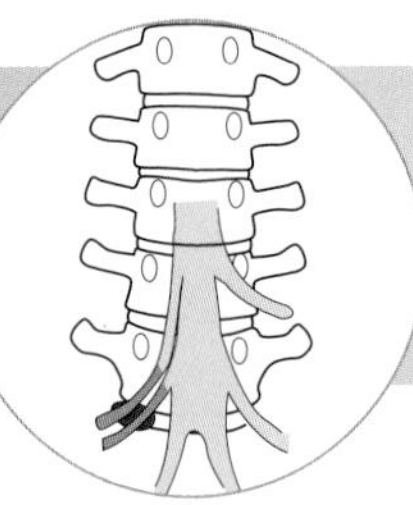
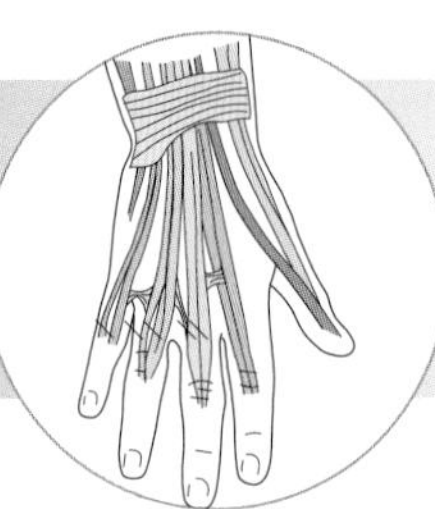

CHAPTER 14

Gait

The Lower Extremity

This section is not intended as a definitive treatise on the lower extremity, but rather it is to serve as the introduction to the lower-extremity physical examination, based on the principles presented in the introductory chapters of this book. This section reviews the more salient aspects of lower-extremity structure, function, and physical examination. Its intended objective is to present the entire lower extremity as a whole. With this perspective, it is hoped that the examiner will become sensitized to the anatomical relationships that place an individual at risk of injury. Its purpose is to provide the examiner (and patient) with the means for identifying, addressing, and avoiding causes of injury.

The linkage and interdependence of articulations and structures of the lower extremity, back, and pelvis must be considered when evaluating and diagnosing complaints of the lower extremity.

The lower extremities are pillars on which the body is supported. They permit and facilitate movement of the body in space. They accomplish this task through a series of linkages: the pelvis, hip, knee, ankle, and foot. Each of these linkages has a unique shape and function. Together they permit the lower extremity to efficiently accommodate varying terrains and contours.

The body's center of gravity is located in the midline, 1 cm anterior to the first sacral vertebra. During bipedal stance, the body's weight is supported equally over each lower limb, creating a downward compression load on the joints of the lower extremities. During the unilateral support phase of gait, however, the body's center of gravity is *medial* to the supporting limb. Therefore, during unilateral support, the hip, knee and ankle of the supporting limb will experience not only a compression load, but also a varus (inward) rotational destabilizing force referred to as a *moment*. This destabilizing force must be counteracted by a muscular effort. Otherwise, the body will fall to the unsupported side (Figure 11.1).

At the base of each pillar is the foot and ankle complex. The ankle and foot are structures uniquely designed to tolerate a lifetime of significant cyclic loads of varying rates while traversing any terrain. The key to the successful functioning of these structures lies in the extraordinary stability of the ankle, and the impact attenuation and surface accommodation properties of the foot. The stability of the ankle may well explain its ability to resist the inevitable mechanical degeneration expected in such a small articulation exposed to such repetitive stress. The ankle structure is that of a keystone recessed into a rigid mortise (Figure 14.1). It is because of this extraordinary stability, unless lost secondary to injury, that the ankle does not demonstrate the normal osteoarthritic changes with aging found in all other synovial joints. This is even more impressive in light of the significant loads that are being supported by the relatively small articular surface of the ankle joint (approximately 40% that of the hip or knee) during weight-bearing activities such as running. However, this stability carries with it an inability to accommodate rotational and angular stresses that would otherwise ultimately lead to compromise of the ankle joint if they were not first buffered by the foot below. The suppleness of the foot articulations, that is, subtalar pronation, accommodates varying surface topographies to reduce these torques. The arches attenuate the repetitive stress of the weight-bearing loads that occur during locomotion. This system of

Musculoskeletal Examination, Fourth Edition. Jeffrey M. Gross, Joseph Fetto and Elaine Rosen.

Companion website: www.wiley.com/go/musculoskeletalexam

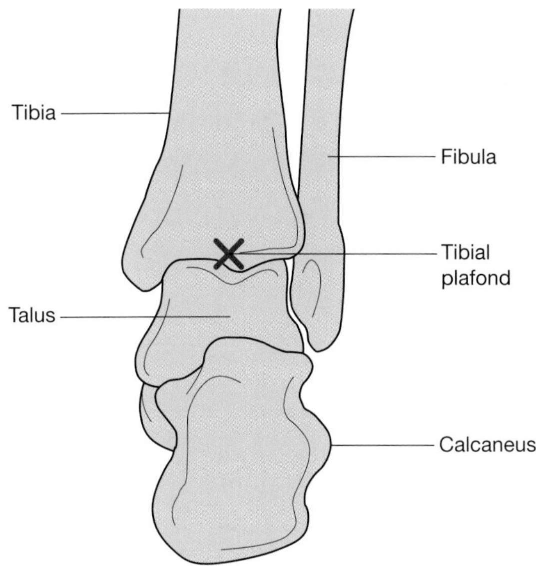

Figure 14.1 The talus is a rectangular bone keystoned within a rigid mortise formed by the medial malleolar process of the tibia, the tibial plafond, and the lateral malleolus.

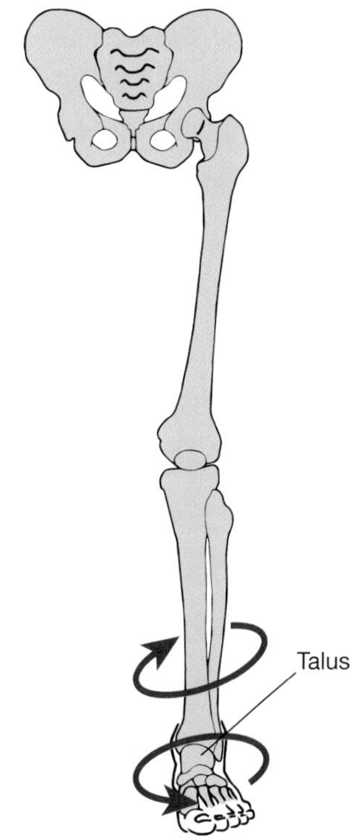

Figure 14.2 Pronation (plantar medial rotation) of the talus results in internal rotation of the leg and supination torque of the middle of the foot.

complementary functions forces recognition of the ankle and foot not as isolated regions, but rather as a single ankle–foot mechanism.

The talus holds the key to the intimate structural and mechanical relationship that exists between the ankle and foot. As the part of the ankle that is held within a rigid mortise, the talus is limited to flexion–extension motion. As a part of the foot, the talus must accommodate medial rotation. This medial rotation is termed *pronation*. Efficient locomotion requires the simultaneous occurrence of both talar functions. The lower extremity must accommodate the internal rotational torque that subtalar pronation creates. It must transmit this force proximally through the rigid ankle mortise during gait. This torque is most efficiently accommodated by a complex combination of knee flexion and internal rotation of the entire lower extremity through the ball-and-socket mechanism of the hip joint. Such a compensatory motion has the potential to place excessive stresses at the structures proximal to the ankle and foot, such as the patellofemoral articulation (Figure 14.2).

Closer inspection of the ankle and foot shows that the body of the talus is supported by the calcaneus, and these bones diverge at 30 degrees in both the coronal and sagittal planes. The result is that the head of the talus is supported by soft tissues (the talocalcaneonavicular or "spring" ligament, and the posterior tibialis tendon). As such, in the presence of soft-tissue or generalized ligamentous laxity or muscular weakness, the head of the talus can experience excessive plantar flexion. This excess movement will force the calcaneus laterally, with an eversion of the hindfoot. During weight bearing, this displacement will force internal rotation of the entire lower extremity about the ball-and-socket articulation of the hip. If unchecked, this situation will create excessive loading at several points along the lower extremity:

1. valgus and medial rotation of the first metatarsophalangeal joint (leading to hallux valgus and bunion formation);
2. excessive stretching and strain of the tibialis posterior muscle and tendon (shin splints);
3. increased internal rotation of the knee, resulting in an apparent increased "Q angle," lateral patellar subluxation stress, increased medial retinacular tension, increased lateral compression loading of the patellofemoral facet, and increased tension in the popliteus muscle; and
4. increased internal rotation of the hip, increased tension/stretch loading of the external rotators of the hip (producing piriformis syndrome and sciatic nerve irritation [sciatica]).

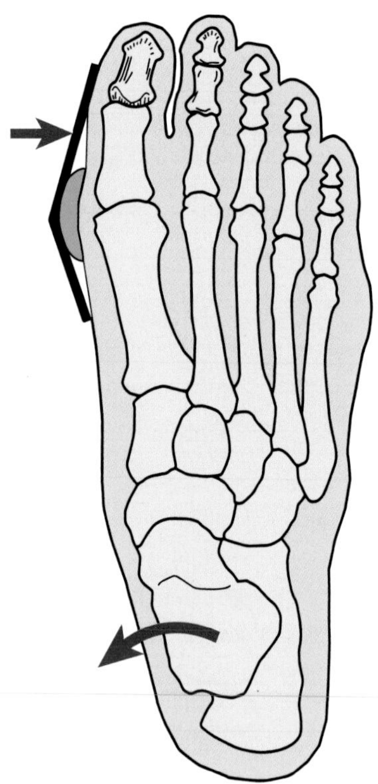

Figure 14.3 Hindfoot pronation may result in valgus stressing of the first metatarsophalangeal joint. Chronic valgus stress can result in the formation of a swelling (bunion) and angulation of this joint (hallux valgus deformity).

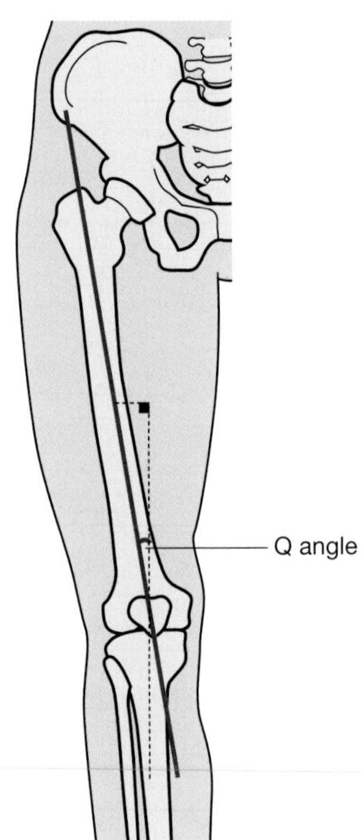

Figure 14.4 The angle formed between the line of the quadriceps musculature and the patellar tendon is termed the Q angle. Contraction of the quadriceps mechanism attempts to resolve the Q angle to 180 degrees. Therefore, the greater the Q angle, the larger the resultant lateral displacement vector force when quadriceps contraction occurs.

As discussed earlier, situations that create excessive repetitive loading may lead to breakdown of tissues and structure (the "vicious cycle of injury"). Each of the pathological conditions listed above is a potential consequence of insufficient subtalar support and resultant excessive pronation, which has produced a biological system failure.

There are several clinical examples of biological system failure secondary to excessive subtalar pronation. The swelling of the medial capsule and resultant accumulation of hard and soft tissues about the first metatarsophalangeal joint of the foot, known as a bunion, is the direct consequence of excessive loading stresses at the medial aspect of the first metatarsophalangeal joint (Figure 14.3). The unsuccessful attempt of the tibialis posterior muscle-tendon to support the subtalar arch results in excessive stretching and stressing of that muscle-tendon unit. This explains the appearance of pain in the posteromedial aspect of the leg and ankle (shin splints) at the location of the muscle's origin, in an insufficiently conditioned runner. The hip, as a ball-and-socket articulation, provides little resistance to inward rotational torques. As such, inward rotation of the entire lower extremity forces the axis of the knee to rotate medially. This inward rotation of the knee will accentuate the valgus alignment of the knee as it flexes. This combination of medial or internal rotation and flexion of the knee creates and increases (apparent) valgus angulation of the knee joint. This valgus in turn creates a greater lateral displacement vector on the patellofemoral mechanism with quadriceps contraction (Figure 14.4). This occurs because the direction of the quadriceps pull attempts to resolve the Q angle to a straight line of 180 degrees. This increased laterally directed vector force on the patella has a direct consequence on the longevity and attrition of patellar articular cartilage. It also creates excessive tension within the medial peripatellar soft tissues. Both situations can result in the painful conditions of patellar chondromalacia and plica syndrome. Attempts to resist or correct this internal rotational torque by muscular effort can be created at several points along the lower extremity. As already mentioned, one mechanism is contraction of the tibialis posterior muscle of the leg. This attempts to counteract talar pronation by supporting the body of the talus against plantar flexion. A second mechanism is that of the popliteus muscle of the posterolateral aspect of the knee, attempting to internally rotate the leg. A third mechanism occurs at the buttocks, posterior to the hip joint. Here, the piriformis and external rotator muscles of the hip are well positioned to exert an external rotation effort on the lower extremity.

However, if these muscles, one or all, are incapable of meeting the demand being made, the result will be breakdown, inflammatory reaction, and pain, with the consequences of initiating a vicious cycle of injury. This inability to meet the demand required might be due to a general lack of proper conditioning (relative overload), or it may be due to a truly excessive load being applied (absolute overload). In either event, injury will result.

At the knee, a breakdown of the popliteus tendon can present as posterolateral knee pain. The symptoms resulting from hip external rotator weakness will present as buttock pain. At the hip, these injuries can also affect adjacent but otherwise uninvolved tissues such as the sciatic nerve. The sciatic nerve lies in close proximity to and, in 15% of people, penetrates the external rotator muscles. Therefore, inflammation and stiffness of the external rotator muscles can create tethering of the sciatic nerve. This in turn can masquerade as an injury to the sciatic nerve or as a referral of symptoms of a more proximal injury (i.e., spinal trauma or intervertebral disk herniation).

It is hoped that this brief discourse on the interrelationships that exist within the lower extremity will prevent the examiner from approaching the lower extremity in a fragmentary fashion. It cannot be emphasized enough that the body, and lower extremity in particular, is a complex system of interdependent and interacting components. This concept is fundamental to the process of accurate diagnosis.

What Is Gait?

Gait is the forward movement of the erect body, using the lower extremities for propulsion. Movement of any mass requires the expenditure of energy. The amount of energy required is a function of the amount of mass to be moved and the amount of displacement of that mass's center of gravity along the X (horizontal), Y (vertical), and Z (anterior–posterior) axes from its point of origin. The body's center of gravity is located in the midline, 1 cm anterior to S1 (first sacral segment) when the patient is erect with the feet placed a few inches apart and the arms at the side.

What Is Normal Gait?

Normal gait is the efficient forward movement of the body. *Efficient* means that energy expenditure is minimized. Any deviation from this minimum can be termed an *abnormal gait pattern.* There are varying degrees of abnormal. *Normal gait* therefore can be defined as the forward locomotion of the body during which the body's center of gravity describes a sinusoidal curve of minimum amplitude in both the Y and X axes (Figure 14.5). An increase in the displacement of the body's center of gravity from this path requires increased energy expenditure, hence creating an increased metabolic demand. The result is decreased efficiency of locomotion and increased fatigue. This is why vaulting over a fused knee and leaning toward one side due to abductor weakness are patterns of abnormal gait. They are each characterized by increased displacement of the center of gravity. In vaulting, there is excessive vertical displacement of the center of gravity, whereas in the lateral list of the Trendelenburg gait, there is increased side-to-side translation of the body's center of gravity.

Gait is a cyclical activity that requires repetitive positioning of the lower extremities. The gait cycle is divided into two phases: stance and swing (Figure 14.6). The stance phase is further subdivided into five discrete periods:

1. Heel-strike
2. Foot flat
3. Midstance
4. Heel-off
5. Toe-off

The stance phase occupies 60% of the time during one cycle of normal gait. The remaining 40% of the gait cycle comprises the swing phase, which is divided into three periods:

1. Initial swing (acceleration)
2. Mid swing
3. Terminal swing (deceleration)

The period when both feet are in contact with the ground is called double support. The step length is the distance between the left heel contact and the right heel contact. The stride length is the distance between one left heel-strike and the next left heel-strike.

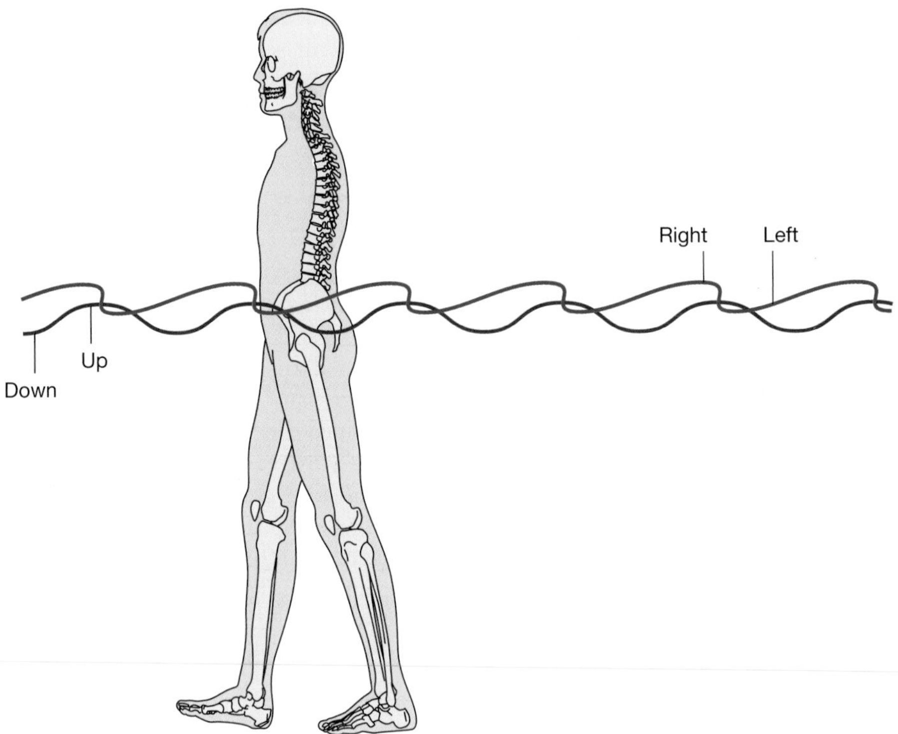

Figure 14.5 During normal gait, the body's center of gravity describes a curve of minimum amplitude in the vertical and horizontal axes.

There are six determinants of gait. These postural accommodations contribute to the efficiency of ambulation by reducing energy expenditure. The first five reduce the vertical displacement of the body. The sixth reduces lateral displacement of the body:

1. Pelvic tilt—about 5 degrees on the swing side
2. Pelvic rotation—about 8 degrees total on the swing side
3. Knee flexion—to about 20 degrees in early stance phase

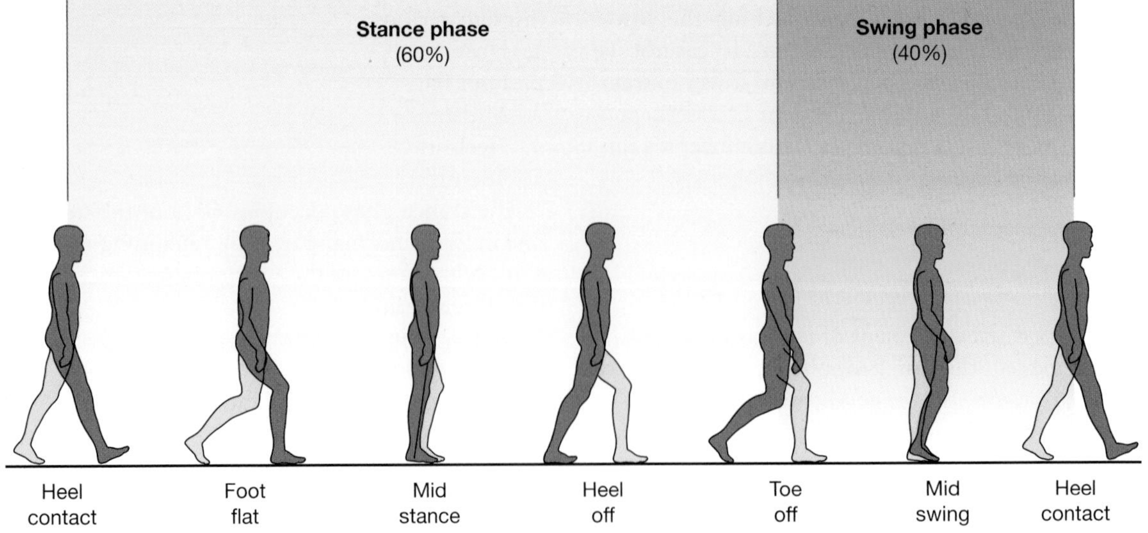

Figure 14.6 The subdivisions of the stance and swing phases of gait.

4. Plantar flexion—to about 15 degrees in early stance phase
5. Plantar flexion—to about 20 degrees in late stance phase
6. Narrow walking base—due to normal knee valgus and foot placement.

During each cycle of gait, gravity is a downward force constantly acting at the body's center of gravity. As such, it causes rotation to occur at each of the joints of the lower extremity. This rotational deformity is called a *moment.* A moment's magnitude is a function of the size of the force acting and the perpendicular distance between the center of gravity and the axis about which the force of gravity is acting (the moment arm) (Figure 14.7). When the moment arm is the Y (vertical) axis, the resulting moments are termed *varus,* for rotation toward the midline, or *valgus,* for rotation away from the midline. When the moment results in the closing of a joint, it is termed a *flexion moment.* For example, at heel-strike, the body's center of gravity is behind the axis of the knee. The moment arm acting at the knee is posterior to the knee joint's center of rotation. The resultant moment of the body weight acting at the knee will close (reduce the angle) the knee joint, causing the knee to flex spontaneously. Therefore, the moment acting at the knee at heel-strike until midstance is a flexion moment (Figure 14.8).

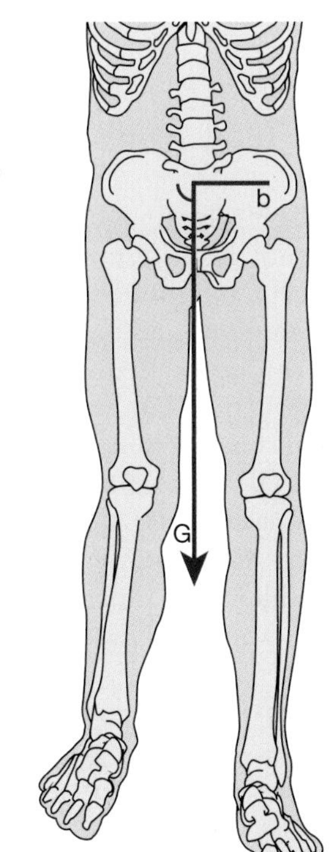

Figure 14.7 The moment of varus (inward) rotation at the hip is the product of the force of gravity, G, acting at the body's center of gravity, and the perpendicular distance, b, from the body's center to the hip: moment of the hip = C × b.

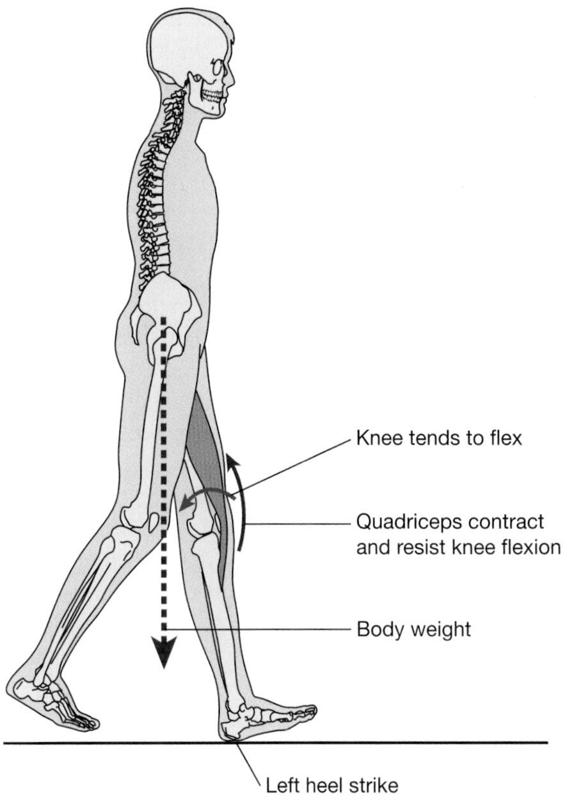

Figure 14.8 At heel-strike, the body's center of gravity is posterior to the axis of the knee joint. There will be a spontaneous tendency for the knee to flex. This is called a flexion moment. This flexion moment is resisted by the active contraction of the knee extensors (quadriceps).

Similarly, at heel-strike, the body's center of gravity is anterior to the hip joint's center of rotation. Therefore, the moment arm with which gravity acts at the hip during heel-strike will cause spontaneous closing (flexion) of the thigh on the torso. Hence, gravity acting on the hip at heel-strike creates a flexion moment.

When the moment acting on the joint creates an opening (increase) in joint angle, it is termed an *extension moment.* An example of an extension moment is the quadriceps contracting. The quadriceps pulling through the patellar tendon acts on a moment arm that is anterior to the axis of knee motion. It therefore opens (increases) the angle of the knee joint. Hence, the quadriceps extends the knee by virtue of the extension moment it creates at the knee when the muscle contracts.

The quadriceps extension moment serves to counteract the spontaneous flexion of the knee that occurs from heel-strike to midstance due to the posterior position of the body's center of gravity relative to the axis of the knee.

By understanding the concept of moment, an analysis can be made for each joint throughout the gait cycle. With such an analysis of the relative positions of the body's center of gravity and the joint in question, it is theoretically possible to predict when a muscular structure must be active and where it should be positioned for optimal effect so as to maintain an equilibrium state of balance (erect posture) during gait. In other words, the muscles function to counteract the effect of gravity on the joints.

Conversely, an inability to maintain this equilibrium state can be analyzed so as to understand what structures are malfunctioning or malpositioned. Such an analysis is fundamental and crucial to the accurate diagnosis and treatment of gait abnormalities.

For example, limping due to hip disease can be analyzed into the gravitational moment acting to rotate the torso inwardly during unilateral stance and the counterbalancing valgus moment created by the abductor muscles (in particular, the gluteus medius). An example of a valgus moment is the action of the gluteus medius acting on the hip at unilateral midstance phase of gait. At this point in the gait cycle, the abductor muscle will contract. Its force vector will pull the pelvis in a valgus (outward) rotation. This will serve to counteract the varus (inward) moment created by the force of gravity. The abductor, however, has a shorter moment arm than does gravity with which to work. Therefore, the abductors must exert a proportionately greater force than that of gravity in order to balance the body across the hip joint. In fact, since the abductor moment arm (a) is about one-half that of the body's (b), the abductor force (A) must be twice that of the weight of the body (B)—the action of gravity pulling at the body's center of gravity. This can be expressed as an equilibrium state equation: $A \times a = B \times b$, knowing $a = b$, then $A = 2B$. With such an analysis of the hip, it is easy to predict the usefulness of a cane held in the opposite hand as a means to assist weak abductor musculature. The cane will prevent the inward rotation of the torso toward the unsupported side caused by gravity and insufficiently resisted by weak abductor muscles (Figure 14.9). Similarly, analysis of the knee will explain how bracing the knee in extension is an effective means of protecting a polio victim with quadriceps paralysis from sudden spontaneous knee flexion and falling during gait.

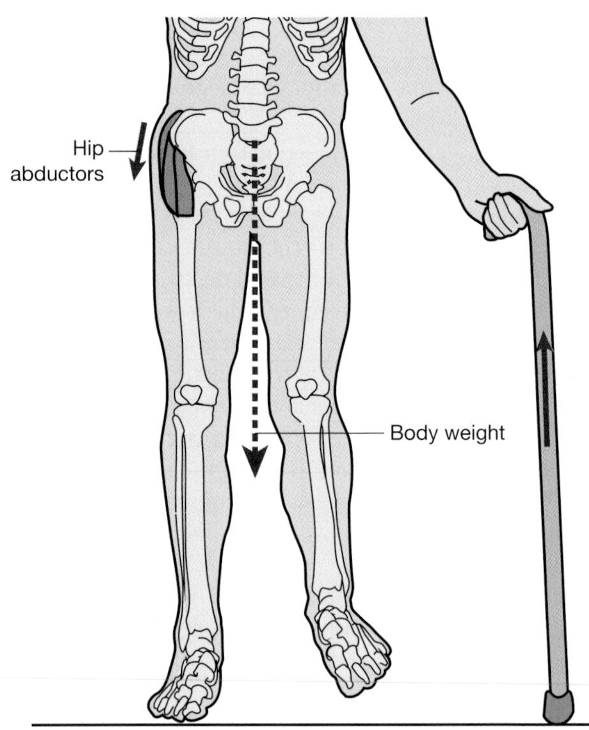

Figure 14.9 A cane held in the contralateral hand assists the hip abductor muscles in resisting the gravitational moment that pulls the body toward the unsupported side during swing phase.

The Examination of Abnormal Gait

As stated above, the evaluation of abnormal gait requires a working knowledge of normal biomechanics. Abnormalities occur as a result of pain, weakness, abnormal range of motion, and leg length discrepancy. These factors can occur separately or together. They are closely interrelated. For example, weakness of a muscle group can result in a painful joint, which would then lose normal range of motion. When isolated, however, pain, weakness, abnormal range of motion, and leg length discrepancy within a particular anatomical region result in a characteristic gait abnormality. Some of these abnormalities were referred to in prior chapters.

Gait disorders due to central nervous system disease or injury, such as spastic, ataxic, or parkinsonian gait, are not described here, as they are beyond the scope of this text.

The key to observing abnormal gait is the ability to recognize symmetry of movement. You should observe the patient walking for some distance. Sometimes it is necessary to watch the patient walk down a long hallway or outdoors. Subtle abnormalities will

Table 14.1 Factors Affecting Gait

Cause of Abnormal Gait	Observable Effect on Gait
Pain	Decreased duration of stance phase. Avoidance of ground contact with the painful part.
Weakness	Increased or decreased motion in the affected joint at the time of the gait cycle when muscle normally contracts. Compensatory motion usually occurs in other joints to prevent falling (by adjusting the location of the center of gravity) and to allow for limb clearance.
Abnormal range of motion and leg length discrepancy	Compensatory movement in other joints to allow for weight bearing, limb clearance, or relocation of the center of gravity over the weight-bearing limb.

not be evident inside the examining room. A patient will walk differently when he or she is "performing" for you. If it is possible, try to observe the patient when he or she is not aware of being watched.

The foot and ankle, knee, and hip should be observed separately for fluidity and degree of motion. The examples that follow are meant to illustrate how pain, weakness, abnormal range of motion, and leg length discrepancy affect the normal symmetry of motion that occurs at the foot and ankle, knee, and hip (Table 14.1).

Foot and Ankle

Antalgic Gait

The patient with pain in the foot or ankle will make every effort to avoid weight bearing on the painful part. For example, if the first metatarsophalangeal joint is painful due to gout, the patient will not want to extend that joint. This results in a flat-footed push-off. The weight is maintained posteriorly on the foot. The patient will also spend less time in the stance phase on the painful foot, causing an asymmetrical cadence (Figure 14.10).

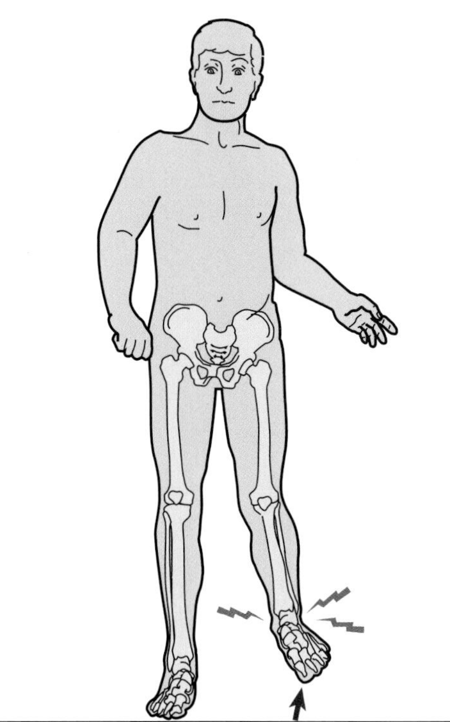

Figure 14.10 An antalgic gait due to pain in the great toe or foot will result in a shortened stance phase.

Weakness

Weakness of the dorsiflexors of the foot due to peroneal nerve injury, for example, will result in a drop foot or steppage gait. Inability to dorsiflex the foot during swing-through will cause the toes to contact the ground. To avoid this from happening, the patient will flex the hip and knee in an exaggerated fashion as if he or she was trying to climb a stair so that the foot will clear the ground during swing-through (Figure 14.11). This is called a *steppage gait* (http://www.youtube.com/watch?v=SWvEU8FYMFc).

Eccentric dorsiflexion of the foot also occurs as the body weight is transferred from the heel to the forefoot following heel-strike. Weakness of the foot dorsiflexors results in a slapping of the foot against the ground following heel-strike, known as *foot slap* (Figure 14.12) (http://www.youtube.com/watch?v=SWvEU8FYMFc).

Abnormal Range of Motion

If the ankle is unable to dorsiflex, as in an equinus deformity (Figure 14.13), the patient lands with each step on the metatarsal heads. This is known as *primary toe-strike* (Figure 14.14) (http://www.youtube.com/watch?v=MMM8Tqntbzo).

Due to the primary toe-strike, the line of force is far in front of the knee and this causes a hyperextension moment at the knee. Therefore, the patient

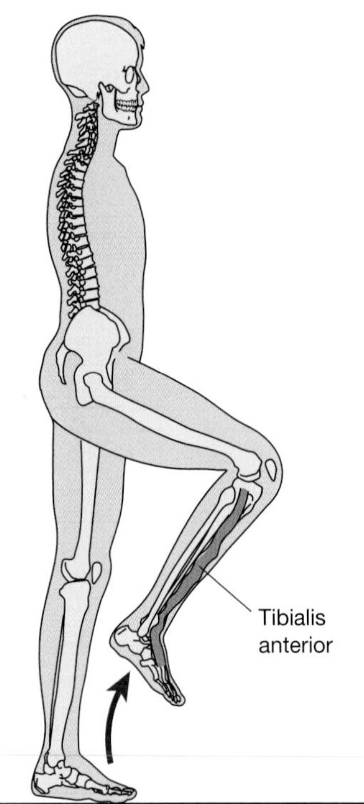

Figure 14.11 Weakness of dorsiflexion results in a steppage gait with increased hip and knee flexion to allow for clearance of the toe during swing-through.

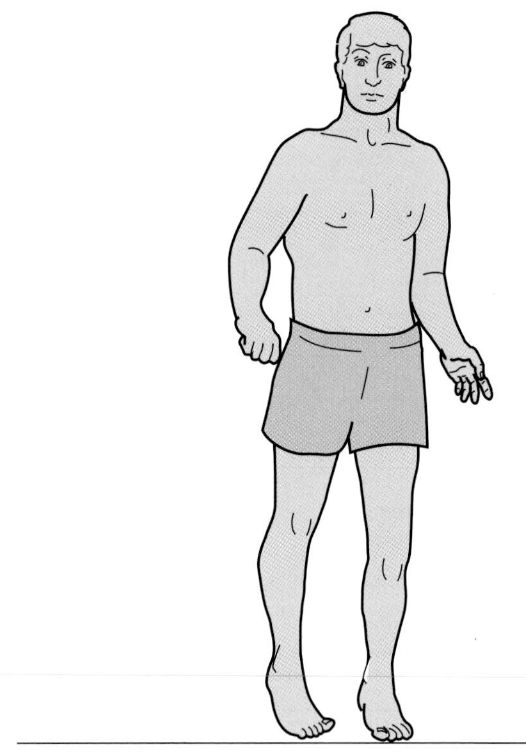

Figure 14.13 A talipes equinus deformity of the foot.

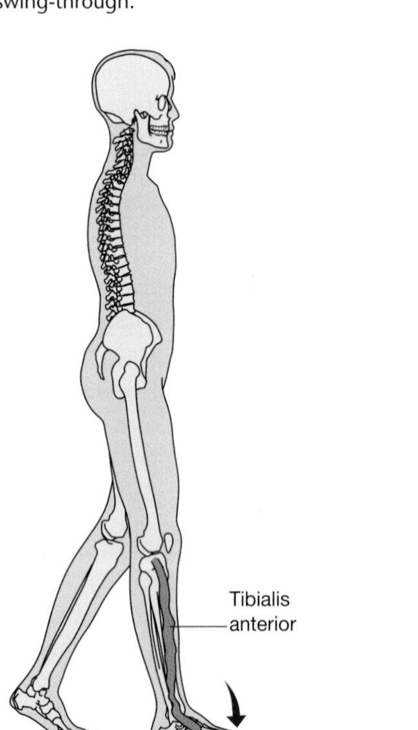

Figure 14.12 After heel-strike, with weakness of foot dorsiflexion, the patient's forefoot slaps against the ground. This is called foot slap.

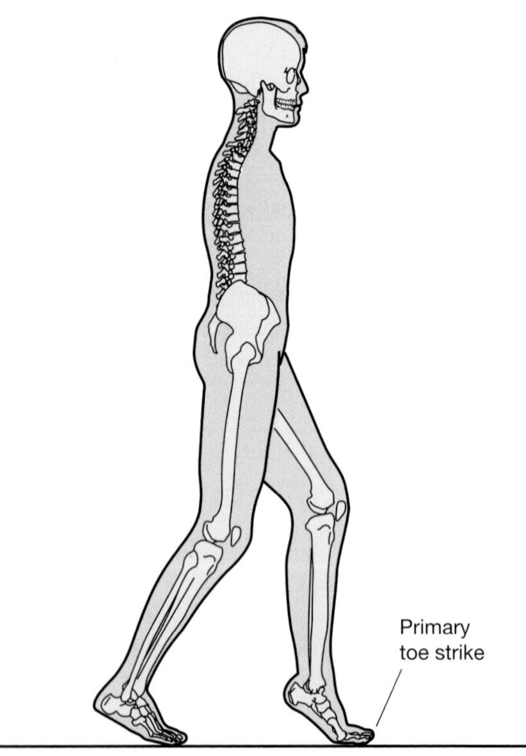

Figure 14.14 With a talipes equinus deformity of the foot, the patient contacts the ground with the ball of the foot instead of the heel. This is called primary toe-strike.

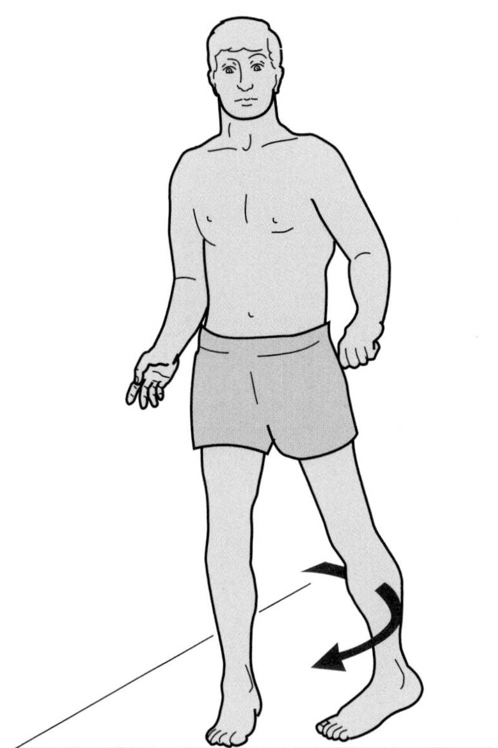

Figure 14.15 An equinus deformity of the foot will result in relative lengthening of the extremity and the patient must circumduct the hip in order to clear the ground.

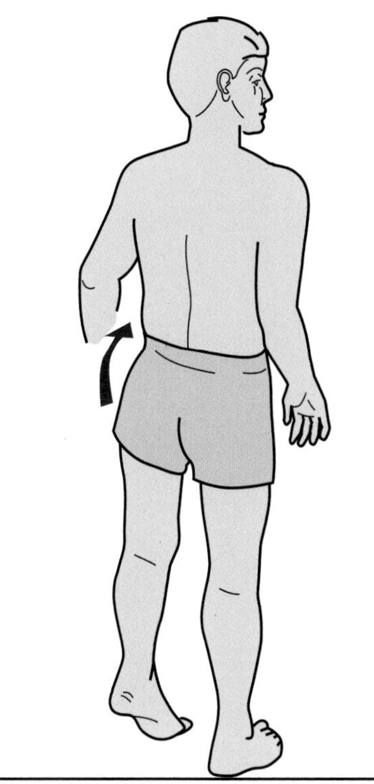

Figure 14.16 The patient may also clear the ground with the relatively lengthened extremity due to an equinus deformity by hip hiking.

may develop genu recurvatum as a result of an equinus deformity. As in the case of foot drop, the patient will again have difficulty preventing the toes from hitting the ground during swing phase. The patient will therefore have to elevate the foot in the air by either increasing knee and hip flexion as in a steppage gait, circumducting the leg at the hip (Figure 14.15), or hiking the extremity up from the hip (Figure 14.16) (http://www.youtube.com/watch?v=t5VJdRUS4 × 0).

These maneuvers effectively shorten the leg and allow for toe clearance during swing-through.

Knee

Antalgic Gait

The patient with a painful knee will walk with less weight on the painful side. Less time will also be spent on that side. The patient will attempt to maintain the knee in flexion if there is an effusion. If the knee is kept in extension, the patient will have to circumduct at the hip or hike the lower extremity upward from the hip in order to clear the ground during swing-through. Heel-strike is painful and will be avoided.

Weakness

Quadriceps weakness is common in patients with poliomyelitis. The gait abnormality that results is hyperextension of the knee following heel-strike. The patient has to try to maintain the weight in front of the knee to create an extension moment. This is effected by throwing the trunk forward following heel-strike. The patient may also attempt to extend the knee by pushing the thigh backward following heel contact (Figure 14.17) (http://www.youtube.com/watch?v=VzcW6oodipk).

Weakness of the quadriceps frequently results in overstretching of the posterior capsule of the knee joint and this causes genu recurvatum.

Abnormal Range of Motion

Loss of full knee extension will result in a functionally shorter extremity. The patient will have to elevate the body on the normal side as that leg tries to swing-through while he or she supports the weight on the abnormal side. This can be accomplished by hip hiking or circumducting the hip on the good side during swing-through. To allow for weight bearing on the

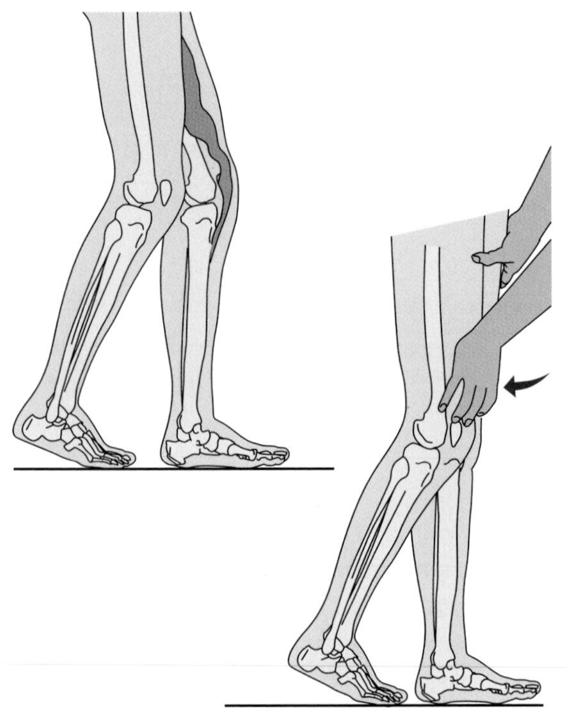

Figure 14.17 Weakness of the quadriceps may be compensated for by the patient pushing the thigh backward following heel-strike when quadriceps function is necessary.

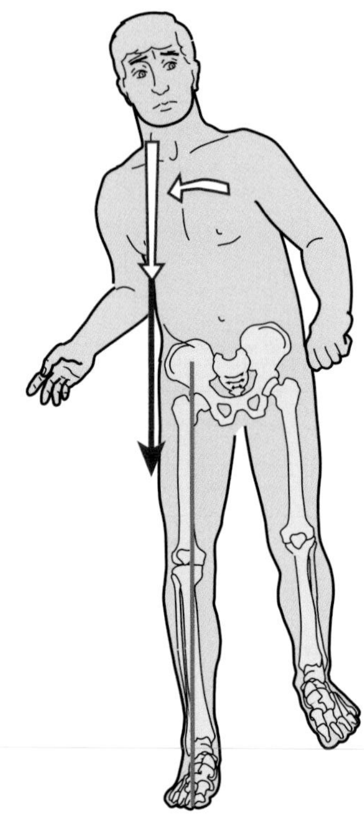

Figure 14.18 The compensated Trendelenburg gait is characterized by the trunk deviating over the hip during stance phase to make up for weakness of hip abduction. This gait pattern may also be noted in patients with a painful hip, in which case the stance phase duration will be markedly reduced.

affected side, the patient will walk on the ball of the foot (primary toe-strike).

Hip

Antalgic Gait

The patient with the painful hip due to osteoarthritis, for example, will make every effort to reduce the amount of time spent weight bearing on that side. The trunk is thrown laterally over the hip during weight bearing. This is done in an effort to reduce the compressive force of the abductor muscles of the hip during weight bearing. This is known as a *compensated Trendelenburg* or *lurch gait* (Figure 14.18) (http://www.youtube.com/watch?v=A85s4HZ8D1w).

The hip is maintained in a relaxed position of external rotation during swing phase. Heel-strike is avoided.

Weakness

Weakness of the hip abductors, seen frequently in patients with poliomyelitis, results in a Trendelenburg gait. This is characterized by abduction of the hip in stance phase. It appears as if the patient is bending the trunk to the side, away from the weak hip during weight bearing (Figure 14.19) (http://www.youtube.com/watch?v=A85s4HZ8D1w).

Some patients may compensate for this by flexing their trunk over the weight-bearing hip. This is called a *compensated Trendelenburg gait.* A compensated Trendelenburg gait results from weakness of hip abduction or a painful hip. You can differentiate the cause of this gait pattern by observing the duration of the stance phase on the abnormal leg. With a painful gait, the stance duration is reduced. Weakness has a lesser effect on stance duration.

Weakness of the hip extensors, seen frequently in myopathies, results in the trunk being thrown posteriorly at heel-strike, when the hip extensors are normally most active.

Abnormal Range of Motion

Loss of hip extension that occurs due to a hip flexion contracture, for example, will cause a functional shortening of the patient's leg. An increase in the lumbar lordosis will develop so that upright posture

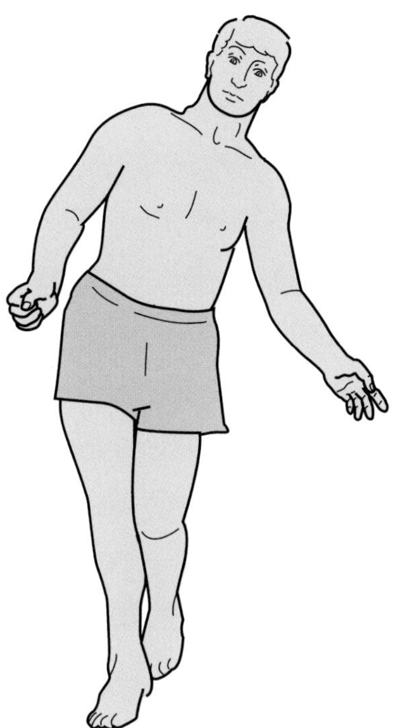

Figure 14.19 The uncompensated Trendelenburg gait is characterized by adduction of the hip, which appears as if the patient is moving the trunk away from the weight-bearing side during the stance phase. This results from weakness of hip abduction.

of the trunk can be maintained. The patient may walk with the foot plantar flexed on the shortened side to increase the functional length of the leg. Increased knee flexion will occur on the contracted side during late stance phase, when the hip is normally in extension.

Leg Length Discrepancy

Leg length discrepancy may be absolute (true) or relative (functional). Absolute leg length discrepancy results from a lengthening or shortening of the extremity due to bony injury or disease. For example, a fracture that unites the femur in a shortened position will result in an absolute shortening of the extremity. A femoral prosthesis that is too long for the patient will result in an absolute lengthening of the extremity.

Relative leg length discrepancy is due to postural abnormalities such as scoliosis, sacroiliac dysfunction, joint contractures, varus and valgus abnormalities, and neuromuscular dysfunction. For example, a hip flexion or knee flexion contracture causes a relative shortening of the extremity. An equinus deformity causes a relative lengthening of the extremity.

When the discrepancy is greater than 1ø in., the patient attempts to lengthen the short limb by walking on the ball of the foot. When the short limb is in the stance phase, the patient must swing-through the long limb without catching the toe on the ground. The patient does this by hip hiking or circumducting the extremity on the swing-through side (see Figure 14.15 and 14.16). When the leg length difference is less than $1\frac{3}{4}$ in., the patient will drop the pelvis on the affected side to functionally lengthen the short extremity. This is accompanied by lowering of the shoulder height on the same side.

SAMPLE EXAMINATION

History: 20-year-old male marathoner presents with a 2-week history of right leg pain which he was initially able to "run through," but now his symptoms prevent him from continuing to run. He has had no prior trauma. He has a past history of hamstring pulls in previous running seasons.

Physical Examination: Well-developed, well-nourished male with good muscle definition. Manual muscle testing 5/5 throughout the lower extremity. There is no tenderness on palpation. He has limited dorsiflexion of the right ankle to 0 degrees and straight leg raise to 50 degrees on the right. All other range of motion was within normal limits. Mobility testing was intact in the ankle and knee.

Presumptive Diagnosis: Acute compartment syndrome secondary to calf inflexibility.

Physical Examination Clues:

1. Male, indicating a possible tendency toward decreased musculoskeletal flexibility.
2. "Good muscle definition" implying a decrease in inherent musculoskeletal flexibility.

Limited dorsiflexion of the ankle further indicates a lack of flexibility. As a result, the tibialis anterior is required not only to act against gravity when actively dorsiflexing the ankle with each stride, but also to overcome the resistance of the tight calf muscles that are inhibiting normal ankle dorsiflexion. This predisposes the patient to suffer an "overuse" failure of the anterior musculature.

Appendices

Appendix A Physical Findings in Abnormal Conditions of the Musculoskeletal System	
Muscle Tendon Injury	
First degree, mild	Tender without swelling, mild spasm No ecchymosis No palpable defect Active contraction and passive stretch are painful
Second degree, moderate	Tender with swelling Mild to moderate ecchymosis Moderate spasm Possibly palpable discontinuity Extremely painful with passive stretching and attempted contraction Joint motion limited
Third degree, complete	Extreme tenderness with swelling May have severe bleeding and possible compartment syndrome with loss of sensation and pulse distally Palpable defect with bunching up of muscle tissue Complete loss of muscle function No change in pain with passive stretch
Ligament Injury	
First degree, mild	Minimal or no swelling Local tenderness Increase in pain with passive and active range of motion Minimal bruising No instability or functional loss expected
Second degree, moderate	Moderate swelling with ecchymosis Very tender, more diffusely tender Range of motion very painful and restricted due to swelling Instability may be recognized Functional loss may result
Third degree, complete	Severe swelling and ecchymosis or hemarthrosis Structural instability with abnormal increase in range of motion Possibly less painful than second-degree tear
Bone Injury	
Contusion	Localized tenderness With or without ecchymosis Subcutaneous swelling No palpable discontinuity
Fracture	Localized to diffuse tenderness Deformity and/or instability Palpable discontinuity in accessible areas Ecchymosis Possible neurovascular compromise
Stress fracture	Localized tenderness with overlying swelling and redness Increased pain with vibration or ultrasound applied to bone Certain locations are very common (i.e., tibia, fibula, metatarsals, femur)

Musculoskeletal Examination, Fourth Edition. Jeffrey M. Gross, Joseph Fetto and Elaine Rosen.

Companion website: www.wiley.com/go/musculoskeletalexam

Appendix A (*Continued*)

Inflammatory joint disease	Swelling, redness of joint, frequently symmetric Synovitis, systemic disease common May see subcutaneous nodules on extensor surface Severe joint deformities are common Valgus deformities are common Extensor tendon ruptures may be noted Compression neuropathy with loss of sensation and muscle strength may be noted Muscle weakness and restricted range of motion Pain worsens with activity
Noninflammatory joint disease	Acute swelling and redness, asymmetrical involvement Hypertrophic joint without destruction Common pattern "capsular," which is painful on range of motion Weakness and tightness of muscles crossing involved joints Pain lessens with activity Stiffness in the morning; fusion of joint may eventually occur Varus deformity may occur
Metabolic joint disease	Abnormal crystals in the joint fluid Very painful, red and swollen joints Loss of range of motion Systemic disease common Joint destruction may be severe
Nerve compression or radiculopathy	Pain, weakness, sensory loss, reflex loss and paresthesias in the dermatomal and/or myotomal distribution of the affected nerve; degree of loss of function may be mild or complete Stretching the nerve may increase pain Tapping over the nerve may result in distal tingling (Tinel's sign), especially if regeneration is occurring
Myofascial pain (trigger points)	Tenderness in a characteristic location of certain muscles Palpation of this location causes referred pain to a distant site A taut band, or sausage-like piece of muscle can often be palpated and may cause a twitch of the muscle when plucked like a guitar string The affected muscle is usually unable to relax fully and therefore passive stretch is limited and painful
Neoplasm	Unremitting pain, often awakens patient from sleep, no comfortable position to relieve pain Palpable mass if accessible and advanced Fracture (pathological) if bone involved Fever, weight loss, and fatigue Possible neurovascular compromise
Infection	Swelling, redness, warmth, and tenderness Fever and fatigue Loss of joint range or motion with characteristic fluid findings in affected joint Painful compression, active and passive range of motion of involved muscle
Reflex Sympathetic Dystrophy	
Acute: Less than 3 months after injury	Pain, warmth, swelling, redness Light touch is very painful Increased hair growth Mild stiffness of joints
Subacute: 4–12 months after injury	Pain is extremely severe Increased joint stiffness with loss of range of motion Passive range of motion is very painful Cool and pale or cyanotic discoloration Less swelling
Chronic: More than 1 year after injury	Less pain (usually) Periarticular fibrosis Marked limitation in range of motion No swelling Pale, dry, and shiny skin

Appendix B Range of Motion of the Extremities

Joint	Motion	Range (degrees)
Shoulder	Flexion	0–180
	Extension	0–60
	Abduction	0–180
	Internal (medial) rotation	0–70
	External (lateral) rotation	0–90
Elbow	Flexion	0–150
	Extension	0
Forearm	Pronation	0–80/90
	Supination	0–80/90
Wrist	Extension	0–70
	Flexion	0–80
	Radial deviation	0–20
	Dinar deviation	0–30
Thumb		
Carpometacarpal	Abduction	0–70
	Adduction	0
	Opposition	Tip of thumb to base or tip of fifth digit
Metacarpophalangeal	Flexion	0–50
	Extension	0
Interphalangeal	Flexion	0–90
	Extension	0–20
Digits 2–5		
Metacarpophalangeal	Flexion	0–80
	Extension	0–45
	Abduction/Adduction	0–20
Proximal interphalangeal	Flexion	0–110
	Extension	0
Distal interphalangeal	Flexion	0–90
	Extension	0–20
Hip	Flexion	0–120
	Extension	0–30
	Abduction	0–45
	Adduction	0–30
	External (lateral) rotation	0–45
	Internal (medial) rotation	0–45
Knee	Flexion	0–135
	Extension	0
Ankle	Dorsiflexion	0–20
	Plantar flexion	0–50
	Inversion	0–35
	Eversion	0–15
Subtalar	Inversion	0–5
	Eversion	0–5
Forefoot	Inversion	0–35
	Eversion	0–15
Toes		
First metatarsophalangeal	Flexion	0–45
	Extension	0–70
First interphalangeal	Flexion	0–40
Second to fifth metatarsophalangeals	Flexion	0–40

Bibliography

Aegerter E, Kirkpatrick JA. *Orthopedic Diseases*, 4th edn. Philadelphia, PA: WB Saunders, 1975.

American Academy of Orthopedic Surgeons. *Joint Motion: Method of Measuring and Recording*. Edinburgh: Churchill Livingstone, 1965.

American Society for Surgery of the Hand. *The Hand: Examination and Diagnosis*, 3rd edn. Edinburgh: Churchill Livingstone, 1990.

Aspinall W. Clinical testing for the craniovertebral hypermobility syndrome. *Journal of Orthopaedic and Sports Physical Therapy* 1990; 12: 47–54.

Backhouse KM, Hutchings RT. *Color Atlas of Surface Anatomy*. Baltimore, MD: Williams & Wilkins, 1986.

Bates B. *A Guide to Physical Examination and History-Taking*, 11th edn. Philadelphia, PA: Lippincott, 2012.

Beasley RW. *Injuries to the Hand*. Philadelphia, PA: WB Saunders, 1981.

Brand P, Hollister A. *Clinical Mechanics of the Hand*. St. Louis, MO: CV Mosby, 1985.

Brashear HR, Raney RB. *Handbook of Orthopedic Surgery*, 10th edn. St. Louis, MO: CV Mosby, 1986.

Bukowski E. Assessing joint mobility. *Clinical Management* 1991; 11:48–56.

Butler DS. *Mobilisation of the Nervous System*. Melbourne: Churchill Livingstone, 1991.

Butler DS. *The Sensitive Nervous System*. Adelaide: Noigroup Publications, 2000.

Cailliet R. *Low Back Pain Syndrome*, 5th edn. Philadelphia, PA: FA Davis, 1995.

Cantu RI, Grodin AJ. *Myofascial Manipulation Theory and Clinical Application*, 3rd edn. Gaithersburg, MD: Aspen, 2011.

Clark CR, Bonfiglio M. *Orthopedics: Essentials of Diagnosis and Treatment*. New York: Churchill Livingstone, 1994.

Cleland J. *Orthopaedic Clinical Examination: An Evidence-Based Approach for Physical Therapists*. Carlstadt, NJ: Icon Learning Systems, 2005.

Corrigan B, Maitland GD. *Practical Orthopaedic Medicine*. London: Butterworth, 1983.

Cyriax J. *Textbook of Orthopaedic Medicine*, 7th edn. Vol. 1: Diagnosis of Soft Tissue Lesions. London: Baillière Tindall, 1982.

Cyriax J. *Textbook of Orthopaedic Medicine*, 11th edn. Vol. 2: Treatment by Manipulation, Massage, and Injection. London: Baillière Tindall, 1984.

Cyriax JH, Cyriax PJ. *Illustrated Manual of Orthopaedic Medicine*, 3rd edn. London: Butterworth, 1996.

D'Ambrosia R. *Musculoskeletal Disorders: Regional Examination and Differential Diagnosis*, 2nd edn. Philadelphia, PA: JB Lippincott, 1986.

Daniels L, Worthington C. *Muscle Testing Techniques of Manual Examination*. Philadelphia, PA: WB Saunders, 1980.

DeGowin E, DeGowin R. *Bedside Diagnostic Examination*, 5th edn. New York: Macmillan, 1987.

DeLisa J, ed. *Rehabilitation Medicine – Principles and Practice*. Philadelphia, PA: JB Lippincott, 1988.

Donatelli R. *Biomechanics of the Foot and Ankle*. Philadelphia, PA: FA Davis, 1990.

Donatelli R, Wooden M. *Orthopedic Physical Therapy*, 4th edn. New York: Churchill Livingstone, 2009.

Downey J, ed. *The Physiological Basis of Rehabilitation Medicine*, 2nd edn. Stoneham, ME: Butterworth–Heinemann, 1994.

Musculoskeletal Examination, Fourth Edition. Jeffrey M. Gross, Joseph Fetto and Elaine Rosen.

Companion website: www.wiley.com/go/musculoskeletalexam

Dutton M. *Dutton's Orthopaedic Examination, Evaluation and Intervention*, 3rd edn. New York: McGraw Hill Medical Publishing Division, 2012.

Edmond SL. *Manipulation and Mobilization Extremity and Spinal Techniques*. St. Louis, MO: Mosby Year Book, 1993.

Epstein O, De Bono DP, Perkin GD, Cookson J. *Clinical Examination*. London: Gower Medical Publishing, 1992.

Esch D, Lepley M. *Evaluation of Joint Motion: Methods of Measurement and Recording*. Minneapolis, MN: University of Minnesota Press, 1976.

Fetto J, Marshall J. Injury to the anterior cruciate ligament producing the pivot-shift sign. *Journal of Bone and Joint Surgery* 1979; 61: 710–714.

Goodgold J, Eberstein A. *Electrodiagnosis of Neuromuscular Diseases*, 3rd edn. Baltimore, MD: Williams & Wilkins, 1983.

Gould J. *Orthopaedic and Sports Physical Therapy*, 2nd edn. St. Louis, MO: CV Mosby, 1990.

Greenman PE. *Greenman's Principles of Manual Medicine*, 4th edn. Philadelphia, PA: Lippincott Williams & Wilkins, 2010.

Grieve GP. *Common Vertebral Joint Problems*. Edinburgh: Churchill Livingstone, 1981.

Groh MM, Herrera J. A comprehensive review of hip labral tears. *Current Reviews in Musculoskeletal Medicine* 2009; 2(2): 105–117.

Harrison AL. The temporomandibular joint. In: Malone TR, McPoil T, Nitz AJ, eds. *Orthopaedic and Sports Physical Therapy*, 3rd edn. St. Louis, MO: Mosby Year Book, 1997.

Hartley A. *Practical Joint Assessment: A Sports Medicine Manual*. St. Louis, MO: Mosby Year Book, 1990.

Hasan SA. Superior Labral Lesions. Available at http://www.emedicine.com/Orthoped/topic317.htm, accessed on January 23, 2006.

Helfet AJ. *Disorders of the Knee*, 2nd edn. Philadelphia, PA: JB Lippincott, 1982.

Hertling D, Kessler RM. *Management of Common Musculoskeletal Disorders, Physical Therapy Principles and Methods*, 4th edn. Philadelphia, PA: Lippincott Williams & Wilkins, 2006.

Hollinshead W. *Textbook of Anatomy*, 3rd edn. Hagerstown, MD: Harper & Row, 1974.

Hoppenfeld S. *Physical Examination of the Spine and Extremities*. New York: Appleton-Century-Crofts, 1976.

Hunter JM, Schneider LH, Mackin EJ, Bell JA, eds. *Rehabilitation of the Hand*. St. Louis, MO: CV Mosby, 1978.

Iglarsh ZA, Snyder-Mackler L. Temporomandibular joint and the cervical spine. In: Richardson JK, Iglarsh ZA, eds. *Clinical Orthopaedic Physical Therapy*. Philadelphia, PA: WB Saunders, 1994.

Isaacs ER, Bookhout MR. *Bourdillon's Spinal Manipulation*, 6th edn. Boston, MA: Butterworth–Heineman, 2002.

Kaltenborn FM. *Manual Mobilization of the Joints: Basic Examination and Treatment Techniques*, 7th edn. Vol. 1: The Extremities. Oslo, Norway: Norli, 2011.

Kaltenborn FM. *Manual Mobilization of the Joints: Basic Examination and Treatment Techniques*, 6th edn. Vol. 2: The Spine. Oslo, Norway: Norli, 2012.

Kapandji IA. *The Physiology of the Joints*, 6th edn. Vol. 1: The Upper Limb. Edinburgh: Churchill Livingstone Elsevier, 2007.

Kapandji IA. *The Physiology of the Joints*, 6th edn. Vol. 3: The Spinal Column, Pelvic Girdle and Head. Edinburgh: Churchill Livingstone Elsevier, 2008.

Kapandji IA. *The Physiology of the Joints*, 6th edn. Vol. 2: The Lower Limb. Edinburgh: Churchill Livingstone Elsevier, 2010.

Kasdan M, ed. *Occupational Medicine – Occupational Hand Injuries*, Vol. 4. Philadelphia, PA: Hanley & Belfus, 1989.

Kendall FP, Provance P, McCreary EK. *Muscles: Testing and Function*, 5th edn. Baltimore, MD: Williams & Wilkins, 2005.

Kenneally M, Rubenach H, Elvey R. The upper limb tension test: the SLR test of the arm. In: Grant R, ed. *Physical Therapy of the Cervical and Thoracic Spine*. Edinburgh: Churchill Livingstone, 1988.

Kisner C, Colby LA. *Therapeutic Exercise: Foundations and Techniques*, 2nd edn. Philadelphia, PA: FA Davis, 1990.

Kottke FJ, Stillwell GK, Lehmann JF, eds. *Krusen's Handbook of Physical Medicine and Rehabilitation*, 3rd edn. Philadelphia, PA: WB Saunders, 1982.

Lehmkuhl L, Smith L. *Brunnstrom's Clinical Kinesiology*. Philadelphia, PA: FA Davis, 1983.

Lichtenstein L. *Diseases of Bone and Joints*, 2nd edn. St. Louis, MO: CV Mosby, 1975.

Lichtman DM. *The Wrist and Its Disorders*. Philadelphia, PA: WB Saunders, 1988.

Magee DJ. *Orthopedic Physical Assessment*, 5th edn. St. Louis, MO: WB Saunders, 2008.

Maitland GD. *Peripheral Manipulation*, 8th edn. Edinburgh: Elsevier Butterworth–Heinemann, 2014a.

Maitland GD, ed. *Maitland's Vertebral Manipulation*, 8th edn. Edinburgh: Elsevier Butterworth–Heinemann, 2014b.

McCarty D. *Arthritis and Allied Conditions*, 10th edn. Philadelphia, PA: Lea & Febiger, 1985.

McKenzie RA. *The Lumbar Spine Mechanical Diagnosis and Therapy*. New Zealand: Spinal Publication, 1981.

McMinn RMH, Hutchings RT. *Color Atlas of Human Anatomy*. Chicago: Yearbook Medical Publishers, 1978.

Melzack R. The McGill pain questionnaire: major properties and scoring methods. *Pain* 1975; 1:277–299.

Mennell JM. *Joint Pain, Diagnosis and Treatment Using Manipulative Techniques*. Boston, MA: Little Brown, 1964.

Mennell JM. *Foot Pain*. Boston, MA: Little Brown, 1969.

Moore KL, Dalley AF. *Clinically Oriented Anatomy*, 4th edn. Philadelphia, PA: Lippincott Williams & Wilkins, 1999.

Norkin CC, White DJ. *Measurement of Joint Motion: A Guide to Goniometry*. Philadelphia, PA: FA Davis, 1985.

Palmer ML, Epler M. *Clinical Assessment Procedures in Physical Therapy*. Philadelphia, PA: JB Lippincott, 1990.

Paris S. *Course Notes: Introduction to Spinal Evaluation and Manipulation*. St. Augustine, FL: Institute of Graduate Physical Therapy, 1991.

Peeler J, Anderson JE. Reliability of the Ely's test for assessing rectus femoris muscle flexibility and joint range of motion. *Journal of Orthopaedic Research* 2008; 26(6):793–799.

Porterfield J, DeRosa C. *Mechanical Low Back Pain Perspectives in Functional Anatomy*. Philadelphia, PA: WB Saunders, 1991.

Porterfield J, DeRosa C. *Mechanical Neck Pain Perspectives in Functional Anatomy*. Philadelphia, PA: WB Saunders, 1995.

Reid D. *Sports Injury Assessment and Rehabilitation*. New York: Churchill Livingstone, 1992.

Richardson J, Iglarsh ZA. *Clinical Orthopaedic Physical Therapy*. Philadelphia, PA: WB Saunders, 1994.

Rocabado M, Iglarsh ZA. *Musculoskeletal Approach to Maxillofacial Pain*. Philadelphia, PA: JB Lippincott, 1991.

Salter R. *Textbook of Disorders and Injuries of the Musculoskeletal System*, 3rd edn. Baltimore, MD: Williams & Wilkins, 1999.

Saunders HD, Saunders RI. *Evaluation and Treatment of Musculoskeletal Disorders*, 3rd edn. Vol. 1: Spine. Chaska, MN: Educational Opportunities, 1994.

Seidel HM. *Mosby's Guide to Physical Examination*. St. Louis, MO: CV Mosby, 1987.

Stanley BG, Tribuzi SM. *Concepts in Hand Rehabilitation*. Philadelphia, PA: FA Davis, 1992.

Tomberlin JP, Saunders HD. *Evaluation and Treatment of Musculoskeletal Disorders*, 3rd edn. Vol. 2: Extremities. Chaska, MN: The Saunders Group, 1995.

Torg J, Shepard RJ. *Current Therapy in Sports Medicine*. Toronto: BC Decker, 1990.

Travell J, Rinzler SI. The myofascial genesis of pain. *Postgraduate Medicine* 1952; 31:425–431.

Travell J, Simons D. *Myofascial Pain and Dysfunction*, 2 nd edn. Vol. 3: The Trigger Point Manual, the Lower Extremities. Baltimore, MD: Williams & Wilkins, 1998.

Tubiana R. *Examination of the Hand and Upper Limb*. Philadelphia, PA: WB Saunders, 1984.

Turek S. *Orthopaedics Principles and Their Application*, 3rd edn. Philadelphia, PA: JB Lippincott, 1977.

Tzannes A, Murrell GA. Clinical examination of the unstable shoulder. *Sports Medicine* 2002; 32(7):1–11.

Wadsworth C. *Manual Examination and Treatment of the Spine and Extremities*. Baltimore, MD: Williams & Wilkins, 1988.

Warwick R, Williams PL. *Gray's Anatomy*, 38th British edn. Philadelphia, PA: WB Saunders, 1998.

Watson HK, Ashmead D 4th, Makhlouf MV. Examination of the scaphoid. *Journal of Hand Surgery* 1988; 13A:657–660.

Whittle M. *Gait Analysis – An Introduction*. Stoneham, MA: Butterworth–Heinemann, 1991.

Wilson F. *The Musculoskeletal System: Basic Processes and Disorders*, 2nd edn. Philadelphia, PA: JB Lippincott, 1983.

Index

Note: Page numbers in *italics* refer to illustrations; those in **bold** refer to tables.

Musculoskeletal Examination, Fourth Edition. Jeffrey M. Gross, Joseph Fetto and Elaine Rosen.

Companion website: www.wiley.com/go/musculoskeletalexam

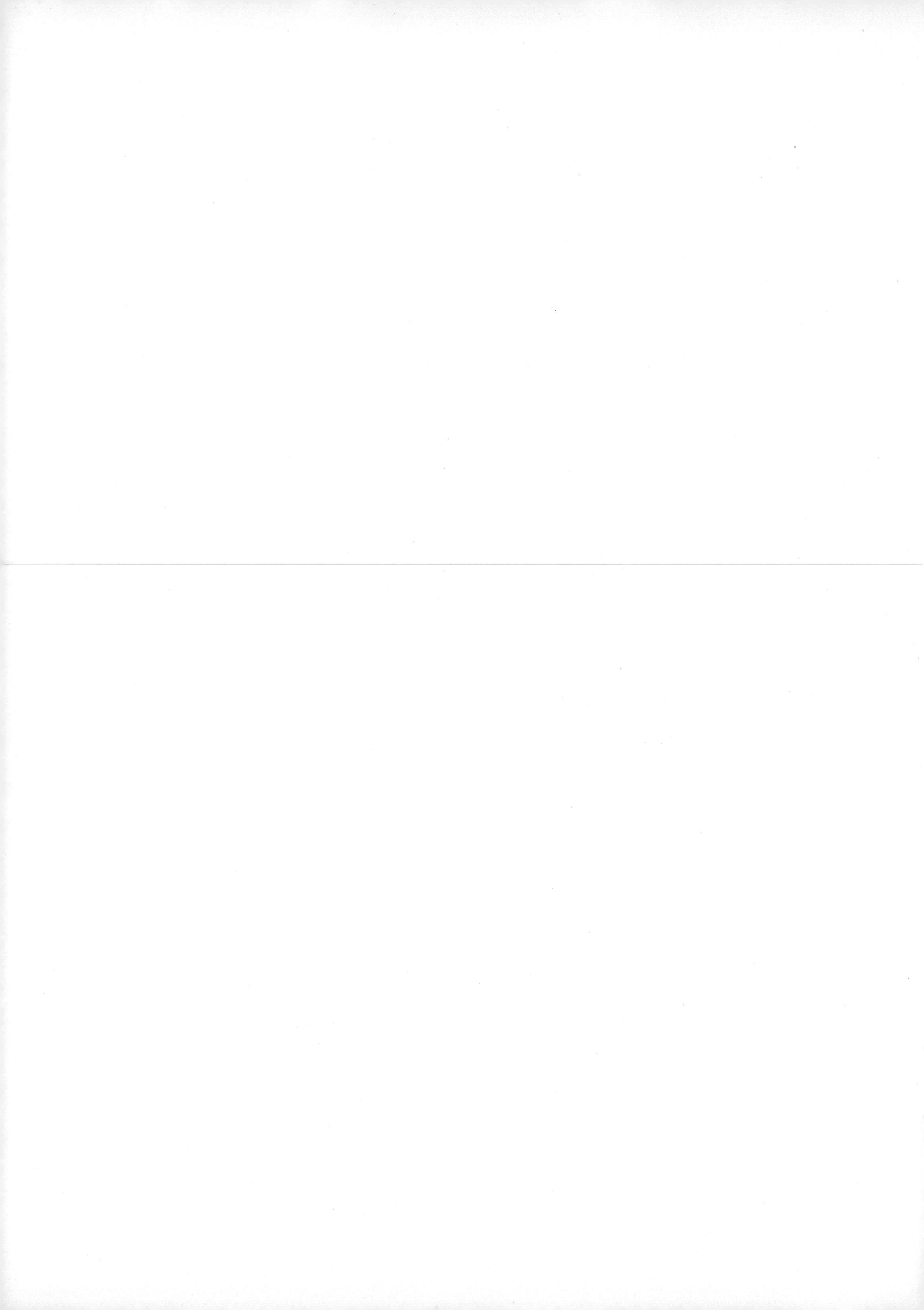